Guidelines for
PERINATAL
CARE   Seventh Edition

American Academy of Pediatrics
DEDICATED TO THE HEALTH OF ALL CHILDREN™

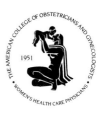

The American College of Obstetricians and Gynecologists
WOMEN'S HEALTH CARE PHYSICIANS

Supported in part by 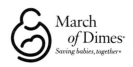 March *of* Dimes·
Saving babies, together®

Guidelines for Perinatal Care was developed through the cooperative efforts of the American Academy of Pediatrics' (AAP) Committee on Fetus and Newborn and the American College of Obstetricians and Gynecologists' (the College) Committee on Obstetric Practice. The guidelines should not be viewed as a body of rigid rules. They are general and intended to be adapted to many different situations, taking into account the needs and resources particular to the locality, the institution, or type of practice. Variations and innovations that improve the quality of patient care are to be encouraged rather than restricted. The purpose of these guidelines will be well served if they provide a firm basis on which local norms may be built.

Library of Congress Cataloging-in-Publication Data

Guidelines for perinatal care / American Academy of Pediatrics [and] the American College of Obstetricians and Gynecologists.—7th ed.
    p. ; cm.
Perinatal care
Includes bibliographical references and index.
ISBN 978-1-58110-734-0 (AAP)—ISBN 978-1-934984-17-8 (ACOG)
I. American Academy of Pediatrics. II. American College of Obstetricians and Gynecologists.
III. Title: Perinatal care.
[DNLM: 1. Perinatal Care—standards—United States—Practice Guideline. WQ 210]

618.3'206—dc23
                    2012009328
ISBN: 978-1-58110-734-0 AAP
ISBN: 978-1-934984-17-8 the College

Orders to purchase copies of *Guidelines for Perinatal Care* or inquiries regarding content can be directed to the respective organizations.

American Academy of Pediatrics
141 Northwest Point Boulevard
PO Box 927
Elk Grove Village, IL 60009-0927

The American College of Obstetricians and Gynecologists
409 12th Street, SW
Washington, DC 20090-6920

12345/65432

Editorial Committee

The College Committee on Obstetric Practice

The College Committee on Obstetric Practice *(continued)*

Members, 2011–2012

George A. Macones, MD, FACOG (Chair)
Jeffrey L. Ecker, MD, FACOG (Vice Chair)
Lindsay S. Alger, MD, FACOG
Heather A. Bankowski, DO, FACOG
Richard H. Beigi, MD, FACOG
Aaron B. Caughey, MD, FACOG
Lorraine Dugoff, MD, FACOG
Rebecca Jackson, MD, FACOG
Sarah Katel, MD, FACOG
Jeffrey C. King, MD, FACOG
Michelle Y. Owens, MD, FACOG
Eva K. Pressman, MD, FACOG
Karla W. Nacion, PhD, CNM
Jeanne Ballard, MD, FACOG (Ex Officio)
Neil S. Silverman, MD, FACOG (Ex Officio)

Liaison Representatives

Vincenzo Berghella, MD, FACOG
May Hsieh Blanchard, MD, FACOG
Jill E. Brown, MD, MPH, FACOG
William M. Callaghan, MD, FACOG
Beth Choby, MD
Joshua A. Copel, MD, FACOG
Craig M. Palmer, MD
Lu-Ann Papile, MD, FAAP
Phillip Price, MD, FACOG
Stuart K. Shapira, MD, PhD
Catherine Y. Spong, MD, FACOG

AAP Committee on Fetus and Newborn

Members, 2009–2010

Lu-Ann Papile, MD, FAAP (Chair)
David Adamkin, MD
Jill E. Baley, MD, FAAP
Vinod K. Bhutani, MD
Waldemar A. Carlo, MD, FAAP
Praveen Kumar, MD, FAAP
Richard A. Polin, MD, FAAP
Rosemarie C. Tan, MD, PhD, FAAP
Kristi L. Watterberg, MD, FAAP

Liaison Representatives

Capt. Wanda D. Barfield, MD, MPH, FAAP
William H. Barth Jr, MD, FACOG
Ann L. Jefferies, MD, FRCPC
Rosalie O. Mainous, PhD, APRN, NNP-BC
Tonse N. K. Raju, MD, DCH, FAAP
Kasper S. Wang, MD, FACS, FAAP

Members, 2010–2011

Lu-Ann Papile, MD, FAAP (Chair)
Jill E. Baley, MD, FAAP
Vinod K. Bhutani, MD
Waldemar A. Carlo, MD, FAAP
James Cummings, MD, FAAP
Praveen Kumar, MD, FAAP
Richard A. Polin, MD, FAAP
Rosemarie C. Tan, MD, PhD, FAAP
Kristi L. Watterberg, MD, FAAP

Liaison Representatives

Capt. Wanda D. Barfield, MD, MPH, FAAP
Ann L. Jefferies, MD, FRCPC
William H. Barth Jr, MD, FACOG
Rosalie O. Mainous, PhD, APRN, NNP-BC
Tonse N. K. Raju, MD, DCH, FAAP
Kasper S. Wang, MD, FACS, FAAP

AAP Committee on Fetus and Newborn *(continued)*

Contents

Preface   xi

Introduction   xiii

chapter 1   *Organization of Perinatal Health Care*   1

Health Care Delivery System   1

Clinical Components of Regionalized and Integrated Delivery of Perinatal Services   6

Workforce: The Distribution and Supply of Perinatal Care Providers   17

chapter 2   *Inpatient Perinatal Care Services*   21

Personnel   21

Physical Facilities   37

chapter 3   *Quality Improvement and Patient Safety*   61

Quality Improvement   62

Patient Safety   67

Quality Improvement and Patient Safety in Neonatal Intensive Care Units   72

chapter 4   *Maternal and Neonatal Interhospital Transfer*   77

Types of Transport   78

Transport Program Components and Responsibilities   79

Personnel   84

Equipment   84
Transport Procedure   87
Outreach Education   91
Program Evaluation   91

chapter 5   *Preconception and Antepartum Care*   95
Preconception Care   95
Antepartum Care   105

chapter 6   *Intrapartum and Postpartum Care of the Mother*   169
Planned Home Birth   170
Underwater Births   170
Admission   170
Labor   175
Analgesia and Anesthesia   182
Delivery   187
Postpartum Maternal Care   195

chapter 7   *Obstetric and Medical Complications*   211
Medical Complications Before Pregnancy   211
Pregnancy-Related Complications   223
Other Medical Complications During Pregnancy   243
Labor and Delivery Considerations and Complications   248

chapter 8   *Care of the Newborn*   265
Delivery Room Care   266
Assessment of the Newborn Infant   280
Transitional Care   283
Neonatal Nutrition   287

Preventive Care   295
Infant Safety   304
Hospital Discharge and Parent Education   306
Follow-up Care   313
Adoption   314

chapter 9   *Neonatal Complications and Management of High-Risk Infants*   321
Neonatal Complications   321
Management of High-Risk Infants   356
Death of a Newborn   367
Hospital Discharge of High-Risk Infants   370
Follow-up Care of High-Risk Infants   376

chapter 10   *Perinatal Infections*   383
Viral Infections   383
Bacterial Infections   414
Spirochetal Infections   427
Parasitic Infections   433

chapter 11   *Infection Control*   439
Definition of Health Care-Associated Infection   439
Prevention and Control of Infections   440
Environmental Control   454

Appendixes   463
A. American College of Obstetricians and Gynecologists' Antepartum Record and Postpartum Form   463
B. Early Pregnancy Risk Identification for Consultation   477
C. Ongoing Pregnancy Risk Identification for Consultation   479
D. Granting Obstetric Privileges   481
E. Glossary of Midwifery Organizations and Terms   491

F. Standard Terminology for Reporting of Reproductive Health Statistics in the United States   497

G. Federal Requirements for Patient Screening and Transfer   513

H. Occupational Safety and Health Administration Regulations on Occupational Exposures to Bloodborne Pathogens   519

I. American Academy of Pediatrics Policy Statements and American College of Obstetrician and Gynecologists' Committee Opinions and Practice Bulletins   531

J. Web Site Resources   545

Index   547

Preface

The seventh edition of *Guidelines for Perinatal Care* is a user-friendly guide that provides updated and expanded information from the sixth edition. Multiple chapters have been reorganized and rewritten. The chapters are supplemented by 10 appendixes (A–J) that provide a wealth of additional information and resources for readers. This edition maintains the focus of the past edition on reproductive awareness and regionally based perinatal care services but with an added focus on patient safety and quality improvement in obstetrics and neonatology, which is highlighted in a new chapter dedicated to this topic.

Guidelines for Perinatal Care represents a cross section of different disciplines within the perinatal community. It is designed for use by all personnel who are involved in the care of pregnant women, their fetuses, and their neonates in community programs, hospitals, and medical centers. An intermingling of information in varying degrees of detail is provided to address their collective needs. The result is a unique resource that complements the educational documents listed in Appendix I, which provide more specific information. Readers are encouraged to refer to the appendix for related documents to supplement those listed at the end of each chapter. A list of web site resources also is included in this edition. The list includes the web sites of relevant health care-related organizations (Appendix J).

Both the American Academy of Pediatrics (AAP) and the American College of Obstetricians and Gynecologists (the College) will continue to update information presented here through policy statements and recommendations that both organizations issue periodically, particularly with regard to rapidly evolving technologies and areas of practice.

Guidelines for Perinatal Care is published as a companion document to the College's *Guidelines for Women's Health Care*, which is in its third edition. Although each book is developed with the aid of a separate committee, the contents are coordinated to provide comprehensive reference to all aspects of women's health care with minimal duplication.

The most current scientific information, professional opinions, and clinical practices have been used to create this document, which is intended to offer guidelines, not strict operating rules. Local circumstances must dictate the way in which these guidelines are best interpreted to meet the needs of a particular hospital, community, or system. (For instance, the term *readily available*, used to designate acceptable levels of care, should be defined by each institution within the context of its resources and geographic location. Therefore, it is reasonable to tailor the time to delivery to local circumstances and logistics.) Emphasis has been placed on identifying those areas to be covered by specific, locally defined protocols rather than on promoting rigid recommendations.

The content of this newest edition of *Guidelines for Perinatal Care* has undergone careful review to ensure accuracy and consistency with the policies of both AAP and the College. The guidelines are not meant to be exhaustive, nor do they always agree with those of other organizations; however, they reflect the latest recommendations of AAP and the College. The recommendations of AAP and the College are based on the best understanding of the data and consensus among authorities in the discipline. The text was written, revised, and reviewed by members of the AAP Committee on Fetus and Newborn and the College Committee on Obstetric Practice; consultants in a variety of specialized areas also contributed to the content. The pioneering efforts of those who developed the previous editions also must be acknowledged. To each and every one of them, our sincere appreciation is extended.

Introduction

Throughout its prior six editions, *Guidelines for Perinatal Care* has focused on improving the outcomes of pregnancies and reducing maternal and perinatal mortality and morbidity by suggesting sound paradigms for providing perinatal care. Its strong advocacy of regionalized perinatal systems, including effective risk identification, care in a risk-appropriate setting, and maternal or neonatal transport to tertiary care facilities when necessary, has had a demonstrable effect on perinatal outcomes. The current edition incorporates evidence-based data to further refine optimal regionalized care, including revised definitions of levels of neonatal care. This edition also includes evidence-based recommendations on the use of safe and effective diagnostic and therapeutic interventions in both maternal–fetal medicine and neonatology.

The full spectrum of high-quality perinatal care is covered by this seventh edition of *Guidelines for Perinatal Care*, from the principles of preconception counseling and the provision of antepartum and intrapartum care in routine and complex settings to guidelines for routine and complex neonatal and postpartum care. The preconception and antepartum care chapter has been expanded to include new information on prenatal care of women with intellectual and developmental disabilities and updated guidelines on immunization, nutrition, diet, weight gain, and the prevention of perinatal group B streptococcal disease. Intrapartum and postpartum information includes coverage of new topics, such as planned home birth and underwater birth, and provides revised postpartum contraception recommendations that are aligned with the *U.S. Medical Eligibility Criteria for Contraception* published by the Centers for Disease Control and Prevention. The chapter on obstetric and medical complications has been expanded with new information and evidence-based recommendations to guide clinical practice in these specialized areas.

The chapters on care of healthy and high-risk infants include updated recommendations on neonatal resuscitation, screening and management of hyperbilirubinemia, and neonatal drug withdrawal. The addition of information on late preterm infants reflects the importance of this group of infants to the rate of prematurity and their increased vulnerability compared with term infants.

Updated recommendations for the conduct of perinatal care in a hospital setting are presented with an emphasis on family-centered and patient-centered care, wherein patients and families are recognized and respected as true partners of their health care team. The roles of hospitalists and laborists are also discussed because these members of the labor management team are increasingly seen in perinatal care centers across the country.

As in previous editions, the concept of quality improvement in all aspects of perinatal care is a focus. Because the data on the importance and effect of quality improvement specific to obstetrics and neonatology has accumulated since the most recent edition, a new chapter entitled "Quality Improvement and Patient Safety" is included. This chapter provides commentary on the need for procedures and policies to ensure effective communication among caregivers and between caregivers and patients because communication remains a critical component of quality perinatal care. The concepts of team training, simulation, and drills and their roles in improving perinatal care are also featured. Quality control and patient safety in the neonatal intensive care unit is highlighted, with information on neonatal intensive care unit data collection, rapid cycle improvement, and quality improvement collaboratives, reflecting the increasing importance of these topics in the field of neonatology.

Achieving the goal of optimal outcomes for newborns and mothers requires a coordinated system of perinatal care, including a multidisciplinary team of physicians working in concert with the patient and within a supportive community. This seventh edition of *Guidelines for Perinatal Care* provides a framework of recommendations based on the best available evidence. Wide implementation of these recommendations will bring health care providers closer to the goal.

Guidelines for

PERINATAL CARE

Seventh Edition

Chapter 1
Organization of Perinatal Health Care

The organization of perinatal health care on a regional basis emerged as an ideal model of health care delivery beginning in the 1970s and 1980s. Regional organization of perinatal care was endorsed in a 1976 report by the March of Dimes Foundation, *Toward Improving the Outcome of Pregnancy*, which was prepared by the Committee on Perinatal Health, an ad hoc committee of representatives appointed by participating professional organizations with support from the March of Dimes Foundation. The importance of regional organization was further emphasized in the second edition and third edition of *Toward Improving the Outcome of Pregnancy* published in 1993 and 2010, respectively. Although a comprehensive, integrated perinatal care delivery system is optimal, this goal has not been attained in many areas of the country, where financial incentives promote competing systems and duplication of services.

Health Care Delivery System

A regionalized system of perinatal care with integrated delivery of services should address the care received by the mother before pregnancy and during pregnancy, the management of labor and delivery, postpartum care, and neonatal care. A health care system that is responsive to the needs of families, and especially women, requires strategies to

- ensure access to services
- identify risks early
- provide linkage to the appropriate level of care
- ensure adherence, continuity, and comprehensiveness of care
- promote efficient use of resources

Structural, financial, and cultural barriers to care need to be identified and eliminated. The regionalized organization and integration of perinatal care must evolve within the framework of the general health care delivery system while avoiding unnecessary duplication of services. Five aspects can be identified as essential responsibilities of the successful perinatal health care system: 1) provide access to comprehensive perinatal health care services, 2) embrace a patient-centered and family-centered approach to health care, 3) deliver culturally and linguistically appropriate care, 4) educate the public about reproductive health, and 5) be accountable for all components of the health care delivery system.

Comprehensive Perinatal Health Care Services

The integration of a spectrum of clinical activities, basic care through subspecialty care, within one system or geographic region potentially provides timely access to care at the appropriate level for the entire population. The primary goal of providing the appropriate level of care is facilitated by early and ongoing risk assessment to prevent, recognize, and treat conditions associated with maternal and neonatal morbidity and mortality. A secondary goal is to improve referral and consultation among institutions that provide different levels of care. When populations that are in need of reproductive health care are widely dispersed, both geographically and economically, a carefully structured, well-organized system of supportive services becomes necessary to ensure access to appropriate care for all pregnant women and newborns. Networks and other forms of vertically integrated systems within a region should be structured to provide all the necessary services, including health care, transportation, public and professional education, research, and outcome evaluations with data organized in standard format. All components are necessary to minimize perinatal mortality and morbidity while using resources efficiently and effectively.

Patient-Centered and Family-Centered Health Care

The perinatal health care system should be oriented toward providing patient-centered and family-centered health care because the family often is the primary source of support for individuals receiving health services. The Institute for Patient- and Family-Centered Care importantly notes that the term family is defined by the patient, as is the degree to which the family is involved in care. The term "family" as it is used here includes the expectant mother and her support system, which may include any or all of the following individuals: a spouse or partner, relatives, and friends. Health care providers should strive to engage the family as co-providers and decision-making partners, as long as this is in accordance with the mother's personal situation, beliefs, and desires.

Every encounter should build on the expectant mother's strengths, preserve her dignity, and enhance her confidence and competence. Such an approach incorporates family perspectives, offers real choices, and respects the decisions made by the family for themselves and their children. All counseling should be sensitive to cultural diversity, and a skilled translator should be used when the primary language of the mother-to-be is not spoken by the health care provider.

Hospital and program leaders should communicate the concepts of patient-centered and family-centered care consistently and clearly to staff, students, families, and communities through statements of vision, mission, and philosophy and through institutional policies and actions. Providing an environment that is supportive of the family's key role in promoting the health of its members is important in successful health promotion. This includes respecting the choices, values, and cultural backgrounds of expectant mothers, new mothers, and other family members; communicating honestly and openly; promoting opportunities for mutual support and information sharing; and collaborating in the development and evaluation of services.

Family-centered practices can help expectant families and new families become nurturing caregivers. Efforts should be made throughout the neonatal course to promote continuous contact between newborns and their families. Economic interests and decisions should never take priority over the best interests of the newborn, the mother, the family, and the community in keeping the family together. When separation of the family unit is necessitated by the requirement for a higher level of care for the mother or newborn, the responsibility for maintaining communication and involvement of the family in decisions relating to care should be shared by the entire health care team. Whenever medically feasible, a mother whose newborn has been transferred to another hospital should be discharged or transferred to the same facility. Staff interactions and unit policies at every level should consistently reinforce the importance of family for the health and well-being of their newborn. Families' strengths and capabilities should be the foundation on which to build competency and confidence in caregiving abilities. Preserving an individual sense of personal responsibility and identity is important for the optimum outcome of pregnancy and family life.

Culturally and Linguistically Appropriate Care

In addition to being family-centered, perinatal health care systems should be culturally and linguistically appropriate. Large perinatal health disparities exist in racial and ethnic minority groups and in low-income level groups, compared with white and high-income level groups. The publication of *National Standards for Culturally and Linguistically Appropriate Services in Healthcare* by the Office of Minority Health of the U.S. Department of Health and Human Services emphasizes the need to address these long-standing disparities through the implementation and evaluation of culturally sensitive and competent health care. These recommendations encourage the coordination of the U.S. Department of Health and Human Services agencies, along with other federal agencies, health care organizations, accreditation bodies, patient communities, and private sector organizations to ensure consistent training for health care providers; increase cultural diversity among health care professionals; and empower minority, vulnerable, and underserved patients to participate as equal partners in the health care process and system.

Education of the Public About Reproductive Health

Insight into the broad social and medical implications of pregnancy and awareness of reproductive risks, health-enhancing behaviors, and family-planning options are essential for improving the outcomes of pregnancy. Education about reproductive health must be integrated more effectively into the health care system and society at large. An Institute of Medicine report, *The Best Intentions, Unintended Pregnancy and the Well-Being of Children and Families*, emphasizes that in the United States

- less than one half of pregnancies are planned.
- approximately 60% of pregnancies are unintended, either mistimed or unwanted altogether.
- unintended pregnancies occur in all segments of society.
- a woman with an unintended pregnancy is less likely to seek early prenatal care and is more likely to expose the fetus to noxious substances.
- a newborn of an unwanted pregnancy is at higher risk of having a low birth weight and other complications throughout childhood.
- approximately one half of unintended pregnancies end in abortion.

Because pregnancy intention and other behavioral health risks—including the use of alcohol, tobacco, and other drugs—occur across all socioeconomic groups, the target group for reproductive education must be all women of childbearing age. Reproductive health screening should be implemented by all health care providers serving women in their reproductive years (see also Chapter 5, "Preconception and Antepartum Care").

Every encounter with the health care system, including those involving adolescents and men, should be viewed as an opportunity to reinforce awareness of reproductive health issues. New messages and marketing techniques regarding responsible reproductive health practices and innovations in marketing techniques may be required to change attitudes and behaviors in women and men.

In communicating with both the patient and the public, it is important to tailor health messages to the appropriate literacy and language level. Low functional literacy or language barriers may compromise the quality of care received, contribute to medical errors and poor health outcomes, and increase the risk of medical liability litigation. This problem can be minimized by consistent use of simplified language on written documents, such as consent forms and patient instructions, and in face-to-face conversation. Whenever necessary, interpreter services must be provided to assist with important discussions if patients are not fluent in English or if they are sensory impaired. Reasonable steps are required to ensure meaningful access to interpreter services, including hiring interpreters as office or hospital staff, using appropriate community resources, or using translation telephone services.

Accountability

Accountability for actions is a fundamental principle of health care provision applicable to all components of a health care delivery system and is a valuable attribute of professional practice that benefits all patients. This accountability includes, but is not limited to, the care of individual patients by individual health care providers. Patients and their support systems have a shared partnership for their health care. Within the perinatal health care delivery system, accountability and responsibility must be required equally of all participants, including patients, families, perinatal health care programs and systems, government agencies, insurers, and health maintenance organizations, all of whose actions and policies influence the delivery of patient care and, thereby, influence outcomes. Accountability includes developing meaningful quality improvement programs, monitoring medical errors, and working to ensure patient safety. Access to high quality care for all patients is a responsibility that requires a coordinated system with involvement, commitment, and accountability of all parties.

Clinical Components of Regionalized and Integrated Delivery of Perinatal Services

A regionalized system that focuses on integrated delivery of graded levels of hospital-based perinatal care has been shown to be effective and to result in improved outcomes for women and their newborns. Integrated perinatal care programs can be extended to encompass preconception evaluation and early-pregnancy risk assessment in both ambulatory and hospital-based settings.

Preconception Care

Preconception care aims to promote the health of women of reproductive age before conception and improve pregnancy outcomes. Integrated perinatal health care programs and systems should place additional emphasis on preconception care through educational programs. All women of childbearing age should have access to preconception care. Health care providers in various disciplines (eg, internal medicine, family medicine, and pediatrics) should be made aware of preconception care recommendations and guidelines. Clinical details of preconception care for perinatal health care providers are presented in Chapter 5.

Ambulatory Prenatal Care

The goals for the coordination of ambulatory prenatal care are to provide appropriate care for all women, to ensure good use of available resources, and to improve the outcome of pregnancies. As recommended by the March of Dimes Foundation in the second edition of *Toward Improving the Outcome of Pregnancy*, prenatal care can be delivered more effectively and efficiently by defining the capabilities and expertise (basic, specialty, and subspecialty) of health care providers and ensuring that pregnant women receive risk-appropriate care (Table 1-1). Developments in maternal–fetal risk assessment and diagnosis, as well as the interventions to change behavior, make early and ongoing prenatal care an effective strategy to improve pregnancy outcomes.

Early and ongoing risk assessment should be an integral component of perinatal care. Early identification of high-risk pregnancies allows prevention and treatment of conditions associated with maternal and fetal morbidity and mortality. Risk assessment facilitates development of a plan of care, including referral and consultation as appropriate, among health care providers of basic, specialty, and subspecialty prenatal care on the basis of the patient's circumstances and the capability of the individual health care providers.

Table 1-1. Ambulatory Prenatal Care Provider Capabilities and Expertise

Level of Care	Capabilities	Health Care Provider Types
Basic	Risk-oriented prenatal care record, physical examination and interpretation of findings, routine laboratory assessment, assessment of gestational age and normal progress of pregnancy, ongoing risk identification, mechanisms for consultation and referral, psychosocial support, childbirth education, and care coordination (including referral for ancillary services, such as transportation, food, and housing assistance)	Obstetricians, family physicians, certified nurse-midwives, certified midwives, and other advanced-practice nurses with experience, training, and demonstrated competence
Specialty	Basic care plus fetal diagnostic testing (eg, biophysical tests, amniotic fluid analysis, basic ultrasonography), expertise in management of medical and obstetric complications	Obstetricians
Subspecialty	Basic and specialty care plus advanced fetal diagnostics (eg, targeted ultrasonography, fetal echocardiography); advanced therapy (eg, intrauterine fetal transfusion and treatment of cardiac arrhythmias); medical, surgical, neonatal, and genetic consultation; and management of severe maternal complications	Maternal-fetal medicine specialists and reproductive geneticists with experience, training, and demonstrated competence

Modified with permission from March of Dimes. Toward improving the outcome of pregnancy: the 90s and beyond. White Plains (NY): March of Dimes Birth Defects Foundation; 1993.

The content and timing of prenatal care should be varied according to the needs and risk status of the woman and her fetus. Use of community-based risk assessment tools, such as a standardized prenatal record (see also Appendix A), by all health care providers within a regionalized perinatal care system helps to ensure the integration of care delivery and appropriate implementation of risk assessment and intervention activities. All prenatal health care providers should be able to identify a full range of medical and psychosocial risks and either provide appropriate care or make appropriate referrals (see also Appendix B and Appendix C).

Prenatal care may involve the services of many types of health care providers, including the early involvement of pediatricians and neonatologists as well as other pediatric subspecialists (eg, cardiologists, surgeons, and geneticists). A consultation with a neonatologist and other appropriate specialists to discuss the pediatric implications with the mother and her partner is particularly important when fetal risks or problems have been identified.

In-Hospital Perinatal Care

In the first edition of *Toward Improving the Outcome of Pregnancy*, the Committee on Perinatal Health of the March of Dimes Foundation designated three levels of perinatal care: I, II, and III. Although these designations remain in use among many institutions and public agencies, such as state maternal–child health programs, the second March of Dimes Foundation Committee on Perinatal Health report in 1993 recommended replacing numerical designations with the functional, descriptive designations of basic, specialty, and subspecialty care. Since then, financial and marketing pressures, as well as community demands, have led some hospitals to raise their perinatal care service-level designation without attention to regional coordination concerns. This tendency conflicts with the traditional concept of regionalized organization, in which single subspecialty care centers had the sole capability to provide complex patient care and usually, but not always, assumed regional responsibilities for transport, outreach education, research, and quality improvement for a specific population or geographic area.

Attempts to share regional responsibilities among hospitals have not been uniformly successful. Sometimes differing levels of perinatal care services have developed within a single hospital—usually a basic or specialty obstetrics service in conjunction with a subspecialty neonatology service. Currently, some hospitals capable of delivering specialty-level obstetric services also provide some elements of neonatal intensive care; such disproportionate service capability is not encouraged. This imbalance or lack of coordination in the provision of services may be a product of a growing competitive health care market and efforts by insurers and health plans to control the costs of health care. Such competitive forces frequently have led to the unnecessary duplication of services within a single community or geographic region, with the potential to result in poorer patient outcomes and, ironically, increased cost.

Systematic review of the published literature over the past three decades demonstrates improved neonatal and posthospital discharge survival among very low birth weight and very preterm infants born in hospitals with neonatal intensive care units. Careful documentation of birth-weight specific neonatal mortality rates by hospital of birth has shown that the chance of survival of premature, very low birth weight infants is highest when births occur in hospitals with higher volume neonatal intensive care units. This finding has been reported in the United States and other countries. In addition, multiple reports regarding the outcomes of neonatal surgery support the concentration of resources and patients in a few highly specialized centers for neonatal surgery. Given the weight of the evidence, it must be emphasized that inpatient perinatal health care services should be organized within individual regions or service areas, in such a manner that there is a concentration of care for the highest-risk pregnant women and their fetuses and neonates who require the highest level of perinatal care.

The determination of the appropriate level of care to be provided by a given hospital should be guided by prevailing local and state health care regulations, national professional organization guidelines, and identified regional perinatal health care service needs. However, state and regional authorities should work with multiple hospitals, clinics, and transportation service providers to determine the appropriate population-based needs in a coordinated system of care. Currently, substantial variation exists among states in the provision of level of care definitions, functional criteria, and regulatory influence.

The expected capabilities of basic, specialty, and subspecialty levels of inpatient perinatal health care services are listed in Table 1-2. Whereas the previous system proposed by the March of Dimes applied to both obstetric and neonatal care, the capabilities outlined in Table 1-2 focus on obstetric care. Table 1-3 outlines the revised and expanded classification system for neonatal care published in 2012 by the American Academy of Pediatrics.

In general, each hospital should have a clear understanding of the categories of perinatal patients that can be managed appropriately in the local facility and those that should be transferred to a higher-level facility. Preterm labor and impending delivery at less than 32 weeks of gestation usually warrant maternal transfer to a facility with neonatal intensive care. In some states, because of geographic distances or demographics, hospitals may be approved for a level of neonatal care higher than that for the perinatal service as a whole. In such circumstances, transfer to a facility with a higher level of perinatal care may be appropriate. An infant, whose mother was unable to be transferred before delivery, usually should be transferred after stabilization of the mother following delivery (see also Chapter 4, "Maternal and Neonatal Interhospital Transfer").

Table 1-2. Capabilities of Health Care Providers in Hospitals Delivering Basic, Specialty, and Subspecialty Perinatal Care*

Level of Care	Capabilities	Health Care Provider Types
Basic	Surveillance and care of all patients admitted to the obstetric service, with an established triage system for identifying patients at high risk who should be transferred to a facility that provides specialty or subspecialty care	Family physicians, obstetricians, laborists, hospitalists, certified nurse-midwives, certified midwives, nurse practitioners, advanced practice registered nurses, physician assistants, surgical assistants, anesthesiologists, and radiologists
	Proper detection and initial care of unanticipated maternal-fetal problems that occur during labor and delivery	
	Capability to begin an emergency cesarean delivery within an interval based on the timing that best incorporates maternal and fetal risks and benefits	
	Availability of appropriate anesthesia, radiology, ultrasonography, and laboratory and blood bank services on a 24-hour basis	
	Care of postpartum conditions	
	Ability to make transfer arrangements in consultation with physicians at higher level receiving hospitals	
	Provision of accommodations and policies that allow families, including their other children, to be together in the hospital following the birth of an infant	
	Data collection, storage, and retrieval	
	Initiation of quality improvement programs, including efforts to maximize patient safety	
Specialty	Provision of all basic care services plus care of appropriate women at high risk and fetuses, both admitted and transferred from other facilities	All basic health care providers, plus sometimes maternal-fetal medicine specialists
Subspecialty	Provision of all basic and specialty care services, plus evaluation of new technologies and therapies	All specialty health care providers, plus maternal-fetal medicine specialists

(continued)

Table 1-2. Capabilities of Health Care Providers in Hospitals Delivering Basic, Specialty, and Subspecialty Perinatal Care* *(continued)*

Level of Care	Capabilities	Health Care Provider Types
Regional subspecialty perinatal health care center	Provision of comprehensive perinatal health care services at and above those of subspecialty care facilities. Responsibility for regional perinatal health care service organization and coordination, including the following areas: • Maternal and neonatal transport • Regional outreach support and education programs • Development and initial evaluation of new technologies and therapies • Training of health care providers with specialty and subspecialty qualifications and capabilities • Analysis and evaluation of regional data, including perinatal complications and outcomes	All subspecialty health care providers, plus other subspecialists, including obstetric and surgical subspecialists

*All institutions providing perinatal care should be capable of neonatal resuscitation and stabilization.

Table 1-3. Definitions, Capabilities, and Health Care Provider Types: Neonatal Levels of Care*

Level of Care	Capabilities	Health Care Provider Types[†]
Level I well newborn nursery	Provide neonatal resuscitation at every delivery Evaluate and provide postnatal care to stable term newborn infants Stabilize and provide care for infants born at 35–37 weeks of gestation who remain physiologically stable Stabilize newborn infants who are ill and those born before 35 weeks of gestation until transfer to a higher level of care	Pediatricians, family physicians, nurse practitioners, and other advanced practice registered nurses

(continued)

Table 1-3. Definitions, Capabilities, and Health Care Provider Types: Neonatal Levels of Care* (continued)

Level of Care	Capabilities	Health Care Provider Types[†]
Level II special care nursery	Level I capabilities plus: Provide care for infants born at 32 weeks of gestation or later and weigh 1,500 g or more who have physiologic immaturity or who are moderately ill with problems that are expected to resolve rapidly and are not anticipated to need subspecialty services on an urgent basis Provide care for infants convalescing after intensive care Provide mechanical ventilation for brief duration (less than 24 hours) or continuous positive airway pressure or both Stabilize infants born before 32 weeks of gestation and weigh less than 1,500 g until transfer to a neonatal intensive care facility	Level I health care providers plus: Pediatric hospitalists, neonatologists, and neonatal nurse practitioners
Level III neonatal intensive care unit	Level II capabilities plus: Provide sustained life support Provide comprehensive care for infants born before 32 weeks of gestation and weigh less than 1,500 g and infants born at all gestational ages and birth weights with critical illness Provide prompt and readily available access to a full range of pediatric medical subspecialists, pediatric surgical specialists, pediatric anesthesiologists, and pediatric ophthalmologists Provide a full range of respiratory support that may include conventional ventilation and/or high-frequency ventilation and inhaled nitric oxide Perform advanced imaging, with interpretation on an urgent basis, including computed tomography, magnetic resonance imaging, and echocardiography	Level II health care providers plus: Pediatric medical subspecialists[‡], pediatric anesthesiologists[‡], pediatric surgeons, and pediatric ophthalmologists[‡]

(continued)

Table 1-3. Definitions, Capabilities, and Health Care Provider Types: Neonatal Levels of Care* *(continued)*

Level of Care	Capabilities	Health Care Provider Types[†]
Level IV regional neonatal intensive care unit	Level III capabilities plus: Located within an institution with the capability to provide surgical repair of complex congenital or acquired conditions Maintain a full range of pediatric medical subspecialists, pediatric surgical subspecialists, and pediatric anesthesiologists at the site Facilitate transport and provide outreach education	Level III health care providers plus: Pediatric surgical subspecialists

*Although the American Academy of Pediatrics uses both functional and numerical designations to describe levels of neonatal care, for the purpose of clarity in this book, functional designations are used to denote levels of perinatal care and numerical designations are used to denote levels of neonatal care.

[†]Includes all health care providers with relevant experience, training, and demonstrated competence

[‡]At the site or at a closely related institution by prearranged consultative agreement

Levels of neonatal care. Policy statement. American Academy of Pediatrics. Committee on Fetus and Newborn. Pediatrics 2012;130:587–97.

Expanded Classification System for Levels of Neonatal Care

The American Academy of Pediatrics published an expanded system for classification of levels of neonatal care in 2004, with a subsequent revision in 2012. The expanded neonatal care classification system, which is illustrated in Table 1-3, builds on the previous categories of basic, specialty, subspecialty, and regional subspecialty perinatal care. Note that each higher level includes the capabilities of the previous level. Although no similar expanded classification system currently exists for obstetric care, women should ideally give birth in an obstetric unit within a facility that provides the level of neonatal care that her newborn is expected to require. Although the American Academy of Pediatrics uses both functional and numerical designations to describe levels of neonatal care, for the purpose of clarity in this book, functional designations will be used to denote levels of perinatal care and numerical designations will be used to denote levels of neonatal care.

Level I Neonatal Care

Level I neonatal care units offer a basic level of newborn care to infants at low risk. These units have personnel and equipment available to perform neonatal resuscitation at every delivery and to evaluate and provide routine postnatal care for healthy term newborn infants. In addition, level I neonatal units have personnel who can care for physiologically stable infants, who are born at or beyond 35 weeks of gestation, and can stabilize ill newborn infants, who are born at less than 35 weeks of gestation, until they can be transferred to a facility where the appropriate level of neonatal care is provided.

Level II Neonatal Care

Level II neonatal care should be reserved for stable or moderately ill newborns born at or beyond 32 weeks of gestation and weigh 1,500 g or more with problems that are expected to resolve rapidly and who would not be anticipated to need subspecialty-level services on an urgent basis. These situations usually occur as a result of relatively uncomplicated preterm labor or preterm rupture of membranes. A facility that provides level II neonatal care has readily available experienced personnel who are capable of providing continuous positive airway pressure or mechanical ventilation for a brief period (less than 24 hours) or both until the infant's condition improves or the infant can be transferred to a higher-level facility (Table 1–3). Level II nurseries must have equipment (eg, portable X-ray equipment, blood gas laboratory) and personnel (eg, physicians, specialized nurses, respiratory therapists, radiology technicians, and laboratory technicians) continuously available to provide ongoing care and to address emergencies. Referral to a higher level of care should occur for all infants when needed for subspecialty surgical or medical intervention.

Level III Neonatal Care

Evidence suggests that infants who are born at less than 32 weeks of gestation or weigh less than 1,500 g at birth or have complex medical or surgical conditions, regardless of gestational age, should be cared for at a level III facility. Designation of level III care should be based on clinical experience, as demonstrated by large patient volume, increasing complexity of care, and availability of pediatric medical subspecialists and pediatric surgical specialists. Subspecialty care services should include expertise in neonatology and, ideally, maternal–fetal medicine if mothers are referred for the management of potential preterm birth. Level III neonatal intensive care units (NICUs) are defined by having continuously available personnel (neonatologists, neonatal nurses, respiratory therapists) and equipment to provide life support for as long as needed. Facilities should have advanced respiratory support and physiologic monitoring equipment, laboratory and imaging facilities, nutrition and pharmacy support with pediatric expertise, social services, and pastoral care. Level III facilities should be able to provide ongoing assisted ventilation for periods longer than 24 hours, which may include conventional ventilation, high-frequency ventilation, and inhaled nitric oxide. Level III facility capabilities also should be based on a region's consideration of geographic constraints, population size, and personnel resources. If geographic constraints for land transportation exist, the level III facility should ensure availability of rotor and fixed-wing transport services to quickly and safely transfer infants requiring subspecialty intervention. Potential transfer to higher-level facilities or children's hospitals, as well as return transport of recovering infants to lower-level facilities, should be considered as clinically indicated.

A broad range of pediatric medical subspecialists and pediatric surgical specialists should be readily accessible on site or by prearranged consultative agreements. Prearranged consultative agreements can be performed using, for example, telemedicine technology, or telephone consultation, or both from a distant location. Pediatric ophthalmology services and an organized program for the monitoring, treatment, and follow-up of retinopathy of prematurity should be readily available in level III facilities. Level III units should have the capability to perform major surgery (including anesthesiologists with pediatric expertise) on site or at a closely related institution, ideally in geographic proximity. Because the outcomes of less complex surgical procedures in children, such as appendectomy or pyloromyotomy, are better when performed by pediatric surgeons compared with general surgeons, it is recommended that pediatric surgical specialists perform all procedures in newborn infants.

Level III facilities should have the capability to perform advanced imaging with interpretation on an urgent basis, including computed tomography, magnetic resonance imaging, and echocardiography. Level III facilities should collect data to assess outcomes within their facility and to compare with other levels.

Level IV Neonatal Care

Level IV units include the capabilities of level III units with additional capabilities and considerable experience in the care of the most complex and critically ill newborn infants and should have pediatric medical and pediatric surgical specialty consultants continuously available 24 hours per day. Level IV facilities also would include the capability for surgical repair of complex conditions (eg, congenital cardiac malformations that require cardiopulmonary bypass with or without extracorporeal membrane oxygenation). Further evidence is needed to assess the risk of morbidity and mortality by level of care for newborn infants with complex congenital cardiac malformations. A recent study by Burstein and colleagues was not able to note a difference in postoperative morbidity or mortality associated with dedicated pediatric cardiac intensive care units versus NICUs and pediatric intensive care units but did not separately assess the newborn and postneonatal periods. Although specific supporting data are not currently available, it is thought that concentrating the care of such infants at designated level IV centers will allow these centers to develop the expertise needed to achieve optimal outcomes.

Not all level IV hospitals need to act as regional centers; however, regional organization of perinatal health care services requires that there be coordination in the development of specialized services, professional continuing education to maintain competency, facilitation of opportunities for transport and return transport, and collection of data on long-term outcomes to evaluate both the effectiveness of delivery of perinatal health care services and the safety and efficacy of new therapies. These functions usually are best achieved when responsibility is concentrated in a single regional center with both perinatal and neonatal subspecialty services.

Maternal and Newborn Postdischarge Care

Perinatal health care at all levels should include ambulatory care of the woman and the neonate after hospital discharge. Increasing economic pressure for early discharge and decreased length of hospital stay after delivery has increased the importance of organization and coordination of continuing care as well as the need for evaluation and monitoring of outcomes. In most cases, healthy term infants discharged before 72 hours of age should be evaluated by a physician within 1–2 days of discharge. Late preterm infants need additional care and monitoring (see also Chapter 8, "Care of the Newborn"). Postdischarge care for an infant who has survived a complicated perinatal course should include care by a pediatrician with expertise and experience in caring for such infants. Infants who have been discharged from the NICU also should be enrolled in an organized follow-up program that tracks and records medical and neurodevelopmental outcomes to allow later analysis. Such a follow-up program is an essential component of level III and level IV neonatal services. Service components for follow-up care for women are discussed in Chapter 6 and for neonates in Chapter 8 and Chapter 9.

Workforce: The Distribution and Supply of Perinatal Care Providers

The distribution and supply of physicians providing perinatal health care services has been changing. Although the number of physicians has increased substantially over the past 20 years, the percentage of all physicians who provide obstetric care has decreased. In addition, obstetricians who provide care for high-risk patients, maternal–fetal medicine specialists, and neonatologists are unevenly distributed among geographic areas and types of facilities. Good data are lacking on the number of obstetricians who provide care for high-risk patients and the number of neonatologists needed to serve a given population. A team approach to perinatal health care delivery is essential to improve the outcome of pregnancy. Certified nurse–midwives, certified midwives, laborists, hospitalists, family practitioners, physician assistants, advanced practice registered nurses, respiratory therapists, perinatal social workers, lactation consultants, and other professionals also are important health care providers of perinatal services.

Strategies aimed at increasing recruitment of perinatal health care providers are needed, particularly in rural and urban medically underserved areas. More than 2,000 federal Health Professional Shortage Areas have been designated; most of the people in need of services in these areas are women of childbearing age and young children. Lack of sufficient funding to support perinatal health care services contributes to the number of underserved women.

Examples of regional programs that have been successfully used to increase access to care include liability cost relief, locum tenens programs, satellite practice models, financial incentives to establish or maintain a practice, innovative approaches to continuing education, and programs to provide technical support. The Health Resources and Services Administration, National Health Service Corps, and state scholarship and loan repayment programs for the education of health care professionals, which include a special requirement for service in underserved areas, provide another important incentive. Such programs should be strengthened, adequately funded, and encouraged to give priority to perinatal health care providers.

Bibliography

Batton DG. Clinical report—Antenatal counseling regarding resuscitation at an extremely low gestational age. Committee on Fetus and Newborn. Pediatrics 2009;124:422–7.

Blackmon LR, Barfield WD, Stark AR. Hospital neonatal services in the United States: variation in definitions, criteria, and regulatory status, 2008. J Perinatol 2009;29: 788–94.

Burstein DS, Jacobs JP, Li JS, Sheng S, O'Brien SM, Rossi AF, et al. Care models and associated outcomes in congenital heart surgery. Pediatrics 2011;127:e1482–9.

Cultural sensitivity and awareness in the delivery of health care. Committee Opinion No. 493. American College of Obstetricians and Gynecologists. Obstet Gynecol 2011;117:1258–61.

Effective patient–physician communication. Committee Opinion No. 492. American College of Obstetricians and Gynecologist. Obstet Gynecol 2011;117(5):1254–7.

Family-centered care and the pediatrician's role. Committee on Hospital Care. American Academy of Pediatrics. Pediatrics 2003;112:691–7.

Engle WA, Tomashek KM, Wallman C. "Late-preterm" infants: a population at risk. Committee on Fetus and Newborn, American Academy of Pediatrics. Pediatrics 2007;120:1390–401.

Howell EM, Richardson D, Ginsburg P, Foot B. Deregionalization of neonatal intensive care in urban areas. Am J Public Health 2002;92:119–24.

Institute for Patient- and Family-Centered Care. Bethesda (MD): IPFCC; 2011. Available at: http://www.ipfcc.org/. Retrieved December 1, 2011.

Institute of Medicine. Health literacy: a prescription to end confusion. Washington, DC: The National Academies Press; 2004.

Institute of Medicine. The best intentions: unintended pregnancy and the well-being of children and families. Washington, DC—National Academies Press; 1995.

Johnson K, Posner SF, Biermann J, Cordero JF, Atrash HK, Parker CS, et al. Recommendations to improve preconception health and health care--United States. A report of the CDC/ATSDR Preconception Care Work Group and the Select Panel on Preconception Care. CDC/ATSDR Preconception Care Work Group; Select Panel on Preconception Care. MMWR Recomm Rep 2006;55(RR-6):1–23.

Lasswell SM, Barfield WD, Rochat RW, Blackmon L. Perinatal regionalization for very low-birth-weight and very preterm infants: a meta-analysis. JAMA 2010;304: 992–1000.

Levels of neonatal care. Policy statement. American Academy of Pediatrics. Committee on Fetus and Newborn. Pediatrics 2012;130:587–97.

March of Dimes. Toward improving the outcome of pregnancy III : enhancing perinatal health through quality, safety and performance initiatives. Committee on Perinatal Health. White Plains (NY): National Foundation--March of Dimes; 2010. Available at: http://www.marchofdimes.com/TIOPIII_FinalManuscript.pdf. Retrieved December 14, 2011.

March of Dimes. Toward improving the outcome of pregnancy : the 90s and beyond. Committee on Perinatal Health. White Plains (NY): National Foundation—March of Dimes; 1993.

March of Dimes. Toward improving the outcome of pregnancy : recommendations for the regional development of maternal and perinatal health services. Committee on Perinatal Health. White Plains (NY): National Foundation—March of Dimes; 1976.

The importance of preconception care in the continuum of women's health care. ACOG Committee Opinion No. 313. American College of Obstetricians and Gynecologists. Obstet Gynecol 2005;106:665–6.

United States. Office of Minority Health. National standards for culturally and linguistically appropriate services in health care: final report. Washington, DC: U.S. Dept. of Health and Human Services; 2001. Available at: http://minorityhealth.hhs.gov/assets/pdf/checked/finalreport.pdf. Retrieved January 19, 2012.

Chapter 2
Inpatient Perinatal Care Services

Inpatient perinatal care services are dependent upon the education, training, and experience of hospital personnel (ie, medical care providers and support staff) as well as the functional capabilities of the physical facilities required for providing care. Regionalized systems are recommended to ensure that each newborn is delivered and cared for in a facility appropriate for his or her health care needs and to facilitate the achievement of optimal outcomes.

Personnel

Factors critical to planning and evaluating the quality and level of personnel required to meet patients' needs in perinatal settings include the mission, philosophy, geographic location, and design of the facility; the patient population; the scope of practice; the qualifications of staff; and obligations for education or research. Perinatal care program personnel include medical care providers (ie, physicians, certified nurse–midwives, and certified midwives), nurse practitioners, physician assistants, and support staff. Medical and nursing directors for obstetric and pediatric services should jointly coordinate perinatal care programs.

Perinatal Medical Care Providers

Perinatal medical care providers include obstetricians, pediatricians, laborists, obstetric–gynecologic and pediatric hospitalists, certified nurse–midwives, and certified midwives.

Obstetricians and Pediatricians

Credentialing and granting privileges to members of its medical staff are among the most important responsibilities of any health care facility. Credentialing is a multifaceted process that involves verification of identification (such as National Provider Identification), licensure, education, training, specialty board certification, medical liability coverage, and experience. Other criteria for effective credentialing include review of official source data, such as the National

Practitioner Data Bank, data from state licensing boards, data from other facilities where the individual has privileges, and references from peers. Hospitals must query the National Practitioner Data Bank at the time of application and every 2 years for clinical privileges, as well as when the hospital wants to expand existing privileges.

The more difficult, yet critical, aspect of the credentialing process is the actual determination of which requested privileges should be granted. The granting of privileges is based on training, experience, and demonstrated current clinical competence. For obstetric providers, care may be stratified into different levels of complexity. New equipment or technology may improve health care outcomes, provided that practitioners and other hospital staff use the tools as specified for the conditions for which they are designed. Problems can arise when physicians or staff perform procedures or use equipment for which they are not trained. Institutions should consider granting privileges for new skills only when the appropriate training has been completed and documented and the competency level has been achieved with adequate supervision (see also Appendix D).

For pediatric providers, the credentials required and the privileges extended will depend on the level of care that is provided. Verification of training, experience, credentialing, and current clinical competence is similar to that for obstetric providers.

Laborists and Hospitalists

The term "laborist" most commonly refers to an obstetrician–gynecologist who is employed by a hospital or physician group and whose primary role is to care for laboring patients and to manage obstetric emergencies. The term "hospitalist" refers to physicians whose primary professional focus is the general medical care of hospitalized patients. Hospitalists help manage the continuum of patient care in the hospital, often seeing patients in the emergency department, following them into the critical care unit, and organizing postacute care. An obstetric–gynecologic hospitalist may provide in-house gynecologic services as well. A pediatric hospitalist is a pediatrician whose responsibilities can include providing neonatal care at deliveries, caring for healthy and moderately ill newborns, and working with neonatologists to assist in the care of critically ill newborns. For both of these types of inpatient providers, guiding principles recommend the maintenance of communication between the laborist or obstetric–gynecologic hospitalist and the obstetrician and between the pediatric hospitalist and the neonatologist or pediatrician primarily responsible for care.

Certified Nurse–Midwives and Certified Midwives

Certified nurse–midwives are registered nurses who have graduated from a midwifery education program accredited by the Accreditation Commission for Midwifery Education and have passed a national certification examination administered by the American Midwifery Certification Board, Inc., formerly the American College of Nurse–Midwives Certification Council, Inc. Certified midwives undergo the same certification process as certified nurse–midwives, but their training does not include education in nursing. They are graduates of a midwifery education program accredited by the Accreditation Commission for Midwifery Education and have successfully completed the American Midwifery Certification Board, Inc. certification examination and adhere to the same professional standards as certified nurse–midwives. Certified nurse–midwives and certified midwives manage the care of low-risk women in the antepartum, intrapartum, and postpartum periods; manage healthy newborns; and provide primary gynecologic services in accordance with state laws or regulations. In collaboration with obstetricians, certified nurse–midwives and certified midwives also may be involved in the care of women with medical or obstetric complications. They work in a variety of settings, including private practice, community health facilities, clinics, hospitals, and accredited birth centers (see also Appendix E).

Capabilities of Perinatal Medical Care Providers

Basic Perinatal Care and Level I Neonatal Care. The perinatal care program at a hospital providing basic care should be coordinated jointly by the chiefs of the obstetric, pediatric, nursing, and midwifery services. This administrative approach requires close coordination and unified policy statements. The coordinators of perinatal care at a hospital who deliver basic care are responsible for developing policy, maintaining appropriate guidelines, and collaborating and consulting with the professional staff of hospitals (including anesthesiologists, radiologists, and laboratory personnel) who provide specialty and subspecialty care in the region. In hospitals that do not separate these services, one person may be given the responsibility for coordinating perinatal care.

Hospitals at this level of care should ensure the availability of skilled personnel for perinatal emergencies. A facility providing level I neonatal care should have the personnel and equipment to perform neonatal resuscitation. At least one person whose primary responsibility is for the newborn and who is capable of initiating neonatal resuscitation should be present at every delivery. Either that person or someone else who is immediately available should have the skills required to perform a complete resuscitation, including endotracheal intubation and administration of medications. This resuscitation should be performed according to the American Heart Association and American Academy of Pediatrics Neonatal Resuscitation Program. When required, one or two additional persons should be available to assist with neonatal resuscitation. (For more information on neonatal resuscitation, see Chapter 8.)

A qualified physician or certified nurse–midwife or certified midwife should attend all deliveries. Collaborative practice involving a multidisciplinary team is encouraged. The team consists of obstetrician–gynecologists and other health-care professionals who function within their educational preparation and scope of practice. These team members work together, utilizing mutually agreed upon guidelines and policies that define the individual and shared responsibilities of each member. Although the responsibilities of obstetrician–gynecologists place them in the role of ultimate authority because of their education and training, the contributions of each team member are valued and important to the quality of patient outcomes. The concept of a team guided by one of its own members and the acceptance of shared responsibility for outcomes promote shared accountability. Facilitation of communication among health care providers is essential for the provision of safe, quality care.

Cesarean delivery may warrant the assistance of an additional physician, a surgical assistant, in order to provide safe surgical care. Although the degree of complexity of cesarean deliveries cannot always be predicted, competent surgical assistants should be available, based on the judgment of the primary obstetric surgeon. Anesthesia personnel with credentials to administer obstetric anesthesia should be available on a 24-hour basis

Specialty Perinatal Care and Level II Neonatal Care. At a hospital providing specialty perinatal care and level II neonatal care, a board-certified obstetrician-gynecologist with special interest, experience, and, in some situations, a subspecialty in maternal–fetal medicine, should be chief of the obstetric service. A board-certified pediatrician with subspecialty certification in neonatal–perinatal medicine should be chief of the neonatal care service. These physicians should coordinate the hospital's perinatal care services and, in conjunction with other medical, anesthesia, nursing, midwifery, respiratory therapy, and hospital administration staff, develop policies concerning staffing, procedures, equipment, and supplies.

Care of neonates at high risk should be provided by appropriately qualified personnel. A facility with a level II special care nursery must have the specialized physicians (eg, pediatricians, pediatric hospitalists, and neonatologists), neonatal nurse practitioners (see also "Perinatal Nurse Practitioners" later in this chapter), and specialized support personnel (eg, respiratory therapists, radiology technicians, and laboratory technicians; see also "Support Health Care Providers" later in this chapter) and equipment (eg, portable chest radiograph and blood gas laboratory) continuously available to provide ongoing care as well as to address emergencies. When an infant is maintained on a ventilator, these specialized personnel should be available on site to manage respiratory emergencies.

A general pediatrician should have the expertise to assume responsibility for acute, although less critical, care of newborns; understand the need for proper continuity of care and be capable of providing it; and share responsibility with a consulting neonatologist for the development and delivery of effective services for newborns at risk in the hospital and community. In collaboration with, or under the supervision of, a physician, care may be provided by qualified advanced practice registered nurses who have completed a formal neonatal educational program and are certified by an accepted national body, such as the National Certification Corporation (see also "Perinatal Nurse Practitioners" later in this chapter).

The director of obstetric anesthesia services should be board certified in anesthesia and should have training and experience in obstetric anesthesia. Anesthesia personnel with privileges to administer obstetric anesthesia should be available according to hospital policy. Policies should be developed regarding the provision of obstetric anesthesia, including the necessary qualifications of personnel who are to administer anesthesia and their availability for both routine and emergency deliveries. Specialized medical and surgical consultation also should be available.

Subspecialty Perinatal Care and Level III and Level IV Neonatal Care. The director of the maternal–fetal medicine service of a hospital providing subspecialty care should be a full-time, board-certified obstetrician with subspecialty certification in maternal–fetal medicine. The director of the neonatal intensive care unit (NICU) should be a full-time, board-certified pediatrician with subspecialty certification in neonatal–perinatal medicine. As co-directors of the perinatal service, these physicians are responsible for maintaining practice guidelines and, in cooperation with nursing and hospital administration, are responsible for developing the operating budget; evaluating and purchasing equipment; planning, developing, and coordinating in-hospital and outreach educational programs; and participating in the evaluation of perinatal care. If they are in a regional center, they should devote their time to providing and supervising patient care services, research, and teaching, and they should coordinate the services provided at their hospital with those provided at institutions delivering lower levels of care in the region or system.

Other maternal–fetal medicine specialists and neonatologists who practice in the subspecialty care facility should have qualifications similar to those of the chief of their service. A maternal–fetal medicine specialist and a neonatologist should be continuously available for consultation 24 hours per day. Personnel qualified to manage the care of mothers or neonates with complex or critical illnesses, including emergencies, should be in-house.

A board-certified anesthesiologist with special training or experience in maternal–fetal anesthesia should be in charge of obstetric anesthesia services at a hospital delivering subspecialty perinatal care. Personnel with privileges in the administration of obstetric anesthesia should be available in the hospital 24 hours per day. In addition, advanced diagnostic imaging facilities with interpretation on an urgent basis should be available 24 hours per day.

A facility providing level III or level IV neonatal care has continuously available personnel and equipment to provide sustained life support and to provide comprehensive care for newborns at extremely high risk and those with complex and critical illnesses. These NICUs provide advanced medical and surgical care. Because of the degree of risk involved, advanced fetal interventions, such as intrauterine fetal transfusions and fetal–placental surgery, should be performed at hospitals capable of providing subspecialty perinatal care with accompanying level III or level IV NICUs.

Level III NICUs require urgent access for consultation to a broad range of pediatric, rather than adult, medical subspecialists, including cardiology, neurology, hematology, genetics, nephrology, metabolism, endocrinology, gastroenterology–nutrition, infectious diseases, pulmonology, immunology, pathology, and pharmacology. Pediatric surgical and anesthesia capability should be available onsite or at a closely related institution for consultation and care. Evidence indicates that management of neonates and young children by adult subspecialists, rather than pediatric subspecialists, results in greater costs, longer hospital stays, and potentially greater morbidity. As previously noted, level IV neonatal units have all the capabilities of a level III NICU as well as the ability to perform surgical repair of complex congenital and medical conditions that require the skills of pediatric surgical subspecialists. Level IV neonatal units often are located within freestanding children's hospitals.

Perinatal Nurse Practitioners

Nursing responsibilities in individual hospitals vary according to the level of care provided by the facility, practice procedures, number of professional registered nurses and ancillary staff, and professional nursing activities in continuing education and research. Intrapartum care requires the same labor intensiveness and expertise as any other intensive care and, accordingly, perinatal units should have the same adequately trained personnel and fiscal support.

Trends in medical management and technologic advances influence and may increase the nursing workload. Each hospital should determine the scope of nursing practice for each nursing unit and specialty department. The scope of practice should be based on national nursing guidelines for the specialty area of practice and should be in accordance with state laws and regulations and the recommended staffing patterns for the particular type of health care provider. The health care provider-to-patient ratio should take into account the role expected at the individual unit, acuity of patients, procedures performed, and participation in deliveries or neonatal transport. A multidisciplinary committee, including representatives from hospital, medical, and nursing administrations, should follow published professional guidelines, consult state nurse practice acts and any accompanying regulations, identify the types and numbers of procedures performed in each unit, delineate the direct and indirect nursing care activities performed, and identify the activities that are to be performed by non-nursing personnel.

Advanced Practice Registered Nurses

Trends in neonatal and maternal care have resulted in the increased use of advanced practice registered nurses. Included in this category are the neonatal, perinatal, and women's health clinical nurse specialist and the neonatal and women's health nurse practitioner (described later in this section). An advanced practice registered nurse is prepared, according to nationally recognized standards, by the completion of an educational program of study and supervised practice beyond the level of basic nursing. As of January 1, 2000, this preparation must include the attainment of a master's degree in the nursing specialty. Nurses without a graduate degree who entered the profession before the year 2000, but are credentialed advanced practice registered nurses or certificate-prepared (nongraduate) nurse practitioners, should be allowed to maintain their practice and are encouraged to complete their formal graduate education. Nationally recognized certification examinations exist for each category of advanced practice nursing. Credentialing is now required on a national level and is no longer governed by individual states.

Clinical Nurse Specialist. A neonatal, perinatal, and women's health clinical nurse specialist is a registered nurse with a master's degree who, through study and supervised practice at the graduate level, has become an expert in the theory and practice of neonatal, perinatal, and women's health nursing. Responsibilities of the clinical nurse specialist include fostering continuous quality improvement in nursing care and developing and educating staff. The clinical nurse specialist models expert nursing practice, participates in administrative functions within the hospital setting, serves as a consultant external to the unit, and applies and promotes evidence-based nursing practice.

Nurse Practitioner. A neonatal or women's health nurse practitioner is a registered nurse who has clinical expertise in neonatal or women's health nursing; has a master's degree or has completed an educational program of study and supervised practice in the specialty; and has acquired supervised clinical experience in the management of patients and their families. Using their acquired knowledge of pathophysiology, pharmacology, and advanced assessment, nurse practitioners exercise independent judgment in the assessment and diagnosis of patients and in the performance of certain procedures. They develop a plan of care, provide treatment, and evaluate outcomes. Similar to the clinical nurse specialist, a nurse practitioner also may be involved in education, administration, consultation, and research.

Neonatal nurse practitioners manage a caseload of neonatal patients in collaboration with a physician, usually a pediatrician or neonatologist. Nurse practitioners caring for neonates in the NICU must demonstrate completion of a formal neonatal educational program and national certification as a neonatal nurse practitioner. Any advanced practice registered nurse caring for neonates must demonstrate completion of a formal neonatal educational program that includes a minimum of 200 neonatal-specific didactic hours and at least 600 supervised clinical hours in the care of the at-risk and critically ill newborn in level II, level III, or level IV NICUs. Nurse practitioners who are not educated as neonatal nurse practitioners and are working as nursing practitioners in the NICU are functioning beyond their scope of practice.

Women's health nurse practitioners manage the care of women in collaboration with a physician, usually an obstetrician–gynecologist or a maternal–fetal medicine specialist. They must demonstrate completion of a formal women's health educational program and national certification as a women's health nurse practitioner. This training includes both didactic and clinical education and includes a demonstrated competency in pharmacology.

Scope of Practice. The spectrum of duties performed by an advanced practice registered nurse will vary according to the institution and may be determined by state regulations. Inpatient care privileges are granted by individual institutions. Each institution should develop a procedure for the initial granting and subsequent maintenance of privileges, ensuring that the proper professional credentials are in place. Each institution must ensure that the advanced practice registered nurse has the formal education to function within the neonatal scope of practice. That procedure is best developed by the collaborative efforts of the nursing administration and the medical staff governing body. The following guidelines are recommended:

- Clinical care by the advanced practice registered nurse for neonates receiving level II, level III, and level IV care is provided in collaboration with, or under the supervision of, a physician, usually a neonatologist. Clinical care by the advanced practice registered nurse for neonates receiving level I neonatal care is provided in collaboration with, or under the supervision of a physician with special interest and experience in neonatal medicine, usually this is a pediatrician or neonatologist.

- Clinical care by the advanced practice registered nurse for women is provided in collaboration with, or under the supervision of, a physician, usually a maternal–fetal medicine specialist.

- Determination of whether the advanced practice registered nurse practices in collaboration with, or under the supervision of, a physician should be determined in accordance with the board of nursing regulations in the state in which the advanced practice registered nurse is practicing.

- The advanced practice registered nurse should be certified by a nationally recognized organization and should maintain that certification.

- The advanced practice registered nurse should maintain clinical expertise and knowledge of current therapy by participating in continuing education and other scholarly activities as recommended by the National Certification Corporation.

- The advanced practice registered nurse should comply with hospital policy regarding credentialing and recredentialing.

Nurse–Patient Ratios

Delivery of safe and effective perinatal nursing care requires appropriately qualified registered nurses in adequate numbers to meet the needs of each patient. The number of staff and level of skill required are influenced by the scope of nursing practice and the degree of nursing responsibilities within an institution. Close evaluation of all factors involved in a specific case is essential for establishing an acceptable nurse–patient ratio. Variables, such as birth weight, gestational age, and diagnoses of patients; patient turnover; acuity of patients' conditions; patient or family education needs; bereavement care; mixture of skills of the staff; environment; types of delivery; and use of anesthesia must be taken into account in determining appropriate nurse–patient ratios.

Levels of Perinatal Nursing Care

Basic Perinatal Care and Level I Neonatal Care. Perinatal nursing care in a facility at this level of care should be under the direction of a registered nurse. The registered nurse's responsibilities include directing perinatal nursing services, guiding the development and implementation of perinatal policies and procedures, collaborating with medical staff, and consulting with hospitals that provide higher levels of care in the region or system.

For perinatal care, it is recommended that there be an on-duty registered nurse whose responsibilities include the organization and supervision of antepartum, intrapartum, and neonatal nursing services. The presence of one or more registered nurses or licensed practical nurses with demonstrated knowledge and clinical competence in the nursing care of women, fetuses, and newborns during labor, delivery, and the postpartum and neonatal periods is suggested. Ancillary personnel, supervised by a registered nurse, may provide support to the patient and attend to her personal comfort.

Intrapartum care should take place under the direct supervision of a registered nurse. Responsibilities of the registered nurse include initial evaluation and admission of patients in labor; continuing assessment and evaluation of patients in labor, including checking the status of the fetus, recording vital signs, monitoring the fetal heart rate, performing obstetric examinations, observing uterine contractions, and supporting the patient; determining the presence or absence of complications; supervising the performance of nurses with less training and experience and of ancillary personnel; and staffing of the delivery room at the time of delivery. A licensed practical nurse or nurse assistant, supervised by a registered nurse, may provide support to the patient and attend to her personal comfort.

Postpartum care of the woman and her newborn should be supervised by a registered nurse whose responsibilities include initial and ongoing assessment, newborn care education, support for the attachment process and breastfeeding, preparation for healthy parenting, preparation for discharge, and follow-up of the woman and her newborn within the context of the family. This registered nurse should have training and experience in the recognition of normal and abnormal physical and emotional characteristics of the mother and her newborn. Again, a licensed practical nurse or nurse assistant, supervised by a registered nurse, may provide support to the mother and attend to her personal comfort in the postpartum period.

Routine newborn care delivered by the registered nurse is provided in collaboration with a pediatrician. The nurse monitors the infant's adaptation to extrauterine life and then, ideally, assists in the transition of the healthy newborn to the mother's room.

Specialty Perinatal Care and Level II Neonatal Care. Hospitals at this level of care should have a director of perinatal and neonatal nursing services who has overall responsibility for inpatient activities in the respective obstetric and neonatal areas. This registered nurse should have demonstrated expertise in obstetric care, neonatal care, or both.

In addition to fulfilling basic perinatal care nursing responsibilities, nursing staff in the labor, delivery, and recovery unit should be able to identify and respond to the obstetric and medical complications of pregnancy, labor, and delivery. A registered nurse with advanced training and experience in routine obstetric care and high-risk obstetric care should be assigned to the labor, delivery, and recovery unit at all times. In the postpartum period, a registered nurse should be responsible for providing support for women and families with newborns who require intensive care and for facilitating visitation and communication with the NICU.

Licensed practical nurses and unlicensed personnel who have appropriate training in perinatal care and are supervised by a registered nurse may provide assistance with the delivery of care, provide support to the patient, assist with lactation support, and attend to the woman's personal comfort.

All nurses caring for ill newborns must possess demonstrated knowledge in the observation and treatment of newborns, including cardiorespiratory monitoring. Furthermore, the registered nursing staff of a level II neonatal unit in a hospital that provides specialty perinatal care takes on a greater responsibility for monitoring the premature newborn or the newborn who is having difficulty in adapting to extrauterine life. The neonatal nurse at this level cares for premature or term newborns who are ill or injured from complications at birth. The neonatal nurse provides the newborn with frequent observation and monitoring and should be able to monitor and maintain the stability of cardio-pulmonary, neurologic, metabolic, and thermal functions, either independently or in conjunction with the physician; assist with special procedures, such as lumbar puncture, endotracheal intubation, and umbilical vessel catheterization; and perform emergency resuscitation. The nurse should be specially trained and able to initiate, modify, or stop treatment when appropriate, according to established protocols, even when a physician or advanced practice nurse is not present. In units where neonates receive mechanical ventilation, medical, nursing, or respiratory therapy staff with demonstrated ability to intubate the trachea, manage assisted ventilation, and decompress a pneumothorax should be available continually. The nursing staff should be formally trained and competent in neonatal resuscitation. The unit's medical director, in conjunction with other personnel, should define and supervise the delegated medical functions, processes, and procedures performed by various categories of personnel.

Subspecialty Perinatal Care and Level III and Level IV Neonatal Care. The director of perinatal and neonatal nursing services at a facility providing this level of care should have overall responsibility for inpatient activities in the maternity–newborn care units. This registered nurse should have experience and training in obstetric nursing, neonatal nursing, or both, as well as in the care of patients at high risk. Preferably, this individual should have an advanced degree.

For antepartum care, a registered nurse should be responsible for the direction and supervision of nursing care. All nurses working with antepartum patients at high risk should have evidence of continuing education in maternal–fetal nursing. An advanced practice registered nurse who has been educated and prepared at the master's degree level should be on staff to coordinate education.

For intrapartum care, a registered nurse should be in attendance within the labor and delivery unit at all times. This registered nurse should be skilled in the recognition and nursing management of complications of labor and delivery.

For postpartum care, a registered nurse should be in attendance at all times. This registered nurse should be skilled in the recognition and nursing management of complications in women and newborns.

Registered nurses in NICUs should have specialty certification or advanced training and experience in the nursing management of neonates at high risk and their families. They also should be experienced in caring for unstable neonates with multiorgan system problems and in specialized care technology. The neonatal nurse provides direct care for the premature or term infant who requires complex care, including neonates requiring intensive life-support techniques, such as mechanical ventilation. In these units, the nurse also should be able to provide care for infants requiring inhaled nitric oxide therapy and high-frequency ventilation as well as care for the chronically technology-dependent infant.

An advanced practice registered nurse should be available to the staff for consultation and support on nursing care issues. Additional nurses with special training are required to fulfill regional center responsibilities, such as outreach and transport (see also "Transport Procedure" and "Outreach Education" in Chapter 4).

The obstetric and neonatal areas may be staffed by a mix of professional and technical personnel. Assessment and monitoring activities should remain the responsibility of a registered nurse or an advanced practice registered nurse in obstetric–neonatal nursing, even when personnel with a mixture of skills are used.

Physician Assistants

Trends in neonatal care also have resulted in an increased use of physician assistants in addition to advanced practice registered nurses. Physician assistants are health care professionals licensed to practice medicine with physician supervision. Within the physician–physician assistant relationship, physician assistants exercise autonomy in medical decision making and provide a broad range of diagnostic and therapeutic services. A physician assistant's responsibilities also may include education, research, and administrative services.

Physician assistants are educated and trained in programs accredited by the Accreditation Review Commission on Education for the Physician Assistant. The length of physician assistant programs averages approximately 26 months, and students must complete more than 2,000 hours of supervised clinical practice before graduation. Graduation from an accredited physician assistant program and passage of the national certifying examination are required for state licensure. A number of postgraduate physician assistant programs also have been established to provide practicing physician assistants with advanced education or master's level education in medical specialties.

The responsibilities of a physician assistant depend on the practice setting, education, and experience of the physician assistant, and on state laws and regulations. Regardless of background training, the following guidelines are recommended:

- Physician supervision should be provided by a neonatologist in subspecialty NICUs. In level I, level II, level III, and level IV neonatal units, a board-certified pediatrician with special interest and experience in neonatal medicine may provide supervision.

- The physician assistant is responsible for maintaining clinical expertise and knowledge of current therapy by participating in continuing medical education and scholarly activities.

- To maintain their national certification, physician assistants must log 100 hours of continuing medical education every 2 years and take a recertification examination given by the National Commission on Certification of Physician Assistants every 6 years.

Support Health Care Providers

All Facilities

Personnel who are capable of determining blood type, crossmatching blood, and performing antibody testing should be available on a 24-hour basis. The hospital's infection control personnel should be responsible for surveillance of infections in women and neonates as well as for the development of an appropriate environmental control program (see also Chapter 11, "Infection Control"). A radiologic technician should be available 24 hours per day to perform portable X-rays. Availability of a postpartum care provider with expertise in lactation is essential. The need for other support personnel depends on the intensity and level of sophistication of the other support services provided. An organized plan of action that includes personnel and equipment should be established for identification and immediate resuscitation of neonates in need of intervention (see also Chapter 8 for information on neonatal resuscitation).

High-Level Care Facilities

The following support personnel should be available to the perinatal care service of hospitals providing specialty and subspecialty perinatal care and level III and level IV neonatal care:

- At least one full-time, master's degree-level, medical social worker for every 30 beds who has experience with the socioeconomic and psychosocial problems of both women and fetuses at high risk, ill neonates, and their families. Additional medical social workers are required when there is a high volume of medical or psychosocial activity.

- At least one occupational or physical therapist with neonatal expertise
- At least one individual skilled in evaluation and management of neonatal feeding and swallowing disorders (eg, speech-language pathologist)
- At least one registered dietitian or nutritionist who has special training in perinatal nutrition and can plan diets that meet the special needs of both women and neonates at high risk
- Qualified personnel for support services, such as diagnostic laboratory studies, radiologic studies, and ultrasound examinations (these personnel should be available 24 hours per day)
- Respiratory therapists who can supervise the assisted ventilation of neonates
- Pharmacy personnel with pediatric expertise who can work to continually review their systems and processes of medication administration to ensure that patient care policies are maintained
- Personnel skilled in pastoral care, available as needed

The hospital's engineering department should include air-conditioning, electrical, and mechanical engineers and biomedical technicians who are responsible for the safety and reliability of the equipment in all perinatal care areas.

Education

In-Service and Continuing Education

The medical and nursing staff of any hospital providing perinatal care at any level should maintain knowledge about and competency in current maternal and neonatal care through joint in-service sessions. These sessions should cover the diagnosis and management of perinatal emergencies, as well as the management of routine problems and family-centered care. The staff of each unit should have regular multidisciplinary conferences at which patient care problems are presented and discussed.

The staff of regional centers should be capable of assisting with the in-service programs of other hospitals in their region on a regular basis. Such assistance may include periodic visits to those hospitals as well as periodic review of the quality of patient care provided by those hospitals. Regional center staff should be accessible for consultation at all times. The medical and nursing staff of hospitals that provide higher level care (ie, beyond basic and level I) should participate in formal courses or conferences. Regularly scheduled conferences may include the following subjects:

- Review of the major perinatal conditions, their medical treatment, and nursing care
- Review of electronic fetal monitoring, including maternal–fetal outcomes, toward a goal of standardizing nomenclature and patient care
- Review of perinatal statistics, the pathology related to all deaths, and significant surgical specimens
- Review of current imaging studies
- Review of perinatal complications and outcomes
- Review of patient satisfaction data, complaints, and compliments

Perinatal Outreach Education

Design and coordination of a program for perinatal outreach education should be provided jointly by neonatal and obstetric physicians and advanced practice registered nurses. Responsibilities should include assessing educational needs; planning curricula; teaching, implementing, and evaluating the program; collecting and using perinatal data; providing patient follow-up information to referring community personnel; writing reports; and maintaining informative working relationships with community personnel and outreach team members.

Ideally, a maternal–fetal medicine specialist, a certified nurse–midwife or certified midwife, an obstetric nurse, a neonatologist, and a neonatal nurse should be members of the perinatal outreach education team. Other professionals (eg, a social worker, respiratory therapist, occupational and physical therapist, or nutritionist) also may be assigned to the team. Each member should be responsible for teaching, consulting with community professionals as needed, and maintaining communication with the program coordinator and other team members.

Each subspecialty care center in a regionalized or integrated system may organize an education program that is tailored to meet the needs of the perinatal health professionals and institutions within the network. The various educational strategies that have been found to be effective include seminars, audiovisual and media programs, self-instruction booklets, and clinical practice rotations. Perinatal outreach education meetings should be held at a routine time and place to promote standardization and continuity of communication among community professionals and regional center personnel. As mandated by the subspecialty boards and the Accreditation Council for Graduate Medical

Education, a facility providing subspecialty care that has a fellowship training program must have an active research program.

Quality Improvement

Support for outcomes measurement, including data collection and membership in a multi-institutional collaborative quality improvement database should be incorporated in the NICU budget. Support also should be available for at least one ongoing, active quality improvement initiative (see also Chapter 3, "Quality Improvement and Patient Safety").

Physical Facilities

The physical facilities in which perinatal care is provided should be conducive to care that meets the unique physiologic and psychosocial needs of newborns and their families (see also "Patient-Centered and Family-Centered Health Care" in Chapter 1). Special facilities should be available when deviations from the norm require uninterrupted physiologic, biochemical, and clinical observation of patients throughout the perinatal period. Labor, delivery, and newborn care facilities should be located in proximity to each other. When these facilities are distant from each other, provisions should be made for appropriate transitional areas.

The following recommendations are intended as general guidelines and should be interpreted with consideration given to local needs. Individual limitations of physical facilities for perinatal care may impede strict adherence to these recommendations. Furthermore, every facility will not have each of the functional units described. Provisions for individual units should be consistent with a regionalized perinatal care system and state and local public health regulations.

Obstetric Functional Units

The patient's personal needs, as well as those of her newborn and family, should be considered when obstetric service units are planned. The service should be consolidated in a designated area that is physically arranged to prohibit unrelated traffic through the service units. The obstetric facility should incorporate the following components of maternity and newborn care:

- Antepartum care for patient stabilization or hospitalization before labor
- Fetal diagnostic testing (eg, nonstress and contraction stress testing, biophysical profile, amniocentesis, and ultrasound examinations)

- Labor observation and evaluation for patients who are not yet in active labor or who must be observed to determine whether labor has actually begun; hospital obstetric services should develop a casual, comfortable area ("false-labor lounge") for patients in prodromal labor
- Labor
- Delivery
- Infant resuscitation and stabilization
- Postpartum maternal and newborn care

Where rooms are suitably sized, located, and equipped, some or all of the components of maternity care listed previously can be combined in one or more rooms. Combining functions into labor, delivery, and recovery rooms maximize economy and flexibility of staff and space. The traditional obstetric program model—with separate rooms for labor, delivery, recovery, and postpartum care—has become obsolete in new construction guidelines, such as the *2010 Guidelines for Design and Construction of Health Care Facilities.*

The following facilities should be available to both the antepartum unit and the postpartum unit and, in appropriate circumstances, may be shared:

- Unit director and head nurse's office
- Nurses' station
- Medical records area with a flat writing surface, computers with access to electronic medical records, or both
- Conference room
- Patient education area
- Staff lounge, locker rooms, and on call sleep rooms
- Examination and treatment room(s)
- Secure area for storage of medications
- Instrument cleanup area
- Soiled workroom and holding room
- Area and equipment for bedpan cleansing
- Kitchen and pantry
- Clean workroom or clean supply room
- Equipment and supply storage area
- Sibling visiting area

The need for care of extremely obese patients is growing for all medical and surgical units in the United States, including maternity units. These patients require more space for antenatal, intrapartum, and postpartum care; staff; and equipment able to support heavier weights. (For more information, see "Obesity and Bariatric Surgery" in Chapter 7.)

The labor and delivery area should be used for nonobstetric patients only during periods of low occupancy. The obstetric department, in conjunction with the hospital administration, should establish written policies according to state and local regulations indicating which nonobstetric patients may be admitted to the labor and delivery suite. Under all circumstances, however, labor and delivery patients must take precedence over nonobstetric patients in this area. Clean gynecologic operations may be performed in the delivery rooms if patients are adequately screened to eliminate infectious cases and if enough personnel are present to prevent any compromise in the quality of obstetric care.

Combined Units

Comprehensive obstetric and neonatal care is optimally provided for women at both low risk and high risk and their healthy newborns in a labor, delivery, and recovery unit that uses another room for mother–baby postpartum care. Alternatively, care can be provided in a conventional obstetric unit that uses different rooms for labor, delivery, recovery, and newborn care. Registered nurses who are cross-trained in antepartum care, labor and delivery care, postpartum care, and neonatal care should staff this unit, increasing the continuity and quality of care.

Each labor, delivery, and recovery room is a single-patient room containing a toilet and shower with optional bathtub. A sink should be located in each room for scrubbing, handwashing, and neonate bathing. A window with an outside view is desirable in the labor, delivery, and recovery room. Each room should contain a birthing bed that is comfortable during labor and can be readily converted to a delivery bed and transported to the cesarean delivery room when necessary. A bassinet for the neonate should be readily available. A designated area within the room, distinct from the laboring woman's area, should be provided for neonatal stabilization and resuscitation and contain a radiant warmer (see also "Neonatal Functional Units" later in this chapter). Separate oxygen, air, and suction facilities for the woman and the neonate should be provided in two separate locations. Gas outlets and wall-mounted equipment should be easily accessible but may be covered with a panel. Either a ceiling mount or a portable delivery light may be used, depending on the preference of the obstetric staff.

Proper care of the woman in labor requires sufficient space for a sphygmomanometer, stethoscope, fetal monitor, infusion pump, regional anesthesia administration, and resuscitation equipment at the head of the bed. Proper care requires access to the newborn from three sides and quick transport to the nursery or NICU should the need arise. The family area should be farthest from the entry to the room, and there should be a comfortable area for the support person.

Equipment needed for labor, delivery, newborn resuscitation, and newborn care should be stored either in the room or in a nearby central storage or supply area and should be immediately available to the labor, delivery, and recovery room. For ease of movement, space below the foot of the bed should be adequate to accommodate staff and equipment brought into the room. Standard major equipment held in this area for delivery should include a fetal monitor, delivery case cart, linen hamper, and portable examination lights. A unit equipped for neonatal stabilization and resuscitation (described in "Neonatal Functional Units" later in this chapter) should be available during delivery.

The workable size of a labor, delivery, and recovery room measures 340 net ft^2 (31.57 m^2), including an infant stabilization and resuscitation area of 40 ft^2 (3.7 m^2) of floor space that is distinct from the mother's area. This room should be able to accommodate six to eight people comfortably during the childbirth process.

Labor. Each labor, delivery, and recovery room should have the following equipment and supplies necessary for women in labor:

- Sterilization equipment (if there is no central sterilization equipment)
- X-ray view box or a computer and monitor to review digital images
- Stretchers with side rails
- Equipment for pelvic examinations
- Emergency drugs
- Suction apparatus, either operated from a wall outlet or portable equipment
- Cardiopulmonary resuscitation cart (maternal and neonatal)
- Protective gear for personnel exposed to body fluids
- Warming cabinets for solutions and blankets

- A labor or birthing bed and a footstool
- A storage area for the patient's clothing and personal belongings
- Sufficient work space for information management systems
- One or more comfortable chairs
- Adjustable lighting that is pleasant for the patient and adequate for examinations
- An emergency signal and intercommunication system
- Adequate ventilation and temperature control
- Equipment to measure and monitor blood pressure
- Mechanical infusion equipment
- Fetal monitoring equipment
- Oxygen outlets
- Adequate electrical outlets
- Access to at least one shower for use by patients in labor
- A writing surface for medical records, computer hookup for medical record purposes, or both
- Storage facilities for supplies and equipment

There should be adequate space for support persons, personnel, and equipment, and room for the patient to ambulate in labor. Design or renovation should include planning for bedside and workstation information management systems and for computer management of medical information.

Patients with significant medical or obstetric complications should be cared for in a labor, delivery, and recovery room that is specially equipped with cardiopulmonary resuscitation equipment and other monitoring equipment necessary for observation and special care. Rooms used for intensive care of patients at high risk in hospitals with no designated high-risk units are best located in the labor and delivery area and should meet the physical standards of any other intensive care room in the hospital, with a minimum of 200 net ft^2 (18.58 m^2) of floor space and at least three oxygen and three suction outlets. When patients with significant medical or obstetric complications receive care in the labor and delivery area, the capabilities of the unit should be identical to those of an intensive care unit.

Delivery. Delivery can be performed in a properly sized and equipped labor, delivery, and recovery room. A comfortable waiting area for families should be adjacent to the labor, delivery, and recovery room, and restrooms should be nearby.

Traditional delivery rooms and cesarean delivery rooms are similar in design to operating rooms. Vaginal deliveries can be performed in a labor, delivery, and recovery room or cesarean delivery room; cesarean delivery rooms are designed especially for that purpose and, therefore, are larger. A cesarean delivery room should measure 440 net ft^2 (40.85 m^2). Each room should be well lit and environmentally controlled to prevent chilling of the woman and the neonate. The World Health Organization recommends that during delivery, rooms be kept at 25°C (77°F) or higher to prevent hypothermia, especially in low birth weight, premature infants. Cesarean deliveries should be performed in the obstetric unit or designated operating unit, and postpartum sterilization capabilities should be available in that area when appropriate. It is recommended that at least one family member is present at the time of delivery.

Each labor, delivery, and recovery room should have the following equipment and supplies necessary for normal delivery and for the management of complications:

- Birthing bed that allows variations in position for delivery
- Instrument table and solution basin stand
- Instruments and equipment for vaginal delivery and repair of lacerations
- Solutions and equipment for the intravenous administration of fluids
- Equipment for administration of all types of anesthesia, including equipment for emergency resuscitation of the patient
- Individual oxygen, air, and suction outlets for the mother and neonate
- An emergency call system
- Good lighting
- Mirrors for patients to observe the birth (optional)
- Wall clock with a second hand or digital clock
- Equipment for fetal heart rate monitoring
- Designated area for neonatal resuscitation and stabilization (as defined in "Neonatal Functional Units" later in this chapter)
- Scrub sinks strategically placed to allow observation of the patient

Trays containing drugs and equipment necessary for emergency treatment of both the mother and the neonate should be kept in the delivery room area.

Equipment necessary for cardiopulmonary resuscitation also should be easily accessible.

A workroom should be available for washing instruments. Instruments should be prepared and sterilized in a separate room; alternatively, these services may be performed in a separate area or by a central supply facility. There also should be a room for the storage and preparation of anesthetic equipment; a room or unit for medication storage, preparation, and distribution; a clean workroom and supply room; and an environmental services room for house-keeping supplies and equipment. Cesarean delivery rooms should additionally have available the following support areas: a control and nurse station, a soiled workroom, and a fluid waste disposal room or area.

Postpartum and Newborn Care. The postpartum unit should be flexible enough to permit the comfortable accommodation of patients when the patient census is at its peak and allow the use of beds for alternate functions when the patient census is low. Ideally, rooms are occupied by a single family and equipped for newborn care, and the patient and her neonate are admitted to the room together. Each room in the postpartum unit should have a handwashing sink and, if possible, a toilet and shower. When this is not possible and it is necessary for patients to use common facilities, patients should be able to reach them without entering a general corridor. When the patient is breastfeeding, the room should have a handwashing sink, a mobile bassinet unit, and supplies necessary for the care of the newborn. Siblings may visit in the patient's room or in a designated space in the antepartum area or postpartum area.

Larger services may have a specific recovery room for postpartum patients and a separate area for patients at high risk. The equipment needed is similar to that needed in any surgical recovery room and includes equipment for monitoring vital signs, suctioning, administering oxygen, and infusing fluids intravenously. Cardiopulmonary resuscitation equipment must be immediately available. Equipment for pelvic examinations also should be available.

Bed Need Analysis

Historically, the calculation of the number of patient rooms needed for all phases of the birth process was based on a simple ratio that involves the number of births, the average length of stay, and the accepted occupancy level. To best estimate patient room needs, each delivery service should thoroughly analyze functions, philosophies, and projections that will determine the types and quantities of rooms needed. An analysis of the present patterns of care should be reviewed, and consideration should be given to the following types of information:

- Projected birth rates
- Projected cesarean delivery rates
- Occupancy projections that address "peaks and valleys" in the census
- Present (and projected) number of women in the unit during peak periods, as well as the length and frequency of the peak periods
- Numbers and types of high-risk births
- Anticipated lengths of stay for women during labor, delivery, and recovery
- Anticipated changes in technology

One planning method is to carefully analyze the activities that will occur in each type of room. For example, labor, delivery, and recovery rooms should not be used routinely to accommodate care, such as outpatient testing, when another room would provide a more appropriate setting. Rooms that allow adequate privacy are recommended for the entire birth process, from labor through discharge.

Planning the number of labor, delivery, and recovery rooms requires that consideration be given to these additional questions:

- Will patients scheduled for cesarean delivery use labor, delivery, and recovery rooms or other types of patient rooms for their preoperative, recovery, and postpartum stays?
- Are the labor, delivery, and recovery rooms to be used for other purposes, such as triage or short-term observation for false labor or antepartum admission? If so, the length of stay and volume of all these activities must be considered in the calculation of bed need.

Once the data have been accumulated, the following normative formula can be used to calculate the number of rooms needed by type of room (note that patient episodes—cases or activities—is used rather than the number of births):

$$\frac{\text{Number of patient episodes (considering all activities, such as admission, observation, and transitional care, in this room)}}{365 \text{ days} \times \text{occupancy for the room type}} \times \text{Mean overall length of stay}$$

This formula will provide, at best, only a crude estimate of bed needs. For more precise estimates, computerized simulation models are available commercially. However, many of these software packages are expensive and require a significant investment of time for adequate training and use. Often this software will be purchased by a hospital planning department and models developed for each service as needed. Alternatively, some expert consulting firms that specialize in maternal–child services can provide an on-site assessment of obstetric capacity and perform a bed need analysis using their own proprietary simulation software.

Neonatal Functional Units

All neonatal services in a birthing hospital should have facilities available to perform the following functions:

- Resuscitation and stabilization
- Admission and observation
- Normal newborn care (in the newborn nursery or, ideally, in the mother's room)
- Isolation
- Visitation
- Supporting service areas

Level II, level III, and level IV NICUs require facilities for intermediate and intensive care. These may be separate or continuous. Consistency of nursing care and efficiency of staffing may be enhanced by having a mix of neonatal patients in a single area. Local circumstances should be considered in the design and management of these care areas.

Resuscitation and Stabilization Area

The resuscitation area should contain the following items:

- Infant warmer or overhead source of radiant heat
- Noncompressible resuscitation and examination mattress that allows access on three sides
- Wall clock with second hand or digital clock
- Flat working surface for medical records
- Table or flat surface for trays and equipment

- Dry, warmed linens
- Stethoscope with neonatal head
- Compressed air and oxygen source
- Oxygen blender with flow meter and tubing
- Pulse oximeter and oximeter probe
- Resuscitation equipment, including bulb syringe, mechanical suction, tubing, and suction catheters; laryngoscope with blades and extra bulbs and batteries; endotracheal tubes and tape; meconium aspirator; ventilation device (self-inflating bag, flow-inflating bag, or T-piece resuscitator that is capable of delivering 90–100% oxygen and continuous positive airway pressure; a self-inflating bag should be available as a back-up for the latter two devices); masks for term neonates and preterm neonates, carbon dioxide detector, and umbilical vessel catheterization supplies
- Syringes, medications (epinephrine, dextrose solution), crystalloid solution for volume expansion, and normal saline for flushes
- Equipment for examination, immediate care, and identification of the neonate
- Protective gear to prevent exposure to body fluids
- Special equipment for surgical care (eg, bowel bag for gastroschisis, donut for neural tube defect) or special circumstances (plastic wrap or bag for very preterm newborns and transport incubator to maintain temperature during the move to the NICU)
- Laryngeal mask airway; oropharyngeal airways
- Task lighting that is capable of providing no less than 2,000 lux at the plane of the infant bed and adjustable so that lighting at less than maximal levels can be provided whenever possible

The resuscitation area usually is within the labor, delivery, and recovery room, although it may be in a designated contiguous, separate room. If resuscitation takes place in the labor, delivery, and recovery room, the area should be large enough to allow for proper resuscitation of the newborn without interference with the care of the mother. Items contaminated with maternal blood, urine, and stool should be kept physically distant from the neonatal resuscitation area. The thermal environment for infant resuscitation should be maintained by use of an infant warmer or overhead source of radiant heat. When delivery of a preterm infant is anticipated, the temperature of the room should be increased. (For more information on neonatal resuscitation, see Chapter 8.)

A resuscitation area should be allotted a minimum of 40 net ft^2 (3.7 m^2) of floor space if it is within a labor, delivery, and recovery room. This space may be used for multiple purposes, including resuscitation, stabilization, observation, examination, or other infant needs. In an operative delivery room, a minimum of 80 net ft^2 (7.5 m^2) of floor space should be provided. A separate resuscitation room should have approximately 150 net ft^2 (13.94 m^2) of floor space. These areas should have adequate suction, oxygen, compressed air, and electrical outlets to accommodate simultaneous resuscitation of twins. A separate resuscitation room also should have an electrical outlet to accommodate a portable X-ray machine, if needed. Electrical outlets should conform to regulations for areas in which anesthetic agents are administered.

Admission and Observation (Transitional and Stabilization Care) Area

The admission and observation area (for evaluating the neonate's condition in the first 4–8 hours after birth) should be near or adjacent to the delivery area and cesarean delivery room and is preferably part of labor, delivery, and recovery room or other area for maternal recovery. Physical separation of the mother and her newborn during this period should be avoided. This evaluation may take place within one or more areas, including the room in which the mother is recovering, the labor, delivery, and recovery room, or the mother–baby unit. No special or separate isolation facilities are required for neonates born at home or in transit to the hospital.

An estimated 40 net ft^2 (3.7 m^2) of floor space is needed for each neonate in the admission and observation area. The capacity required depends on the size of the delivery service and the duration of close observation. The number of observation stations required depends on the birth rate and the length of stay in the observation area. There should be a minimum of two observation stations. The admission and observation area should be well lit and should contain a wall clock and emergency resuscitation equipment similar to that in the designated resuscitation area. Outlets also should be similar to those in the resuscitation area.

The health care providers' assessment of the neonate's condition determines the subsequent level of care. When the admission and observation is in a labor, delivery, and recovery room, the neonate remains in the room with the mother for breastfeeding. Healthy neonates are never separated from their healthy mothers, and they are kept with their mothers in the labor, delivery, and recovery room at all times. In facilities where the mother must be transferred from the delivery room to a postpartum room, the newborn also is admitted to the postpartum room. Some neonates require transfer to an intermediate or intensive care area.

Neonatal Care Units

Within each perinatal care facility there may be several types of units for newborn care. These units are defined by the content and complexity of care required by a specific group of infants. As in the resuscitation and stabilization area and the admission and observation area, equipment for emergency resuscitation is required in all neonatal care areas. Recommendations regarding the intensity of care are made in the following paragraphs.

Newborn Nursery. In most cases, care for healthy term neonates can be provided in the mother's room. A separate newborn nursery is available for infants who require closer observation or whose mothers cannot care for them. In addition to providing care for healthy term infants, a level I neonatal unit can provide care for late preterm infants born at 35–37 weeks of gestation who are physiologically stable. These neonates are not ill but may require frequent feeding and more hours of nursing care than healthy term neonates. Level I units in hospitals without higher level units also have the equipment and personnel to stabilize newborns who are ill or are born at less than 35 weeks of gestation until they can be transferred to a higher level facility.

Because relatively few staff members are needed to provide care in the newborn nursery and bulky equipment is not needed, 24 net ft^2 (2.23 m^2) of floor space for each neonate should be adequate. Bassinets should be at least 3 ft (approximately 1 m) apart in all directions, measured from the edge of one bassinet to the edge of the neighboring bassinet. In this type of setting, one neonatal registered nurse is recommended for every 6–8 neonates requiring routine care, and the nurse should be available in each newborn-occupied area at all times (see also "Nurse–Patient Ratios" earlier in this chapter). During decreased patient occupancy, central nurseries use nursing staff inefficiently. Direct care of those newborns remaining in the nursery may be provided by licensed practical nurses and unlicensed nursing personnel under the registered nurse's direct supervision.

The newborn nursery should be well lit, have a large wall clock and a sink for handwashing, and be equipped for emergency resuscitation. One pair of wall-mounted electrical outlets is recommended for every two neonatal stations. One oxygen outlet, one compressed-air outlet, and one suction outlet are recommended for every four neonatal stations. Cabinets and counters should be available within the newborn care area for storage of routinely used supplies, such as diapers, formula, and linens. If circumcisions are performed in the nursery, an appropriate table with adequate lighting is required. Electrical outlets to power portable X-ray machines are highly recommended.

Special Care Nursery. Sick neonates who do not require intensive care but who require 6–12 hours of nursing care each day should be cared for in a special care nursery. A special care unit also may be used for convalescing neonates who have returned to specialty facilities from an intensive care unit in an outside facility or have been transferred from a higher level of care within the institution. The special care area may be separate from, adjacent to, or combined with a level III or level IV NICU in hospitals where these exist.

The neonatal special care area is optimally close to the delivery area, cesarean delivery room, and the intensive care area (if there is one in the same facility) and away from general hospital traffic. It should have radiant heaters or incubators for maintaining body temperature, as well as infusion pumps, cardiopulmonary monitors, and oximeters.

In facilities with both level II and level III units, infants who need assisted ventilation should be cared for in the level III unit. In facilities where the special care unit is the highest level of neonatal care, equipment should be available to provide continuous positive airway pressure and, in some units, equipment may be available to provide short-term (less than 24 hours) assisted ventilation. In that case, newborns requiring complex care or prolonged assisted ventilation should be transferred to a facility with a level III or level IV NICU.

When care is provided in single-family rooms, at least 150 net ft^2 (14 m^2) of floor space is needed for singleton births and at least 240 net ft^2 (22.4 m^2) of floor space is needed for twin births. At least 120 net ft^2 (11.2 m^2) of floor space is needed for each patient station when care is provided in multipatient rooms, and there should be at least 8 ft (2.4 m) between each incubator, warmer, bassinet, or crib. Aisles should be at least 4 ft wide to accommodate passage of personnel and equipment. Space needed for other purposes (eg, desks, counters, cabinets, corridors, and treatment rooms) should be added to the space needed for patients. In multipatient rooms, each room should accommodate some multiple of three to four newborn stations because one registered neonatal nurse is required for every three to four neonates who require intermediate care. Large rooms allow greater flexibility in the use of equipment and assignment of personnel but offer less privacy for family involvement in newborn care. Staffing requirements may be increased if patients are in individual rooms.

Twenty simultaneously accessible electrical outlets, three oxygen outlets, three compressed-air outlets, and three suction outlets should be provided for each patient. In addition, the area should have a special outlet to power the neonatal unit's portable X-ray machine. All electrical outlets for each patient station should be connected to both regular and auxiliary power. An oxygen tank for emergency use should be stored but readily available for each newborn receiving wall-supplied oxygen. All equipment and supplies for resuscitation should be immediately available within the intermediate care unit. These items may be conveniently placed on an emergency cart.

Neonatal Intensive Care Unit. Constant nursing and continuous cardiopulmonary and other support for severely ill newborns should be provided in the intensive care unit. Because emergency care is provided in this area, laboratory and radiologic services should be readily available 24 hours per day. The results of blood gas analyses should be available shortly after sample collection. In many centers, a laboratory adjacent to the intensive care unit provides this service.

The neonatal intensive care area should ideally be located near the delivery area and cesarean delivery room(s) and should be easily accessible from the hospital's ambulance entrance. It should be located away from routine hospital traffic. Intensive care may be provided in individual patient rooms, in a single area, or in two or more separate rooms.

The number of nursing, medical, and surgical personnel required in the neonatal intensive care area is greater than that required in less acute perinatal care areas. The nurse-to-patient ratio should be 1:2 or 1:1, depending on acuity. In some cases, such as during extracorporeal life support, additional nursing personnel are required. In addition, the amount and complexity of equipment required also are considerably greater. In multipatient rooms, there should be at least 120 ft^2 of floor space for each neonate, beds should be separated by at least 8 ft, and aisles should be 4 ft (1.22 m) wide. Single-patient rooms should have 150 net ft^2 (13.94 m^2) of floor space for each neonate and 8-ft (2.44 m) wide aisles, plus space for desks, cabinets, computers, and corridors. In addition, the educational responsibilities of a neonatal intensive care facility require that the design include space for instructional activities and, for those facilities also serving as regional centers, office space for files on the region's perinatal experience.

Each patient station needs at least 20 simultaneously accessible electrical outlets, 3–4 oxygen outlets, 3–4 compressed-air outlets, and 3–4 vacuum outlets. Like those in the intermediate care area, all electrical outlets for each patient station should be connected to both regular and auxiliary power. In addition, each room should have a special outlet to power the portable X-ray machine housed in the NICU. An oxygen tank for emergency use should be stored but readily available for each newborn receiving wall-supplied oxygen. If wireless transmission is not available, provisions should be made at each bedside to allow data transmission from cardiorespiratory monitors to a remote location.

Equipment and supplies in the intensive-care area should include all those needed in the resuscitation and intermediate-care areas. Immediate availability of emergency oxygen is essential. In addition, equipment for long-term ventilatory support should be provided. Ventilators should be equipped with nebulizers or humidifiers with heaters. Equipment for manual-assisted ventilation, including appropriately sized face masks and flow-inflating or self-inflating bags should be available at each bed space. Continuous, online monitoring of oxygen concentrations, body temperature, heart rate, respiration, oxygen saturation, and blood pressure measurements should be available for each patient. Supplies should be kept close to the patient bed space so that nurses are not away from the neonate unnecessarily and may use their time and skills efficiently. A central modular supply system can enhance efficiency.

In some cases, certain surgical procedures (eg, ligation of a patent ductus arteriosus) are performed in an area in or adjacent to the NICU. Specific policies should address preparatory cleaning, physical preparation of the unit, presence of other newborns and staff, venting of volatile anesthetics, and quality assessment. Ideally, equipment, facilities, and supplies for this area, as well as procedures, should be comparable to those required for similar procedures in the surgical department of the hospital.

Supporting Service Areas

Milk and Formula Preparation Areas. Unless performed elsewhere in the hospital (eg, in a milk bank), a specialized area or room to prepare feedings should be provided in the NICU, away from the bedside, to accommodate mixing of additives to human milk or formula. This area should be equipped with a hands-free handwashing station, counter workspace, and storage areas for supplies, formula, and both refrigerated and frozen human milk.

Utility Rooms. Both clean and soiled utility rooms are needed in neonatal care areas. Separate storage areas should be available for foodstuffs, medications, and clean supplies. Clean utility rooms should not have direct lighting because some of the formulas, medications, and supplies may be light sensitive. The maintenance of soiled utility rooms should conform to the guidelines and state regulations of the Facility Guidelines Institute.

Storage Areas. A three-zone storage system is desirable. The first storage area should be the central supply department of the hospital. The second storage area should be adjacent to the patient care areas or within the patient care areas. In this area, routinely used supplies and clean utilities, such as diapers, formula, linen, cover gowns, medical records, and information booklets, may be stored. Generally, space is required in this area only for the amount of each item used between deliveries from the hospital's central supply department (eg, daily or three times weekly). The third area is needed for the storage of items frequently used at the neonate's bedside. There should be a bedside cabinet storage area for each bed–patient unit in the mother–baby unit or newborn nursery, intermediate care area, and intensive care area. The newborn nursery requires secondary storage of items such as linen and formula. In the resuscitation and stabilization area, the admission and observation area, the intermediate care area, and the intensive-care areas, there should be space for secondary storage of syringes, needles, intravenous infusion sets, and sterile trays needed in procedures, such as umbilical vessel catheterization, lumbar puncture, and thoracostomy.

Large equipment items (eg, bassinets, incubators, warmers, radiant heaters, phototherapy units, and infusion pumps) should be stored in a clean, enclosed storage area in close proximity to, but not within, the immediate patient care area. Easily accessible electrical outlets are desirable in this area for recharging equipment.

Treatment Rooms. Many facilities have developed areas for resuscitation and stabilization, admission and observation, intermediate care, and intensive care in which each patient station constitutes a treatment area. This largely has eliminated the need for a separate treatment room for procedures, such as lumbar punctures, intravenous infusions, venipuncture, and minor surgical procedures. A separate treatment area may be necessary, however, if neonates in the newborn nursery or postpartum mother–baby unit are to undergo certain procedures (eg, circumcision). The facilities, outlets, equipment, and supplies in the treatment area should be similar to those of the resuscitation area. The amount of space required depends on the procedures performed.

Scrub Areas

At the entrance to each neonatal care area, there should be a scrub area that can accommodate all personnel and families entering the area. It should have a sink that is large enough to prevent splashing, with faucets operated by hands-free controls. A backsplash should be provided to prevent standing or retained water. Waterless antiseptics also often are available at these sinks. Sinks for handwashing should not be built into counters used for other purposes. Soap and towel dispensers and appropriate trash receptacles should be available. The scrub areas also should contain racks, hooks, or lockers for storing clothing and personal items, as well as cabinets for clean gowns, a receptacle for used gowns, and a large wall clock with a sweep second hand, or digital clock, to time handwashing.

Scrub sinks should have hands-free faucets and should be large enough to control splashing and to prevent retained water. These hands-free sinks should be provided at a minimum ratio of one for at least every eight patient stations in the newborn nursery. In the intermediate care or intensive care areas, every bed should be within 20 ft (6.10 m) of a hands-free washing station. In addition, one scrub sink is needed in the resuscitation and stabilization area, and one is needed for every three to four patient stations in the admission and observation area. Alcohol-based hand hygiene solutions should be available at all entry points and at each bed space.

Nursing Areas

Space should be provided at the bedside not only for patient care but also for instructional and medical record activities. For electronic documentation, computer terminals should be readily accessible, and policies should be in place to ensure cleaning of keyboards. If manual documentation is performed, a flat writing surface (eg, a clipboard or loose leaf notebook) is needed.

A nurses' area or desk for tasks, such as compiling more detailed records, completing requisitions, and handling specimens is useful. Primary care providers also may perform medical record and clerical activities in this area. However, in level III or level IV and many level II care units, documentation needs to take place at or near the bedside. Maintaining medical records should be considered an unclean procedure, and personnel who have been working on medical records should perform hand hygiene before they have further contact with a neonate.

The unit director or nurse manager should have an office close to the newborn care areas. Nurses' dressing rooms preferably should be adjacent to a lounge and should contain lockers, storage for clean and soiled scrub attire (in hospitals that provide and launder staff scrubs), a dressing area, toilets, and showers.

Education Areas

A conference room suitable for educational purposes is highly desirable, particularly for facilities with level II, level III, and level IV units. It should be in or adjacent to the maternal–newborn areas.

Clerical Areas

The control point for patient-care activities is the clerical area. It should be located near the entrance to the neonatal care areas so that personnel can supervise traffic and limit unnecessary entry into these areas. It should have telephones and communication devices that connect to the various neonatal care areas and the delivery suite. In addition, patients' medical records, computer terminals, and hospital forms may be located in the clerical area.

General Considerations

Disaster Preparedness and Evacuation Plan

An overall disaster preparedness plan is essential for all areas of the hospital and all personnel. A plan addressing natural and terrorist disasters should be in place for each perinatal care area (ie, antepartum care, labor and delivery care, postpartum care, routine neonatal care, intermediate care, and intensive care). This should include an evacuation plan; a relocation plan; triage principles; immediate measures for utilities and water supply; emergency supply of medical gases, essential medications, and equipment; and the role of each staff member in the plan. A floor plan that indicates designated evacuation routes should be posted in a conspicuous place in each unit. The policy and floor plan should be reviewed with the staff at least annually.

Safety and Environmental Control

Because of the complexities of environmental control and monitoring, a hospital environmental engineer must ensure that all electrical, lighting, air composition, and temperature systems function properly and safely. A regular maintenance program should be specified to ensure that systems continue to function as designed after initial occupancy.

The environmental temperature in newborn care areas should be independently adjustable, and control should be sufficient to prevent hot and cold spots, particularly when heat-generating equipment (eg, a radiant warmer) is in use. The air temperature should be kept at 22–26°C (72–78°F). Humidity should be kept between 30% and 60% and should be controlled through the heating and air-conditioning system of the hospital. Condensation on wall and window surfaces should be avoided.

A minimum of six air changes per hour is recommended, and a minimum of two changes should be outside air. The ventilation pattern should inhibit particulate matter from moving freely in the space, and intake and exhaust vents should be placed so as to minimize drafts on or near the patient beds. Ventilation air delivered to the NICU should be filtered at 90% efficiency, or as specified in the most current edition of the Facilities Guidelines Institute's *Guidelines for Design and Construction of Health Care Facilities*. Filters should be located outside the infant care area so that they can be changed easily and safely. Fresh-air intake should be located at least 25 ft (7.6 m) from exhaust outlets of ventilating systems, combustion equipment stacks, medical or surgical vacuum systems, plumbing vents, or areas that may collect vehicular exhausts or other noxious fumes.

Radiation exposure to newborns, families, and staff is another safety concern (see also Chapter 9, "Radiation Risk"). Radiation exposure to personnel is negligible at a distance of more than 1 ft (0.30 m) lateral to the primary vertical roentgen beam. Care should be taken to ensure that only the patient and the area of interest being examined is in the primary beam and staff needed to assist in patient positioning should wear appropriate shielding. It is unnecessary for families or personnel to leave the area during the roentgen exposure.

Illumination

Ambient lighting levels in all infant care areas should be adjustable. Both natural and artificial light sources should have controls that allow immediate darkening of any bed position sufficient for transillumination or ultrasonography when necessary. Artificial light sources should have a color rendering index of no less than 80, and a full-spectrum color index of no less than 55. Artificial light sources should have a visible spectral distribution similar to that of daylight but should avoid unnecessary ultraviolet or infrared radiation by the use of appropriate lamps, lenses, or filters. Newly constructed or renovated NICUs should be able to provide ambient lighting at levels recommended by the Illuminating Engineering Society. Separate procedure lighting should be available at each patient care station. Procedure lighting should minimize shadows and glare, and it should be controlled with a rheostat so that it can be provided at less than maximal levels whenever possible. Light should be highly framed so that newborns at adjacent bed stations will not experience any increase in illumination.

Illumination of support areas within the NICU, including medical records areas, medication preparation areas, reception desks, and handwashing areas, should conform to the specifications of the Illuminating Engineering Society. Illumination should be adequate in the areas of the NICU where staff perform important or critical tasks. In locations where these functions overlap with patient care areas (eg, proximity of the nurse documentation area to patient beds), the design should permit separate light sources with independent controls so that the very different needs of sleeping newborns and working nurses can be accommodated to the greatest possible extent.

Windows

Windows may provide an important psychological benefit to staff and families in the NICU. Properly designed natural light is the most desirable illumination for nearly all nursing tasks, including updating medical records and evaluating newborn skin tone. However, placing newborns too close to external windows can cause serious problems with temperature control and glare, so providing windows in the NICU requires careful planning and design.

At least one source of natural light should be visible from each patient care area. External windows in patient care rooms should be glazed with insulating glass to minimize heat gain and loss. They should be situated at least 2 ft (0.60 m) away from any part of a patient bed to minimize radiant heat loss from the newborn. All external windows should be equipped with shading devices that are easily controlled to allow flexibility at various times of day. These shading devices should be either contained within the window or easily cleanable. Windows in neonatal care areas should have opaque shades that make it possible to darken the area to reduce inappropriate radiant heat gain or loss, or for procedures that require reduced light, such as transillumination or ultrasonography examination.

Wall Surfaces

Wall surfaces should be easily cleanable, provide protection at point of contact with moveable equipment, and be free of substances known to be teratogenic, mutagenic, carcinogenic, or otherwise harmful to human health.

Oxygen and Compressed-Air Outlets

Newborn care areas should have oxygen and compressed air piped from a central source at a pressure of 50–60 psi. An alarm system that warns of any critical reduction in line pressure should be installed. Reduction valves and mixers should produce adjustable concentrations of 21–100% oxygen at atmospheric pressure for head hoods and 50–60 psi for mechanical ventilators.

Acoustic Characteristics

Infant rooms (including airborne infection isolation rooms), staff work areas, family areas, staff lounge, sleeping areas, and spaces opening into them should be designed to produce minimal background noise and to contain and absorb much of the transient noise that arises within them. The ventilation system, monitors, incubators, suction pumps, mechanical ventilators, and staff produce considerable noise, and the noise level should be monitored intermittently. Mechanical systems and equipment in infant rooms and adult sleep rooms should conform to noise criteria 25. The construction and redesign of neonatal care areas and adult sleep areas should include acoustic absorption units or other means to ensure that the combination of continuous background sound and transient sound in any bed space or patient care area does not exceed an hourly L_{eq} of 45 dB and an hourly L_{10} of 50 dB, both A-weighted slow response. Transient sounds or L_{max}, should not exceed 65 dB, A-weighted slow response. Staff members should take particular care to avoid noise pollution in enclosed patient spaces (eg, incubators). Care should be taken to avoid spaces shaped so as to focus or amplify sound levels, thus creating "hot spots" that exceed the maximum recommended noise levels. In staff work areas, staff lounge areas, and family areas, the combination of continuous background and operational sound should not exceed an hourly L_{eq} of 50 dB and an hourly L_{10} of 55 dB, both A-weighted slow response. The transient sounds should not exceed 70 dB, A-weighted slow response in these areas.

Electrical Outlets and Electrical Equipment

All electrical outlets should be attached to a common ground. All electrical equipment should be checked for current leakage and grounding adequacy when first introduced into the neonatal care area, after any repair, and periodically while in service. Current leakage allowances, preventive maintenance standards, and equipment quality should meet the standards developed by the Joint Commission. There should be both emergency and normal power for all electrical outlets per National Fire Protection Association recommendations. Personnel should be thoroughly and repeatedly instructed on the potential electrical hazards within the neonatal care areas.

Bibliography

Late-preterm infants. ACOG Committee Opinion No. 404. American College of Obstetricians and Gynecologists. Obstet Gynecol 2008;111:1029–32.

American College of Obstetricians and Gynecologists. Statement on surgical assistants. ACOG Committee Opinion 240. Washington, DC: ACOG; 2000.

American Nurses Association, National Association of Neonatal Nurses. Neonatal nursing: scope and standards of practice. Washington, D.C.; ANA; Glenview (IL): NANN; 2004.

Dilaura DL, Houser KW, Mistrick RG, Steffy GR, editors. The lighting handbook: reference and application. 10th ed. New York (NY): Illuminating Engineering Society of North America; 2011.

Facility Guidelines Institute. Guidelines for design and construction of health care facilities. 2010. Chicago (IL): American Society for Healthcare Engineering of the American Hospital Association; 2010.

Illuminating Engineering Society of North America. Lighting for hospitals and health care facilities. New York (NY): IESNA; 2006.

Joint statement of practice relations between obstetrician–gynecologists and certified nurse–midwives/certified midwives. American College of Nurse–midwives and American College of Obstetricians and Gynecologists. Washington, DC: American College of Obstetricians and Gynecologists; 2011.

Lathrop JK, Bielen RP, editors. Health care facilities code: NFPA 99. 8th ed. Quincy (MA): National Fire Prevention Association; 2011.

Levels of neonatal care. Policy statement. American Academy of Pediatrics. Committee on Fetus and Newborn. Pediatrics 2012;130:587–97.

National Association of Neonatal Nurses. Minimum staffing in NICUs. Position Statement #3009. Glenview (IL): NANN; 1999. Available at: http://www.nann.org/pdf/08_3009_rev.pdf. Retrieved December 2, 2011.

National Association of Neonatal Nurses. Requirements for advanced neonatal nursing practice in neonatal intensive care units. Position Statement #3042. Glenview (IL): NANN; 2009. Available at: http://www.nann.org/pdf/10req_annp.pdf. Retrieved December 1, 2011.

Percelay JM, Strong GB. Guiding principles for pediatric hospitalist programs. American Academy of Pediatrics Section on Hospital Medicine. Pediatrics 2005;115:1101–2.

Rea M, Deng L, Wolsey R. Light sources and color. NlPIP Lighting Answers 2004;8:1–38. Available at: http://www.lrc.rpi.edu/programs/nlpip/lightinganswers/lightsources/abstract.asp. Retrieved December 1, 2011.

Reynolds EW, Bricker JT. Nonphysician clinicians in the neonatal intensive care unit: meeting the needs of our smallest patients. Pediatrics 2007;119:361–9.

Robbins ST, Meyers R, editors. Infant feedings: guidelines for preparation of formula and breastmilk in health care facilities. Pediatric Nutrition Practice Group. 2nd ed. Chicago (IL): American Dietetic Association; 2011. p. 136.

Wallman C. Advanced practice in neonatal nursing. American Academy of Pediatrics Committee on Fetus and Newborn. Pediatrics 2009;123:1606–7.

Weinstein L. The laborist: a new focus of practice for the obstetrician. Am J Obstet Gynecol 2003;188:310–2.

White RD. Recommended standards for the newborn ICU. J Perinatol 2007;27 Suppl 2: S4–19.

Chapter 3
Quality Improvement and Patient Safety

The Institute of Medicine (IOM) and other organizations have stressed the urgency of "transforming hospitals into places where each patient receives the best quality care, every single time." In studies of progress in quality improvement (QI) and patient safety, a recurring theme emerges: hospitals need to change systems to increase reliability. Obstetric and neonatal services share many of the characteristics of high reliability organizations in other industries, such as the aviation industry and nuclear power plants. The success of these types of organizations depends on an awareness of the high-risk nature of the organization's activities, a commitment to resilience after failure, sensitivity to issues facing health care providers immediately involved with care and finally, development of a culture of safety. The latter is paramount. Individuals must feel comfortable drawing attention to potential hazards or actual failures without fear of censure from management and peers.

In its report, *Crossing the Quality Chasm*, the IOM set forth a list of performance characteristics that, if addressed and improved, would lead to better health and function for the people of the United States (see "Bibliography" in this chapter). The following are the six specific qualities of good care, according to the IOM, that can be helpful in designing a QI program:

1. Safe—avoiding injuries to patients from the care that is intended to help

2. Effective—providing services based on scientific knowledge to all who could benefit and refraining from providing services to those not likely to benefit (avoiding underuse and overuse)

3. Patient centered—providing care that is respectful of and responsive to individual patient preferences, needs, and values, and ensuring that patient values guide all the clinical decisions

4. Timely—reducing waiting times and sometimes harmful delays for those who receive and those who provide care

5. Efficient—avoiding waste, in particular, waste of equipment, supplies, ideas, and energy
6. Equitable—providing care that does not vary in quality because of personal characteristics, such as gender, ethnicity, geographic location, and socioeconomic status

Quality Improvement

Over the years, the focus of QI efforts has shifted from a punitive approach to an educational one. The QI process assists all health care providers at all levels of care. Ongoing monitoring and evaluation of clinical patient care should be implemented through a process known as QI. Quality improvement is an approach to quality management that builds upon traditional quality assurance methods by emphasizing the organization and systems. It focuses on the process rather than the individual, recognizes both internal and external customers, and promotes the need for objective data to analyze and improve processes. The QI process must focus on the total care delivered to the patient by an institution, thus involving outpatient care leading up to hospital admission and the patient's discharge and transition of care to outpatient facilities; care from physicians, midwives, nurses, and support staff; administration; and all components of care that contribute to a patient's hospital experience. However, it does not eliminate individual responsibility and accountability for care, when appropriate.

Quality improvement starts from the premise that although most medical care is good, it always can be better. The goal is to reduce variations in care and improve performance. Quality improvement accepts that good care depends upon more than just the judgment of the individual. Important components of a well-designed QI program include leadership, peer review, methods to reduce variation, quality measures and indicators, and data collection and analysis.

Leadership

A QI program requires effective, responsive leadership from both medical staff and administration. The chair of the department is ultimately responsible for QI activities. However, with the growing awareness of obstetric and neonatal care units as high reliability organizations and with increased reporting requirements of local, state, and national organizations, the responsibilities related to patient safety and quality in perinatal health care are substantial. Larger departments may benefit from designation of a patient safety officer and quality reporting directly to the department chair. When physicians accept these leadership positions, their primary purpose is to establish an environment in which quality and a culture of patient safety can thrive.

Peer Review

Peer review is a quality assessment process in which a retrospective analysis of cases is undertaken using outcomes data to assess adherence to guidelines or other standards of care. Although initial screening may be performed by non-physicians, peer review is performed by peer physicians with similar background and training. Peer review may result in recommendations of individual practice changes or more systems and process changes as an outcome of the QI process.

A departmental peer review committee should be multidisciplinary and may include the following members, with consideration given to the vice chair of the department who serves as the committee chair:

- Representative physicians with varying levels of clinical experience (junior and senior staff) within the department
- Representative subspecialists, when available
- House staff member, when appropriate
- The department chair (ex officio)

Small hospitals may face difficulty conducting peer review because of competitive interests or interpersonal problems that have a real or perceived effect on the efficacy of the review. Therefore, it may be helpful to develop a relationship with another hospital or outside independent reviewer or consultant to conduct peer review. In either case, it is important to remember that responsibility for peer review and QI rests with the hospital medical staff and, ultimately, the governing board. The focus of peer review should not be punitive but instead directed toward system and process improvements that lead to better patient outcomes.

Reducing Variation

Experts suggest that substantial QIs can be achieved by eliminating unnecessary variation in treatment plans. One approach to reducing variation is the development and implementation of clinical protocols. The Institute for Clinical Systems Improvement defines *protocols* as step-by-step statements of a procedure routinely used in the care of individual patients to ensure that the intended effect is reliably achieved. Protocols tend to be very directive and provide the physician or health care providers with a clear path in care management that is problem-specific. The QI committee can develop a draft protocol that addresses a particular issue with the entire staff and amend it to meet the staffs' needs. Once the protocol has been finalized, staff should be reminded that they may deviate from the protocol as long as the medical record reflects awareness of the protocol and documents the critical thinking for not following it.

Quality Measures and Indicators

Quality improvement programs must focus on measurable dimensions of care when selecting indicators to track for identifying processes in need of improvement. The Agency for Healthcare Research and Quality maintains an updated list of possible quality measures, including those in obstetrics and neonatology. Their National Quality Measures Clearinghouse is available at http://www.qualitymeasures.ahrq.gov/. Sample quality indicators proposed by the American College of Obstetricians and Gynecologists (the College) are shown in Box 3-1. Pragmatic considerations in developing and deploying valid measures of quality and safety in obstetrics are addressed in the College's resource, *Quality and Safety in Women's Health Care*, second edition.

Data Collection and Analysis

The QI process requires accurate collection and analysis of outcomes data. Outcomes have been a concern of perinatal health care providers for decades. Care has been monitored and improved by focusing on specific outcomes, such as maternal, newborn, and neonatal mortality. Significant progress has been made in methods for collecting data and gathering vital statistics (eg, prenatal records, linked birth and death certificate data, linked birth and hospital discharge data). It is recommended that all states follow the most current National Center for Health Statistics requirements for issuing standard certificates and reports for birth, death, and fetal death. The 2003 revision included new recommendations for reporting antenatal treatment (eg, corticosteroids) and postnatal care (eg, NICU admission) (Appendix F). Another revision was proposed in 2011. The concept of key indicators has been used to signal inadequate access to early and continuous perinatal care and to predict or measure poor pregnancy outcome. For example, rates of unintended pregnancy; use of prenatal care services; and fetal, neonatal, and maternal mortality are possible measures of access and outcome at different points along the continuum of perinatal health care delivery. Many states now use the Centers for Disease Control and

Prevention's Pregnancy Risk Assessment Monitoring System or similar surveys to measure population-based health indicators before, during, and after pregnancy (available at http://www.cdc.gov/prams/).

Box 3-1. Sample Clinical Indicators of Quality and Safety in Perinatal Care

Maternal Indicators

1. Maternal mortality
2. Elective delivery at less than 39 weeks of gestation
3. Unplanned maternal readmission within 14 days
4. Maternal cardiopulmonary arrest, resuscitated
5. In-hospital initiation of antibiotics 24 hours or more following term vaginal delivery
6. Unplanned removal, injury, or repair of organ during operative procedure
7. Excessive maternal blood loss
   a. Required transfusion
   b. Postpartum anemia hematocrit less than 22%, hemoglobin less than 7 g (decline of antepartum hematocrit of 11% or hemoglobin decline of 3.5 g)
8. Maternal length of stay in excess of 1 day greater than the local standard after vaginal or cesarean delivery
9. Eclampsia
10. Delivery unattended by the responsible physician*
11. Unplanned postpartum return to the delivery room or operating room for management
12. Cesarean delivery for uncertain fetal status
13. Cesarean delivery for failure to progress

Neonatal Indicators

1. Deaths of infants weighing 500 g or more subcategorized by intrahospital neonatal deaths, total stillborn fetuses, and intrapartum stillborn fetuses
2. Delivery of an infant at less than 32 weeks of gestation in an institution without a neonatal intensive care unit
3. Transfer of a neonate to a neonatal intensive care unit

*To be defined by each institution
Modified from American College of Obstetricians and Gynecologists. Quality and Safety in Women's Health Care. 2nd ed. Washington, DC. American College of Obstetricians and Gynecologists; 2010. p. 17.

New and improved tools in evaluative clinical sciences should be used to monitor performance and provide the basis for improvement in clinical care and outcomes. Perinatal health care providers and facilities must play an active role by participating in regional data collection, developing standardized data collection tools, supporting analysis, benchmarking, and using the resulting information for individual, institutional, and professional QI. Thorough and systematic collection of data on long-term outcomes is essential to evaluate changes in perinatal care delivery systems as well as new technologies and therapies.

In addition to the efforts of individual hospitals and perinatal care systems to track outcomes and mortality sentinel events, the National Fetal and Infant Mortality Review (NFIMR) program provides an opportunity for QI efforts to review fetal, infant, and maternal deaths. The NFIMR process is a broad type of analysis that is valuable at the community level. The program brings together key members of the community, including prenatal and pediatric providers, public health professionals, social service agency representatives, grief professionals, consumer advocates, consumers, and others. They review de-identified information from individual cases of fetal and infant death to identify factors associated with those deaths, determine if they represent service system problems that require change, develop recommendations for change, and assist in the implementation of change. A national evaluation of NFIMR has documented that the process is an effective perinatal-systems initiative. Currently, NFIMR is being implemented in 200 communities in 40 states, the District of Columbia, the U.S. Virgin Islands, and the Commonwealth of Puerto Rico. The entire NFIMR evaluation report can be viewed on the Johns Hopkins University web site (http://www.jhsph.edu/wchpc/projects/fimr.html). The NFIMR program is a collaborative effort between the College and the federal Maternal and Child Health Bureau, Health Resources and Services Administration to refine and promote the NFIMR process. (For more information about the NFIMR process or to learn if there is a NFIMR program in your community, go to www. nfimr.org.)

Although maternal deaths attributable to pregnancy remain relatively rare, it is important that each death be identified and carefully reviewed at the state level. The lessons learned from reviews of these deaths need to be shared with those who have the opportunity to influence policies and practices related to the systems of care in place for women in the preconception, antepartum, and postpartum periods.

Patient Safety

Patient safety shares many characteristics with a well-designed QI model. However, patient safety emphasizes a systems analysis of medical errors and minimizes individual blame and retribution while still maintaining individual accountability. Patient safety is an explicit principle that must be embraced as a core value in patient care. This is an ongoing process that requires health care professionals to continually strive to learn from problems, identify system deficiencies, redesign processes, and implement change in their daily practice. Patient-centered care, open communication, and teamwork provide the foundation for optimal patient care and safety.

National Patient Safety Goals

The Joint Commission recognizes the importance of patient safety. Beginning in 2003, The Joint Commission created the first set of National Patient Safety Goals (see "Bibliography" in this chapter). These goals, derived from Sentinel Event Alerts and other sources, are designed to be explicit, evidence based, and measurable. Each year, existing goals are modified based on public comment and the experience of reviewers and new goals are added. In this way, over time, The Joint Commission will develop a compendium of recommended practices that will improve patient safety.

Patient Safety Principles

The College and the American Academy of Pediatrics also have a long-standing commitment to patient safety and quality. To improve patient care and reduce medical errors, they encourage all health care providers to promote the following four principles in all practice settings, which are discussed in the following paragraphs:

1. Commit to a culture of patient safety
2. Implement safe medication practices
3. Reduce the likelihood of surgical errors
4. Improve communication

Culture of Patient Safety

A culture of patient safety continuously evolves and should be the framework for every effort to reduce medical errors. Patient safety focuses on systems of care, not individuals. Confidential reporting and analysis of errors and near misses will reveal areas that require remediation to provide improved patient safety. State and federal laws may have an effect on the level of confidentiality and the manner of reporting. A culture of patient safety starts at the top with strong leadership that provides the necessary human and financial resources to achieve patient safety.

Additionally, a culture of safety recognizes the importance of team function in optimizing individual performance. A culture of patient safety fosters open communication and welcomes input from team members at every level. Care must be taken to ensure that hierarchical systems do not hamper free communication among physicians. Competing clinical demands, interruptions, and distractions are inherent in clinical practice. It requires specific effort to ensure that issues are understood and that meaningful information is transferred. Certain clinical communications should be verified, such as reading back medication orders. Inaccurate information and missing clinical data can result in serious medical errors and patient injury. Relevant communications should be documented appropriately.

Safe Medication Practices

Medication errors are one of the most common types of preventable adverse events. Automated systems for prescribing and dispensing medication can greatly reduce these errors, but there are many low technical support solutions that can be implemented rapidly with minimal cost, such as the following:

- Improve the legibility of written orders.
- Avoid the use of nonstandard abbreviations, as recommended by the Joint Commission (see "Bibliography" in this chapter).
- Always use a leading 0 for doses less than 1 unit (eg, 0.1 not .1) and never use a trailing 0 after a decimal point (eg, 1 mg not 1.0 mg): "always lead, never follow."
- Require that all verbal orders be written by the individual receiving the order and then read back to the prescriber. An effort should be made to eliminate verbal orders.

Reduce the Likelihood of Surgical Errors

The College and the American Academy of Pediatrics, along with other specialty societies and other organizations, have endorsed The Joint Commission's

Universal Protocol to Prevent Wrong Site, Wrong Procedure, and Wrong Patient Surgery. The Joint Commission now requires this protocol as part of a preoperative time out, which involves all members of the operating room team, including the patient (see "Bibliography" in this chapter). In obstetrics, the time out process does not need to be limited to patient identification and planned procedure, but also may provide an opportunity to ensure the completion of other patient safety or clinical recommendations, such as administration of antibiotics before cesarean delivery, communication of critical neonatal information with pediatricians or the possible need for and availability of blood products, or at the completion of vaginal delivery to ensure the absence of retained vaginal sponges. A time out also is required for all invasive procedures performed in the NICU.

Communication

Physicians should be aware that complete and accurate communication of medical information is critical in reducing preventable medical errors. Improving communication skills merits the same attention as improving clinical skills. According to information gathered from The Joint Commission, in collecting sentinel event information, the most common cause of preventable adverse outcomes is communication error. Optimal communication to improve patient safety has many dimensions including the following:

- Communication with the patient and the family
- Communication among all those caring for the patient
- Availability of information necessary for coordination of care

Physician–Patient Communication. The key to a good physician–patient relationship is the ability to listen, explain, and empathize. This is particularly important if the patient is under stress, which negatively affects her ability to grasp important messages. The U.S. Preventive Services Task Force defines *shared decision making* as a process in which both the patient and physician share information, participate in the decision-making process, and agree on a course of action (see "Bibliography" in this chapter).

Another factor potentially limiting communication is health literacy, which is unrelated to level of education or social status. In order to have a meaningful discussion with an individual about her health care, it is imperative that one recognize and address the patient's level of understanding and knowledge.

Consider the following options to improve communication, increase the level of understanding, and improve health literacy:

- Actively listen to the patient and understand her concerns and issues.
- Learn to recognize when the patient does not comprehend.
- Have the patient bring a family member or friend when difficult and crucial discussions are held.
- Have the patient recount her understanding of the information that was presented to her.
- Use several formats and repeat material and information in different ways to increase understanding and comprehension.
- Do not rush encounters.

A very important part of physician–patient communication is when and how to disclose medical errors. The Joint Commission requires that accredited hospitals inform patients of adverse events. According to the Joint Commission Standard RI.01.02.01, "the licensed independent practitioner responsible for managing the patient's care, treatment, and services, or his or her designee, informs the patient about unanticipated outcomes of care, treatment and services." When an error contributed to the injury, the patient and the family or representative should receive a truthful and compassionate explanation about the error and the remedies available to the patient. They should be informed that the factors involved in the injury will be investigated so that steps can be taken to reduce the likelihood of similar injury to other patients. Improving the disclosure process through policies, programmatic training, and available resources will enhance patient satisfaction, strengthen the physician–patient relationship, potentially decrease litigation, and most importantly promote higher quality health care.

Patient Handoffs. Physician-to-physician handoff of patient information is one of the most important factors to focus on to prevent discontinuity of care, eliminate preventable errors, and provide a safe patient environment. Certain clinical communications should be verified, such as reading back medication orders. Inaccurate information and missing clinical data can result in serious medical errors and patient injury. Relevant communications should be documented appropriately.

Physician Fatigue and Patient Safety

Individuals who are tired are more likely to make mistakes. Reducing fatigue may improve patient care and safety as well as improve a health care provider's performance satisfaction and increase communication. Although there are no current guidelines placing any limits on the volume of deliveries and procedures performed by a single physician or the length of time physicians may be on call and still perform procedures, it is imperative that physicians recognize their limitations caused by fatigue.

The National Sleep Foundation recommends 8 hours of sleep per night for an adult. Sleep deprivation can result from insufficient sleep, fragmented sleep, or both. Recovery from a period of insufficient sleep generally requires at least two or three full nights of adequate uninterrupted sleep. The following recommendations adapted from the National Highway Traffic Safety Administration guidelines offer some guidance that may assist obstetric and neonatal care providers in achieving a balance between work schedules and continuity of patient care:

- Arrange work schedules to take advantage of circadian influences.

- Recognize that the urge to sleep is very strong between 2:00 AM and 9:00 AM, and especially between 3:00 AM and 5:00 AM.

- Sleep when sleepy.

- Provide backup coverage during times that impairment is likely.

- Go to sleep immediately after working a night shift to maximize sleep length.

- Apply good sleep habits. The sleep environment should be quiet and dark. It should have adequate ventilation and a comfortable temperature.

- Use naps strategically. A 2-hour nap before a night shift will help prevent sleepiness. If a 2-hour nap cannot be scheduled, sleep no more than 45 minutes to avoid deep sleep and difficulty with arousal.

Individual practitioners and group practices should examine their sleeping habits and work schedules to ensure an optimal balance between fatigue and continuity of patient care. Although there may be an economic effect of such considerations, patient safety should take precedence.

Drills and Simulator Training

The principle that standardized care can result in safe care applies to emergencies as well as to routine care. Thus, each service should consider a protocol for management of common emergencies. This training may use a sophisticated simulated environment, but it also may use the everyday workspace in a mock event. Protocols also can be reinforced by being prominently displayed as posters, pocket cards, or other aids.

Using drills to train physicians to respond to emergencies has several theoretical advantages. Adult learning theory supports the importance of experiential learning. Emergencies occur in a specific physical setting and may involve a group of nurses, physicians, and other health care providers attempting to respond. By conducting a drill in a realistic simulator or in the actual patient care setting, issues related to the physical environment become obvious.

Emergency drills also allow physicians and others to practice principles of effective communication in a crisis. Many aspects of the medical environment work against effective communication, including the often hierarchical hospital structure, and the nature of the training, work setting, and the different educational backgrounds and levels of understanding of the health care team. Many physicians are accustomed to talking to nurses. Effective teamwork requires talking with each other. It requires that there be a team leader coordinating the response, but it also should empower all members of the team to share information. By practicing together, barriers hindering communication and teamwork can be overcome. Effective drills may lead to improved standardization of response, health care provider satisfaction, and patient outcomes.

Simulator training also may be beneficial with respect to identifying common clinical errors made during emergencies and correcting those deficiencies. Although this is promising, there are limited data to suggest that improved proficiency with simulation models correlates with increased proficiency during actual emergencies.

Quality Improvement and Patient Safety in Neonatal Intensive Care Units

Similar principles of QI and patient safety apply to the management of high-risk infants who require neonatal care. In its report, *Toward Improving the Outcome of Pregnancy III*, the March of Dimes outlined QI and patient safety recommendations for NICUs. The guidelines recommend that each NICU implement QI projects that incorporate the following essential principles:

- Timely and clinically useful feedback on measurable goals
- Transparency that results in sharing outcomes with all stakeholders
- Evidence-based practices to provide safe and effective patient care
- Reliability of care, which is fostered through teamwork and effective nonhierarchical communication, objective identification and analysis of errors, and identification of system characteristics that are vulnerable to error

Ideally, NICUs should participate in regional or national QI collaboratives that can help foster the QI process through shared learning, simultaneous testing of multiple strategies, and competition among NICUs. In addition, the March of Dimes advocates the application of tools and strategies across a group of NICUs and comparison of performance data to both increase the desired outcome and decrease the variability among processes, group outcomes, or both.

As with perinatal care, ensuring a culture of patient safety is essential in the NICU, including an emphasis on nonhierarchical team culture. Because of the acuity and complexity of neonatal conditions encountered in the NICU and the shift changes of multiple personnel who provide care, accurate transfer of information about each patient is essential. The March of Dimes recommends that these patient handoffs be face-to-face, structured, uninterrupted, and provide opportunity for clarification of information between participants. Standardized verbal tools, electronic tools, or both are important aids in this process.

Another essential indicator of safe patient care in the NICU is the ability of the clinical team to respond appropriately to relatively infrequent life-threatening events, such as the need to perform cardiopulmonary resuscitation. The March of Dimes recommends the use of simulation-based training with debriefing to provide realistic exercises of conditions that may be encountered in the NICU without involving actual patients. Teams including obstetric care providers can be used to practice simulated high-risk events in labor and delivery.

Bibliography

American College of Obstetricians and Gynecologists. Quality and safety in women's health care. 2nd ed. Washington, DC: American College of Obstetricians and Gynecologists; 2010.

Communication strategies for patient handoffs. Committee Opinion No. 517. American College of Obstetricians and Gynecologists. Obstet Gynecol 2012;119:408–11.

Congressional Budget Office. Factors contributing to the infant mortality ranking of the United States. CBO Staff Memorandum. Washington, DC: CBO; 1992. Available at: http://www.cbo.gov/ftpdocs/62xx/doc6219/doc05b.pdf. Retrieved December 7, 2011.

Disclosure and discussion of adverse events. Committee Opinion No. 520. American College of Obstetricians and Gynecologists. Obstet Gynecol 2012;119:686–9.

Effective patient-physician communication. Committee Opinion No. 492. American College of Obstetricians and Gynecologists. Obstet Gynecol 2011;117:1254–7.

Evaluation of Fetal and Infant Mortality Review (FIMR) Programs Nationwide. The Women's and Children's Health Policy Center. Johns Hopkins University. Available at: http://www.jhsph.edu/wchpc/projects/fimr.html. Retrieved January 13, 2012.

Facts about the official "do not use" list. Oakbrook Terrace (IL): The Joint Commission; 2011. Available at: http://www.jointcommission.org/assets/1/18/Official_do_not_use_list_6_111.pdf. Retrieved December 20, 2011.

Fatigue and patient safety. Committee Opinion No. 519. American College of Obstetricians and Gynecologists. Obstet Gynecol 2012;119:683–5.

Health literacy. Committee Opinion No. 491. American College of Obstetricians and Gynecologists. Obstet Gynecol 2011;117:1250–3. Establish a rapid response team. Cambridge (MA): IHI; 2011. Available at: http://www.ihi.org/knowledge/Pages/Changes/EstablishaRapidResponseTeam.aspx. Retrieved December 14, 2011.

Hines S, Luna K, Lfthus J, Marquardt M, Stelmokas D. Becoming a high reliability organization: operational advice for hospital leaders. Rockville (MD): Agency for Healthcare Research and Quality; 2008. Available at: http://www.ahrq.gov/qual/hroadvice/hroadvice.pdf. Retrieved December 7, 2011.

Institute for Clinical Systems Improvement. Prevention of unintentionally retained foreign objects during vaginal deliveries. Health Care Protocol, 3rd ed. Bloomington (MN): ICSI; 2009. Available at: http://www.icsi.org/retained_foreign_objects_during_vaginal_deliveries/retained_foreign_objects_during_vaginal_deliveries__prevention_of_untentionally__protocol_.html. Retrieved December 22, 2011.

Institute of Medicine (US). Crossing the quality chasm : a new health system for the 21st century. Washington, DC: National Academy Press; 2001.

March of Dimes. Toward improving the outcome of pregnancy III : enhancing perinatal health through quality, safety and performance initiatives. Committee on Perinatal Health. White Plains (NY): National Foundation--March of Dimes; 2010. Available at: http://www.marchofdimes.com/TIOPIII_FinalManuscript.pdf. Retrieved December 14, 2011.

Martin JA, Osterman MJ, Sutton PD. Are preterm births on the decline in the United States? Recent data from the National Vital Statistics System. NCHS Data Brief 2010;(39)(39):1–8.

Martin JA, Kirmeyer S, Osterman M, Shepherd RA. Born a bit too early: recent trends in late preterm births. NCHS Data Brief 2009;(24):1–8.

National Patient Safety Goals. Oakbrook Terrace (IL): The Joint Commission; 2011. Available at: http://www.jointcommission.org/standards_information/npsgs.aspx. Retrieved December 20, 2011.

National Sleep Foundation. Arlington (VA): National Sleep Foundation; 2011. Available at: http://www.sleepfoundation.org/. Retrieved December 20, 2011.

National Transportation Safety Board. Factors that affect fatigue in heavy truck accidents. Safety Study NTSB/SS-95/01. Washington, DC: NTSB; 1995.

Partnering with patients to improve safety. ACOG Committee Opinion No. 320. American College of Obstetricians and Gynecologists. Obstet Gynecol 2005;106:1123–5.

Patient safety in obstetrics and gynecology. ACOG Committee Opinion No. 447. American College of Obstetricians and Gynecologists. Obstet Gynecol 2009;114:1424–7.

Patient safety in the surgical environment. Committee Opinion No. 464. American College of Obstetricians and Gynecologists. Obstet Gynecol 2010;116:786–90.

Preparing for clinical emergencies in obstetrics and gynecology. Committee Opinion No. 487. American College of Obstetricians and Gynecologists. Obstet Gynecol 2011;117:1032–4.

Sheridan SL, Harris RP, Woolf SH. Shared decision making about screening and chemoprevention. a suggested approach from the U.S. Preventive Services Task Force. Shared Decision-Making Workgroup of the U.S. Preventive Services Task Force. Am J Prev Med 2004;26:56-66. Available at: http://www.uspreventiveservicestaskforce.org/3rduspstf/shared/sharedba.htm. Retrieved December 20, 2011.

The Joint Commission. Comprehensive accreditation manual for hospitals : CAMH. Oakbrook Terrace (IL): The Commission; 2010.

The Joint Commission. Introduction to the Universal Protocol for preventing wrong site, wrong procedure, and wrong person surgery. In: Comprehensive accreditation manual for hospitals : CAMH. Oakbrook Terrace (IL): The Commission; 2010. p. NPSG-19-NPSG-24.

Resources

Clinical practice improvement and patient safety. Chicago (IL): AMA; 2011. Available at: http://www.ama-assn.org/ama/pub/physician-resources/clinical-practice-improvement.page. Retrieved December 14, 2011.

Managing obstetrical risk efficiently: MOREob. Society of Obstetricians and Gynaecologists of Canada; Healthcare Insurance Reciprocal of Canada. London, Ontario: Salus Global Corporation; 2011. Available at: http://moreob.com/. Retrieved December 14, 2011.

National Fetal and Infant Mortality Review Program. Available at: http://www.nfimr.org. Retrieved January 13, 2012.

National Quality Measures Clearinghouse. Rockville (MD): Agency for Healthcare Research and Quality; 2011. Available at: http://www.qualitymeasures.ahrq.gov/. Retrieved December 20, 2011.

Pregnancy Risk Assessment Monitoring System (PRAMS): home. Atlanta (GA): CDC; 2011. Available at: http://www.cdc.gov/prams/. Retrieved December 7, 2011.

Chapter 4
Maternal and Neonatal Interhospital Transfer

The primary goal of regionalized perinatal care is for women and neonates at high risk to receive care in facilities that provide the required level of specialized care. Neonates born to women transported during the antepartum period have better survival rates and decreased risks of long-term sequelae than those transferred after birth. Delivery in a center providing high level neonatal care offers availability of pediatric subspecialists for early diagnosis and treatment of life-threatening conditions. Antepartum transport avoids separation of mother and infant in the immediate postpartum period, allows mothers to communicate directly with neonatal intensive care unit (NICU) health care providers, and supports the goal of family-centered health care. Because all hospitals cannot provide all levels of perinatal and neonatal care, interhospital transport of pregnant women and neonates is an essential component of a regionalized perinatal health care system.

Both facilities and professionals providing health care to pregnant women need to understand their obligations under federal and state law. The Emergency Medical Treatment and Labor Act defines the responsibilities of both transferring and receiving facilities and practitioners. Federal law requires all Medicare-participating hospitals to provide an appropriate medical screening examination for any individual seeking medical treatment at an emergency department to determine whether the patient has an emergency medical condition (Appendix G). Some states have similar statutory requirements. These laws also place strict requirements on the transfer of these patients. However, there have been misinterpretations of these laws that have been barriers to optimal health care. For example, the medical condition of a woman having contractions is not considered an emergency if there is adequate time for her safe transfer before delivery or if the transfer will not pose a threat to the health or safety of the woman or the fetus.

Types of Transport

There are three types of perinatal patient transport: 1) maternal transport, 2) neonatal transport, and 3) return transport. Maternal and neonatal transport programs are typically considered separately because they each have particular characteristics, requirements, and are generally overseen by their respective specialists.

Maternal Transport

Maternal transport refers to the transport of a pregnant woman during the antepartum period or intrapartum period for special care of the woman, the neonate, or both. Occasionally, the same system is used to transport a postpartum woman so that the mother can either be with her baby or receive a higher level of care for severe postpartum complications. Depending on the severity of the maternal illness, a team from the receiving hospital may go to the referring hospital to pick up the patient, or the patient may be sent by one-way ambulance from the referring hospital to the receiving hospital.

All attempts should be made to ensure that women and infants at high risk receive care in a facility that provides the required level of specialized obstetric and newborn care. If a woman is receiving obstetric care in a hospital with a low level of NICU care and she is found to be at risk of adverse outcome or premature delivery, transfer of care to a hospital with a high level of NICU care is indicated, whenever safely possible. Delivery hospitals that do not have a level III or level IV NICU should develop affiliation(s) with facilities that provide higher levels of care. Formal transfer agreements should be in place that clearly outline the responsibilities of each facility. The American Academy of Pediatrics has developed general guidance based on neonatal gestational age and potential complications to help determine the most optimal level of NICU care for a given gestational age and estimated fetal weight (see Table 1-3 in Chapter 1).

Neonatal Transport

The interhospital transfer of a newborn infant who requires specialized or intensive care generally proceeds according to one of the following approaches:

- A team is sent from one hospital, often a regional center, to the referring hospital to evaluate and stabilize the infant at the referring hospital and then transfer the infant to the team's hospital.
- A team is sent from the referring hospital with an infant who is being transferred to another hospital for specialized or intensive care.

- A team is sent from one hospital to the referring hospital to evaluate and stabilize the infant and then transfer the infant to a third hospital. Such a transfer may be necessary because of bed constraints or the need for specialized care available only at the third hospital. (For more information, see "Expanded Classification System for Levels of Neonatal Care" in Chapter 1 and the American Academy of Pediatrics' resource *Guidelines for Air and Ground Transport of Neonatal and Pediatric Patients.*)

Return Transport

After receiving intensive or specialized care at a referral center, a woman or her infant, may be returned to the original referring hospital or to a local hospital for continuing care after the problems that required the transfer have been resolved. This should be done in consultation with the referring physician.

Transport Program Components and Responsibilities

Components

To ensure optimal care of patients at high risk, the following components should be part of a regional referral program:

- Formal transfer plans for mothers and infants with receiving hospitals that are established by facilities that provide lower levels of care
- A method of risk identification and assessment of problems that are expected to benefit from consultation and transport
- Assessment of the perinatal capabilities and determination of conditions necessitating consultation, referral, transfer, and return transfer of each participating hospital
- Resource management to maximize efficiency, effectiveness, and safety
- Adequate financial and personnel support
- A reliable, accurate, and comprehensive communication system between participating hospitals and transport teams
- Determination of responsibility for each of these functions

An interhospital transport program should provide 24-hour service. It should include a receiving or program center responsible for ensuring that patients at high risk receive the appropriate level of care, a dispatching unit to coordinate the transport of patients between facilities, an appropriately equipped transport vehicle, and a specialized transport team. The program also should have a system for providing a continuum of care by various health care providers, including the personnel and equipment required for the level of care needed, as well as outreach education and program evaluation.

Responsibilities

Each of the functional components of an interhospital transport program has specific responsibilities. If the transport is done by the referring hospital, the referring physician and hospital retain responsibility until the transport team arrives with the patient at the receiving hospital. If the transport team is sent by the receiving hospital, the receiving physician or designee assumes responsibility for patient care from the time the patient leaves the referring hospital. It should be emphasized that during the preparation for transport by the transport team, the referring physician and hospital retain responsibility for the patient unless there have been other prior agreements. Transport services should work with their referring hospital to delineate clearly the primary medical responsibility for the patient when the patient is still within the referring hospital but is being cared for by the transport team. Regardless of the site of origin of the transport team, qualified staff should accompany the patient to the receiving hospital.

Medical–Legal Aspects

Many legal details of perinatal transport are not well defined and are subject to interpretation. In addition, many transport teams provide service in more than one state and therefore must comply with the laws of the state in which they are practicing and cannot be guided solely by their home state or area. Legal consult should be sought when developing a service to ensure compatibility with existing laws, and periodic review is encouraged to maintain compliance with laws and regulations. It is clear that all involved parties (eg, the referring hospital and personnel, the receiving hospital and personnel, and the transportation carriers or corporations) assume a number of responsibilities for which they are accountable:

- Each transport system must comply with the standards and regulations set forth by local, state, and federal agencies.
- Informed consent for transfer, transport, and admission to and care at the receiving hospital should be obtained before the transport team moves the patient. All federal and state laws regulating patient transfer must be followed. The completed consent form should be signed by the patient or

parent or guardian and witnessed; a copy should be placed in the patient's medical record. If the neonatal patient requires an emergency procedure before the parents' arrival at the receiving facility, the informed consent for this procedure should be obtained before departure from the referring facility if this action will not adversely delay the transport.

• Consent for any surgical procedures needed for the infant should be obtained by the surgical staff by telephone if parents are not at the receiving facility.

• Formal protocols should be developed by hospitals that provide lower levels of care to outline procedures for transport and to clarify responsibilities for care of the patient being transported

• Hospital medical staff policies should delineate the level of capability of their perinatal units, which conditions should prompt consultation, and which patients should be considered for transfer.

• Relevant personal identification must be provided for the patient to wear during transport.

• Patient care guidelines, standing orders, and verbal communication with the designated supervising transport physician are to be used to initiate and maintain patient-care interventions during transport.

The professional qualifications and actions of the transport team are the responsibility of the institution that employs the team. Insurance must be adequate to protect both patients and transport team members.

Director

The director of the transport programs (maternal or neonatal) should be either a subspecialist in maternal–fetal medicine or neonatology, respectively, or, in selected cases, an obstetrician–gynecologist or pediatrician, respectively, with special expertise in these subspecialty areas. As noted previously, typically the programs are organized and directed separately. The program director's responsibilities include the following:

• Training and supervising staff

• Ensuring appropriate review of all transport records

• Developing and implementing protocols for patient care

• Developing and maintaining standardized patient records and a database to track the program

• Establishing a program for performance quality

- Identifying trends and effecting improvements in the transport system by regularly reviewing the following elements:
  — Reviewing operational aspects of the program, such as response times, effectiveness of communications, and equipment issues
  — Reviewing evaluation forms completed by the referring and receiving hospitals soon after each transport
- Developing protocols for programs that use multiple modes of transport (ground, helicopter, and airplane)
- Determining which mode of transport should be used and any conditions, such as weather, that would preclude the use of a particular form of transport
- Developing alternative plans for care of the patient if a transport cannot be accomplished
- Ensuring that proper safety standards are followed during transport
- Requiring the transportation services to follow established guidelines regarding maintenance and safety

The director may delegate specific responsibilities to other persons or groups but retains the responsibility of ensuring that these functions are addressed appropriately.

Referring Hospital

Referring physicians should be familiar with the transport system, including how to gain access to its services and appropriately use its services. The referring physician is responsible for evaluating the patient's condition and initiating stabilization procedures before the transport team arrives. Within the referring hospital, the transport team continues resuscitation and care in collaboration with the referring physician and staff. Transfer generally is performed when the patient is clinically stable, although there are circumstances when ongoing stabilization is necessary during the transfer to the accepting hospital.

When being transferred, each patient should be accompanied by a maternal or neonatal transport form. This form should contain general information about the patient, including the reason for referral, the transport mode, and any additional information that may enhance understanding of the patient's needs. Also provided should be relevant patient medical information that maximizes the opportunity for appropriate and timely care and minimizes duplication of tests and diagnostic procedures at the receiving hospital.

The newborn must have appropriate identification bands in place, and the following items should be sent with the neonate:

- Properly labeled, red-topped tubes of clotted maternal and umbilical cord blood with label identification consistent with the newborn identification bands

- Copies of all relevant maternal antepartum, intrapartum, and postpartum records

- All recent or new diagnostic or clinical information for the neonate, including imaging studies

Responsibility for care of the newborn should be delineated between the referring team and the transport team. Parental consent should be obtained for transfer to and treatment of the neonate at the receiving hospital. The referring physician should personally transfer care to the transport team or should designate another physician to transfer care. A report on the neonate's care should be provided by the referring hospital's nursing staff to the appropriate transport team member.

Receiving Center

The receiving center is responsible for the overall coordination of the regional program. It should ensure that interhospital transport is organized in a way that ensures that patients will receive the appropriate level of care. The receiving hospital for maternal transports typically decides whether the woman's condition warrants a team going to pick her up or if she can be safely transported by one-way ambulance. Programs that use one-way ambulances must have procedures in place that identify the ambulance company, level of ambulance, and how to initiate the transport.

Contingency plans should be in place to avoid a shortage of beds for patients needing tertiary or quaternary care. These plans should include provisions for accepting or transferring patients among the cooperating centers or to an alternate receiving center, rather than only the receiving center affiliated with the referral center, when special circumstances warrant (eg, patient census or need for specialized services, such as extracorporeal membrane oxygenation).

The receiving center is responsible for providing referring physicians with the following services:

- Access by telephone on a 24-hour basis to communicate with receiving obstetric and neonatal units

- Follow-up on the patient by telephone, letter, or fax, provided all federal, state, and local requirements are met
- A complete summary, including diagnosis, an outline of the hospital course, and recommendations for ongoing care for each patient at discharge
- Ongoing communication and follow-up

Dispatching Units

Dispatching units are responsible for the following activities:

- Providing rapid coordination of vehicles and staff
- Serving as a communication link between the transport team and the referring and receiving hospitals
- Communicating the transport team's estimated time of arrival at the referring hospital to pick up the patient so that any planned therapeutic or diagnostic interventions can be completed in time
- Communicating the patient's estimated time of arrival at the receiving center so that all resources can be mobilized and ready
- Coordinating any connections that need to be made between air transport and ground ambulances

Personnel

The transport teams should have the expertise necessary to provide supportive care for a wide variety of emergency conditions that can arise with pregnant women and neonates at high risk. Team members may include physicians, neonatal nurse practitioners, registered nurses, respiratory therapists, and emergency medical technicians. The composition of the transport team should be consistent with the expected level of medical need of the patient being transported. Transport personnel also should be thoroughly familiar with the transport equipment to ensure that any malfunction en route can be handled.

Equipment

Safe and successful patient transfer depends on the equipment available to the transport team. The kinds and amounts of equipment, medications, and supplies needed by the transport team depend on the type of transport (maternal or neonatal), the distance of the transfer, the type of transport vehicle used, and the resources available at the referring medical facility. The transport equipment and supplies should be based on the needs of the most seriously ill patients to be transported and should include essential medications and special supplies needed during stabilization and transfer.

The transport team generally needs the following items to perform its functions:

- Equipment for monitoring physiologic functions (heart rate, blood pressure levels [invasive or noninvasive], temperature [skin or axillary], respiratory rate, and noninvasive pulse oximetry

- Resuscitation and support equipment (intravenous pumps, suction apparatus, mechanical ventilators) and newborn incubators for neonatal transport

- Portable medical gas tanks attached to a flowmeter, with a blender that can be easily integrated with vehicle or building sources of pressurized gas during transport, if patients dependent on ventilators are transported

Electrical equipment that is capable of alternating current operation, extended direct-current operation, or both and is compatible with the sources in the transport vehicle or medical facility. Additional specialized equipment and supplies may be needed for individual clinical situations.

The performance characteristics of transport equipment should be tested for the most severe environmental conditions of air or ground transport that may be encountered. Equipment performance may be altered by a harsh electromagnetic environment, altitude changes, vibration, forces of acceleration, or extremes of temperature and humidity. Hospital-based equipment may cause electromagnetic interference with aircraft navigation or communication systems. Altered performance of medical or aircraft systems could affect the safety of the transport team and the patient.

All equipment should be tested to ensure accuracy and safety in flight. The Federal Aviation Administration and the U.S. Food and Drug Administration have no known comprehensive testing guidelines. The Federal Aviation Administration has guidance for operators of emergency medical services/ helicopters on what may be used. The United States Department of Defense has discovered flaws in hospital-based medical equipment that could affect safety when used in air transport. The Department of Defense has comprehensive testing guidelines for electronic and electric component parts and electromagnetic interference characteristics of subsystems and equipment. ASTM International (formerly known as the American Society for Testing and

Materials) has developed standards for fixed and rotary wing aircraft operating as air ambulances.

The following organizations also can offer assistance in choosing medical equipment suitable for use in aircraft:

Association of Air Medical Services
909 N. Washington Street, Suite 410
Alexandria, VA 22314
Tel: (703) 836-8732, Fax: (703) 836-8920
www.aams.org

Emergency Care Research Institute
5200 Butler Pike
Plymouth Meeting, PA 19462-1298
Tel: (610) 825-6000, Fax: (610) 825-1275
www.ecri.org

Federal Aviation Administration
800 Independence Avenue, SW
Washington, DC 20591
Tel: (866) 835-5322
www.faa.gov

National Aeronautics and Space Administration
Washington, DC 20546-0001
Tel: (202) 358-0001, Fax: (202) 358-4338
www.nasa.gov

Several factors should be considered in selecting vehicles for an interhospital transport system. Ground transportation is most appropriate for short-range transport. The use of airplanes allows for coverage of a large referral area but is more expensive, requires skilled operators and specially trained crews, and may actually prolong the time required for response and transport over relatively short distances because of the time needed to prepare for flight and the time required for transport to and from the airport. Helicopters can shorten response and transport times over intermediate distances or in highly congested areas but are very expensive to maintain and operate.

The decision to use an aircraft in a patient-transport system requires special commitments from the director and members of the transport team. The pilot's decision needs to be based solely on flight safety. Therefore, the pilot should be included in appropriate decision making and should have the authority to change, modify, or cancel the mission for safety reasons.

Transport Procedure

Interhospital transport should be considered if the necessary resources or personnel for optimal patient outcomes are not available at the facility currently providing care. The resources available at both the referring and the receiving hospitals should be considered. The risks and benefits of transport, as well as the risks and benefits associated with not transporting the patient, should be assessed. Transport may be undertaken if the physician determines that the well-being of the woman, the fetus, or the infant will not be adversely affected or that the benefits of transfer outweigh the foreseeable risks. The staff of the referring hospital should consult with the receiving hospital as soon as the need for the transport of a woman or her neonate is considered.

Transportation of patients to an alternate receiving center solely because of third-party payer issues (eg, conflicts between managed care plans and referring and receiving hospital affiliations) should be strongly discouraged and may be illegal in certain situations. All transfers should be based on medical need. When faced with preterm labor or preterm premature rupture of membranes, transport of the mother in labor is recommended if time allows. Preterm labor is a valid reason for transport within the context of the Emergency Medical Treatment and Labor Act.

If the patient to be transported is pregnant, pretreatment evaluation should include the following:

- Maternal vital signs
- Fetal assessment via electronic fetal monitoring or Doppler, depending on gestational age
- Fetal position
- Maternal cervical examination, if contracting

It may be necessary to stabilize the mother before transport. Initiation of blood pressure medication, intravenous fluids, or tocolytics may be started at the referring hospital. The level of care to be provided in the referring hospital is dependent on the time required for transport, method of transport, and maternal medical condition. This level of care should be determined locally between the referring and receiving hospitals' medical personnel.

If the patient to be transferred is a neonate, the family should be given an opportunity to see and touch the neonate before the transfer. A transport team member should meet with the family to explain what the team will be doing en route to the receiving hospital. The patient, personnel, and all equipment should be safely secured inside the transport vehicle.

Patient Care and Interactions

The following important components of patient care needed for either a maternal patient or a neonate during transport should be implemented:

- Patients should be observed continuously.
- Vital signs should be monitored and recorded.
- Intravenous fluids and medications should be given, monitored, and recorded as required.

The following components of care are specific for either a maternal patient or a neonate:

Maternal patients

- Uterine activity of maternal patients and fetal heart rates should be monitored before and after transport; continuous uterine activity or fetal heart rate monitoring during transport should be individualized.

Neonates

- Neonates should be kept in a neutral thermal environment and should receive appropriate respiratory support and additional monitoring, such as assessment of oxygen saturation and blood glucose, as clinically indicated.
- If ventilator support is needed, ventilator parameters and inspired oxygen percentages should be monitored.
- The team should be prepared to perform lifesaving invasive procedures, such as placement of a chest tube and intubation.

On arrival at the receiving hospital, the following activities are recommended:

- The receiving staff should be prepared to address any unresolved problems or emergencies that involved the transported patient.
- The transport team should report the patient's history and clinical status to the receiving staff.
- The receiving staff should inform the patient's family, as well as the referring physician and staff at the referring hospital, of the condition of the patient on arrival to the receiving hospital and periodically thereafter.

- On completion of the patient transfer, the transport team or other designated personnel should immediately restock and re-equip the transport vehicle in anticipation of another call.

Transfer for Critical Care

The care of any pregnant women requiring intensive care unit services should be managed in a facility with obstetric adult and neonatal intensive care unit capabilities. Guidelines for perinatal transfer have been published and follow the federal Emergency Medical Treatment and Labor Act guidelines. General recommendations include antenatal rather than neonatal transfer. In the event that maternal transport is unsafe or impossible, alternative arrangements for neonatal transfer may be necessary. In the event of imminent delivery, transfer should be held until after delivery.

The minimal monitoring required for a critically ill patient during transport includes continuous pulse oximetry, electrocardiography, and regular assessment of vital signs. All critically ill patients must have secure venous access before transfer. Patients who are mechanically ventilated must have endotracheal tube position confirmed and secured before transfer. In the obstetric patient, left uterine displacement and supplemental oxygen should be applied routinely during transport. The utility of continuous fetal heart rate monitoring or tocodynamic monitoring is unproven; therefore, its use should be individualized.

Return Transport

Infants whose conditions have stabilized and who no longer require specialized services should be considered for return transport. Transporting the patient back to the referring hospital is important for the following reasons:

- It allows the family to return to their home, often permitting more frequent interactions between the family and the infant.
- It involves the health care providers who ultimately will be responsible for the continuing care of the infant earlier in the care process.
- It preserves specialized services for patients who require them and allows for a better distribution of resources.
- It enhances the integrity of the regionalized care system and emphasizes the partnership between the hospitals in the system.

Economic barriers, including those imposed by managed care organizations, that restrict or raise barriers to this movement of neonates are detriments to optimal patient care. Every effort should be made to eliminate these artificial constraints.

Transfer is best accomplished after detailed communication between physicians and nursing services at both hospitals outlining the infant's care requirements and the anticipated course of the patient to ensure that the hospital receiving the return transport can provide the needed services. These services must not only be available but they must be provided in a consistent fashion and be of the same quality as those that the infant is receiving in the regional center. Further, if special equipment or treatment is required at the hospital receiving the infant, arrangements for these should be made before the infant is transferred. Lastly, there also must be an understanding that if problems arise that cannot be managed in an appropriate manner at the receiving hospital, the infant will be returned to the regional center, or the regional center will participate in developing an alternative care plan.

It is important that parents consent to the return transfer of the infant and understand the benefits to them and their infant. Their comfort with this process will be enhanced if they realize that the regional center and the referring hospital are working together in a regionalized system of care, that there is frequent communication between the staffs of the two hospitals, that there will be continuing support after the return transport, and that the patient will be returned to the regional center if necessary. It also may be helpful if parents visit the facility to which the infant will be transported before transfer.

A comprehensive plan for follow-up of the infant after return transfer and after discharge from the hospital should be developed. This plan should outline the required services and identify the party bearing the responsibility for follow-up.

To ensure optimal care during a return transfer, the following guidelines are recommended:

- The parents' informed consent for return transfer should be obtained.
- Return transfer should be accomplished via an adequately equipped vehicle with trained personnel so that the level of care received by the neonate remains the same during transport.
- Staffing at both hospitals should be adequate to ensure a safe transition of care.
- The family should be notified of the transfer so that they may be present at the accepting facility when the transfer occurs.

- Appropriate records, including a summary of the hospital course, diagnosis, treatments, recommendations for ongoing care, and follow-up, should accompany the infant.

- The transport team should call the referring hospital and the infant's parents to inform them of the completion of the transport and to report the neonate's condition.

- The center that provided the higher level of care should provide easily accessible consultation on current or new problems to professional staff at the return transfer facility.

Outreach Education

Critical to the appropriate use of a regional referral program is a program to educate the public and users about its capabilities. The receiving center and receiving hospitals should participate in efforts to educate the public about the kinds of services available and their accessibility.

Outreach education should reinforce cooperation between all individuals involved in the interhospital care of perinatal patients. Receiving hospitals should provide all referring hospitals with information about their response times and clinical capabilities and should ensure that health care providers know about the specialized resources that are available through the perinatal care network. Primary physicians should be informed as changes occur in indications for consultation and referral of perinatal patients at high risk and for the stabilization of their conditions. Each receiving hospital also should provide continuing education and information to referring physicians about current treatment modalities for high-risk situations. Effective outreach programs will improve the care capabilities of referring hospitals and may allow for some patients either to be retained or, if transferred, to be returned earlier in their course of care.

Program Evaluation

Ideally, the director of a regional program should coordinate program evaluation based on patient outcome data and logistic information. Program monitoring should include the following information:

- Unexpected neonatal morbidity (eg, hypothermia or tension pneumothorax) or mortality during transport

- Deliveries during transport or immediately after arriving at the receiving hospital

- Morbidity or mortality of patients at the receiving hospital
- Frequency of failure to transfer patients generally considered to require tertiary care (eg, newborns born at less than 32 weeks of gestation)
- Availability of all the services that may be needed by the perinatal patient
- Accessibility of services, capability to connect the patient quickly and appropriately with the services needed, and programs to promote patient and community awareness of available and appropriate regional referral programs

These data should be tracked as part of the ongoing quality improvement programs of the transport team and the receiving hospital (see also Chapter 3, "Quality Improvement and Patient Safety").

Bibliography

American Academy of Pediatrics. Guidelines for air and ground transport of neonatal and pediatric patients. 3rd ed. Elk Grove Village (IL): AAP; 2007.

American College of Obstetricians and Gynecologists. Guidelines for women's health care: a resource manual. 3rd ed. Washington, DC: ACOG; 2007.

ASTM International. Standard specification for fixed wing basic life support, advanced life support, and specialized medical support air ambulances. Designation: F2319–04. West Conshohocken (PA): ASTM International; 2004.

ASTM International. Standard specification for rotary wing basic life support, advanced life support, and specialized medical support air ambulances. Designation: F2318-04. West Conshohocken (PA): ASTM International; 2004.

Federal Aviation Administration. Advisory circular: emergency medical services/helicopeter. AC No.: 135-14A. Washington, DC: FAA; 1991.

March of Dimes. Toward improving the outcome of pregnancy: the 90s and beyond. Committee on Perinatal Health. White Plains (NY): National Foundation—March of Dimes; 1993.

March of Dimes. Toward improving the outcome of pregnancy III: enhancing perinatal health through quality, safety and performance initiatives. Committee on Perinatal Health. White Plains (NY): National Foundation—March of Dimes; 2010. Available at: http://www.marchofdimes.com/TIOPIII_FinalManuscript.pdf. Retrieved December 14, 2011.

Section on Transport Medicine. American Academy of Pediatrics. Elk Grove Village (IL): American Academy of Pediatrics; 2011. Available at: http://www2.aap.org/sections/transmed/default.cfm. Retrieved December 20, 2011.

U.S. Department of Defense. Department of Defense interface standard: requirements for the control of electromagnetic interference characteristics of subsystems and equipment. MIL-STD-461E. Wright-Patterson AFB (OH); DOD: 1999.

U.S. Department of Defense. Department of Defense test method standard: electronic and electrical component parts. MIL-STD-202G. Columbus (OH); DOD: 1999.

Warren J, Fromm RE, Jr, Orr RA, Rotello LC, Horst HM. Guidelines for the inter- and intrahospital transport of critically ill patients. American College of Critical Care Medicine. Crit Care Med 2004;32:256-62. Available at: http://www.learnicu.org/docs/guidelines/inter-intrahospitaltransport.pdf. Retrieved December 20, 2011.

Woodward GA, Insoft RM, Kleinman ME, editors. Guidelines for air and ground transport of neonatal and pediatrics. American Academy of Pediatrics. Section on Transport Medicine. 3rd ed. Elk Grove Village (IL): American Academy of Pediatrics; 2007.

Resources

Association of Air Medical Services (AAMS). Alexandria (VA): AAMS; 2011. Available at: http://www.aams.org/. Retrieved December 20, 2011.

ECRI Institute. Plymouth Meeting (PA): ECRI Institute; 2011. Available at: https://www.ecri.org/Pages/default.aspx. Retrieved December 20, 2011.

Federal Aviation Administration (FAA). Washington, DC: FAA; 2011. Available at: http://www.faa.gov/. Retrieved December 20, 2011.

National Aeronautics and Space Administration (NASA). Washington, DC: NASA; 2011. Available at: http://www.nasa.gov/. Retrieved December 20, 2011.

Chapter 5
Preconception and Antepartum Care

A comprehensive antepartum care program involves a coordinated approach to medical care, continuous risk assessment, and psychosocial support that optimally begins before conception and extends throughout the postpartum period and interconceptional period. Health care professionals should integrate the concept of family-centered care into antepartum care (see also "Patient-Centered and Family-Centered Health Care" in Chapter 1). The Institute for Patient- and Family-Centered Care importantly notes that the term family is defined by the patient, as is the degree to which the family is involved in care. As the term is used here, it includes the expectant mother and her support system (which can include any or all of the following individuals: a spouse or partner, blood relatives, and friends). Care should include an assessment of the expectant mother's attitude toward her pregnancy (as well as the family's attitudes, if this is so desired by the expectant mother) the support systems available, and the need for parenting education. To the extent it is desired by the expectant mother, she and her family should be encouraged to work with her caregivers in order to make well-informed decisions about pregnancy, labor, delivery, the postpartum period, and the interconceptional period. The health care team should assess the level of support for each woman and refer her appropriately to agencies if the expectant mother does not have a spouse, partner, or other individuals with whom to share this experience and to provide support.

Preconception Care

Optimizing a woman's health, health behaviors, and knowledge before she plans and conceives a pregnancy is known as preconception care. Preconception care is a component of a larger health care goal—optimizing the health of every woman. Because reproductive capacity spans almost four decades for most women, optimizing women's health before and between pregnancies is an ongoing process that requires access to and the full participation of all segments of the health care system. Increasingly it is apparent that few women seek a specific visit before conception for preconception counseling, which would be the ideal situation. Therefore, all health encounters during a woman's reproductive years should include counseling on appropriate medical care and behavior to optimize pregnancy outcomes. However, women should still be encouraged to seek a specific preconception visit if they are planning a pregnancy.

Questions, such as "Are you considering pregnancy?" or "Could you possibly become pregnant?" can initiate several preconception care interventions, including those listed as follows:

• A dialogue regarding the patient's readiness for pregnancy
• An evaluation of her overall health and opportunities for improving her health
• Education about the significant effect that social, environmental, occupational, behavioral, and genetic factors have on pregnancy
• Identification of women at high risk of an adverse pregnancy outcome, with interventions recommended to improve her risk profile before conception

Preconception Counseling and Interventions

During episodic or focused health care visits in women who could become pregnant, in addition to performing a physical exam and obtaining her obstetric and gynecologic histories, there are core topics in preconception care that should be addressed. The following topics may serve as the basis for such counseling (Table 5-1):

• Family planning and pregnancy spacing
• Immunity and immunization status
• Risk factors for sexually transmitted infections (STIs)
• Substance use, including alcohol, tobacco, and recreational and illicit drugs
• Exposure to violence and intimate partner violence
• Medical, surgical, and psychiatric histories
• Current medications (prescription and nonprescription)
• Family history
• Genetic history (both maternal and paternal)
• Nutrition
• Teratogens; environmental and occupational exposures
• Assessment of socioeconomic, educational, and cultural context

Table 5-1. Health Screening for Women of Reproductive Age

Selective Reproductive Health Screening	Done	Referred
Reproductive awareness		
Pregnancy prevention counseling	❏	❏
Prepregnancy and nutrition counseling	❏	❏
Medical diseases (counsel regarding effects on future pregnancies)		
Diabetes mellitus	❏	❏
Hypertension	❏	❏
Epilepsy	❏	❏
Other chronic illness	❏	❏
Infectious diseases (counsel, test, or refer)		
Sexually transmitted diseases, including human immunodeficiency virus (HIV)	❏	❏
Hepatitis A	❏	❏
Hepatitis B (immunize if at high risk)	❏	❏
Rubella (test; if nonimmune, immunize)	❏	❏
Varicella	❏	❏
Teratogens and genetics (counsel regarding effects on future pregnancies)		
Hemoglobinopathy	❏	❏
Medication and vitamin use (eg, isotretinoin and vitamin A [retinoic acid])	❏	❏
Self or prior child with congenital defect	❏	❏
Family history of genetic disease	❏	❏
Environmental exposure at home or in workplace	❏	❏
Behavior (counsel regarding effects on future pregnancies)		
Alcohol use	❏	❏
Tobacco use	❏	❏
Use of illicit substances (eg, cocaine)	❏	❏
Social support		
Safety (eg, domestic violence)	❏	❏
Personal resources (eg, transportation or housing)	❏	❏

Modified with permission from March of Dimes Birth Defects Foundation, Committee on Perinatal Health. Toward improving the outcome of pregnancy: the 90s and beyond. White Plains (NY): March of Dimes Birth Defects Foundation; 1993.

In addition, women should be counseled regarding the benefits of maximizing their personal health status; maintaining a menstrual calendar to assist with estimating the conception date; and practicing safe sex to avoid STIs, including human immunodeficiency virus (HIV).

Reproductive Health Plan

Physicians should encourage women to formulate a reproductive health plan and discuss it in a nonjudgmental way at each visit. Such a plan would address the individual's or couple's desire for a child or children (or desire not to have children); the optimal number, spacing, and timing of children in the family; and age-related changes in fertility. Because many women's plans change over time, creating a reproductive health plan requires an ongoing conscientious assessment of the desirability of a future pregnancy, determination of steps that need to be taken either to prevent or to plan for and optimize a pregnancy, and evaluation of current health status and other issues relevant to the health of a pregnancy. If pregnancy is not desired, a woman's current contraceptive use and options should be discussed to assist in the identification of the most appropriate and effective method for her. If a woman's request for care is in conflict with her primary caregiver's recommendations or preferences, consultation or referral may be indicated.

Preconception Immunization

Preconception care offers the opportunity to review immunization status. Although there is no evidence of adverse fetal effects from vaccinating pregnant women with an inactivated virus or bacterial vaccines or toxoids, ideally vaccinations should be administered before conception in order to avoid unnecessary exposure to the fetus. Live vaccines do pose a theoretical risk for the fetus. Women who receive a live-virus vaccination should be advised to avoid pregnancy for at least 1 month after vaccination.

The Advisory Committee on Immunization Practices of the Centers for Disease Control and Prevention (CDC) recommends vaccination with the inactivated influenza vaccine for all women who will be pregnant through the influenza season (October through May in the United States). No study to date has shown an adverse consequence of the inactivated influenza vaccine in pregnant women or their offspring. Vaccination early in the season and regardless of gestational age is optimal, but unvaccinated pregnant women should be immunized at any time during the influenza season as long as the vaccine supply lasts. In addition, women who have not been immunized with the tetanus toxoid, reduced diphtheria toxoid, and acellular pertussis vaccine (Tdap) or women whose vaccine status is unknown should be offered immunization with Tdap.

In addition, vaccination(s) should be offered to women found to be at risk of or susceptible to measles, mumps, rubella, varicella, hepatitis A, hepatitis B, meningococcus, and pneumococcus. Additionally, the human papillomavirus (HPV) vaccination can be offered to appropriate nonpregnant women. However, because the vaccine is not recommended during pregnancy, completion of the vaccine series may need to be delayed until the postpartum period.

Sexually Transmitted Infections

Chlamydia trachomatis and *Neisseria gonorrhea* have been strongly associated with ectopic pregnancy, infertility, and chronic pelvic pain. Annual screening of chlamydial infection for all sexually active women aged 25 years or younger is recommended, as is screening of older women with risk factors (eg, those who have a new sex partner or multiple sex partners). Targeted screening for gonorrhea is recommended for women younger than 25 years who are at increased risk of infection (eg, women with previous gonorrhea, other STIs, new or multiple sex partners, and inconsistent condom use; those who engage in commercial sex work and drug use; women in certain demographic groups; and those living in communities with a high prevalence of disease). Women who have a positive test result for gonorrhea, chlamydial infection, or both should be treated in accordance with current CDC guidelines (see also "Chlamydial Infection" and "Gonorrhea" in Chapter 10). Syphilis during pregnancy might result in fetal death or substantial physical and developmental disabilities, including intellectual disabilities and blindness. Preconception HIV testing can be considered to allow the woman to make informed decisions regarding treatment and timing of pregnancy.

Substance Use and Abuse

Behavioral counseling can be particularly effective during the preconception period and antenatal period. Preconception women who smoke cigarettes or use any other form of tobacco product should be identified and encouraged and supported in an effort to quit. Importantly, tobacco cessation at any point during pregnancy yields substantial health benefits for the expectant mother and newborn. There is a strong association between smoking during pregnancy and sudden infant death syndrome. Children born to mothers who smoke during pregnancy are at increased risk of asthma, infantile colic, and childhood obesity. Cessation of smoking is recommended before pregnancy. Patients who are willing to try to quit smoking benefit from a brief counseling session, such as the 5-A intervention (Box 5-1), which has been proven to be effective when initiated by health care providers. Training in the use of the 5-A smoking cessation tool and knowledge of health care support systems, including the National Cancer Institute's Smoking Quitline (1-877-44U-QUIT or 1-877-448-7848) and pharmacotherapy add to the techniques health care providers can use to support perinatal smoking cessation.

Other important behavioral issues to address include alcohol use and misuse and the abuse of prescription and nonprescription recreational drugs. All women should be asked about the quantity and frequency of their alcohol use. Women who are trying to become pregnant should be counseled to completely refrain from all alcohol use. Referral relationships with appropriate resources should be established and used as needed to assist women with these issues. Women who are counseled concerning their alcohol or drug use should be followed up to assess adherence to recommendations.

Chronic Medical Conditions
Certain chronic medical conditions, such as such as diabetes, thyroid disease, and maternal phenylketonuria (PKU), should be controlled before pregnancy. It has been shown that achieving preconception and early pregnancy blood sugar control can decrease the risk of spontaneous abortion, birth defects, and macrosomia. By achieving a hemoglobin A_{1C} level at or below 6.0 mg/dL or normal range preconceptionally, the risk of birth defects in the offspring of a pregestational diabetic woman is reduced to those of her age-related cohort. Women with either hyperthyroidism (most often Graves disease) or hypo-

---

**Box 5-1. U.S. Preventive Services Task Force:
5-A Tool for Smoking Cessation**

1. Ask about tobacco use.
2. Advise to quit through clear, personalized messages.
3. Assess willingness to quit.
4. Assist to quit.
5. Arrange follow up and support.

Modified from Treating tobacco use and dependence: 2008 update. Clinical Practice Guideline. Rockville (MD): U.S. Department of Health and Human Services, Public Health Service; 2008. Available at: http://www.ahrq.gov/path/tobacco.htm. Retrieved May 16, 2012.

thyroidism should be appropriately treated so that they are euthyroid before attempting pregnancy. Inadequately treated hyperthyroidism or hypothyroidism is associated with adverse pregnancy outcomes, including miscarriage and preterm delivery. Women in whom PKU was diagnosed and treated during infancy and childhood are at risk of having children with mental retardation and other birth defects if they do not adhere to a low-phenylalanine diet before conception and during pregnancy. Other chronic medical conditions that should be addressed preconceptionally include asthma, hemoglobinopathies, inherited thrombophilias, obesity, a history of bariatric surgery, and hypertension. (For more information, see "Medical Complications Before Pregnancy" in Chapter 7.)

Medication Use

All medications (prescription and over the counter), supplements and herbal therapies should be noted. In general, using the lowest effective dose of only necessary medications is recommended. The use of known or potential teratogenic medications should be addressed. Some common teratogenic medications include the oral anticoagulant warfarin, the antiseizure drugs valproic acid and carbamazepine, isotretinoin, and angiotensin-converting enzyme inhibitors. Physician and patient information about known teratogenic medications, as well as other teratogenic exposures, can be found on the Organization of Teratology Information Specialists' web site, available at http://www.otispregnancy.org.

Preconception Genetic Screening

Preconception visits are a reasonable time to offer screening for genetic disorders based on racial and ethnic background. Testing both partners preconceptionally is often more straightforward and less stressful than doing so in pregnancy, although insurance carriers may decline to reimburse for this testing. Carrier screening for specific genetic conditions often is determined by an individual's ancestry. It is recommended that Caucasians be tested for cystic fibrosis and that carrier screening for the Ashkenazi Jewish population be done for Tay–Sachs disease, Canavan disease, cystic fibrosis, and familial dysautonomia (see also "Antepartum Genetic Screening and Diagnosis" later in this chapter), and African Americans for sickle cell disease and thalassemias.

Physicians also may perform preconception screening for other genetic disorders on the basis of family history (eg, fragile X syndrome for individuals with a family history of nonspecific, predominantly male-affected mental retardation; Duchenne muscular dystrophy).

Preconception Nutritional Counseling

Consumption of a balanced diet with the appropriate distribution of the basic food pyramid groups is especially important during pregnancy. Diet can be affected by food preferences, cultural beliefs, and eating patterns. A woman who is a vegan or who has special dietary restrictions secondary to medical illnesses, such as diabetes mellitus, inflammatory bowel disease, renal disease or PKU, will require special dietary measures as well as vitamin and mineral supplements. Women who frequently diet to lose weight, fast, skip meals, or have eating disorders or unusual eating habits should be identified and counseled. Additional risk factors for nutritional problems include adolescence, tobacco and substance abuse, history of pica during a previous pregnancy, high parity, and mental illness. Women who have undergone bariatric surgery should be assessed as well because some of these surgical procedures affect vitamin absorption and B_{12} production. The patient's access to food and the ability to purchase food can be pertinent.

Ideally, women should be advised to achieve a near-normal body mass index (BMI) before attempting conception because infertility as well as both maternal and fetal complications are associated with abnormal BMI (see also "First-Trimester Patient Education" later in this chapter). All women should be encouraged to exercise at least 30 minutes on most days of the week. Obese women should be advised regarding their increased risk of adverse perinatal outcomes, including difficulty becoming pregnant, conception of a fetus with a variety of birth defects, preterm delivery, diabetes, cesarean delivery, hypertensive disease, and thromboembolic disease. Weight loss before pregnancy reduces these risks.

Dietary supplements are particularly important during the preconception period (Table 5-2). Folic acid (also known as folate) should be recommended to all women who could become pregnant in order to improve the health of the woman and to decrease the risk of certain birth defects, including neural tube defects (NTDs), such as open spina bifida and anencephaly; congenital heart disease; and cleft lip and palate.

Folic acid supplementation is recommended before pregnancy and during pregnancy, despite the fortification of fortified grain products in the United States, because the amount of folic acid consumed in fortified grain products may be less than the amount recommended to prevent NTDs. The CDC and the U.S. Public Health Service recommend the daily intake of 400 micrograms of folic acid for all women who could become pregnant. The CDC urges women to start this daily intake at least 1 month before getting pregnant to help reduce major birth defects of the baby's brain and spine (anencephaly and spina bifida) by 50–70%. Women planning a pregnancy who have previously had a fetus or baby with an NTD should be advised to follow the 1991 U.S. Public Health Service guideline, which recommends the daily consumption of 4,000 micrograms of folic acid beginning 1 month before trying to conceive and continuing through the first 3 months of pregnancy. This dosage should be prescribed and monitored by the health care provider.

Table 5-2. Recommended Daily Dietary Allowances and Tolerable Upper Intake Levels* for Nonpregnant Adolescents and Women

Nutrient (unit)	14–18 years	19–30 years	31–50 years
Fat-soluble vitamins			
Vitamin A (µg/d)[†]	700	700	700
UL*,[‡]	2,800	3,000	3,000
Vitamin D (µg/d)[§]	15	15	15
UL*	100	100	100
Vitamin E (mg/d)[ǁ]	15	15	15
UL*,[¶]	800	1,000	1,000
Vitamin K (µg/d)[#]	75	90	90
UL*	–	–	–
Water-soluble vitamins			
Folate (µg/d)**	400	400	400
UL*,[¶]	800	1,000	1,000
Niacin (mg/d)[††]	14	14	14
UL*,[¶]	30	35	35
Riboflavin (mg/d)	1.0	1.1	1.1
UL*	–	–	–
Thiamin (mg/d)	1.0	1.1	1.1
UL*	–	v	–
Vitamin B$_6$ (mg/d)	1.2	1.3	1.3
UL*	80	100	100
Vitamin B$_{12}$ (µg/d)	2.4	2.4	2.4
UL*	–	–	–
Vitamin C (mg/d)	65	75	75
UL*	1,800	2,000	2,000

(continued)

Table 5-2. Recommended Daily Dietary Allowances and Tolerable Upper Intake Levels* for Nonpregnant Adolescents and Women *(continued)*

Nutrient (unit)	14–18 years	19–30 years	31–50 years
Minerals			
Calcium (mg/d)	1,300	1,000	1,000
UL*	3,000	2,500	2,500
Iodine (μg/d)	150	150	150
UL*	900	1,100	1,100
Iron (mg/d)	15	18	18
UL*	45	45	45
Phosphorus (mg/d)	1,250	700	700
UL*	4,000	4,000	4,000
Selenium (μg/d)	55	55	55
UL*	400	400	400
Zinc (mg/d)	9	8	8
UL*	34	40	40

*UL = tolerable upper intake level. This is the highest level of daily nutrient intake that is likely to pose no risk of adverse effects to almost all individuals in the general population. Unless otherwise specified, the UL represents total intake from food, water, and supplements. Due to lack of suitable data, ULs could not be established for vitamin K, thiamin, riboflavin, and Vitamin B_{12}. In the absence of ULs, extra caution may be warranted in consuming levels above recommended intakes. Members of the general population should be advised not to routinely exceed the UL. The UL is not meant to apply to individuals who are treated with the nutrient under medical supervision or to individuals with predisposing conditions that modify their sensitivity to the nutrient.

†As retinol activity equivalents.

‡As preformed vitamin A only.

§1) Under the assumption of minimal sunlight. 2) As cholecalciferol; 1 microgram cholecalciferol = 40 international units of vitamin D.

‖As α-tocopherol.

¶The ULs for vitamin E, niacin, and folate apply to synthetic forms obtained from supplements, fortified foods, or a combination of the two.

#Recommendations measured as Adequate Intake (AI) instead of Recommended Daily Dietary Allowance (RDA). An AI is set instead of an RDA if insufficient evidence is available to determine an RDA. The AI is based on observed or experimentally determined estimates of average nutrient intake by a group (or groups) of healthy people.

**As dietary folate equivalents (DFE). 1 DFE = 1 microgram food folate = 0.6 micrograms of folic acid from fortified food or as a supplement consumed with food = 0.5 micrograms of a supplement taken on an empty stomach. In view of the evidence linking folate intake with neural tube defects in the fetus, it is recommended that all women capable of becoming pregnant consume 400 micrograms from supplements or fortified foods in addition to intake of food folate from a varied diet.

††As niacin equivalents.

Modified with permission from Institute of Medicine. Dietary reference intakes. The essential guide to nutrient requirements. Washington, DC: The National Academies Press; 2006 and Dietary Reference Intakes for Calcium and Vitamin D. Washington, DC: The National Academies Press; 2010.

Women also should assess their diets and dietary supplements to confirm that they are meeting the recommended daily doses for calcium, iron, vitamin D, vitamin A, vitamin B_{12}, and other nutrients, minerals and vitamins (Table 5-2). The U.S. Department of Agriculture and the U.S. Department of Health and Human Services recommend that women who could become pregnant consume foods that supply heme iron (which is more readily absorbed by the body), additional iron sources, and foods that enhance iron absorption, such as those rich in vitamin C (eg, citrus fruits, strawberries, broccoli, and tomatoes).

Assisted Reproductive Therapy

Over the past two decades, the use of assisted reproductive technology (ART) has increased dramatically worldwide and has made pregnancy possible for many infertile couples. The American Society for Reproductive Medicine defines ART as treatments and procedures involving the handling of human oocytes and sperm, or embryos, with the intent of establishing a pregnancy. By this definition, ART includes in vitro fertilization with or without intracyto-plasmic sperm injection, but it excludes techniques, such as artificial insemination and superovulation drug therapy.

Perinatal risks that may be associated with ART include high-order multiple pregnancy, prematurity, low birth weight, small for gestational age, perinatal mortality, cesarean delivery, placenta previa, placental abruption, preeclampsia, and birth defects. It is still unclear to what extent these adverse outcomes are specifically related to ART procedures versus any underlying factors within the couple, such as coexisting maternal disease, the cause of infertility, or differences in behavioral risk (eg, smoking). Before initiating ART procedures, it is important to counsel patients about the risks associated with treatment and complete a thorough medical evaluation to ensure that they are in good health. To reduce the risk of high-order multiple gestation and associated perinatal complications, it is recommended that ART procedures be performed in accordance with updated American Society for Reproductive Medicine and Society for Assisted Reproductive Technology guidelines on limiting the number of embryos that can be transferred.

Antepartum Care

Women who receive early and regular prenatal care are more likely to have healthier infants. Prenatal care includes a process of ongoing risk identification and assessment in order to develop appropriate care plans. This plan of care should take into consideration the medical, nutritional, psychosocial, cultural and educational needs of the patient and her family, and it should be periodically reevaluated and revised in accordance with the progress of the pregnancy.

Health care providers of antepartum care must be able to either primarily provide or easily refer to others to provide a wide array of services to pregnant women. These services include the following:

- Readily available and regularly scheduled obstetric care, beginning in early pregnancy and continuing through the postpartum period
- Access to unscheduled visits or emergency visits on a 24-hour basis. Timing of access varies depending on the nature of the problem
- Timely transmittal of prenatal records to the site of the patient's planned delivery so that her records are readily accessible at the time of delivery
- Medical interpretation services exclusive of family members for women with limited English language ability
- Referral network of reliable, competent, culturally sensitive, accessible social service, mental health, and specialist medical care providers.

Prenatal Care Visits

The first visit for prenatal care typically occurs in the first trimester. The frequency of follow-up visits is determined by the individual needs of the woman and an assessment of her risks.

Frequency

The frequency of obstetric visits should be individualized. Women with poor pregnancy outcomes in earlier pregnancies, known medical problems, vaginal bleeding before initiation of routine prenatal care, and those who achieved a pregnancy through infertility treatments and are known to be carrying multiple gestations should be seen as early as possible.

Typically, a woman with an uncomplicated first pregnancy is examined every 4 weeks for the first 28 weeks of gestation, every 2 weeks until 36 weeks of gestation, and weekly thereafter. Women with medical or obstetric problems, as well as women at the extremes of reproductive age will likely require close surveillance; the appropriate intervals between scheduled visits are determined by the nature and severity of the problems (see also Appendix B and Appendix C). Likewise, parous women with prior normal pregnancy outcomes and without medical and obstetric problems during the current pregnancy may be able to be seen less frequently as long as additional visits on an as-needed basis are available.

The frequency and regularity of scheduled prenatal visits should be sufficient to enable health care providers to accomplish the following activities:

- Assess the well-being of the woman and her fetus
- Provide ongoing, timely, and relevant prenatal education
- Complete recommended health screening studies and review results
- Detect medical and psychosocial complications and institute indicated interventions
- Reassure the woman

First Visit

Unless there was a recent preconception visit, risk assessment, and patient education begin with the first prenatal visit, at which time the physician or nurse begins to compile an obstetric database. Appendix A contains a format for documenting information and the database recommended by the American College of Obstetricians and Gynecologists (the College). Whatever format is used, the record should be designed to record the large amount of data in a longitudinal manner that is clear and concise, to prompt the health care provider to complete the evaluations and screening steps appropriate for that patient, and to communicate the results in a clear fashion to the users of the chart.

During the first prenatal visit the following general information should be discussed with each patient:

- Scope of care that is provided in the office
- Laboratory studies and their indications
- Expected course of the pregnancy
- Signs and symptoms to be reported to the physician (eg, vaginal bleeding, rupture of membranes, or decreased fetal movements) and how to do so
- Role of the members of the health care provider team
- Anticipated schedule of visits
- Physician or midwife schedule and labor and delivery coverage
- Cost to the patient of prenatal care and delivery (eg, insurance plan participation)

- Practices to promote health maintenance (eg, use of safety restraints, including lap and shoulder belts)
- Risk counseling, including substance use and abuse
- Psychosocial topics in pregnancy and the postpartum period

Patient education early in pregnancy also includes specialized counseling on topics, such as nutrition, exercise, nausea and vomiting, vitamin and mineral toxicity, and teratogens, dental care, working, and air travel (see also "First-Trimester Patient Education" later in this chapter).

Routine Visits

During each regularly scheduled visit, the health care provider should evaluate the woman's blood pressure, weight, uterine size for progressive growth and consistency with the estimated date of delivery (EDD), and presence of fetal heart activity at appropriate gestational ages. After the patient reports quickening and at each subsequent visit, she should be asked about fetal movement. She should be queried about contractions, leakage of fluid, or vaginal bleeding,

The time-honored inclusion of routine urine dipstick assessment for all pregnant women can be modified according to site-specific protocols. A baseline screen for urine protein content to assess renal status is recommended. However, in the absence of risk factors for urinary tract infections, renal disease, and preeclampsia (such as diabetes, hypertension, and autoimmune disorders) and in the absence of symptoms of urinary tract infection, hypertension or unusual edema, there has not been shown to be a benefit in routine urine dipstick testing during prenatal care for women at low risk.

Later in pregnancy, important topics to discuss with patients during routine visits include childbirth education classes, choosing a newborn care provider, anticipating labor, preterm labor, options for intrapartum care, umbilical cord banking, breastfeeding, choice of a postpartum contraception method, and preparation for hospital discharge (see also "Second-Trimester and Third-Trimester Patient Education" later in this chapter).

Group Prenatal Care

Group, or shared, medical visits have been in use in a variety of medical settings during the past two decades and have been associated with improved health outcomes for patients. Currently, there are several models of group prenatal care in use that show promise.

In group prenatal care, health care providers deliver prenatal health services and information to groups of patients during regularly scheduled shared visits. The group visits are begun after the first prenatal assessment and physical examination, and groups usually comprise women with similar estimated delivery dates. The typical group visit includes 8–12 women and lasts longer than the traditional prenatal visit, usually 1–2 hours. The visit usually begins with physical assessments, including fundal height measures, fetal heart tones, maternal–fetal well-being questions, and appropriate testing. Individual issues may be raised at this time. The physical assessment is followed by an informational group discussion facilitated by an obstetrician–gynecologist, a certified nurse–midwife, or a family medicine practitioner. Health care providers are assisted by a variety of other health care professionals, who may serve as a co-facilitator or a guest for a specific topic. Visits are billed as traditional prenatal visits.

The group model is a promising innovation in prenatal care delivery, but additional research and evaluation of patient outcomes are needed. Practitioners should approach group prenatal care with deliberate planning and research. Resources are available in the literature as well as on the Internet.

Routine Antepartum Care

Estimated Date of Delivery

An accurately assigned EDD is among the most important results of evaluations and history-taking early in prenatal care. In addition to the planning aspects for the pregnant woman herself, this information is vital for the scheduling and interpretation of certain antepartum tests, determination of appropriateness of fetal size estimates in order to risk-assess accurately, and designing interventions to prevent preterm births, postterm births, and related morbidities.

The first date of the last menstrual period, when known, should be recorded in the chart, as well as documentation regarding the reliability of this date. Factors, such as maternal uncertainty, use of hormonal contraceptives within the past 6 months, irregular cycles, and recent pregnancy or lactation should be noted. In general, ultrasound-established dates should take preference over menstrual dates when the discrepancy is greater than 7 days in the first trimester and greater than 10 days in the second trimester. Reassigning gestational age based on a third-trimester ultrasonography should be done with caution because the accuracy of ultrasonography is within 3–4 weeks. Once the dates are established by a last menstrual period with consistent ultrasound examination or an early ultrasonography alone, the final estimated delivery date should not be altered. Changing the EDD on the basis of serial examinations should be avoided.

Fetal Ultrasound Imaging

Ultrasonography is the most commonly used fetal imaging tool and is an accurate method of determining gestational age, fetal number, viability, and placental location. Ultrasonography should be performed only by technologists or physicians who have undergone specific training and only when there is a valid medical indication for the examination. Physicians who perform, evaluate, and interpret diagnostic obstetric ultrasound examinations should be licensed medical practitioners with an understanding of the indications for such imaging studies, the expected content of a complete obstetric ultrasound examination, and a familiarity with the limitations of ultrasound imaging. A physician is responsible for the interpretation of all studies; ultrasonographers may not interpret the studies nor bill for them.

The timing and type of ultrasonography performed should be such that the clinical question being asked is answered. In order to select the best time for a particular patient to receive her scan, health care providers must balance the types and accuracy of information to be gained at different gestational ages with the financial reality of limitations to the number of scans many insurance carriers will pay for. The optimal timing for a single ultrasound examination in the absence of specific indications for first-trimester examinations is at 18–20 weeks of gestation.

Each type of ultrasound examination should be performed only when indicated and should be appropriately documented. A first-trimester ultrasound examination is an ultrasound examination performed before 13 weeks and 6 days of gestation. Scanning in the first trimester can be performed transabdominally or transvaginally. Indications for performing first-trimester ultrasound examinations are listed in Box 5-2. Second-trimester and third-trimester ultrasound examinations include the following three types:

1. Standard—Evaluation of fetal presentation, amniotic fluid volume, cardiac activity, placental position, fetal biometry, and fetal number, plus an anatomic survey.

2. Limited—A limited examination does not replace a standard examination and is performed when a specific question, such as fetal presentation or amniotic volume assessment, requires investigation.

3. Specialized—A detailed or targeted anatomic examination is performed when an anomaly is suspected on the basis of history, laboratory abnormalities, or the results of either the limited examination or standard examination.

Patients with an abnormal fetal ultrasound examination result should be referred for evaluation and management of fetal anomalies to a health care provider who can accurately and thoroughly assess the fetus, communicate the findings to the patient and health care provider, and coordinate further management if needed. The care of a multidisciplinary team may be helpful. Some conditions may require the involvement of a maternal–fetal medicine subspecialist, geneticist, pediatrician, neonatologist, anesthesiologist, or other medical specialist in the evaluation, counseling, and care of the patient. Relationships with appropriate maternal–fetal care team should be developed.

Fetal Magnetic Resonance Imaging

If additional imaging modalities are required prenatally, magnetic resonance imaging may be chosen. Fetal magnetic resonance imaging does not involve

---

Box 5-2. Indications for First-Trimester Ultrasonography

- To confirm the presence of an intrauterine pregnancy
- To evaluate a suspected ectopic pregnancy
- To evaluate vaginal bleeding
- To evaluate pelvic pain
- To estimate gestational age
- To diagnosis or evaluate multiple gestations
- To confirm cardiac activity
- As adjunct to chorionic villus sampling, embryo transfer, or localization and removal of an intrauterine device
- To assess for certain fetal anomalies, such as anencephaly, in patients at high risk
- To evaluate maternal pelvic or adnexal masses or uterine abnormalities
- To screen for fetal aneuploidy (nuchal translucency)
- To evaluate suspected hydatidiform mole

American College of Radiology. ACR practice guideline for the performance of obstetrical ultrasound. In: ACR practice guidelines and technical standards, 2007. Reston (VA): ACR; 2007. p. 1025–1033.

radiation exposure. The most common use of fetal magnetic resonance imaging is to further delineate a fetal anomaly or rule out placenta accreta identified or suspected on ultrasound examination results. Although the safety of ultrasonography has been established, comparatively few studies have analyzed the safety of magnetic resonance imaging; however, this technology is being used with increasing frequency in pregnant patients, and there are no known risks.

Routine Laboratory Testing in Pregnancy

Certain laboratory tests should be performed routinely in pregnant women in order to identify conditions that may affect the outcome of the pregnancy for the mother or fetus. The results of these tests should be reviewed in a timely manner, communicated to the patient, and documented in the medical record. Abnormal test results should prompt some action on the part of the health care provider.

Early in Pregnancy. The CDC recommends screening all pregnant women for HIV, hepatitis B, syphilis, and chlamydial infection during the first prenatal visit. In addition, the CDC recommends that, when indicated, pregnant women should be screened for *N. gonorrhoeae* at the first prenatal visit. Women a high risk of tuberculosis also should be screened early in pregnancy. Other laboratory tests that are routinely performed early in pregnancy are listed in Table 5-3 and Appendix A (College Antepartum Record). Table 5-3 also suggests actions to be considered if results are abnormal. Recommended intervals for additional tests that are indicated after the first prenatal visit are detailed in the College Antepartum Record (see also Appendix A). A more detailed explanation of the CDC recommendations is provided as follows:

- Human immunodeficiency virus—Pregnant women universally should be tested for HIV infection, with patient notification, as part of the routine battery of prenatal blood tests unless they decline the test (ie, opt-out approach), as permitted by local and state regulations. Refusal of testing should be documented. In some states, it is necessary to obtain the woman's written authorization before disclosing her HIV status to health care providers who are not members of her health care team (see also "Human Immunodeficiency Virus" in Chapter 10). Women at high risk of HIV infection (eg, women who use illicit drugs, have STIs during pregnancy, have multiple sex partners during pregnancy, live in areas with high HIV prevalence, or have HIV-infected partners) should be retested during the third trimester, ideally before 36 weeks of gestation. Repeat testing in patients from high-HIV-prevalent areas and

Table 5-3. Routine Laboratory Tests Early in Pregnancy

Laboratory Test	Potential Actions for Abnormal Results
Blood type	There is no abnormal result here. Blood type is documented for information only, should urgent blood transfusion be necessary at a later time and in order to communicate to the pediatric care provider the risk of ABO blood incompatibility in the neonatal period.
D (Rh) type	Patients who are Rh negative are at risk of developing isoimmunization to D antigen. Further steps depend on results of the antibody screening. Weak rhesus-positive (formerly Du-positive) patients are not at risk of isoimmunization.
Antibody screen	Any positive antibody test result requires obtaining a titer and further action by the health care provider.
Complete blood count (Hematocrit/hemoglobin/ MCV/and platelets)	Women with microcytic anemia should be evaluated further for iron deficiency, or treated with supplemental iron, or both, and retested in 3–4 weeks. Women who are of African descent, Asian, or Mediterranean should have a hemoglobin electrophoresis test performed to rule out thalassemia or sickle cell disease. Further testing may be warranted pending the results of these interventions and tests.
VDRL/RDR (nontreponemal tests)	Evaluate to confirm active syphilis status with treatment as needed. False-negative serologic tests results may occur in early primary infection, and infection after the first prenatal visit is possible. False-positive nontreponemal test results can be associated with various medical conditions unrelated to syphilis; therefore, persons with a reactive VDRL or RDR test result should receive a treponemal test to confirm the diagnosis of syphilis.
Urine culture (if performed)	Treat asymptomatic bacteriuria and then do a test of cure.* If results are positive for GBS bacteriuria, document this on the patient's chart and do not perform third-trimester GBS screening but administer prophylactic antibiotics in labor instead.
Urine screening	Obtain baseline screening for urine protein content (dipstick) to assess renal status.
HBsAg	If positive, counsel patient regarding her health risks; document clearly in the chart so that the infant's physicians know to treat the infant with hepatitis B vaccination and hepatitis B immune globulin.
HIV counseling/testing	Affirm your state's laws. If the patient is HIV positive, counsel and refer her to an infectious disease clinic or maternal–fetal medicine specialist for further management. Discuss safe-sex practices.

(continued)

Table 5-3. Routine Laboratory Tests Early in Pregnancy *(continued)*

Laboratory Test	Potential Actions for Abnormal Results
Chlamydia	Women found to have chlamydial infection during the first trimester should be retested within approximately 3–6 months, preferably in the third trimester.
Gonorrhea (when indicated)	Pregnant women found to have gonococcal infection during the first trimester should be retested within approximately 3–6 months, preferably in the third trimester. Uninfected pregnant women who remain at high risk for gonococcal infection also should be retested during the third trimester.
Mantoux tuberculin skin test or interferon-gamma release assay (when indicated)	Women with a positive or intermediate test result should be evaluated with a chest X-ray and review of their pertinent history to determine the need for additional evaluation.

Abbreviations: GBS, group B streptococci; HBsAg, hepatitis B surface antigen; HIV, human immunodeficiency virus; MCV, mean corpuscular volume; RPR, rapid plasma reagin; VDRL, venereal disease research laboratory.

*In this case, test of cure refers to retesting the patient's urine after completion of antibiotic therapy to determine if the bacteria have been eliminated. Although this practice is recommended in the literature, more data are needed to determine the effectiveness of this strategy.

using rapid HIV testing in patients with unknown HIV status in labor and delivery also should be considered. State laws vary and should be followed.

- Hepatitis B—All pregnant women should be routinely tested for hepatitis B surface antigen during the first trimester, even if they have been previously vaccinated or tested. Women who were not screened prenatally, those who engage in behaviors that put them at high risk of infection (eg, having had more than one sex partner in the previous 6 months, evaluation or treatment for an STI, recent or current injection-drug use, and a hepatitis B surface antigen-positive sex partner) and those with clinical hepatitis should be retested at the time of admission to the hospital for delivery. Pregnant women at risk of hepatitis B infection also should be vaccinated (see also "Hepatitis B Virus" in Chapter 10).

- Syphilis—A serologic test for syphilis should be performed on all pregnant women at the first prenatal visit. Women who are at high risk of syphilis, live in areas of high syphilis morbidity, or are previously untested should be screened again early in the third trimester (at approximately 28 weeks of gestation) and at delivery, as well as after exposure to an infected partner. Some states require all women to be screened at delivery. Infants should not be discharged from the hospital unless the syphilis serologic status of the mother has been determined at least one time during pregnancy and preferably again at delivery. Any woman who gives birth to a stillborn fetus should be tested for syphilis (see also "Syphilis" in Chapter 10).

• Chlamydial infection—All pregnant women should be routinely screened for *Chlamydia trachomatis* during the first prenatal visit. Women aged 25 years or younger and those at increased risk of chlamydia (eg, women who have a new sex partner or more than one sex partner) should be retested during the third trimester to prevent maternal postnatal complications and chlamydial infection in the infant. Women found to have chlamydial infection during the first trimester should be retested within approximately 3–6 months, preferably in the third trimester (see also "Chlamydial Infection" in Chapter 10).

• Gonorrhea—All pregnant women at risk of gonorrhea or living in an area in which the prevalence of *N. gonorrhoeae* is high should be screened for *N. gonorrhoeae* at the first prenatal visit. Women aged 25 years or younger are at highest risk of gonorrhea infection as are those of black, Hispanic, and American Indian or Alaska Native ethnicity. Other risk factors for gonorrhea include a previous infection of gonorrhea, other STIs, new or multiple sex partners, inconsistent condom use, commercial sex work, and drug use. Pregnant women found to have gonococcal infection during the first trimester should be retested within approximately 3–6 months, preferably in the third trimester. Uninfected pregnant women who remain at high risk of gonorrhea also should be retested during the third trimester (see also "Gonorrhea" in Chapter 10).

• Tuberculosis—Women at high risk of tuberculosis (TB) should be screened early in pregnancy with a TB skin test. Screening women at low risk is not indicated. High risk factors include the following:

— Known HIV infection

— Close contact with individuals known or suspected to have TB

— Medical risk factors known to increase the risk of disease if infected (such as diabetes, lupus, cancer, alcoholism, and drug addiction)

— Birth in or emigration from high-prevalent countries

— Being medically underserved

— Homelessness

— Living or working in long-term care facilities, such as correctional institutions, mental health institutions, and nursing homes

The Mantoux tuberculin skin test should be used and read by a health professional within 48–72 hours, although it can be accurately read up to 7 days after the test is applied. In the United States, induration (not erythema) measuring greater than 10 mm in diameter is a positive test result except in patients who have HIV, have received an organ transplant, are immunosuppressed, or have had recent close contact with others with infectious TB; in these individuals, induration greater than 5 mm is a positive test result. A TB blood test is also available and has the added advantage of not requiring the patient to return to have the test read. A positive or intermediate test result should be evaluated by obtaining three induced sputum cultures or with a chest X-ray.

- Third trimester—Early in the third trimester, measurement of hemoglobin or hematocrit levels should be repeated. Tests for STIs may be repeated in the third trimester if the woman has specific risk factors for these diseases. These tests may be mandated by local and state regulations.

- Antibody testing—Antibody tests should be repeated in unsensitized, D-negative patients at 28–29 weeks of gestation (see also "Isoimmunization in Pregnancy" in Chapter 7). These patients also should receive anti-D immune globulin at a dose of 300 micrograms prophylactically at that time. In addition, any patient who is unsensitized and D-negative should receive anti-D immune globulin at the time of any of the following:

  — Ectopic gestation

  — Abortion (either threatened, spontaneous, or induced)

  — Procedures associated with possible fetal-to-maternal bleeding, such as chorionic villus sampling (CVS) or amniocentesis

  — Conditions associated with fetal–maternal hemorrhage (eg, abdominal trauma or abruptio placentae)

  — Unexplained vaginal bleeding during pregnancy

  — Delivery of a newborn who is D-positive

- Diabetes mellitus screening—All pregnant women should be screened for gestational diabetes mellitus (GDM), whether by patient history, clinical risk factors, or a laboratory screening test to determine blood glucose levels. In most women, glucose screening should be performed at 24–28 weeks of gestation and can be done in the fasting state or fed state. A 50-g oral glucose challenge test is given followed in 1 hour by a plasma test for glucose level. Different screening thresholds (ranging from 130 mg/dL to 140 mg/dL) are utilized, and those meeting or exceeding this threshold undergo a 100-g, 3-hour diagnostic oral glucose tolerance test (see also "Gestational Diabetes Mellitus Diagnosis and Management" in Chapter 7).

• Group B streptococcal disease—In its 2010 updated guidelines for the prevention of perinatal group B streptococcal disease, the CDC continues to recommend screening of all women at 35–37 weeks of gestation (see the complete recommendations at http://www.cdc.gov/groupbstrep/guidelines/guidelines.html). Testing is conducted by obtaining a single swab specimen (not by speculum examination) from the lower vagina (introitus) and rectum (through the anal sphincter), placing the swab in transport media, and using selective broth media. This includes patients expected to have planned cesarean deliveries because onset of labor or rupture of membranes may occur before the recommended administration of prophylactic antibiotics. Cultures for group B streptococci (GBS) are not required in women who have group B streptococcal bacteriuria during the current pregnancy or who have previously given birth to a neonate with early-onset group B streptococcal disease because these women should receive intrapartum prophylactic antibiotics. Because GBS carriage is intermittent, women who had GBS colonization during a previous pregnancy require culture evaluation for GBS with each pregnancy. In addition, these women do not need intrapartum prophylactic antibiotics unless there is an indication for GBS prophylaxis during the current pregnancy (see also "Group B Streptococci" in Chapter 10).

Antepartum Immunizations

A routine assessment of each pregnant woman's immunization status is recommended, with appropriate immunization if indicated. There is no evidence of risk from vaccinating pregnant women with an inactivated virus or bacterial vaccines or toxoids, and these should be administered if indicated. However, live vaccines do pose a theoretic risk to the fetus and generally should be avoided during pregnancy. The benefits of vaccines outweigh any unproven potential concerns about traces of thimerosal preservative. When deciding whether to immunize a pregnant woman with a vaccine not routinely recommended in pregnancy, the risk of exposure to disease as well as the benefits of vaccination for reducing the deleterious effects on the woman and the fetus must be balanced against unknown risks of the vaccine. All vaccines administered should be fully documented in the patient's permanent medical record. Information on the safety of vaccines given during pregnancy is frequently updated and may be verified from the CDC web site at www.cdc.gov/vaccines. Additional information on immunization during pregnancy can be found on the College's Immunization for Women web site, available at http://www.immunizationforwomen.org/.

The influenza vaccine should be recommended to all women who will be pregnant during the influenza season, regardless of their stage of pregnancy. Pregnant women with medical conditions that increase their risk of complications from influenza should be offered the vaccine before the influenza season. Administration of the injectable, inactivated influenza vaccine is considered safe at any stage of pregnancy. In contrast, the intranasal influenza vaccine contains a live attenuated virus and should not be used in pregnant women.

Other vaccines that are recommended in pregnancy, if indicated, include Tdap; hepatitis A; hepatitis B; and pneumococcal (recommended for pregnant patients with prior splenectomy or functional asplenia). According to the CDC, pregnancy should not preclude vaccination with the meningococcal polysaccharide vaccine, if indicated. In studies of meningococcal vaccination with the meningococcal polysaccharide vaccine during pregnancy, adverse effects have not been documented in either pregnant women or newborns. However, no data are available on the safety of meningococcal conjugate vaccines during pregnancy.

Although the use of either the bivalent or quadrivalent HPV vaccine during pregnancy is not recommended, no teratogenic effects have been reported in animal studies. The manufacturer's pregnancy registry should be contacted if pregnancy is detected during the vaccination schedule. Completion of the series should be delayed until pregnancy is completed. It is not known whether vaccine antigens or antibodies found in the quadrivalent vaccine are excreted in human milk. Lactating women can receive the quadrivalent HPV vaccine because inactivated vaccines, such as the HPV vaccine do not affect the safety of breastfeeding for mothers or infants.

Both the varicella and the measles–mumps–rubella vaccine are contraindicated during pregnancy. Pregnant women should be assessed for evidence of varicella and rubella immunity. The CDC recommends that women who do not have evidence of immunity should receive the first dose of varicella vaccine and the measles–mumps–rubella vaccine during the postpartum period before discharge from the health care facility. (For more information on immunization during pregnancy, see Chapter 10.)

Antepartum Genetic Screening and Diagnosis

There are ever-increasing ways to screen pregnant women for fetal birth defects or genetic abnormalities and to provide diagnostic testing for those who desire it. Obstetric care providers must be knowledgeable about the choices available to patients in general and either provide that screening themselves or have established referral sources for doing so. It is the responsibility of the health care provider to educate the patient and make her aware of available options.

Genetic Screening. Pretest counseling should be provided to couples who will be offered screening. Pretest counseling may consist of the review of standardized printed material. Ideally, this information may be provided by trained support staff in the ambulatory practice setting. Videos, Internet resources, and interactive computer programs also may be developed for this purpose. The information about genetic screening should be provided in a nondirective manner. If the partner does not accompany a woman to her prenatal or preconception visit, a copy of the printed educational materials should be provided for her to give to her partner. Referral to a geneticist, genetic counselor, or perinatologist may be necessitated by the complexities of determining risks, evaluating a family history of such abnormalities, interpreting laboratory test results, or providing counseling.

Family history plays a critical role in assessing risk of inherited medical conditions and single gene disorders. Several methods have been established to obtain family medical histories, each with its own advantages and disadvantages. A common tool used in general practice is the family history questionnaire or checklist. Any positive responses on the questionnaire should be followed up by the health care provider to obtain more detail, including the relationship of the affected family member(s) to the patient, exact diagnosis, age of onset, and severity of disease. Another family history assessment tool, commonly used by genetics professionals, is the pedigree. The health care provider may decide to complete a detailed pedigree or refer to a genetics professional for further evaluation. A pedigree ideally shows at least three generations using standardized symbols, clearly marking individuals affected with a specific diagnosis to allow for easy identification. The pedigree may visibly assist in determining the size of the family and the mode of inheritance of a specific condition, and may facilitate identification of members at increased risk of developing the condition. The screening tool selected should be tailored to the practice setting and patient population, taking into consideration patient education level and cultural competence. Whether the pedigree or questionnaire is used, it is important to review and update the family history periodically for new diagnoses within the family and throughout pregnancy as appropriate. Screening can be offered for the following:

- Single-gene (mendelian inheritance) disorders—Disorders inherited as autosomal dominant or recessive disorders of single genes are typically referred to as mendelian inheritance disorders. Health care providers should be aware that many single-gene disorders are discovered each year and may be tracked using Internet databases, such as Online Mendelian Inheritance in Man (www.ncbi.nlm.nih.gov/omim). One way to screen for these disorders is to ask for family history and to determine the patient's ethnic background. The same information should be gained about the father of the baby. Certain disorders are more common in different ethnic groups, although it is essential to note that there are no disorders found uniquely in a certain ethnic or racial group and that many families may be interracial and not have an obvious predominant ethnicity.

  If carrier testing is to be done on the basis of ethnicity only, it is reasonable to offer this to the preconception or pregnant woman first and then test the father only if the mother is positive. If testing is being considered on the basis of an affected relative, offer it to the family member of the affected individual first. Table 5-4 includes recommendations for genetic testing based solely on a patient's ethnic identity. Some health care providers choose to offer cystic fibrosis (CF) carrier testing to all women rather than on a selective basis and this is acceptable. Given that CF screening has been a routine part of reproductive care for women since 2001, it is prudent to determine if the patient has been previously screened before ordering CF screening that may be redundant. If a patient has been screened previously, CF screening results should be documented but the test should not be repeated.

- Aneuploidy—Down syndrome and other trisomies are primarily the result of meiotic nondisjunction, which increases with maternal age (Table 5-5). Fetuses with aneuploidy may have major anatomic malformations that often are discovered during an ultrasound examination that is performed for another indication. Abnormalities involving a major organ or structure, with a few notable exceptions, or the finding of two or more minor structural abnormalities in the same fetus indicate increased risk of fetal aneuploidy.

Table 5-4. Recommended Prenatal Genetic Carrier Screening Tests Based on Ethnic Background

Ethnic Background	Screening Tests to Offer	Additional Screening Tests to Make Available
Caucasian	Cystic fibrosis	
African descent (African, African-American, African-Caribbean)	Sickle hemoglobinopathies, beta-thalassemia, alpha-thalassemia	Cystic fibrosis
Ashkenazi Jewish (European Jewish)	Tay–Sachs disease, familial dysautonomia, cystic fibrosis, Canavan disease	Mucolipidosis IV, Niemann–Pick disease type A, Fanconi anemia group C, Bloom syndrome, Gaucher disease
Southeast Asian	Beta-thalassemia, alpha-thalassemia (if microcytic anemia)	Cystic fibrosis
French Canadian and Cajun	Tay–Sachs disease	Cystic fibrosis
Mediterranean	Beta-thalassemia	Cystic fibrosis

Screening and invasive diagnostic testing for aneuploidy should be offered to all women who seek prenatal care before 20 weeks of gestation regardless of maternal age. Women should be counseled regarding the differences between screening and invasive diagnostic testing. Regardless of which screening tests your patients are offered, information about the detection and false-positive rates, advantages, disadvantages, and limitations, as well as the risks and benefits of diagnostic procedures, should be available to patients so that they can make informed decisions. In couples in which the male partner is 45 years or older, counseling also should address the increased risk of new onset autosomal dominant disorders (such as neurofibromatosis or Marfan syndrome) that are associated with increased paternal age. Some patients may benefit from a more extensive discussion with a genetics professional or a maternal–fetal medicine specialist, especially if there is a family history of a chromosome abnormality, genetic disorder, or congenital malformation.

Laboratories that report aneuploidy screening test results generally provide the physician with numerical information regarding the patient's revised risk of aneuploidy using maternal age, the serum analyte levels, and nuchal translucency measurement if available as well as other factors, such as maternal weight, diabetes status, and ethnicity.

Table 5-5. Down Syndrome Screening Tests and Detection Rates
(5% Positive Screen Rate)

Screening Test	Detection Rate (%)
First trimester	
NT measurement	64–70*
NT measurement, PAPP-A, free or total β-hCG[†]	82–87*
Second trimester	
Triple screen (MSAFP, hCG, unconjugated estriol)	69*
Quadruple screen (MSAFP, hCG, unconjugated estriol, inhibin A)	81*
First plus second trimester	
Integrated (NT, PAPP-A, quad screen)	94–96*
Serum integrated (PAPP- A, quad screen)	85–88*
Stepwise sequential	95*
First-trimester test result:	
Positive: diagnostic test offered	
Negative: second-trimester test offered	
Final: risk assessment incorporates first and second results	
Contingent sequential	88–94[‡]
First-trimester test result:	
Positive: diagnostic test offered	
Negative: no further testing	
Intermediate: second-trimester test offered	
Final: risk assessment incorporates first and second results	

Abbreviations: hCG, human chorionic gonadotropin; MSAFP, maternal serum alpha-fetoprotein; NT, nuchal translucency; PAPP-A, pregnancy-associated plasma protein A; quad, quadruple.

*From the FASTER trial (Malone F, Canick JA, Ball RH, Nyberg DA, Comstock CH, Buckowski R, et al. First-trimester or second-trimester screening, or both, for Down's syndrome. First- and Second-Trimester Evaluation of Risk (FASTER) Research Consortium. N Engl J Med 2005;353:2001–11.)

[†]Also referred to as combined first-trimester screen.

[‡]Modeled predicted detection rates (Cuckle H, Benn P, Wright D. Down syndrome screening in the first and/or second trimester: model predicted performance using meta-analysis parameters. Semin Perinatol 2005;29:252–7.)

Screening for fetal chromosomal abnormalities. ACOG Practice Bulletin No. 77. American College of Obstetricians and Gynecologists. Obstet Gynecol 2007;109:217–27.

Communicating a numerical risk assessment after screening enables women and their partners to balance the consequences of having a child with the particular disorder against the risk of an invasive diagnostic test. It is often useful to contrast this risk with the general population risk and their age-related risk before screening.

There are many strategies available to screen for chromosomal abnormalities (Table 5-5). These incorporate maternal age and a variety of first-trimester and second-trimester ultrasonography and biochemical markers that include nuchal translucency measurement and pregnancy-associated plasma protein A, human chorionic gonadotropin, maternal serum alpha-fetoprotein (MSAFP), estriol, and inhibin levels. The choice of screening test depends on many factors, including gestational age at first prenatal visit, number of fetuses, previous obstetric history, family history, availability of nuchal translucency measurement, test sensitivity and limitations, risk of invasive diagnostic procedures, desire for early test results, and reproductive options. The goal is to offer screening tests with high detection rates and low false-positive rates that also provide patients with the diagnostic options they might want to consider. Ideally, patients seen early in pregnancy can be offered first-trimester aneuploidy screening or integrated or sequential aneuploidy screening that combines first-trimester and second-trimester testing. Each has its own detection and false positive rates (Table 5-5). The options for women who are first seen during the second trimester are limited to quadruple (or "quad") screening and ultrasound examination.

When a first-trimester screening test is performed and followed by a separate second-trimester screening test, the results are interpreted independently and there is a high Down syndrome detection rate (94–98%); however, the false-positive rates are additive, leading to many more unnecessary invasive procedures (11–17%). For this reason, women who have had first-trimester screening for aneuploidy should not undergo independent second-trimester serum screening in the same pregnancy. Instead, women who want a higher detection rate can have an integrated or a sequential screening test, which combines both first-trimester and second-trimester screening results.

The integrated approach to screening uses both the first-trimester and second-trimester markers to adjust a woman's age-related risk of having a child with Down syndrome. The results are reported only after both first-trimester and second-trimester screening tests are completed. Integrated screening best meets the goal of screening by providing the highest sensitivity with the lowest false-positive rate. The lower false-positive rate results in fewer invasive tests and, thus, fewer procedure-related losses of normal pregnancies. Concerns about integrated screening include possible patient anxiety generated by having to wait 3–4 weeks between initiation and completion of the screening and the loss of the opportunity to consider CVS if the first-trimester screening indicates a high risk of aneuploid. The possibility that patients might fail to complete the second-trimester portion of the screening test after performing the first-trimester component is another potential disadvantage because the patient would be left with no screening results.

Sequential screening has a high detection rate of integrated screening but identifies very high-risk patients early in gestation, after the first-trimester component of the testing. In the stepwise sequential screening women determined to be at high risk (Down syndrome risk above a predetermined cutoff) after the first-trimester screening are offered genetic counseling and the option of invasive diagnostic testing, and women below the cutoff are offered second-trimester screening. The sequential approach takes advantage of the higher detection rate achieved by incorporating the first-trimester and second-trimester results with only a marginal increase in the false-positive rate.

Women found to have an increased risk of aneuploidy with first-trimester screening should be offered genetic counseling and diagnostic testing by CVS or a second-trimester genetic amniocentesis. Neural tube defect screening should be offered in the second trimester to patients who elected to have only first-trimester screening for aneuploidy or who have had a normal result from CVS; this is best performed between 16–18 weeks of gestation with an MSAFP level. Neural tube defect screening may include second-trimester serum alpha-fetoprotein screening, targeted second-trimester ultrasonography, or both. Patients who have a fetal nuchal translucency measurement of 3.5 mm or greater in the first trimester, despite a negative test result on an aneuploidy screening, normal fetal chromosomes, or both, should be offered a targeted ultrasound examination, fetal echocardiogram, or both, because such fetuses are at a significant risk of nonchromosomal anomalies, including congenital heart defects and some genetic syndromes.

Patients with abnormal first-trimester serum markers or an increased nuchal translucency measurement also may be at increased risk of an adverse pregnancy outcome, such as spontaneous fetal loss before 24 weeks of gestation, fetal demise, low birth weight, or preterm birth. At the present time, there are no data indicating whether or not fetal surveillance in the third trimester will be helpful in the care of these patients.

- Neural tube defects—The results of second-trimester MSAFP testing may be used to screen for NTD and other open fetal defects. The use of a standard screening cutoff (2.5 multiples of the median) will detect approximately 80% of cases of open spina bifida and 90% of cases of anencephaly. Patients with increased MSAFP levels are evaluated by ultrasonography to detect identifiable causes of false–positive test results (eg, fetal death, multiple gestation, underestimation of gestational age) and for targeted study of fetal anatomy for NTDs and other defects associated with increased MSAFP values (eg, omphalocele or gastroschisis). Amniocentesis may be recommended to confirm the presence of open defects or to obtain a fetal karyotype. Amniocentesis may be offered even when ultrasound examination results do not reveal an identifiable defect or cause for the increased MSAFP level, particularly if the ultrasound examination was suboptimal because of maternal obesity or abdominal scarring. Under ideal circumstances, second-trimester ultrasonography will detect approximately 100% of anencephaly and 95% of spina bifida anomalies.

Diagnostic Testing. In the woman who chooses to have a diagnostic test for aneuploidy, rather than a screening, there are two primary options: 1) Chorionic villus sampling and 2) amniocentesis. Less commonly, placental biopsy testing (usually in the third trimester) and fetal umbilical cord blood sampling can be performed:

- Chorionic villus sampling—Chorionic villus sampling is a technique for removing a small sample (5–40 mg) of placental tissue (chorionic villi) for performing chromosomal, metabolic, or DNA studies. It generally is performed between 10 weeks and 12 weeks of gestation, either by a transabdominal or a transcervical approach. Chorionic villi, however, cannot be used for the prenatal diagnosis of NTDs. Therefore, women who have undergone cytogenetic testing by CVS should be offered MSAFP, detailed ultrasound examinations, or both for the detection of NTD. Most prospective studies have shown that the procedure-related risk of pregnancy loss after CVS is not significantly different from the pregnancy loss rate after amniocentesis.

- Amniocentesis—Amniocentesis is the technique most commonly used for obtaining fetal cells for genetic studies. This well-established, safe, and reliable procedure usually is offered between 15 weeks and 20 weeks of gestation. The cells obtained via amniocentesis can be used for blood typing or cytogenetic, metabolic, microbiologic, chemical, or DNA testing.

Alpha-fetoprotein and acetylcholinesterase levels can be measured in the supernatant amniotic fluid to detect open fetal NTDs.

Many large, multicenter studies have confirmed the safety of genetic amniocentesis as well as its cytogenetic diagnostic accuracy (greater than 99%). Studies suggest that the procedure-related loss rate is as low as 1 in 300–500. Complications include transient vaginal spotting or amniotic fluid leakage in approximately 1–2% of all cases and chorioamnionitis in less than 1 in 1,000 cases.

Early amniocentesis performed from 11 weeks to 13 weeks of gestation has been widely studied, and the technique is similar to traditional amniocentesis; however, performing early amniocentesis results in significantly higher rates of pregnancy loss and complications than performing traditional amniocentesis. For these reasons, early amniocentesis (at less than 14 weeks of gestation) should not be performed.

Invasive Diagnostic Testing in Women Who Are Rh D Negative. Because both amniocentesis and CVS can result in fetal-to-maternal bleeding, the administration of anti-D immune globulin is indicated for women who are Rh-D negative, unsensitized, and undergo either of these procedures. Chorionic villus sampling should not be performed in women who are red cell antibody sensitized because it may worsen the antibody response.

Psychosocial Risk Screening and Counseling

Psychosocial issues are nonbiomedical factors that affect mental and physical well-being. Screening for psychosocial risk factors may help predict a woman's attentiveness to personal health matters, her use of prenatal services, and the health status of her offspring. Such screening should be done for all pregnant women and should be performed regardless of social status, educational level, race, and ethnicity. The reason for this is that past obstetric events and infant outcomes, medical considerations in a current pregnancy, beliefs about and experience with breastfeeding, and family circumstances (among other factors) influence the experience of labor, delivery, and early neonatal and postpartum adjustment. Additionally, some women experience social, economic, and personal difficulties in pregnancy. Given the sensitive nature of psychosocial assessment, every effort should be made to screen patients in private. Even then, patients may not be comfortable discussing problems with physicians until a trusting relationship has been formed. Other clinical staff may be trained to provide this screening, with results communicated to the physician.

Addressing the broad range of psychosocial issues with which pregnant women are confronted is an essential step toward improving women's health and birth outcomes. An effective system of referrals will be helpful in augmenting the screening and brief intervention that can be carried out in an office setting. Although some psychosocial issues are present before pregnancy, others arise during the course of pregnancy or may not be disclosed early on. To increase the likelihood of successful interventions, psychosocial screening should be performed on a regular basis and documented in the patient's prenatal record. Screening should include assessment of patients' desire for pregnancy, tobacco use, substance use, depression, safety, intimate partner violence, stress, barriers to care, unstable housing, communication barriers, and nutrition.

When screening is completed, every effort should be made to identify areas of concern, validate major issues with the patient, provide information, and, if indicated, make suggestions for possible changes. Screening positive for a condition often necessitates a referral to resources outside the practice for further evaluation or intervention. Physicians should be aware of individuals and community agencies to which patients can be referred for additional counseling and assistance when necessary.

Desire for Pregnancy. Assess all patients' desire for pregnancy. If the patient indicates that the pregnancy is unwanted, she should be fully informed in a balanced manner about all options, including raising the child herself, placing the child for adoption, and abortion. The information conveyed should be appropriate to the gestational age. The health care professional should make every effort to avoid introducing personal bias. Some patients may feel more comfortable having a discussion of this type with someone who is not involved with their ongoing medical care. The physician should evaluate the patient's available psychosocial support and refer her to appropriate counseling or other supportive services. Physicians often may best fulfill their obligations to patients through referral to other professionals who have the appropriate skills and expertise to address these difficult issues.

Substance Use and Abuse. All pregnant women should be screened at their first prenatal visit about their past and present use of tobacco, alcohol, and other drugs, including the recreational use of prescription and over-the-counter medications and herbal remedies. Use of validated screening questionnaires, along with the assurance of confidentiality improves patient–physician communication and may increase the veracity of patient responses. If a woman acknowledges the use of tobacco, alcohol, cocaine, opioids, amphetamines, or other mood-altering drugs or if chemical dependence is suspected, she should be counseled about the perinatal implications of their use during pregnancy and offered referral to an appropriate treatment program.

To reinforce and encourage continued abstinence, periodic health care provider follow-up is important. With the patient's consent, drug or metabolite testing may be indicated for a pregnant woman who reports substance use before or during pregnancy. Testing of the mother, the neonate, or both also may be indicated in some clinical situations, including the presence of unexplained intrauterine growth restriction, third-trimester stillbirth, unexpected preterm birth, or abruptio placentae in a woman not known to have hypertensive disease. Because positive test results have implications for patients that transcend their health, patients should give informed consent before testing. The requirements for consent to test vary from state to state, and practitioners should be familiar with the testing and the reporting requirements in their states.

- *Tobacco.* Inquiry into tobacco use and smoke exposure should be a routine part of the prenatal visit. Patients should be strongly discouraged from smoking. Multiple studies have demonstrated a clear association between maternal smoking and perinatal morbidity and mortality. This includes intrauterine growth restriction, placenta previa, abruptio placentae, preterm premature rupture of membranes, low birth weight, perinatal mortality, ectopic pregnancy, and sudden infant death syndrome. Children born to mothers who smoke during pregnancy are at increased risk of asthma, infantile colic, and childhood obesity. Secondhand prenatal exposure to tobacco smoke also increases the risk of having an infant with low birth weight by as much as 20%.

  The U.S. Preventive Services Task Force has concluded that the use of nicotine replacement products or other pharmaceuticals for smoking cessation aids during pregnancy and lactation have not been sufficiently evaluated to determine their efficacy or safety. Therefore, the use of nicotine replacement therapy should be undertaken with close supervision and after careful consideration and discussion with the patient of the known risks of continued smoking and the possible risks of nicotine replacement therapy. If nicotine replacement is used, it should be with the clear resolve of the patient to quit smoking. An office-based protocol that systematically identifies pregnant women who smoke and offers treatment or referral has been proved to increase smoking cessation rates. A short counseling session with pregnancy-specific educational materials and a referral to the smokers' quit line is an effective smoking cessation strategy. The 5A's is an office-based intervention developed to be used under the guidance of trained practitioners to help pregnant women quit smoking (See Box 5-1).

- *Alcohol.* Alcohol is a teratogen. Women should be advised to remain abstinent from alcohol consumption during pregnancy because there is no known safe threshold. Health care providers should advise women that low-level consumption of alcohol in early pregnancy is not an indication for pregnancy termination. However, women who have already consumed alcohol during a current pregnancy should be advised to stop in order to minimize further risk.

  Patients should be informed that prenatal alcohol consumption is a preventable cause of birth defects, including intellectual disability and neurodevelopmental deficits. Fetal alcohol syndrome is characterized by three findings: 1) growth restriction, 2) facial abnormalities, and 3) central nervous system dysfunction. Even moderate alcohol consumption during pregnancy may alter psychomotor development, contribute to cognitive defects, and produce emotional and behavioral problems in children.

- *Mood-Altering Drugs.* Large numbers of women of childbearing age abuse potentially addictive and mood-altering drugs. Use of cocaine, marijuana, diazepam, opioids (including morphine, heroin, codeine, meperidine, methadone, and oxycodone), other prescription drugs, and approximately 150 other substances can lead to chemical dependency. Depending on geographic location, it is estimated that 1–40% of pregnant women have used one of these substances during pregnancy. Data suggest that approximately 1 in 10 neonates are exposed to one or more mood-altering drugs during pregnancy; the number varies only slightly for publicly versus privately insured patients.

  Chemical dependency is a chronic, relapsing, and progressive disease. Many drug-dependent pregnant women do not seek early prenatal care and, therefore, are at increased risk of medical and obstetric complications. Drug-exposed neonates often go unrecognized and are discharged from the newborn nursery to homes where they are at increased risk of a complex of medical and social problems, including abuse and neglect.

  Warning signs of drug abuse include nonadherence to prenatal care (eg, late entry to care, multiple missed appointments, episodic or no prenatal care), evidence of poor nutrition, encounters with law enforcement, and marital and family disputes during the pregnancy. Screening of all patients at the time of delivery is not recommended. Screenings at delivery are likely to have a negative result when drugs were used early in pregnancy, and a urine screening can have a negative result even when women have taken certain drugs during the 48 hours before delivery. Toxicologic analysis of hair and meconium have been reported to be more sensitive methods of identifying illicit drug use, although urine remains the most frequently used specimen for screening. Because the components of urine toxicology screenings vary among laboratories, physicians should verify with their laboratory which metabolites are included in its screening.

The information gained by toxicologic testing should be used to assist the pregnant woman or new mother to receive the treatment she needs and not as a vehicle for punishment. Practitioners also should be aware that laws in some states consider in utero drug exposure to be a form of child abuse or neglect under civil child-welfare statutes and require that positive drug test results in pregnant women or their newborns be reported to the state's child protection agency. States vary in their requirements for the evidence of drug exposure to the fetus or newborn in order to report a case to the child welfare system. Legally mandated testing and reporting puts the therapeutic relationship between the obstetrician–gynecologist and the woman at risk, potentially placing the physician in an adversarial relationship with the patient. To identify drug-exposed neonates, the child's physician should obtain a thorough maternal history from all new mothers in a nonthreatening, organized manner.

Clinical Depression. Clinical depression is common in reproductive-aged women. A recent retrospective cohort analysis in a large U.S. managed care organization found that one in seven women was treated for depression between the year before pregnancy and the year after pregnancy. According to the World Health Organization, depression is the leading cause of disability in women, which accounts for $30–50 billion in lost productivity and direct medical costs in the United States each year.

Screening for, diagnosing, and treating depression have the potential to benefit a woman and her family. Infants of mothers who are depressed display delayed psychologic, cognitive, neurologic, and motor development. Furthermore, children's mental and behavioral disorders improve when maternal depression is in remission. Women with current depression or a history of major depression warrant particularly close monitoring and evaluation. Pregnancy and the postpartum period represent an ideal time during which consistent contact with the health care delivery system will allow women at risk to be identified and treated. There are multiple depression screening tools available for use. These tools usually can be completed in less than 10 minutes. Examples of highly sensitive screening tools include the Edinburgh Postnatal Depression Scale, Postpartum Depression Screening Scale, and Patient Health Questionnaire-9.

Women who have been receiving treatment for depression before pregnancy should receive counseling concerning management options during pregnancy. Consultation with the prescribing psychiatrist is recommended regarding antidepressant medication dosing and safety.

Intimate Partner Violence. Risk assessment during pregnancy should include identification of women who are victims of intimate partner violence, which has been identified as a significant public health problem, affecting millions of American women each year. Screening should occur at the first prenatal visit, at least once per trimester, and at the postpartum checkup. Trauma, including trauma caused by intimate partner violence, is one of the most frequent causes of maternal death in the United States. There is no single profile of an abused woman. Victims come from all ages, sexual orientations, and backgrounds. The prevalence of abuse, particularly sexual abuse, may be greater in pregnant adolescents versus adult pregnant women.

Research indicates that most abused women continue to be victimized during pregnancy. Violence against women also may begin or escalate during pregnancy and affects both maternal and fetal well-being. The prevalence of violence during pregnancy ranges from 1% to 20%, with most studies identifying rates between 4% and 8%. The presence of violence between intimate partners also affects the children in the household. Studies demonstrate that child abuse occurs in 33–77% of families in which there is abuse of adults. In women who are being abused, 27% have demonstrated abusive behavior toward their children while living in the violent environment.

Abuse may involve threatened or actual physical, sexual, verbal, or psychologic abuse. The fundamental issues at play are power, control, and coercion. There is no clearly established set of symptoms that signal abuse. However, some of the obstetric presentations of abused women include the following:

• Unwanted pregnancy
• STIs
• Late entry into prenatal care or missed appointments
• Substance abuse or use

- Poor weight gain and nutrition
- Multiple, repeated somatic complaints

With the possible exception of preeclampsia, intimate partner violence is more prevalent than any major medical condition detected through routine prenatal screening. Detection may be possible by discussing with the patient that pregnancy sometimes places increased stress on a relationship and then asking how the woman and her partner resolve their differences. In many cases, however, women will not disclose their abuse unless asked directly. Abused women usually are forthright when asked directly in a caring, nonjudgmental manner. The likelihood of disclosure increases with repeated inquiries.

Screening should be conducted in private with only the patient present. Translation services may be helpful in inquiring about these issues with women who have limited English proficiency. It is important to avoid using a family member or friend as an interpreter. If a patient confides that she is being abused, verbatim accounts of the abuse should be recorded in the patient's medical record. The physician should inquire about her immediate safety and the safety of her children. Physicians should become familiar with local resources, and referrals to appropriate counseling, legal, and social-service advocacy programs should be made. Additionally, physicians should be familiar with state laws that may require reporting of intimate partner violence. Child abuse is always reportable. When the physician suspects abuse, whether or not it is corroborated by the woman, supportive statements should be offered, and the need for follow-up should be addressed. It is important to encourage women who are victims of violence, with the assistance of social services, to begin to create an escape plan, with a reliable safe haven for retreat, particularly if they believe the violence is escalating.

First-Trimester Patient Education

Patient education is an essential element of prenatal care. Topics for specialized counseling include nutrition, exercise, dental care, nausea and vomiting, vitamin and mineral toxicity, teratogens, and air travel.

Nutrition. Both fetal and maternal outcomes can be affected by maternal nutritional status during pregnancy. Nutrition counseling is an integral part of perinatal care for all patients. Dietary counseling and intervention based on special or individual needs usually are most effectively accomplished by referral to a nutritionist or registered dietitian. All women should receive information that is focused on a well-balanced, varied, nutritional food plan that is consistent with the patient's access to food and food preferences. Special attention should be given to low-income and minority women who are more likely to be in higher BMI categories, consume diets of poor nutritional quality, and get less exercise before pregnancy. If a patient is financially unable to meet nutritional needs, she should be referred to federal food and nutrition programs, such as the Special Supplemental Nutrition Program for Women, Infants, and Children.

The recommended dietary allowances for most vitamins and minerals increase during pregnancy (Table 5-6). The National Academy of Sciences recommends 27 mg of iron supplementation (present in most prenatal vitamins) be given to pregnant women daily because the iron content of the standard American diet and the endogenous iron stores of many American women are not sufficient to provide for the increased iron requirements of pregnancy. The U.S. Preventive Services Task Force recommends that all pregnant women be routinely screened for iron-deficiency anemia. The treatment of frank iron deficiency anemia requires dosages of 60–120 mg of elemental iron each day. Iron absorption is facilitated by or with vitamin C supplementation or ingestion between meals or at bedtime on an empty stomach.

Women should supplement their diets with folic acid before and during pregnancy (see also "Preconception Nutritional Counseling" in this chapter). Current U.S. dietary guidelines recommend that women who are pregnant consume 600 micrograms of dietary folate equivalents daily from all sources (Table 5-6).*

During pregnancy, severe maternal vitamin D deficiency has been associated with biochemical evidence of disordered skeletal homeostasis in the newborn, congenital rickets and fractures. Recent evidence suggests that vitamin D deficiency is common during pregnancy especially in high-risk groups, including vegetarians, women with limited sun exposure (eg, those who live in cold climates, reside in northern latitudes, or wear sun and winter protective clothing), and ethnic minorities, especially those with darker skin. In 2010, the Food and Nutrition Board at the Institute of Medicine of the National Academies established that an adequate intake of vitamin D during pregnancy and lactation was 15 micrograms daily (or 600 international units per day) (see Table 5-6).

---

*Dietary Folate Equivalents (DFE) adjust for the difference in bioavailability of food folate compared with synthetic folic acid. 1 DFE = 1 microgram of food folate = 0.6 micrograms of folic acid from supplements and fortified foods taken with meals. U.S. Department of Agriculture. Dietary Guidelines for Americans, 2010. Available at: http://www.cnpp.usda.gov/Publications/DietaryGuidelines/2010/PolicyDoc/PolicyDoc.pdf. Retrieved January 13, 2012.

Table 5-6. Recommended Daily Dietary Allowances and Tolerable Upper Intake Levels* for Pregnant and Lactating Adolescents and Women

Nutrient (unit)	Pregnant			Lactating		
	14–18 years	19–30 years	31–50 years	14–18 years	19–30 years	31–50 years
Fat-soluble vitamins						
Vitamin A (μg/d)[†]	750	770	770	1,200	1,300	1,300
UL*, [‡]	2,800	3,000	3,000	2,800	3,000	3,000
Vitamin D (μg/d)[§]	15	15	15	15	15	15
UL*	100	100	100	100	100	100
Vitamin E (mg/d)[‖]	15	15	15	19	19	19
UL*, [¶]	800	1,000	1,000	800	1,000	1,000
Vitamin K (μg/d)[#]	75	90	90	75	90	90
UL*	–	–	–	–	–	–
Water-soluble vitamins						
Folate (μg/d)**	600	600	600	500	500	500
UL*, [¶]	800	1,000	1,000	800	1,000	1,000
Niacin (mg/d)[††]	18	18	18	17	17	17
UL*, [¶]	30	35	35	30	35	35
Riboflavin (mg/d)	1.4	1.4	1.4	1.6	1.6	1.6
UL*	–	–	–	–	–	–
Thiamin (mg/d)	1.4	1.4	1.4	1.4	1.4	1.4
UL*	–	–	–	–	–	–
Vitamin B_6 (mg/d)	1.9	1.9	1.9	2	2	2
UL*	80	100	100	80	100	100
Vitamin B_{12} (μg/d)	2.6	2.6	2.6	2.8	2.8	2.8
UL*	–	–	–	–	–	–
Vitamin C (mg/d)	80	85	85	115	120	120
UL*	1,800	2,000	2,000	1,800	2,000	2,000

(continued)

Table 5-6. Recommended Daily Dietary Allowances and Tolerable Upper Intake Levels* for Pregnant and Lactating Adolescents and Women *(continued)*

Nutrient (unit)	Pregnant			Lactating		
	14–18 years	19–30 years	31–50 years	14–18 years	19–30 years	31–50 years
Minerals						
Calcium (mg/d)	1,300	1,000	1,000	1,300	1,000	1,000
UL*	3,000	2,500	2,500	3,000	2,500	2,500
Iodine (µg/d)	220	220	220	290	290	290
UL*	900	1,100	1,100	900	1,100	1,100
Iron (mg/d)	27	27	27	10	9	9
UL*	45	45	45	45	45	45
Phosphorus (mg/d)	1,250	700	700	1,250	700	700
UL*	3,500	3,500	3,500	4,000	4,000	4,000
Selenium (µg/d)	60	60	60	70	70	70
UL*	400	400	400	400	400	400
Zinc (mg/d)	12	11	11	13	12	12
UL*	34	40	40	34	40	40

*UL = tolerable upper intake level. This is the highest level of daily nutrient intake that is likely to pose no risk of adverse effects to almost all individuals in the general population. Unless otherwise specified, the UL represents total intake from food, water, and supplements. Due to lack of suitable data, ULs could not be established for vitamin K, thiamin, riboflavin, and Vitamin B$_{12}$. In the absence of ULs, extra caution may be warranted in consuming levels above recommended intakes. Members of the general population should be advised not to routinely exceed the UL. The UL is not meant to apply to individuals who are treated with the nutrient under medical supervision or to individuals with predisposing conditions that modify their sensitivity to the nutrient.

[†]As retinol activity equivalents (RAE). 1 RAE = 3.3 international units.

[‡]As preformed vitamin A only.

[§]1) Under the assumption of minimal sunlight. 2) As cholecalciferol; 1 microgram cholecalciferol = 40 international units of vitamin D.

[||]As α-tocopherol.

[¶]The ULs for vitamin E, niacin, and folate apply to synthetic forms obtained from supplements, fortified foods, or a combination of the two.

[#]Recommendations measured as Adequate Intake (AI) instead of Recommended Daily Dietary Allowance (RDA). An AI is set instead of an RDA if insufficient evidence is available to determine an RDA. The AI is based on observed or experimentally determined estimates of average nutrient intake by a group (or groups) of healthy people.

(continued)

Table 5-6. Recommended Daily Dietary Allowances and Tolerable Upper Intake Levels* Pregnant and Lactating Adolescents and Women *(continued)*

**As dietary folate equivalents (DFE). 1 DFE = 1 microgram food folate = 0.6 micrograms of folic acid from fortified food or as a supplement consumed with food = 0.5 micrograms of a supplement taken on an empty stomach. In view of the evidence linking folate intake with neural tube defects in the fetus, it is recommended that all women capable of becoming pregnant consume 400 micrograms from supplements or fortified foods in addition to intake of food folate from a varied diet.

††As niacin equivalents.

Modified with permission from Institute of Medicine. Dietary reference intakes. The essential guide to nutrient requirements. Washington, DC: The National Academies Press; 2006 and Dietary Reference Intakes for Calcium and Vitamin D. Washington, DC: The National Academies Press; 2010.

Most prenatal vitamins typically contain 10 micrograms (400 international units) of vitamin D per tablet. For pregnant women thought to be at increased risk of vitamin D deficiency, maternal serum 25-hydroxyvitamin D levels can be considered and should be interpreted in the context of the individual clinical circumstance. When vitamin D deficiency is identified during pregnancy, most experts agree that 25–50 micrograms (1,000–2,000 international units) per day of vitamin D is safe. Higher dose regimens used for treatment of vitamin D deficiency have not been studied during pregnancy. Recommendations concerning routine vitamin D supplementation during pregnancy beyond that contained in a prenatal vitamin should await the completion of ongoing randomized clinical trials.

Weight Gain. Ideally, women should have a normal BMI before conception and then adjust their diets during pregnancy in order to gain a recommended amount of weight and to obtain the appropriate nutrition for both maternal and fetal benefit. Increasingly, however, women are becoming pregnant when they are obese, they gain more weight than is necessary during pregnancy, and retain the weight postpartum.

The Institute of Medicine guidelines for maternal weight gain based on prepregnancy BMI are listed in Table 5-7. These same recommendations are made for adolescents, short women, and women of all racial and ethnic groups. Empiric recommendations for weight gain with twin gestations in women include: normal BMI: 37–54 lb; overweight women: 31–50 lb; and obese women 25–42 lb. Progress toward meeting these weight gain goals should be monitored and specific individualized counseling provided if significant deviations are noted.

The Institute of Medicine guidelines provide physicians with a basis for practice. Health care providers caring for pregnant women should determine a

Table 5-7. Institute of Medicine Weight Gain Recommendations for Pregnancy

Prepregnancy Weight Category	BMI* (kg)/[height (m)]²	Recommended Total Weight Gain Range (lb)	Recommended Rates of Weight Gain† Second and Third Trimesters (Mean Range, lb/wk)
Underweight	Less than 18.5	28-40	1 (1-1.3)
Normal weight	18.5-24.9	25-35	1 (0.8-1)
Overweight	25.0-29.9	15-25	0.6 (0.5-0.7)
Obese (includes all classes)	30.0 or greater	11-20	0.5 (0.4-0.6)

*BMI, body mass index. To calculate BMI, go to http://www.nhlbisupport.com/bmi.
†Calculations assume a 1.1-4.4 lb (0.5-2 kg) weight gain in the first trimester.
Modified with permission from Institute of Medicine (US). Weight gain during pregnancy: reexamining the guidelines. Washington, DC. National Academies Press; 2009. ©2009 National Academy of Sciences.

woman's BMI at the initial prenatal visit (an online BMI calculator is available at http://www.nhlbisupport.com/bmi.) It is important to discuss appropriate weight gain, diet, and exercise, both at the initial visit and periodically throughout the pregnancy. Individualized care and clinical judgment is necessary in the management of the obese and overweight woman who wishes to gain, or is gaining, less weight than recommended but has an appropriately growing fetus. Balancing the risks of fetal growth (both large and small), obstetric complications, and maternal weight retention are essential until research provides evidence to further refine the recommendations for gestational weight gain. Postpartum and interconceptional care should include advice and recommendations to help the woman to return to her prepregnancy weight, or lower if necessary to achieve a normal BMI, in the first year after the delivery.

Exercise. In the absence of either medical or obstetric complications, 30 minutes or more of moderate exercise per day on most, if not all, days of the week is recommended for pregnant women. Generally, participation in a wide range of recreational activities appears to be safe during pregnancy; however, each sport should be reviewed individually for its potential risk, and activities with a high risk of falling or those with a high risk of abdominal trauma should be avoided. Pregnant women also should avoid supine positions during exercise as much as possible. Recreational and competitive athletes with uncomplicated pregnancies can remain active during pregnancy and should modify their usual exercise routines as medically indicated. Pregnant competitive athletes may require close obstetric supervision. Women should not take up a new strenuous sport during pregnancy, and previously inactive women and those with medical or obstetric complications should be evaluated before recommendations for physical activity participation during pregnancy are made. Additionally, a physically active woman with a history of or risk of preterm delivery or intrauterine growth restriction may be advised to reduce her activity in the second trimester and third trimester.

Warning signs to terminate exercise while pregnant include the following:

- Chest pain
- Vaginal bleeding
- Dizziness
- Headache
- Decreased fetal movement
- Amniotic fluid leakage
- Muscle weakness
- Calf pain or swelling
- Regular uterine contractions

The following medical conditions are absolute contraindications to aerobic exercise in pregnancy:

- Hemodynamically significant heart disease
- Restrictive lung disease
- Cervical insufficiency or cerclage
- Persistent second-trimester or third-trimester bleeding
- Placenta previa confirmed after 26 weeks of gestation
- Current premature labor
- Ruptured membranes
- Preeclampsia or pregnancy-induced hypertension

Dental Care. It is very important that pregnant women continue usual dental care in pregnancy. This dental care includes routine brushing and flossing, scheduled cleanings, and any medically needed dental work. The patient should be aware that pregnant women's gums do bleed more easily. Caries, poor dentition, and periodontal disease may be associated with an increased risk of preterm delivery. Dental health should be addressed preconceptionally.

If dental X-rays are necessary during pregnancy, the American Dental Association advises the use of a leaded apron to minimize exposure to the abdomen and the use of a leaded thyroid collar. The American Dental Association guidelines recommend timing elective dental procedures to occur during the second trimester or first half of the third trimester and postponing major surgery and reconstructive procedures until after delivery. Many dentists will require a note from the obstetrician stating that dental care requiring local anesthesia, antibiotics, or narcotic analgesia is not contraindicated in pregnancy.

Nausea and Vomiting. Nausea and vomiting of pregnancy affects more than 70% of pregnant women and can diminish the woman's quality of life. For women with prior pregnancies complicated by nausea and vomiting, it is reasonable to recommend preconceptional and early pregnancy use of a multivitamin because studies show this reduces the risk of vomiting requiring medical attention. First-line therapy for nausea and vomiting should be vitamin B_6 with or without doxylamine. Other effective nonpharmacologic treatments for mild cases include increasing protein consumption and taking powdered ginger capsules daily, which has been found to be effective in reducing episodes of vomiting. Acupressure treatments have shown mixed results. Effective and safe treatments for more serious cases include antihistamine H1-receptor blockers, phenothiazines, and benzamides. The most severe form of pregnancy-associated nausea and vomiting is hyperemesis gravidarum, which occurs in less than 2% of pregnancies. This may require more intense therapy, including hospitalization; additional medications; intravenous hydration and nutrition; and, if refractory, total parenteral nutrition.

Vitamin and Mineral Toxicity. Although vitamin A is essential, excessive vitamin A (more than 10,000 international units per day) may be associated with fetal malformations. The amount of vitamin A in standard prenatal vitamins is considered the maximum recommended dose before and during pregnancy (see Table 5-6) and is well below the probable minimum human teratogenic dose. Dietary intake of vitamin A in the United States is adequate to meet the needs of most pregnant women throughout gestation. Therefore, additional supplementation besides a prenatal vitamin during pregnancy is not recommended except in women in whom the dietary intake of vitamin A may not be adequate, such as strict vegetarians. Vitamin tablets containing 25,000 international units or more of vitamin A are available as over-the-counter preparations; however, pregnant women or those planning to become pregnant who use high doses of vitamin A supplements (and topical retinol) should be cautioned about the potential teratogenicity because excess vitamin A is associated with anomalies of bones, the urinary tract, and the central nervous system. The use of beta carotene, the precursor of vitamin A found in fruits and vegetables, has not been shown to produce vitamin A toxicity.

Excessive vitamin and mineral intake (ie, more than twice the recommended dietary allowances) should be avoided during pregnancy. For example, excess iodine is associated with congenital goiter. There also may be toxicity from excessive use of other fat-soluble vitamins (vitamin D, vitamin E, and vitamin K; see Table 5-6).

Fish provides a source of easily digestible protein with high biologic value in terms of vitamins, amino acids and minerals. Also many fish are a uniquely rich food source of long chain omega-3 fatty acids and long-chain polyunsaturated fatty acids. There is strong evidence to suggest that these fatty acids are important in central nervous system development and that maternal consumption of these fatty acids benefits fetal development and provides good nutrition for the mother.

Some large fish, such as shark, swordfish, king mackerel, and tilefish are known to contain high levels of methylmercury, which is known to be teratogenic. As such, pregnant women and women in the preconceptional period and lactation period should avoid these fish.

To gain the benefits of consuming fish, while avoiding the risks of methylmercury consumption, pregnant women should be encouraged to enjoy a variety of other types of fish, including up to 12 ounces (2 average meals) a week of a variety of fish and shellfish that are lower in mercury. Five of the most commonly eaten fish that are low in mercury are shrimp, canned light tuna, salmon, pollock, and catfish. White (albacore) tuna has more mercury than canned light tuna and should be limited to no more than 6 ounces per week.

Pregnant and nursing women also should check local advisories about the safety of fish caught in local lakes, rivers, and coastal areas. If no advice is available, they should consume no more than 6 ounces (one average meal) per week of fish caught in local waters and no other fish during that week.

To prevent pregnancy-related listeria infections, pregnant women are advised not to eat hot dogs or luncheon meats unless they are steaming hot and to avoid unpasteurized soft cheeses. Maternal infection has been associated with preterm delivery and other obstetric and neonatal complications. For more information on listeriosis and its prevention during pregnancy, see "Listeriosis" in Chapter 10 and the CDC web site at http://www.cdc.gov/ncbddd/pregnancy_gateway/infections-listeria.html.

Teratogens. Major birth defects occur in 2–3% of the general population. The possible occurrence of a major birth defect is a frequent cause of anxiety among pregnant women. Many patient inquiries concern the teratogenic potential of environmental exposures. There is little scientifically valid information on which a risk estimate in human pregnancy can be based. Patients should be counseled that relatively few agents have been identified that are known to cause malformations in exposed pregnancies. Relatively few patients are exposed to agents that are known to be associated with increased risk of fetal malformations or mental retardation. The health care provider may wish to consult with or refer such patients to health care professionals with special knowledge or experience in teratology and birth defects. The Organization of Teratology Information Specialists provides information on teratology issues and exposures in pregnancy (www.otispregnancy.org).

Prenatal lead exposure has known adverse effects on maternal health and infant outcomes across a wide range of maternal blood lead levels. In 2010, the CDC issued the first guidelines regarding the screening and management of pregnant and lactating women who have been exposed to lead (available at http://www.cdc.gov/nceh/lead/publications/leadandpregnancy2010.pdf). Routine blood lead testing of all pregnant women is not recommended. Obstetric health care providers should consider the possibility of lead exposure in individual pregnant women by evaluating risk factors for exposure as part of a comprehensive health risk assessment and perform blood lead testing if a single risk factor is identified.

Although most medications are not known to be teratogens, patients should consult with their health care providers before using prescription and nonprescription medications or herbal remedies (see also "Medication Use" earlier in this chapter). Importantly, patients and health care providers should be reminded that alcohol and hyperglycemia are more common teratogens than medications. Physician and patient information about known teratogenic medications, as well as other teratogenic exposures, can be found on the Organization of Teratology Information Specialists' web site. Health care providers also can refer patients to the CDC's web page on medication use during pregnancy, available at http://www.cdc.gov/features/medicationspregnancy/ for more information on medication safety.

Many patients raise questions about the methods of detecting birth defects related to drug exposure. Amniocentesis or CVS for chromosome analysis is not helpful for the diagnosis of birth defects caused by teratogens. Although obstetric ultrasonography has been the mainstay of surveillance for teratogen-induced congenital anomalies, its sensitivity varies with the experience and skill of the imager as well as the specific anatomic abnormality. However, even in expert hands, the overall sensitivity of ultrasonography in the detection of fetal anatomic anomalies is in the range of 50–70%.

Concerns frequently are expressed over the teratogenic potential of diagnostic imaging modalities used during pregnancy, including X-ray, nuclear imaging, contrast agents, and magnetic resonance imaging. The imaging modality that causes the most anxiety for both the obstetrician and the patient is X-ray or ionizing radiation. Much of this anxiety is secondary to a general misperception that any radiation exposure is harmful and may result in injury to or anomaly of the fetus. This anxiety may lead to inappropriate therapeutic abortion. In fact, most diagnostic X-ray procedures are associated with few, if any, risks to the fetus. Exposure to less than 5 rads has not been associated with an increase in fetal anomalies or pregnancy loss. Moreover, according to the American College of Radiology, no single diagnostic X-ray procedure results in radiation exposure to a degree that would threaten the well-being of a developing preembryo, embryo, or fetus.

Concern about radiation exposure during pregnancy should not prevent medically indicated diagnostic X-ray studies when these are important for the care of the woman. When such a study is indicated, the minimal dose of radiation should be used. Because magnetic resonance imaging does not use ionizing radiation, it may be the preferred test. Both spiral computed tomography and ventilation–perfusion scanning expose the fetus to only small amounts of radiation. However, most centers avoid the use of iodinated contrast agents in pregnancy because of the risk of neonatal hypothyroidism. Patients concerned about previously performed or planned diagnostic studies should have counseling to allay these concerns.

Most diagnostic studies in which radioisotopes are used are not hazardous to the fetus and result in low levels of radiation exposure. A typical technetium Tc-99m scan results in a fetal dose of less than 0.5 rads, and a thallium 201 scan also results in a low dose. Many of these isotopes are excreted in the urine.

Therefore, women should be advised to drink plenty of fluids and to void frequently after a radionuclide study.

One important exception is the use of iodine 131 for the treatment of Graves disease. The fetal thyroid gland begins to incorporate iodine actively by the end of the first trimester. Administration of iodine 131 after this time can result in concentration of the radiation within, and destruction of, the fetal thyroid gland. Therefore, iodine 131 is contraindicated for therapeutic use during pregnancy. By comparison, there are few reports on the safety of radioisotope imaging of the maternal thyroid during pregnancy, and such studies should be undertaken only after careful consideration of the risks and benefits of the procedure.

Because significant elevation of core body temperature may be associated with fetal anomalies, pregnant women might reasonably be advised to remain in saunas for no more than 15 minutes and hot tubs for no more than 10 minutes. As an additional precaution, it is best for women to ensure their head, arms, shoulders and upper chest are not submerged in a hot tub so there will be less surface area to absorb heat and more surface area to radiate it.

Air Travel. Occasional air travel during pregnancy is generally safe. Recent cohort studies suggest no increase in adverse pregnancy outcomes for occasional air travelers. Most commercial airlines allow pregnant women to fly up to 36 weeks of gestation. Some restrict pregnant women from international flights earlier in gestation and some require documentation of gestational age. For specific airline requirements, women should check with the individual carrier. Civilian and military aircrew members who become pregnant should check with their specific agencies for regulations or restrictions to their flying duties.

Air travel is not recommended at any time during pregnancy for women who have medical or obstetric conditions that may be exacerbated by flight or that could require emergency care. The duration of the flight also should be considered when planning travel. Pregnant women should be informed that the most common obstetric emergencies occur in the first trimester and third trimester.

In-craft environmental conditions, such as changes in cabin pressure and low humidity, coupled with the physiologic changes of pregnancy, do result in adaptations, including increased heart rate and blood pressure and a significant decrease in aerobic capacity. The risks associated with long hours of air travel immobilization and low cabin humidity, such as lower extremity edema and venous thrombotic events, have been the focus of attention for all air travelers.

Despite the lack of evidence of such events during pregnancy, certain preventive measures can be used to minimize these risks, eg, use of support stockings and periodic movement of the lower extremities, avoidance of restrictive clothing, occasional ambulation, and maintenance of adequate hydration.

In pregnant women the seat belt should be belted low on the hipbones, between the protuberant abdomen and pelvis. Several precautions may ease discomfort for pregnant air travelers. For example, gas-producing foods or drinks should be avoided before scheduled flights because entrapped gases expand at altitude. Preventive antiemetic medication should be considered for women with increased nausea.

Antepartum Tests of Fetal Well-Being

Fetal surveillance techniques, including fetal heart rate monitoring and ultrasonography, can identify the fetus that is either suboptimally oxygenated or, with increasing degrees of placental dysfunction, acidemic. Identification of suspected fetal compromise provides the opportunity to intervene before progressive metabolic acidosis can lead to fetal death. Although there have been no randomized clinical trials that clearly demonstrate improved perinatal outcome with the use of antepartum testing or that determine the optimal time to initiate testing, certain tests have become an integral part of the clinical care of pregnancies suspected to be at increased risk of fetal demise due to uteroplacental insufficiency. Indications for initiating antenatal testing can be thought of in categories of maternal conditions and pregnancy-related or fetal conditions and are listed below.

Maternal conditions

- Antiphospholipid syndrome
- Cyanotic heart disease
- Systemic lupus erythematosus
- Chronic renal disease
- Insulin-treated diabetes mellitus
- Hypertensive disorders

Pregnancy-related or fetal conditions

- Pregnancy-induced hypertension
- Decreased fetal movement

- Oligohydramnios and polyhydramnios
- Intrauterine growth restriction
- Postterm pregnancy
- Isoimmunization (moderate to severe)
- Previous fetal demise (unexplained)
- Multiple gestation (with significant growth discrepancy)
- Monochorionic diamniotic multiple gestation

Antenatal Testing Strategy

Devising the appropriate antenatal testing strategy—what test to use, when to start testing, and how frequently to re-test—requires balancing several considerations. The prognosis for neonatal survival, the severity of maternal disease, the risk of fetal death, and the potential for iatrogenic prematurity as a complication from false-positive test results all must be taken into account when considering antenatal testing. Antepartum testing is intended for use in pregnancies at risk of fetal demise. There are risks of false-positive test results, including unnecessary delivery of a healthy baby. As with any screening test, false positive test results are more common in populations at low risk of the disease intended to be identified. Hence antepartum surveillance should be reserved for high risk pregnancies.

In general, antepartum testing should not begin before a gestational age at which the health care provider is willing to intervene and should be targeted at the gestational age at which the increased risk of stillbirth is likely. Therefore, the College supports initiating antenatal testing at 32–34 weeks of gestation for most pregnancies with increased risk of stillbirth. However, for pregnancies with particularly high-risk conditions or multiple complicating factors, testing may begin earlier. The following tests are commonly used in clinical practice to assess fetal status and are described in detail later in this section (see also "Assessment and Management of Fetal Pulmonary Maturation" in Chapter 7):

- Assessment of fetal movement (eg, kick counts)
- Nonstress test (NST)
- Acoustic stimulation
- Biophysical profile (BPP)
- Modified biophysical profile (NST plus amniotic fluid index [AFI])

- Contraction stress test (CST) or oxytocin challenge test
- Doppler ultrasonography of umbilical artery blood flow velocity

Repeat antenatal testing should be performed when the condition that initiated testing persists. Typically the NST, CST, and BPP are repeated at weekly intervals. However, in the presence of certain conditions, such as postterm pregnancy, intrauterine growth restriction, or pregnancy-induced hypertension, some investigators perform twice-weekly antenatal testing. In addition, any significant deterioration in maternal condition or new decrease in fetal activity requires fetal testing independent of time elapsed from previous testing. For the indication of decreased fetal movement, usually only one antenatal testing episode is indicated.

A normal test is highly reassuring. The false-negative rate is defined as the incidence of a stillbirth occurring within 1 week of a normal test. The risk of a fetal death within 7 days of a reassuring testing is as follows (rates expressed per 1,000 fetuses): NST, 1.9; CST, 0.3; BPP, 0.8; modified BPP, 0.8.

Interpretation of abnormal test results must take into consideration the overall clinical picture and the possibility that the test result is falsely positive. An abnormal NST or modified BPP should be further evaluated by using either a CST or full BPP. Decisions regarding serial testing or proceeding with delivery should be made in the context of the gestational age, and the maternal and fetal condition. Certain maternal conditions, such as diabetic ketoacidosis, pneumonia with hypoxemia, or general anesthesia can result in abnormal test results. In these circumstances, stabilization of the maternal condition and retesting the fetus may be appropriate. If delivery is planned, in the absence of obstetric indications, an induction of labor with continuous fetal heart rate monitoring may be attempted, with a plan for cesarean delivery in the case of repetitive late decelerations.

Assessment of Fetal Movement

A decrease in the maternal perception of fetal movement may, but does not invariably, precede fetal death. This observation provides the rationale for fetal movement assessment by the mother (kick counts) as a means of antepartum fetal surveillance in all women, not just those at increased risk of stillbirth. Multiple studies have demonstrated that women who report decreased fetal movement are at increased risk of adverse perinatal outcome. Although fetal kick counting is an inexpensive test of fetal well being, the effectiveness in preventing stillbirth is uncertain. Neither the ideal number of kicks nor the ideal duration of daily movement count assessment has been defined. Perhaps more important than any single quantitative guideline is the mother's perception of a decrease in fetal activity relative to a previous level.

One strategy for fetal movement counts is the use of "10 movements in 2 hours" using focused counting. The perception of 10 distinct movements in a period of up to 2 hours is considered normal. After 10 movements have been perceived, the count can be discontinued for that day. In the absence of 10 movements in 2 hours, additional fetal evaluation is warranted.

Nonstress Test

A nonstress test uses fetal heart rate patterns and accelerations as an indicator of fetal well-being. Fetal heart rate accelerations occur via a link between fetal peripheral movements and a cardioregulatory center in the midbrain, which requires intact peripheral, central, and autonomic neural in-flow and out-flow pathways. These pathways mature as the fetus matures, such that criteria for accelerations differ based on gestational age.

To perform an NST, the fetal heart rate is monitored with an external transducer for at least 20 minutes. The tracing is observed for fetal heart rate accelerations. The testing can be continued for an additional 40 minutes or longer to take into account the typical fetal sleep–wake cycle. Fetal heart rate accelerations that peak at 15 beats per minute above the baseline and persist for 15 seconds are associated with an extremely low risk of fetal acidosis and, thus, are considered reassuring. Because fetal heart rate reactivity is a function of fetal maturity, if a nonstress test is performed at an early gestational age it is more likely to be nonreactive in the absence of fetal compromise. Before 32 weeks of gestation, accelerations that peak at 10 beats per minute and persist for 10 seconds (from baseline to baseline) are as reassuring as the 15 beat criteria for those fetuses beyond 32 weeks of gestation.

The results of an NST are considered reactive (reassuring) if two or more fetal heart rate accelerations are detected within a 20-minute period, with or without fetal movement discernible by the mother. A nonreactive tracing is one without sufficient fetal heart rate accelerations in a 40-minute period and requires further testing for confirmation of fetal reassurance. An NST may be nonreactive for a variety of reasons, including fetal sleep-cycles, maternal ingestion of sedatives, fetal cardiac or central nervous system abnormalities, or a lack of fetal movement as an adaptive mechanism for conservation of energy and metabolism in the context of hypoxemia (detection of the latter being the specific aim of antepartum testing).

Perinatal outcomes after a reactive tracing provoked with acoustic stimulation are comparable to those associated with a spontaneously reactive NST. The use of acoustic stimulation decreases false nonreactive NSTs and reduces overall testing time. Stimulation is delivered for 1–2 seconds using a specially designed artificial larynx that is placed on the maternal abdomen. It can be repeated up to three times, each for a maximum duration of 2 seconds, to elicit fetal heart rate accelerations.

Contraction Stress Test

Formerly known as an oxytocin challenge test, CST involves subjecting the fetus to the physiologic stress of uterine contractions. Relative contraindications to inducing contractions for CSTs include preterm labor, pregnancies with a high risk of preterm delivery, preterm premature rupture of membranes, known placenta previa, or history of classical uterine scar.

To perform a CST, the fetal heart rate is obtained using an external transducer, and uterine contraction activity is monitored with a tocodynamometer. A baseline tracing is obtained for 10–20 minutes. If at least three contractions of 40 seconds or more are present in a 10-minute period, uterine stimulation is not necessary. If the contractions are not present, they are induced with either nipple stimulation or intravenously administered oxytocin. Intravenous infusion of low-dose oxytocin can be initiated, usually at a rate of 0.5–1 microunit/min, and increased every 15–20 minutes until an adequate contraction pattern occurs (ie, three contractions in 10 minutes). The results of the CST can be categorized as follows:

- Negative—No late or significant variable decelerations
- Positive—Late decelerations are present following 50% or more of contractions, even if the frequency of contractions is less than three in 10 minutes
- Equivocal—Intermittent late or significant variable decelerations
- Unsatisfactory—Fewer than three contractions within 10 minutes or a tracing that cannot be interpreted

Both oxytocin and nipple stimulation can produce tachysystole. If fetal heart rate decelerations occur in the presence of tachysystole, retesting is appropriate to ensure a correct interpretation. The presence of variable decelerations may prompt examination of amniotic fluid volume. Equivocal testing may be repeated in 24 hours or sooner unless an intervening indication for delivery arises or may prompt admission for closer observation. As with all antepartum testing, the management of a positive (or nonreassuring) CST requires individualized decision making based on other parameters of fetal reassurance and gestational age.

Biophysical Profile

A biophysical profile consists of assessment of five fetal variables. The five components of a reassuring BPP are as follows:

1. NST reactive—Because the probability of fetal well-being is identical with scores of 10 out of 10 and 8 out of 10

2. Fetal breathing movements—At least one or more episodes of rhythmic fetal breathing movements of 30 seconds or more within 30 minutes

3. Fetal movement—Three or more discrete body or limb movements within 30 minutes

4. Fetal tone—One or more episodes of fetal extremity extension with return to flexion, or opening or closing of a hand within 30 minutes

5. Amniotic fluid volume—A pocket of amniotic fluid that measures at least 2 cm in two planes perpendicular to each other

The combination of the aforementioned parameters accounts for both acute changes in fetal reserve (NST, breathing, flexion, and extension) as well as changes that are influenced over a more chronic time course (amniotic fluid volume and fetal tone).

A BPP is scored from 0–10 with a score of either 2 (present) or 0 (absent) being assigned to each of the five observations. Before a 0 can be given for any of the ultrasound variables the fetus must be observed for 30 minutes. A score of 8 or 10 is reassuring. A score of 6 is equivocal and a decision to re-test within 12–24 hours or proceed with delivery must be made within the context of gestational age and weighed against the risk of prematurity. A score of 4 or less is nonreassuring and warrants further evaluation and consideration of delivery. Irrespective of the overall score, except in the setting of premature rupture of membranes, the finding of oligohydramnios may warrant consideration of delivery in term pregnancies or more frequent antepartum testing in the case of preterm gestations.

Modified Biophysical Profile

Another approach to fetal surveillance, the modified BPP, combines the use of an NST as a short-term indicator of fetal status with the assessment of AFI as an indicator of long-term placental function. Nonstress test changes are thought to be one of the early manifestations of fetal hypoxia, whereas amniotic fluid volume likely changes more slowly over time as the fetus preferentially shunts cardiac output to the heart and brain while decreasing renal perfusion and, thus, fetal urine output. The AFI is a semiquantitative, four-quadrant assessment of amniotic fluid depth. To appropriately perform an AFI, the maternal abdomen is divided into four quadrants. The deepest vertical pocket of amniotic fluid is measured with the ultrasound probe directly at 90 degrees to the maternal abdomen (and with care not to include fetal parts or the umbilical cord). The sum of all four measurements is totaled to obtain the AFI. A value of less than or equal to five is considered indicative of oligohydramnios. The modified BPP is less cumbersome than complete BPP assessment and appears to be as predictive of fetal well-being as other approaches of biophysical fetal surveillance.

Doppler Ultrasonography of Umbilical Artery

The umbilical arteries arise from the common iliac arteries in the fetus and comprise the main outflow tract of fetal blood back to the placental bed. Normal placental physiology is such that vascular resistance decreases as gestational age progresses and, more specifically, high velocity forward diastolic flow in the umbilical arteries is maintained. Umbilical artery Doppler flow ultrasonography uses these hemodynamic characteristics to assess resistance to blood flow in the placenta, which may be altered in certain pathologic conditions, such as intrauterine growth restriction. Umbilical artery Doppler ultrasonography is not a screening test for detecting fetal compromise in the general population, but it can be used in conjunction with other biophysical tests in high-risk pregnancies associated with suspected intrauterine growth restriction. The index most commonly used to quantify the flow velocity waveform is the systolic/diastolic ratio. As placental resistance increases, the systolic/diastolic ratio increases, the end diastolic flow decreases and may become absent or reversed.

Serial Doppler studies can be performed in the growth-restricted fetus and can be used in conjunction with other measures of fetal well-being (such as amniotic fluid volume, NST, or BPP) to guide the timing of delivery. The finding of abnormal umbilical artery Doppler studies also may be used to guide the administration of corticosteroids in anticipation of delivery.

Special Populations and Considerations

All pregnant women should receive the best appropriate care. However, each of the following groups is potentially more vulnerable to poor pregnancy outcomes or barriers to health care and has unique circumstances that require additional attention.

Adolescents

Minors typically have legal rights protecting their privacy regarding the diagnosis and treatment of pregnancy. Once the gestational age is determined, she should be fully informed in a balanced manner about all options, including continuation of the pregnancy, either with the intent of raising the child herself or placing the child for adoption, or termination of the pregnancy. The physician should assess the adolescent's ability to understand the implications of the diagnosis of pregnancy and the options available.

The patient should be encouraged to return for visits as needed and helped to understand the importance of a timely decision. She should be encouraged to include her parents or guardian and the father of the fetus in her decisions, if appropriate. The patient's right to decide the outcome of the pregnancy and who should be involved should be respected. Many states have laws regarding adolescent rights, and the physician should be aware of these state laws when making health care decisions.

If the adolescent chooses to continue the pregnancy, she should be referred for psychosocial support. There is an increased incidence of delivery of low birth weight neonates, neonatal death, preterm delivery, preeclampsia, anemia, and STIs in pregnant adolescents necessitating increased monitoring and appropriate medical management. Pregnant adolescents should be counseled about the effects of STIs on themselves and their fetuses. They should receive repetitive reinforcement that condoms should be used during pregnancy for STI protection. Rapid repeat pregnancy is common in adolescents. Plans for postpartum contraception should be discussed during prenatal care visits and the patient's contraceptive method should be provided before discharge.

Incarcerated Women

Generally, pregnant inmates, because of their disadvantaged background, are at a higher risk of poor pregnancy outcomes than the general population. Upon entry into a prison or jail, every woman of childbearing age should be assessed for pregnancy risk by inquiring about menstrual history, heterosexual activity, and contraceptive use and tested for pregnancy, as appropriate, to enable the provision of adequate perinatal care and abortion services. Incarcerated women who wish to continue their pregnancies should have access to readily available and regularly scheduled obstetric care, beginning in early pregnancy and continuing through the postpartum period, although many facilities do not offer it. Incarcerated pregnant women also should have access to unscheduled or emergency obstetric visits on a 24-hour basis.

Because of high rates of substance abuse and HIV infection in incarcerated women, prompt screening for these conditions in pregnant women is important. All pregnant women should be questioned about their past and present use of alcohol, tobacco, and other drugs, including the recreational use of prescription and over-the-counter medication. Substance abuse can continue during incarceration despite efforts to prevent drugs from entering correctional facilities. Effective drug and alcohol treatment programs are essential. Incarcerated pregnant women also should be screened for depression or mental stress and for postpartum depression after delivery and be appropriately treated.

Although maintaining adequate safety is critical, correctional officers do not need to routinely be present in the room while a pregnant woman is being examined or in the hospital room during labor and delivery unless requested by medical staff or the situation poses a danger to the safety of the medical staff or others. Delivery services for incarcerated pregnant women should be provided in a licensed hospital with facilities for high-risk pregnancies when available. It is important to avoid separating the mother from the infant to allow for the formation of maternal–child bonds during a critical period of infant development. Breastfeeding should be encouraged. Incarcerated pregnant women often have short jail or prison stays and may not give birth while incarcerated. Postpartum contraceptive options should be discussed and provided during incarceration to decrease the likelihood of an unintended pregnancy during and after release from incarceration.

The use of physical restraints on pregnant incarcerated women may not only compromise health care, but is demeaning and rarely necessary. Shackling of pregnant and postpartum women (within 6 weeks postpartum) during transportation to medical care facilities and during the receipt of health services should occur only in exceptional circumstances after a strong consideration of the health effects of restraints by the physician providing care. Exceptions include when there is imminent risk of escape or harm. If restraint is needed, it should be the least restrictive possible to ensure safety and should never include restraints that interfere with leg movement or the ability of the woman to break a fall. The woman should be allowed to lie on her side, not flat on her back or stomach. Pressure should not be applied either directly or indirectly to the abdomen. Correctional officers should be available and required to remove the shackles immediately upon request of medical personnel. Women should never be shackled during evaluation for labor and delivery. If restraint is used, a report should be filed by the Department of Corrections and reviewed by an independent body. There should be consequences for individuals and institutions when use of restraints was unjustified.

Homeless Women

It has been estimated that as many as 14% of individuals living in the United States have been homeless at some time and as many as 3.5 million people (1% of the U.S. population, or 10% of the poor population) experience homelessness in a given year. Domestic and sexual violence is the leading cause of homelessness for women and families, and 20–50% of all homeless women and children become homeless as a direct result of fleeing domestic violence. Homeless women are far more likely to experience violence of all sorts compared with women who are not homeless because of a lack of personal security when living outdoors or in shelters.

Homeless women are less likely to receive prenatal care than women who are not homeless, and adverse birth outcomes are substantially higher in homeless women compared with the general population. A Canadian study found that compared with women who are not homeless, homeless women were 2.9 times more likely to have a preterm delivery, 6.9 times more likely to give birth to an infant who weighed less than 2,000 grams, and 3.3 times more likely to have a small for gestational age newborn, even after adjustment for risk factors, such as maternal age, number of previous pregnancies, and smoking. In the United States, preterm birth rates and low birth weight rates in homeless women exceed national averages.

It is important for physicians to identify patients within the practice who are (or are at risk of becoming) homeless by asking questions about living conditions, nutrition, substance abuse, and intimate partner violence; provide health care, including preventive care, for homeless women without bias; and not withhold treatment based on concerns about lack of adherence. Health care professionals are advised to simplify medical regimens and address barriers, including transportation needs for follow-up health care visits. In addition, physicians should become familiar with and inform patients who are (or at risk of becoming) homeless about appropriate community resources, including local substance abuse programs, intimate partner violence services, and social service agencies.

Women With Disabilities

Physical, intellectual and developmental, sensory, and psychiatric impairments may affect both the quality and availability of health care services for women. With all disabilities, consideration of the history of the disability, the number and severity of limitations, and its expected progression is critical in meeting the health care needs and concerns of women. Health care providers may be unfamiliar with the individual's specific disability and its consequences on health, sexual functioning, and reproductive potential. This information may be accessible through various means, such as consultation with rehabilitation physicians or other disability health care providers, further investigation of medical literature, disability organizations, and through discussion with the woman and her family. Many women are well informed about their disabilities and the resources available to them.

Language and educational differences between women and their health care providers are barriers to effective care. Women with disabilities may have additional challenges. Knowledge of the women's mode of communication and patience in the process is critical to ensure informed health care delivery. Women with disabilities also may need extra time allotted for their appointment. When scheduling appointments, asking patients about the need for extra time or services in a nonjudgmental and nonstigmatizing fashion may be one way of accommodating such needs. Creativity and flexibility on the part of each staff member can go a long way in ameliorating these challenges and establishing mutually rewarding and respectful services.

Physical Disabilities. Pregnancy and parenting for women with physical disabilities may pose unique medical and social challenges but rarely are precluded by the disability itself. Few, if any, physical disabilities directly limit fertility. Health care professionals have the responsibility to provide appropriate reproductive health services to these women or arrange adequate consultation or referral. Nonbiased preconception counseling for couples in which one partner has a physical disability may decrease subsequent psychosocial and medical complications of pregnancy. Screening and provision of disability-specific information, such as condition-appropriate genetic counseling and folate supplementation for women who have spina bifida, is highly desirable (see also "Preconception Nutritional Counseling" earlier in this chapter).

Once pregnancy occurs, the patient should have early contact with a physician. Detailed pregnancy care plans should be developed in negotiation with managed care plans and other insurers to increase access to and use of prenatal care services, ensure appropriate postpartum hospital length of stay, and arrange postpartum home care services, if necessary. Assessment of the need for additional assistance during pregnancy to ambulate, perform safe transfers, and maintain hygiene and household activities is recommended. Regular consultation or referral may be required to achieve the optimum outcome.

Intellectual and Developmental Disabilities. In caring for pregnant women with intellectual and developmental disabilities, it is important to consider the following psychosocial factors: whether the individual lives at home or in a domiciliary care setting; whether there is a reliable caregiver present; previous history of sexual abuse; and cognitive factors, including her ability to relay a personal or family history of disease and symptoms. Genetic screening is particularly important for pregnant women with Down syndrome. First-trimester alpha-fetoprotein testing and ultrasound examinations focused on nuchal translucency, cardiac malformations, and other fetal indications of Down syndrome should be offered (see also "Antepartum Genetic Screening and Diagnosis" earlier in this chapter).

Before examination, it should be determined who will give consent for the examination and any consequential treatment. It also is important at this time to ascertain if the patient is competent to understand findings and health recommendations or whether this information needs to be transmitted to an identified guardian or caregiver. For women with intellectual and developmental disabilities, making materials available in pictorial formats or in simple, straightforward language can facilitate communication greatly. It often is helpful, with the patient's consent, to have a companion with whom the patient is familiar accompany her to the examination room. Additionally, health care providers who care for patients with intellectual and developmental disabilities may find it helpful to provide a short summary of the patient's medical problems for the patient or guardian to keep in their billfold along with the name of a contact person and their primary medical provider. This will help emergency room personnel, new health care providers, or consulting physicians when records are not available.

Consent and Power of Attorney

Obtaining informed consent for medical treatment is an ethical requirement that is partially reflected in legal doctrines and requirements. Seeking informed consent expresses respect for the patient as an individual. It not only ensures the protection of the patient against unwanted medical treatment, but it also makes possible the patient's active involvement in her medical planning and care. Communication is necessary if informed consent is to be realized, and physicians can and should help to find ways to facilitate communication not only in individual relations with patients but also in the structured context of medical care institutions. When informed consent by the patient is impossible, a surrogate decision maker should be identified to represent the patient's wishes or best interests. In emergency situations, medical professionals may have to act according to their perceptions of the best interests of the patient; in rare instances, they may have to forgo obtaining consent because of some other overriding ethical obligation, such as protecting the public health.

An advance directive is the formal mechanism by which a patient may express her values regarding her future health status. It may take the form of a proxy directive or an instructional directive or both. Proxy directives, such as the durable power of attorney for health care, designate a surrogate to make medical decisions on behalf of the patient who is no longer competent to express her choices. Instructional directives, such as living wills, focus on the types of life-sustaining treatment that a patient would or would not choose in various clinical circumstances.

Although courts at times have intervened to impose treatment on a pregnant woman, currently there is general agreement that a pregnant woman who has decision-making capacity has the same right to refuse treatment as a nonpregnant woman. When a pregnant woman does not have decision-making capacity, however, legislation frequently limits her ability to refuse treatment through an advance directive. Statutes that prohibit pregnant women from exercising their right to determine or refuse current or future medical treatment are unethical.

Second-Trimester and Third-Trimester Patient Education

Important topics to discuss with women before delivery include working, childbirth education classes, choosing a newborn care provider, anticipating labor, preterm labor, breech presentation at term, trial of labor after cesarean delivery, elective delivery, cesarean delivery on maternal request, umbilical cord blood banking, breastfeeding, preparation for discharge, and neonatal interventions.

Working

A woman with an uncomplicated pregnancy usually can continue to work until the onset of labor. Women with medical or obstetric complications of pregnancy may need to make adjustments based on the nature of their activities, occupations, and specific complications. It also has been reported that pregnant women whose occupations require standing or repetitive, strenuous, physical lifting have a tendency to give birth earlier and have small for gestational age infants.

A period of 4–6 weeks after delivery generally is required for a woman's physiologic condition to return to normal; however, the patient's individual circumstances should be considered when recommending resumption of full activity. It also is important for the development of children and the family unit that adequate family leave be available for parents to be able to participate in early childrearing. The federal Family and Medical Leave Act and state laws should be consulted to determine the family and medical leave that is available.

Childbirth Education Classes and Choosing a Newborn Care Provider

Pregnant women should be referred to appropriate educational literature and urged to attend childbirth education classes. Studies have shown that childbirth education programs can have a beneficial effect on patient experience in labor and delivery. The prenatal period should be used to expose the prospective parents to information about labor and delivery, pain relief, obstetric complications and procedures, breastfeeding, normal newborn care, and postpartum adjustment. Other family members also should be encouraged to participate in childbirth education programs. Adequate preparation of family members may benefit the mother, the neonate, and, ultimately, the family unit. Many hospitals, community agencies, and other groups offer such educational programs. The participation of physicians, certified nurse–midwives, and hospital obstetric nurses in educational programs is desirable to ensure continuity of care and consistency of instruction. National organizations are available for assistance as well. Integration of parenting education in prenatal education is beneficial in facilitating transition to parenthood.

Sometime in the third trimester, it should be determined if the patient has a newborn care provider. If she does not have one, she should be referred to the appropriate resources to identify her newborn care provider before delivery, if possible.

Anticipating Labor

Most women will give birth near term. As pregnancy progresses, patients should be advised when and how to contact the health care provider should symptoms of labor or membrane rupture occur. If a patient has a birth plan, she should be encouraged to review it with her health care provider before labor. A detailed discussion should take place during the third trimester regarding analgesic and anesthetic options available for labor and delivery.

Solid foods should be avoided in patients who are in labor. The oral intake of modest amounts of clear liquids may be allowed for patients with uncomplicated labor. The patient without complications undergoing elective cesarean delivery may have modest amounts of clear liquids up to 2 hours before induction of anesthesia. Particulate containing fluids should be avoided. Patients with risk factors for aspiration (eg, morbid obesity, diabetes, and difficult airway), or patients at increased risk of operative delivery may require further restrictions of oral intake, determined on a case-by-case basis. Pregnant women are at highest risk of aspiration pneumonitis when stomach contents are greater than 25 mL and when the pH of those contents is less than 2.5. Pregnancy slows gastric emptying, and labor can delay it further. The type of aspiration pneumonitis that produces the most severe physiologic and histologic alteration is partially digested food.

Preterm Labor

Preterm labor generally can be defined as regular contractions that occur before 37 weeks of gestation and are associated with changes in the cervix. Toward the end of the second trimester, signs and symptoms of preterm birth, ruptured membranes, and vaginal bleeding should be reviewed with the patient and she should be encouraged to contact the health care provider should these symptoms occur. Patients should be given a telephone number to call where assistance is available 24 hours per day. Short-term interventions to allow for steroid administration and transfer of the pregnant woman to an appropriate level of hospital for her situation are possible if a woman is seen early enough after onset of symptoms (see also "Preterm Birth" in Chapter 7).

Breech Presentation at Term

If the fetus persists in a breech presentation at 36–38 weeks of gestation, women should be offered an external cephalic version if appropriate. Contraindications to the procedure include multifetal gestation, nonreassuring fetal testing, müllerian duct anomalies, and suspected placental abruption or placenta previa. Relative contraindications include intrauterine growth restriction and oligohydramnios. The success rate of external cephalic version ranges from 35–86%, with an average success rate of approximately 58%. Planned cesarean delivery is the most common and safest route of delivery for singleton fetuses at term in breech presentations. However, planned vaginal delivery of a term singleton breech may be reasonable under hospital-specific protocol guidelines for both eligibility and labor management if the health care provider is experienced in vaginal breech deliveries. Before embarking on a plan for a vaginal breech delivery, women should be informed that the risk of perinatal or neonatal mortality or short-term serious neonatal morbidity might be somewhat higher than if a cesarean delivery is planned. Informed consent for vaginal delivery should be obtained and documented. In those instances in which breech vaginal deliveries are pursued, great caution should be used.

Trial of Labor After Cesarean Delivery

The enthusiasm to consider trial of labor after cesarean delivery (TOLAC) varies greatly among women, and this variation is at least partly related to the differences in the way individuals value the potential risks and benefits. Accordingly, potential benefits and risks of both TOLAC and elective repeat cesarean delivery should be discussed and documented. Discussion should consider individual characteristics that affect the chances of vaginal birth after cesarean delivery (VBAC) and TOLAC-associated complications so that a patient can choose her intended route of delivery based on data that are most personally relevant.

A discussion of VBAC early in a woman's prenatal care course, if possible, will allow the most time for her to consider options for TOLAC or elective repeat cesarean delivery. Many of the factors that are related to the chance of VBAC or uterine rupture are known early in pregnancy. If the type of previous hysterotomy is in doubt, reasonable attempts should be made to obtain the patient's medical records. As the pregnancy progresses, if other circumstances arise that may change the risks or benefits of TOLAC (eg, need for induction), these should be addressed. Counseling also may include consideration of intended family size and the risk of additional cesarean deliveries, with the recognition that the future reproductive plans may be uncertain or change.

Counseling also should consider the resources available to support women electing TOLAC at their intended delivery site, and whether such resources match those recommended for caring for women electing TOLAC. Available data support that TOLAC may be safely undertaken in both university and community hospitals and facilities with and without residency programs.

After counseling, the ultimate decision to undergo TOLAC or a repeat cesarean delivery should be made by the patient in consultation with her health care provider. Global mandates for TOLAC are inappropriate because individual risk factors are not considered. Documentation of counseling and the management plan should be included in the medical record (see also "Vaginal Birth After Cesarean Delivery" in Chapter 6).

Elective Delivery

An elective delivery is a delivery that is performed without medical indication. Deliveries before 39 weeks of gestation should not be done without a maternal or fetal indication. If an elective delivery is planned after 39 weeks of gestation, then accuracy of the gestational age, cervical status, and consideration of any potential risks to the mother or fetus are paramount in any discussion of a nonmedically indicated delivery. Term gestation should be confirmed using the following criteria:

- Ultrasound measurement at less than 20 weeks of gestation supports gestational age of 39 weeks or greater
- Fetal heart tones have been documented as present for 30 weeks by Doppler ultrasonography
- It has been 36 weeks since a positive serum or urine hCG test

(See also "Induction of Labor and Cervical Ripening" in Chapter 6 for more information.)

Cesarean Delivery on Maternal Request

When a woman desires a cesarean delivery on maternal request, her health care provider should consider her specific risk factors, such as age, body mass index, accuracy of estimated gestational age, reproductive plans, personal values, and cultural context. Critical life experiences (eg, trauma, violence, poor obstetric outcomes) and anxiety about the birth process may prompt her request. If her main concern is a fear of pain in childbirth, then prenatal childbirth education, emotional support in labor, and anesthesia for childbirth should be offered (see also "Cesarean Delivery" in Chapter 6).

Umbilical Cord Blood Banking

Prospective parents may seek information regarding umbilical cord blood banking. Balanced and accurate information regarding the advantages and disadvantages of public versus private banking should be provided. Discussion might include information regarding maternal infectious disease and genetic testing, the ultimate outcome of use of poor quality units of umbilical cord blood, and a disclosure that demographic data will be maintained on the patient. The remote chance of an autologous unit being used for a child or family member should be disclosed (about 1/2,700 individuals). Directed donation of umbilical cord blood should be considered when there is a specific diagnosis of a disease known to be treatable by a hematopoietic transplant for an immediate family member. Umbilical cord blood donation should be encouraged when the umbilical cord blood is stored in a bank for public use. Some states have passed legislation requiring physicians to inform their patients about umbilical cord blood banking options. Physicians should consult their state medical associations for more information regarding state laws.

Breastfeeding

During prenatal visits, the woman should be counseled regarding the nutritional advantages of human breast milk and encouraged to breastfeed her infant. Human milk supports optimal growth and development of the infant while decreasing the risk of a variety of acute and chronic diseases. Prenatal counseling and education regarding methods of newborn feeding may allow correction of misperceptions about feeding methods. Women should be educated about the benefits of breastfeeding at the practice site or referred to other locations for such education (see also "Breastfeeding" in Chapter 8).

Preparation for Discharge

Prospective parents should be aware of the timing of hospital discharge after delivery. The couple should be encouraged to prepare for discharge by setting up required resources for home health services and acquiring a newborn car seat, newborn clothing, and a crib that meets standard safety guidelines. The prospective parents should be apprised of proper newborn positioning during sleep. Reports have shown a significant reduction in the incidence of sudden infant death syndrome in newborns that are placed on their backs (as opposed to the prone position) during sleep (see also Chapter 8, "Care of the Newborn"). The patient's plan for postpartum contraception should be confirmed and needed supplies and counseling provided before discharge (see also "Postpartum Contraception" in Chapter 6).

Neonatal Interventions

During prenatal visits, the topic of neonatal interventions also should be discussed, including male circumcision, administration of vitamin K, conjunctival eye care, and hepatitis B immunization. For more information, see Chapter 8, "Care of the Newborn."

Bibliography

2010 Guidelines for the prevention of perinatal Group B Streptococcal disease. Atlanta (GA): CDC; 2010. Available at: http://www.cdc.gov/groupbstrep/guidelines/guidelines.html. Retrieved December 20, 2011.

Adoption. Committee Opinion No. 528. American College of Obstetricians and Gynecologists. Obstet Gynecol 2012;119:1320–4.

Air travel during pregnancy. ACOG Committee Opinion No. 443. American College of Obstetricians and Gynecologists. Obstet Gynecol 2009;114: 954–5.

Alto WA. No need for glycosuria/proteinuria screen in pregnant women. J Fam Pract 2005;54:978–83.

American College of Medical Genetics. Technical standards and guidelines for CFTR mutation testing. 2006 ed. Bethesda (MD): ACMG; 2006. Available at: http://www. acmg.net/Pages/ACMG_Activities/stds-2002/cf.htm. Retrieved December 20, 2011.

American College of Obstetricians and Gynecologists. Access to reproductive health care for women with disabilities. In: Special issues in women's health. Washington, DC: ACOG; 2005. p. 39–59.

American College of Obstetricians and Gynecologists. Antepartum fetal surveillance. ACOG Practice Bulletin 9. Washington, DC: ACOG; 1999.

American College of Obstetricians and Gynecologists. External cephalic version. ACOG Practice Bulletin 13. Washington, DC: ACOG; 2000.

American College of Obstetricians and Gynecologists, American College of Medical Genetics. Preconception and prenatal carrier screening for cystic fibrosis : clinical and laboratory guidelines. Washington, DC; ACOG; Bethesda (MD): ACMG; 2001.

American College of Radiology. Practice guideline for the performance of obstetrical ultrasound. In: ACR practice guidelines and technical standards, 2007. Reston (VA): ACR; 2007. Available at: http://www.acr.org/SecondaryMainMenuCategories/quality_safety/guidelines/us/us_obstetrical.aspx. Retrieved October 15, 2009; December 20, 2011.

American Dental Association. Women's oral health issues. Chicago (IL): ADA; 2006. Available at: http://www.ada.org/sections/professionalResources/pdfs/healthcare_womens.pdf. Retrieved December 20, 2011.

At-risk drinking and alcohol dependence: obstetric and gynecologic implications. Committee Opinion No. 496. American College of Obstetricians and Gynecologists. Obstet Gynecol 2011;118:383–8.

Atrash HK, Johnson K, Adams M, Cordero JF, Howse J. Preconception care for improving perinatal outcomes: the time to act. Matern Child Health J 2006;10(suppl):S3–11.

Briggs GG, Freeman RK, Yaffe SJ. Drugs in pregnancy and lactation: a reference guide to fetal and neonatal risk. 9th. Philadelphia (PA): Wolters Kluwer: Lippincott Williams & Wilkins; 2011.

Castles A, Adams EK, Melvin CL, Kelsch C, Boulton ML. Effects of smoking during pregnancy. Five meta-analyses. Am J Prev Med 1999;16:208–15.

Circumcision. ACOG Committee Opinion No. 260. American College of Obstetricians and Gynecologists. Obstet Gynecol 2001;98:707–8.

Controversies concerning vitamin K and the newborn. American Academy of Pediatrics Committee on Fetus and Newborn. Pediatrics 2003;112:191–2.

Counseling and interventions to prevent tobacco use and tobacco-caused disease in adults and pregnant women: U.S. Preventive Services Task Force reaffirmation recommendation statement. U.S. Preventive Services Task Force. Ann Intern Med 2009;150:551–5.

Cuckle H, Benn P, Wright D. Down syndrome screening in the first and/or second trimester: model predicted performance using meta-analysis parameters. Semin Perinatol 2005;29:252–7.

Cuckle HS, Wald NJ, Thompson SG. Estimating a woman's risk of having a pregnancy associated with Down's syndrome using her age and serum alpha-fetoprotein level. Br J Obstet Gynaecol 1987;94:387–402.

Cunniff C. Prenatal screening and diagnosis for pediatricians. American Academy of Pediatrics Committee on Genetics. Pediatrics 2004;114:889–94.

Dietz PM, England LJ, Shapiro-Mendoza CK, Tong VT, Farr SL, Callaghan WM. Infant morbidity and mortality attributable to prenatal smoking in the U.S. Am J Prev Med 2010;39:45–52.

Exercise during pregnancy and the postpartum period. ACOG Committee Opinion No. 267. American College of Obstetricians and Gynecologists. Obstet Gynecol 2002;99:171–3.

Family history as a risk assessment tool. Committee Opinion No. 478. American College of Obstetricians and Gynecologists. Obstet Gynecol 2011;117:747–50.

Gribble RK, Fee SC, Berg RL. The value of routine urine dipstick screening for protein at each prenatal visit. Am J Obstet Gynecol 1995;173:214–7.

Guttmacher Institute. Substance abuse during pregnancy. State Policies in Brief. New York (NY): Guttmacher Institute; 2011. p. 1-2. Available at: http://www.guttmacher.org/statecenter/spibs/spib_SADP.pdf. Retrieved December 20, 2011.

Hook EB. Rates of chromosome abnormalities at different maternal ages. Obstet Gynecol 1981;58:282–5.

Health care for pregnant and postpartum incarcerated women and adolescent females. ACOG Committee Opinion No. 511. American College Obstetricians and Gynecologists. Obstet Gynecol 2011;118:1198–202.

Ickovics JR, Kershaw TS, Westdahl C, Magriples U, Massey Z, Reynolds H, et al. Group prenatal care and perinatal outcomes: a randomized controlled trial. Obstet Gynecol 2007;110:330–9.

Ickovics JR, Kershaw TS, Westdahl C, Rising SS, Klima C, Reynolds H, et al. Group prenatal care and preterm birth weight: results from a matched cohort study at public clinics. Obstet Gynecol 2003;102:1051–7.

Influenza vaccination during pregnancy. Committee Opinion No. 468. American College of Obstetricians and Gynecologists. Obstet Gynecol 2010;116:1006–7.

Informed consent. ACOG Committee Opinion No. 439. American College of Obstetricians and Gynecologists. Obstet Gynecol 2009;114:401–8.

Intimate partner violence. Committee Opinion No. 518. American College of Obstetricians and Gynecologists. Obstet Gynecol 2012;119:412–7.

Invasive prenatal testing for aneuploidy. ACOG Practice Bulletin No. 88. American College of Obstetricians and Gynecologists. Obstet Gynecol 2007;110:1459–67.

Klein JD. Adolescent pregnancy: current trends and issues. American Academy of Pediatrics Committee on Adolescence. Pediatrics 2005;116:281–6.

Lead screeening during pregnancy and lactation. Committee Opinion No. 533. American College of Obstetricians and Gynecologists. Obstet Gynecol 2012;120:416–20.

Malone FD, Canick JA, Ball RH, Nyberg DA, Comstock CH, Bukowski R, et al. First-trimester or second-trimester screening, or both, for Down's syndrome. First- and Second-Trimester Evaluation of Risk (FASTER) Research Consortium. N Engl J Med 2005;353:2001–11.

Management of diabetes from preconception to the postnatal period: summary of NICE guidance. Guideline Development Group. BMJ 2008;336(7646):714–7.

March of Dimes. Toward improving the outcome of pregnancy : the 90s and beyond. Committee on Perinatal Health. White Plains (NY): National Foundation--March of Dimes; 1993.

McDonald SD, Walker MC, Ohlsson A, Murphy KE, Beyene J, Perkins SL. The effect of tobacco exposure on maternal and fetal thyroid function. Eur J Obstet Gynecol Reprod Biol 2008;140:38–42.

Methamphetamine abuse in women of reproductive age. Committee Opinion No. 479. American College of Obstetricians and Gynecologists. Obstet Gynecol 2011;117:751–5.

Mode of term singleton breech delivery. ACOG Committee Opinion No. 340. American College of Obstetricians and Gynecologists. Obstet Gynecol 2006;108:235–7.

Morris JK, Wald NJ, Mutton DE, Alberman E. Comparison of models of maternal age-specific risk for Down syndrome live births. Prenat Diagn 2003;23:252–8.

Murray N, Homer CS, Davis GK, Curtis J, Mangos G, Brown MA. The clinical utility of routine urinalysis in pregnancy: a prospective study. Med J Aust 2002;177:477–80.

Nausea and vomiting of pregnancy. ACOG Practice Bulletin No. 52. American College of Obstetricians and Gynecologists. Obstet Gynecol 2004;103:803–14.

Newborn screening. Committee Opinion No. 481. American College of Obstetricians and Gynecologists. Obstet Gynecol 2011;117:762–5.

Obesity in pregnancy. ACOG Committee Opinion No. 315. American College of Obstetricians and Gynecologists. Obstet Gynecol 2005;106:671–5.

Obstetric management of patients with spinal cord injuries. ACOG Committee Opinion: No. 275. American College of Obstetricians and Gynecologists. Obstet Gynecol 2002;100:625–7.

Opioid abuse, dependence, and addiction in pregnancy. Committee Opinion No. 524. American College of Obstetricians and Gynecologists. Obstet Gynecol 2012;119:1070–6.

Oral intake during labor. ACOG Committee Opinion No. 441. American College of Obstetricians and Gynecologists. Obstet Gynecol 2009;114:714.

Otten JJ, Hellwig JP, Meyers LD, editors. DRI, dietary reference intakes : the essential guide to nutrient requirements. Institute of Medicine. Washington, D.C.: National Academies Press; 2006.

Perinatal risks associated with assisted reproductive technology. ACOG Committee Opinion No. 324. American College of Obstetricians and Gynecologists. Obstet Gynecol 2005;106:1143–6.

Preconception and prenatal carrier screening for genetic diseases in individuals of Eastern European Jewish descent. ACOG Committee Opinion No. 442. American College of Obstetricians and Gynecologists. Obstet Gynecol 2009;114:950–3.

Prenatal and perinatal human immunodeficiency virus testing: expanded recommendations. ACOG Committee Opinion No. 418. American College of Obstetricians and Gynecologists. Obstet Gynecol 2008;112:739–42.

Rasmussen KM, Yaktine AL, editors. Weight gain during pregnancy: reexamining the guidelines. Institute of Medicine. Washington, DC: National Academies Press; 2009.

Ross AC, Taylor CL, Yaktine AL, Del Valle HB, editors. Dietary reference intakes: calcium vitamin D. Committee to Review Dietary Reference Intakes for Vitamin D and Calcium, Food and Nutrition Board, Institute of Medicine. Washington, D.C.: National Academies Press; 2011.

Screening and diagnosis of gestational diabetes mellitus. Committee Opinion No. 504. American College of Obstetricians and Gynecologists. Obstet Gynecol 2011;118:751–3.

Screening for fetal chromosomal abnormalities. ACOG Practice Bulletin No. 77. American College of Obstetricians and Gynecologists. Obstet Gynecol 2007;109:217–27.

Smoking cessation during pregnancy. Committee Opinion No. 471. American College of Obstetricians and Gynecologists. Obstet Gynecol 2010;116:1241–4.

Spinillo A, Nicola S, Piazzi G, Ghazal K, Colonna L, Baltaro F. Epidemiological correlates of preterm premature rupture of membranes. Int J Gynaecol Obstet 1994;47:7–15.

Subclinical hypothyroidism in pregnancy. ACOG Committee Opinion No. 381. American College of Obstetricians and Gynecologists. Obstet Gynecol 2007;110:959–60.

Substance abuse reporting and pregnancy: the role of the obstetrician-gynecologist. Committee Opinion No. 473. American College of Obstetricians and Gynecologists. Obstet Gynecol 2011;117:200–1.

The importance of preconception care in the continuum of women's health care. ACOG Committee Opinion No. 313. American College of Obstetricians and Gynecologists. Obstet Gynecol 2005;106:665–6.

Toriello HV, Meck JM. Statement on guidance for genetic counseling in advanced paternal age. Professional Practice and Guidelines Committee. Genet Med 2008;10:457–60.

Treating tobacco use and dependence: 2008 update. Clinical Practice Guideline. Rockville (MD): U.S. Department of Health and Human Services; 2008. Available at: http://www.ahrq.gov/path/tobacco.htm. Retrieved May 16, 2012.

U.S. Dept. of Health and Human Services Public Health Service Office of the Surgeon General. The health consequences of smoking: a report of the Surgeon General. Washington, D.C.: USDHHS; 2004. Available at: http://www.cdc.gov/tobacco/data_statistics/sgr/2004/complete_report/index.htm. Retrieved December 21, 2011.

Ultrasonography in pregnancy. ACOG Practice Bulletin No. 101. American College of Obstetricians and Gynecologists. Obstet Gynecol 2009;113:451–61.

Umbilical cord blood banking. ACOG Committee Opinion No. 399. American College of Obstetricians and Gynecologists. Obstet Gynecol 2008;111:475–7.

Update on carrier screening for cystic fibrosis. Committee Opinion No. 486. American College of Obstetricians and Gynecologists. Obstet Gynecol 2011;117:1028–31.

Update on immunization and pregnancy: tetanus, diphtheria, and pertussis vaccination. Committee Opinion No. 521. American College of Obstetricians and Gynecologists. Obstet Gynecol 2012;119:690–1.

Vaginal birth after previous cesarean delivery. Practice Bulletin No. 115. American College of Obstetricians and Gynecologists. Obstet Gynecol 2010;116:450–63.

Villar J, Say L, Shennan A, Lindheimer M, Duley L, Conde-Agudelo A, et al. Methodological and technical issues related to the diagnosis, screening, prevention, and treatment of pre-eclampsia and eclampsia. Int J Gynaecol Obstet 2004;85 Suppl 1S28–41.

Vitamin D: screening and supplementation during pregnancy. Committee Opinion No. 495. American College of Obstetricians and Gynecologists. Obstet Gynecol 2011;118:197–8.

Wapner R, Thom E, Simpson JL, Pergament E, Silver R, Filkins K, et al. First-trimester screening for trisomies 21 and 18. First Trimester Maternal Serum Biochemistry and Fetal Nuchal Translucency Screening (BUN) Study Group. N Engl J Med 2003;349:1405–13.

Resources

Aim for a healthy weight. Calculate your body mass index. BMI calculator. Bethesda (MD): NHLBI; 2011. Available at: http://www.nhlbisupport.com/bmi/. Retrieved December 21, 2011.

American Psychiatric Association (APA). Arlington (VA): APA; 2011. Available at: http://www.psych.org/. Retrieved December 20, 2011.

Calculate your body mass index. National Heart, Lung, and Blood Institute. National Institutes of Health. Bethesda (MD): NIH; 2012. Available at: http://www.nhlbisupport.com/bmi/. Retrieved January 13, 2012.

Immunization for women. Washington, DC: American College of Obstetricians and Gynecologists; 2011. Available at: http://immunizationforwomen.org/. Retrieved December 20, 2011.

Institute for Patient- and Family-Centered Care (IPFCC). Bethesda (MD): IPFCC; 2011. Available at: http://www.ipfcc.org/. Retrieved December 20, 2011.

Listeriosis (Listeria) and pregnancy. Atlanta, GA: CDC; 2011. Available at: http://www.cdc.gov/ncbddd/pregnancy_gateway/infections-listeria.html. Retrieved December 20, 2011.

Medications and pregnancy. Atlanta (GA): CDC; 2011. Available at: http://www.cdc.gov/ncbddd/pregnancy_gateway/meds/index.html. Retrieved December 20, 2011.

Medication use during pregnancy. Atlanta (GA): CDC; 2011. Available at: http://www.cdc.gov/features/medicationspregnancy/. Retrieved December 20, 2011.

National Center for Complementary and Alternative Medicine. National Institutes of Health. Bethesda (MD): NIH; 2011. Available at: http://nccam.nih.gov/. Retrieved December 21, 2011.

Online Mendelian Inheritance in Man (OMIM). Baltimore (MD): Johns Hopkins University School of Medicine; 2011. Available at: http://www.ncbi.nlm.nih.gov/omim. Retrieved December 21, 2011.

Organization of Teratology Information Services (OTIS). Tucson (AZ): 2010. Available at: http://www.otispregnancy.org. Retrieved December 21, 2011.

OTIS fact sheets. Tucson (AZ): OTIS; 2010. Available at: http://www.otispregnancy.org/otis-fact-sheets-s13037#1. Retrieved December 21, 2011.

Preconception care. Atlanta (GA): CDC; 2011. Available at: http://www.cdc.gov/ncbddd/preconception/. Retrieved December 20, 2011.

United States. Dietary Guidelines Advisory Committee. Dietary guidelines for Americans. 7th. Washington, D.C.: U.S. Dept. of Agriculture; U.S. Dept. of Health and Human Services; 2010. Available at: http://www.cnpp.usda.gov/Publications/DietaryGuidelines/2010/PolicyDoc/PolicyDoc.pdf Retrieved December 21, 2011.

Vaccines and Immunizations. Atlanta (GA): CDC; 2011. Available at: http://www.cdc.gov/vaccines/. Retrieved December 21, 2011.

Chapter 6

Intrapartum and Postpartum Care of the Mother

The goal of all labor and delivery units is a safe birth for mothers and their newborns. At the same time, staff should attempt to make the patient feel welcome, comfortable, and informed throughout the labor and delivery process. Ongoing risk assessment should determine appropriate care for each woman. The father, partner, or other primary support person should be made to feel welcome and should be encouraged to participate throughout the labor and delivery experience.

Labor and delivery is a normal physiologic process that most women experience without complications. Obstetric staff can greatly enhance this experience for the woman and her family by exhibiting a caring attitude and helping them understand the process. Efforts to promote healthy behaviors can be as effective during labor and delivery as they are during antepartum care. Physical contact between the newborn and the parents in the delivery room should be encouraged. Every effort should be made to foster family interaction and to support the desire of the family to be together.

Because intrapartum complications can arise, sometimes quickly and without warning, ongoing risk assessment and surveillance of the mother and the fetus are essential. A hospital, birthing center within a hospital complex, or a freestanding birthing center that meets the standards of the Accreditation Association for Ambulatory Health Care, The Joint Commission, or the American Association of Birth Centers provides the safest setting for labor, delivery, and the postpartum period. This setting ensures accepted standards of safety that cannot be matched in a home-birthing situation. The collection and analysis of data on the safety and outcome of deliveries in other settings have been problematic. The development of approved, well-designed research protocols, prepared in consultation with obstetric departments and their related institutional review boards, is appropriate to assess safety, feasibility, and birth outcomes in such settings.

Planned Home Birth

Although the American College of Obstetricians and Gynecologists believes that hospitals and birthing centers are the safest setting for birth, it respects the right of a woman to make a medically informed decision about the delivery. Women inquiring about planned home birth should be informed of its risks and benefits based on recent evidence. Specifically, they should be informed that although the absolute risk may be low, planned home birth is associated with a twofold to threefold increased risk of neonatal death when compared with planned hospital birth. Importantly, women should be informed that the appropriate selection of candidates for home birth; the availability of a certified nurse–midwife, certified midwife, or physician practicing within an integrated and regulated health system; ready access to consultation; and assurance of safe and timely transport to nearby hospitals are critical to reducing perinatal mortality rates and achieving favorable home birth outcomes.

Underwater Births

Over the past 25 years, underwater birth has become more popular in certain parts of the world despite a paucity of data demonstrating that it is either beneficial or safe. Underwater birth occurs either intentionally or accidentally after water immersion for labor, a procedure promoted primarily as a means of decreasing maternal discomfort. Although there is no suggested benefit of underwater birth to the newborn, the morbidities identified in clinical reports have raised concerns that this mode of delivery may not be safe. Numerous case reports have associated underwater birth with respiratory distress, hyponatremia, infections, hypoxic ischemic encephalopathy, ruptured umbilical cords, seizures, tachycardia and fever (related to water temperature of the bath), and near drowning in newborns or fetuses. There is no convincing evidence of benefit to the neonate but some concern for serious harm. Therefore, underwater birth should be considered an experimental procedure that should not be performed except within the context of an appropriately designed randomized controlled trial after informed parental consent.

Admission

Pregnant women may come to a hospital's labor and delivery area not only for obstetric care, but also for evaluation and treatment of nonobstetric illnesses. However, a nonobstetric condition, such as highly transmissible infectious diseases (eg, varicella), is best treated in another area of the hospital. The obstetric department should establish policies, in consultation with other hospital units or personnel, for coordinated care of pregnant women. Departments should agree on the conditions that are best treated in the labor and delivery area and those that should be treated in other hospital care units. Qualified obstetric care providers should evaluate patients with medical or surgical conditions that could reasonably be expected to cause obstetric complications. The priority of that evaluation and the site where it is best performed should be determined by the patient's needs (including gestational age of the fetus) and the care unit's ability to provide for those needs. The obstetric department also should establish policies for the admission of nonobstetric patients according to state regulations. Federal and state regulations address the management and treatment of patients in hospital acute-care areas, including labor and delivery (see also Appendix G).

Written departmental policies regarding triage of patients who come to a labor and delivery area should be reviewed periodically for compliance with appropriate regulations. A pregnant woman who comes to the labor and delivery area should be evaluated in a timely fashion. Obstetric nursing staff may perform this initial evaluation, which should minimally include assessment of the following:

- Maternal vital signs
- Fetal heart rate
- Uterine contractions

The responsible obstetric provider should be informed promptly if any of the following findings are present or suspected:

- Vaginal bleeding
- Acute abdominal pain
- Temperature of (100.4°F) or higher
- Preterm labor
- Preterm premature rupture of membranes (PROM)
- Hypertension
- Category II or category III (nonreassuring) change throughout fetal heart rate pattern (see also "Fetal Heart Rate Monitoring" in this chapter)

Any patient who is suspected to be in labor, has rupture of the membranes, or has vaginal bleeding should be evaluated promptly in an obstetric service area.

Whenever a pregnant woman is evaluated for labor, the following factors should be assessed and recorded in the patient's permanent medical record:

- Maternal vital signs
- Frequency and duration of uterine contractions
- Documentation of fetal well-being
- Cervical dilatation and effacement, unless contraindicated (eg, placenta previa, preterm PROM) or cervical length as ascertained by transvaginal ultrasonography
- Fetal presentation and station of the presenting part
- Status of the membranes
- Date and time of the patient's arrival and of notification of the health care provider
- Estimation of fetal weight and assessment of maternal pelvis

If the patient is in prodromal or early labor and has no complications, admission to the labor and delivery area may be deferred after initial evaluation and documentation of fetal well-being (see also Appendix G). A patient with a transmissible infection should be admitted to a site where isolation techniques may be followed according to hospital policy.

If a woman has received prenatal care and a recent examination has confirmed the normal progress of pregnancy, her admission evaluation may be limited to an interval history and physical examination directed at the presenting condition. Previously identified risk factors should be recorded in the medical record. If no new risk factors are found, attention may be focused on the following historic factors:

- Time of onset and frequency of contractions
- Status of the membranes
- Presence or absence of bleeding
- Fetal movement
- History of allergies
- Time, content, and amount of the most recent food or fluid ingestion
- Use of any medication

Serologic testing for hepatitis B virus surface antigen may be necessary, as described in Chapter 10. Women who have not received prenatal care, had episodic prenatal care, or who received care late in pregnancy are more likely to have sexually transmitted infections and substance abuse problems. Social problems, such as poverty and family conflict, also may affect patients' health. Because of these factors, a shortened obstetric hospital stay poses even greater problems for patients who have had no prenatal care. Routine obstetric screening tests (eg, hemoglobin level, blood type, and Rh factor), social intervention, and additional education may be needed within this limited period. Women with unidentified alcohol or drug dependence often opt for early postpartum discharge or leave the hospital against medical advice putting themselves and their infants in danger.

If no complications are detected during initial assessment in the labor and delivery area and if contraindications have been ruled out, qualified nursing personnel may perform the initial pelvic examination. Once the results of the examination have been obtained and documented, the health care provider responsible for the woman's care in the labor and delivery area should be informed of her status. The health care provider can make a decision regarding her management. The timing of the health care provider's arrival in the labor area should be based on this information and hospital policy. If epidural, spinal, or general anesthesia is anticipated, or if conditions exist that place the patient at risk of requiring rapid institution of an anesthetic, anesthesia personnel should be informed of the patient's presence soon after her admission. If a preterm delivery, infected or depressed newborn, or newborn with a prenatally diagnosed congenital anomaly is expected, the pediatric provider who will assume responsibility for the newborn's care should be informed. When the patient has been examined and instructions regarding her management have been given and noted on her medical record, all necessary consent forms should be signed and incorporated into the medical record.

By 36 weeks of gestation, preregistration for labor and delivery at the hospital should be confirmed and a copy of the prenatal medical record, which includes information pertaining to the patient's antepartum course (see also Appendix A), should be on file in the hospital's labor registration area. If electronic medical records are used, the electronic prenatal records should be accessible. Consideration should be given to providing periodic updates to the prenatal medical record on file.

At the time of a patient's admission to the labor and delivery area, pertinent information from the prenatal record should be noted in the admission records. Because labor and delivery is a dynamic process, all entries into a patient's medical record should include the date and time of occurrence. Blood typing and screening tests need not be repeated if they were performed during the antepartum period and no antibodies were present, provided that the report is in the hospital records. If the results of the woman's antenatal laboratory evaluation are not known and cannot be obtained, blood typing, Rh D type determination, hepatitis B virus antigen testing, and serologic testing for syphilis should be performed before the woman is discharged. State laws governing testing of umbilical cord blood may vary. Serologic testing for human immunodeficiency virus (HIV) infection and other tests should be encouraged and performed according to state law. Rapid HIV testing can be done in labor if the mother's HIV status is unknown (see also "Routine Laboratory Testing in Pregnancy" in Chapter 5 and "Human Immunodeficiency Virus" in Chapter 10). Collection of umbilical cord blood may be useful for subsequent evaluation of ABO incompatibility if the mother is type O. Policies should be developed to ensure expeditious preparation of blood products for transfusion if the patient is at increased risk of hemorrhage or if the need arises.

At all times in the hospital labor and delivery area, the safety and well-being of the mother and the fetus are the primary concern and responsibility of the obstetric staff. This concern, however, should not unnecessarily restrict the activity of women with uncomplicated labor and delivery, or exclude people who are supportive of her. The woman should have the option to stay out of bed during the early stages of labor, to ambulate, and to rest in a comfortable chair as long as the fetal status is reassuring. Practices such as showers during labor, placement of intravenous lines, use of fetal heart rate monitoring, and restrictions on ambulation should be reviewed in departmental policies. These policies should take into consideration physicians' preferences as well as patients' desires for comfort, privacy, and a sense of participation. Likewise, the use of drugs for relief of pain during labor and delivery should depend on the needs and desires of the woman. The development of a birth plan that has been discussed previously with a woman's health care provider and placed in her medical record may promote her participation in and satisfaction with her care.

The woman's health care team should communicate regarding all factors that may pose a risk to her, her fetus, or her newborn. Obstetric department policies should include recommendations for transmitting to the nursery those maternal and fetal historical and laboratory data that may affect the care of the newborn. Information on conditions that may influence neonatal care should be communicated, as well. The lack of such data, perhaps because of a lack of prenatal care, also should be made known to the nursery personnel. The physician who will care for the newborn should be identified on the maternal medical record (see Appendix A). Health care professionals who provide anesthesia should be notified of women who may be at significant risk of complications from anesthetic procedures (eg, women with hypertension, morbid obesity, or receiving anticoagulation).

Labor

The onset of true labor is established by observing progressive change in a woman's cervix in the setting of regular, phasic, uterine contractions. This may require two or more cervical examinations that are separated by an adequate period of time to observe change. Even a well-prepared woman may arrive at the hospital labor and delivery area before true labor has begun. A policy that both allows for adequate evaluation of patients for the presence of labor and prevents unnecessary admissions to the labor and delivery unit is advisable (see also Appendix G).

False Labor at Term

Uterine contractions in the absence of cervical change are commonly referred to as false labor. Treatment for this condition should be based on individual circumstances. Patients who are having uterine contractions and are not yet in active labor may be observed for evidence of cervical change in a casual, comfortable area. The patient may be discharged, after observation and evaluation by appropriate hospital-designated personnel and assurance of fetal well-being (see also Appendix G).

Premature Rupture of Membranes at Term

The definition of *PROM* is rupture of membranes before the onset of labor. Membrane rupture that occurs before 37 weeks of gestation is referred to as preterm PROM (see also "Premature Rupture of Membranes" in Chapter 7). At term, PROM complicates approximately 8% of pregnancies and generally is followed by the onset of spontaneous labor and delivery. Although term PROM results from the normal physiologic process of progressive membrane weakening, preterm PROM can result from a wide array of pathologic mechanisms acting individually or in concert. The gestational age and fetal status at membrane rupture have significant implications in the etiology and consequences of PROM. Management may be dictated by the presence of overt intrauterine infection, advanced labor, or fetal compromise. When such factors are not present, especially with preterm PROM, obstetric management may have a significant effect on maternal and infant outcomes. The most significant maternal risk of term PROM is intrauterine infection, a risk that increases with the duration of membrane rupture. Fetal risks associated with term PROM include umbilical cord compression and ascending infection. An accurate assessment of gestational age and knowledge of the maternal, fetal, and neonatal risks are essential to appropriate evaluation, counseling, and care of patients with PROM.

The diagnosis of PROM is established by history, physical examination, and laboratory test result confirmation. Diagnosis based on history alone is correct in some patients. Nevertheless, all patients reporting symptoms that suggest ruptured membranes should be examined with a sterile speculum as soon as possible to confirm this diagnosis. In any labor occurring after rupture of membranes, vaginal examinations should be limited in number and attention paid to clean technique. Gross pooling of amniotic fluid in the vagina usually is diagnostic of PROM. Supportive laboratory testing includes vaginal pH, fern testing, and ultrasound estimation of amniotic fluid volume. The obstetric providers who perform the examination to confirm or rule out PROM should be aware of the causes of false-positive and false-negative test results that occur with the use of pH and fern testing. These causes include leakage of alkaline urine, cervical mucus, bacterial vaginosis, and blood. Given equivocal findings, exclusion of PROM remote from term may require an amniocentesis with instillation of indigo carmine dye.

In all patients with PROM, gestational age, fetal presentation, and well-being should be determined. Delivery, usually by induction of labor, is recommended when PROM occurs at or beyond 34 weeks of gestation. However, at any gestational age, a patient with evident intrauterine infection, abruptio placentae, or evidence of fetal compromise is best cared for by expeditious delivery. In the absence of an indication for immediate delivery, swab specimens for diagnosis of *Chlamydia trachomatis* and *Neisseria gonorrhoeae* may be obtained from the cervix, if appropriate. The need for group B streptococcal intrapartum prophylaxis should be determined if preterm PROM occurs.

Management of Labor

Ideally, every woman admitted to the labor and delivery area should know who her principal, designated health care provider will be. Members of the obstetric team should observe the patient to follow the progress of labor, record her vital signs and the fetal heart rate in her medical record at regular intervals, and make an effort to ensure her understanding of the events that are occurring. The health care provider principally responsible for the patient's care should be kept informed of her progress and notified promptly of any abnormality. When the patient is in active labor, that health care provider should be readily available (see also "Cesarean Delivery" later in this chapter).

Patients in active labor should avoid oral ingestion of solid foods, but modest intake of clear liquids is acceptable in an uncomplicated laboring patient. Ideally, intravenous access should be secured when the active phase of labor begins. The progress of labor should be evaluated by periodic vaginal examinations, and the obstetric provider should be notified of the patient's labor progress. Sterile, water-soluble lubricants may be used to reduce discomfort during vaginal examinations. Antiseptics, such as povidone-iodine and hexachlorophene, have not been shown to decrease infections acquired during the intrapartum period. Furthermore, these agents may produce local irritation and are absorbed through maternal mucous membranes.

Evaluation of the quality of the uterine contractions and pelvic examinations should be sufficient to detect abnormalities in the progress of labor. Vital signs should be recorded at regular intervals of at least every 4 hours. This frequency may be increased, particularly as active labor progresses, according to clinical signs and symptoms, and is increased in the presence of complications, such as infection or preeclampsia. Documentation of the course of a woman's labor may include, but need not be limited to, the presence of physicians, midwives, or nurses, position changes, cervical status, oxygen and drug administration, blood pressure levels, temperature, amniotomy or spontaneous rupture of membranes, color of amniotic fluid, and Valsalva maneuver.

Fetal Heart Rate Monitoring

Either electronic fetal heart rate (FHR) monitoring or intermittent auscultation may be used to determine fetal status during labor. Obstetric unit guidelines should clearly delineate the procedures to be followed for using these techniques according to the phase and stage of labor.

The method of FHR monitoring for fetal surveillance during labor may vary depending on the risk assessment at admission, the preferences of the patient and obstetric staff, and departmental policy. If no risk factors are present at the time of the patient's admission, a standard approach to fetal surveillance is to determine, evaluate, and record the FHR every 30 minutes in the active phase of the first stage of labor and at least every 15 minutes in the second stage of labor.

If risk factors are present at admission or appear during labor, there is no difference in perinatal outcome between intermittent auscultation and continuous fetal monitoring if one of the following methods for FHR monitoring is used:

- During the active phase of the first stage of labor, the FHR should be determined, evaluated, and recorded at least every 15 minutes, preferably before, during, and after a uterine contraction, when intermittent auscultation is used. If continuous electronic FHR monitoring is used, the heart rate tracing should be evaluated at least every 15 minutes.

- During the second stage of labor, the FHR should be determined, evaluated, and recorded at least every 5 minutes if auscultation is used. If continuous electronic FHR monitoring is used, the tracing should be evaluated at least every 5 minutes.

The appropriate use of electronic FHR monitoring includes recording and interpreting the tracings. Nonreassuring findings should be noted and communicated to the physician or certified nurse–midwife so that the appropriate intervention can occur. When a change in the rate or pattern has been noted, it also is important to document a subsequent return to reassuring findings. The nomenclature used to describe electronic FHR monitoring and contraction patterns should be consistent with the guidelines developed at the 2008 *Eunice Kennedy Shriver* National Institute of Child Health and Human Development Workshop. This terminology should be used in both medical record entries and in verbal communication among obstetric personnel. Uterine contractions should be described as normal (five contractions or fewer in 10 minutes) or tachysystole (more than five contractions in 10 minutes) averaged over a 30-minute window. Fetal heart rate patterns are described by baseline rate, variability, accelerations, and decelerations, which can be early, late, or variable. Based on these characteristics of FHR monitoring, tracings can be categorized using a three-tier system (Box 6-1). Category I FHR tracing results are normal and may be monitored in a routine manner, and no specific action is required. Category II tracing results are indeterminate, requiring evaluation and continued surveillance and re-evaluation. Category III tracing results are abnormal and require prompt evaluation and management because they are predictive of abnormal fetal acid–base status.

Internal FHR monitoring and internal uterine pressure monitoring may be used when needed to gain further information about fetal status and uterine contractility, respectively. Relative contraindications to internal fetal monitoring include maternal HIV infection and other high-risk factors of fetal infection, including herpes simplex virus and hepatitis B virus or hepatitis C virus. However, if there are indications for fetal scalp monitoring, it is reasonable in a woman who has a history of a recurrence of herpes simplex virus and no active lesions.

Box 6-1. Three-Tiered Fetal Heart Rate Interpretation System

Category I

Category I FHR tracings include all of the following:

- Baseline rate: 110–160 beats per minute
- Baseline FHR variability: moderate
- Late or variable decelerations: absent
- Early decelerations: present or absent
- Accelerations: present or absent

Category II

Category II FHR tracings include all FHR tracings not categorized as Category I or Category III. Category II tracings may represent an appreciable fraction of those encountered in clinical care. Examples of Category II FHR tracings include any of the following:

Baseline rate

- Bradycardia not accompanied by absent baseline variability
- Tachycardia

Baseline FHR variability

- Minimal baseline variability
- Absent baseline variability with no recurrent decelerations
- Marked baseline variability

Accelerations

- Absence of induced accelerations after fetal stimulation

Periodic or episodic decelerations

- Recurrent variable decelerations accompanied by minimal or moderate baseline variability
- Prolonged deceleration more than 2 minutes but less than 10 minutes
- Recurrent late decelerations with moderate baseline variability
- Variable decelerations with other characteristics, such as slow return to baseline, overshoots, or "shoulders"

(continued)

Box 6-1. Three-Tiered Fetal Heart Rate Interpretation System
(continued)

Category III

Category III FHR tracings include either:

• Absent baseline FHR and any of the following:

 —Recurrent late decelerations

 —Recurrent variable decelerations

 —Bradycardia

• Sinusoidal pattern

Abbreviation: FHR, fetal heart rate.
Macones GA, Hankins GD, Spong CY, Hauth J, Moore T. The 2008 National Institutes of Child Health and Human Development workshop report on electronic fetal heart monitoring: update on definitions, interpretation, and research guidelines. Obstet Gynecol 2008;112:661–6.

Fetal scalp or acoustic stimulation that results in acceleration of the FHR is reassuring when the FHR pattern is difficult to interpret. If electronic FHR monitoring is used, all FHR tracings should be identified with the patient's name, hospital number, and the date and time of admission. All FHR tracings should be easily retrievable from storage so that the events of labor can be studied in proper relationship to the tracings.

Induction of Labor and Cervical Ripening

The goal of induction of labor is to achieve vaginal delivery by stimulating uterine contractions before the spontaneous onset of labor. Generally, induction of labor has merit as a therapeutic option when the benefits of expeditious delivery outweigh the risks of continuing the pregnancy. The benefits of labor induction must be weighed against the potential maternal and fetal risks associated with this procedure.

Methods used for induction of labor include administration of oxytocic agents, membrane stripping, and amniotomy. If the cervix is unfavorable for induction, cervical ripening may be beneficial and should be considered. Cervical ripening facilitates the process of cervical softening, thinning, and dilating with resultant reduction in the rate of failed induction and induction-to-delivery time. Effective methods for cervical ripening include the use of mechanical cervical dilators and administration of synthetic prostaglandin E_1 and prostaglandin E_2.

Indications for induction of labor are not absolute but should take into account maternal and fetal conditions, gestational age, cervical status, and other factors. Elective inductions should not be performed before 39 weeks of gestation. The individual patient and clinical situation should be considered in determining when induction of labor is contraindicated. Generally, the contraindications to labor induction are the same as those for spontaneous labor and vaginal delivery.

The patient should be counseled regarding the indications for induction, the agents and methods of labor stimulation, and the possible need for repeat induction or cesarean delivery. Additional requirements for cervical ripening and induction of labor include assessment of the cervix, pelvis, fetal size, and presentation. Monitoring FHR and uterine contractions is recommended for any high-risk patient in active labor.

Each hospital's department of obstetrics and gynecology should develop written protocols for preparing and administering oxytocin solution or other agents for labor induction or augmentation. Indications for induction and augmentation of labor should be stated. Personnel who are familiar with the effects of the agents used and who are able to identify both maternal and fetal complications should be in attendance during administration of the induction agent(s). The qualifications of personnel authorized to administer oxytocic agents for this purpose should be described. The methods for assessment of the woman and the fetus before and during administration of these agents should be specified. A physician capable of performing a cesarean delivery should be readily available.

Amnioinfusion

The transcervical infusion of sterile, balanced salt solutions during labor (amnioinfusion) may be used to ameliorate severe, variable decelerations in the FHR tracing that are suspected to be caused by umbilical cord compression. Meta-analysis confirms that amnioinfusion lowers caesarean delivery rates in the setting of oligohydramnios with repetitive variable FHR decelerations. There is no proven benefit of amnioinfusion for other FHR abnormalities, such as late decelerations, and the resultant increase in uterine tone may exacerbate underlying uteroplacental vascular insufficiency. Because it is possible to introduce fluid into the uterus at too rapid a rate, each obstetric unit should establish a protocol for intrauterine pressure monitoring during amnioinfusion, or limitations of the volume and infusion rate when the technique is used. Based on the totality of published data, routine prophylactic amnioinfusion for meconium-stained amniotic fluid is not indicated. However, amnioinfusion is a reasonable approach to treatment of repetitive, variable decelerations irrespective of amniotic fluid meconium status.

Analgesia and Anesthesia

Management of discomfort and pain during labor and delivery is an essential part of good obstetric practice. It is the responsibility of the physician or certified nurse–midwife, in consultation with the anesthesiologist, if appropriate, to develop the most appropriate response to the woman's request for analgesia or anesthesia. Analgesia or anesthesia during labor and delivery has no lasting effect on the physiologic status of the neonate. No evidence exists that suggests that the administration of analgesia or anesthesia during childbirth per se has an effect on the child's later mental and neurologic development. In the absence of a medical contraindication, maternal request is a sufficient medical indication for pain relief during labor.

Some patients tolerate the pain of labor by using techniques learned in childbirth preparation programs. Although specific techniques vary, classes usually seek to relieve pain through the general principles of education, support, relaxation, paced breathing, focusing, and touch. The staff at the bedside should be knowledgeable about these pain management techniques and should be supportive of the patient's decision to use them.

Available Methods of Analgesia and Anesthesia

Available methods of obstetric analgesia and anesthesia include parenteral agents and regional, general, and local anesthesia. The choice and availability of analgesic and anesthetic techniques depends on the experience and judgment of the obstetrician and anesthesiologist, the physical condition of the patient, the circumstances of labor and delivery, and the personal preferences of the patient.

Parenteral Agents

Various opioid agonists and opioid agonist–antagonists are available for systemic analgesia and can be administered during prodromal and early labor to allow the patient to rest. These agents can be given in intermittent doses on patient request or via patient-controlled administration. The decision to use parenteral agents to manage labor pain should be made in collaboration with the patient after a careful discussion of the risks and benefits.

Reports suggest that the analgesic effect of parenteral agents used in labor is limited, and a primary mechanism of action is sedation. Although regional analgesia provides superior pain relief, some women are satisfied with the level of analgesia provided by narcotics when adequate doses are used. Patients exposed to high doses of narcotics are at increased risk of aspiration and respiratory arrest. High doses potentially are depressing to the woman, fetus, and particularly the newborn immediately after delivery. All patients receiving parenteral narcotics should be closely monitored.

Parenteral pain medications for labor pain decrease FHR variability and may limit the obstetrician's ability to interpret the FHR tracing. Therefore, considerations should be given to other agents for pain management in the setting of minimal or absent FHR variability. There has been some concern about fetal safety with the use of nalbuphine hydrochloride; however, there is insufficient evidence at this time to recommend a change in practice with the use of this medication.

Regional Anesthesia

Regional (neuraxial) anesthesia is another option for management of pain, and several methods of administration are available: epidural, spinal, and combined spinal–epidural. In obstetric patients, regional analgesia refers to a partial to complete loss of pain sensation below the T8–T10 level. In addition, a varying degree of motor blockade may be present, depending on the agents used. Ambulation to some extent may be possible when using regional analgesia, depending on the technique used, the experience of the anesthesiologist, and the patient's response. Data indicate that low-dose neuraxial analgesia administered in early labor does not increase the rate of cesarean delivery and some techniques may shorten the duration of labor for some patients. Thus, there seems to be little justification to withhold this form of pain relief from women in early labor until an arbitrary cervical dilation is achieved (ie, 4-cm cervical dilation).

When regional anesthesia is administered during labor, the patient's vital signs should be monitored at regular intervals by a qualified member of the health care team. It also should be noted that a low-grade maternal fever might be associated with a normal epidural anesthetic reaction in the absence of infection. If the temperature is greater than (100.4°F), it may be difficult to differentiate this benign febrile response from the temperature elevation associated with chorioamnionitis. In the absence of intra-amniotic infection, neonatal surveillance blood cultures in patients exhibiting this response are negative, indicating no evidence of infection.

Epidural. Epidural analgesia offers one of the most effective forms of intrapartum pain relief and is used in some form by most women in the United States. A catheter is placed in the epidural space, allowing for a continuous infusion or intermittent injection of pain medication during labor. The advantage of this method of analgesia is that the medication may be titrated over the course of labor as needed. In addition, epidural catheters placed for labor may be dosed and used for cesarean delivery, postpartum tubal ligation, postcesarean pain control, or for repair of obstetric lacerations following vaginal delivery, if needed.

Spinal. Spinal techniques usually involve a single injection of medication into the cerebrospinal fluid and can provide excellent surgical anesthesia for procedures of limited duration, such as cesarean delivery or postpartum tubal ligation, as well as analgesia of limited duration during labor. Spinal labor analgesia using primarily opioids with very low doses of local anesthetics can provide excellent analgesia with rapid onset during labor. Placement of a catheter directly into the subarachnoid space can be used to provide continuous spinal analgesia. Because of the relatively high incidence of postdural puncture headache after this technique, it usually is used only for specific indications.

Use of higher-dose local anesthetics can provide sensory anesthesia and motor blockade for vaginal delivery. Such higher dose techniques typically result in profound sensory and motor blockade, which may impair maternal expulsive efforts. Therefore, spinal anesthesia usually is not administered until delivery is imminent or the physician has made a decision to perform an operative delivery.

Combined Spinal-Epidural. Combined spinal–epidural analgesia offers the advantages of the rapid onset of spinal analgesia along with the ability to use the indwelling epidural catheter to prolong analgesia and titrate medication throughout labor. The technique also may be used and dosed to provide anesthesia for a cesarean delivery and the catheter dosed for postcesarean pain control before being removed.

General Anesthesia

Because general anesthesia results in a loss of maternal consciousness, it must be accompanied by airway management by trained anesthesia personnel. General anesthesia is rarely used or necessary for vaginal delivery and should be used only for specific indications.

Local Anesthesia

Local anesthesia is another possible method of pain control. At the time of delivery, local anesthetics may be injected into the tissues of the perineum and the vagina to provide anesthesia for episiotomy, and repair of vaginal and perineal lacerations. Local anesthetics also may be injected to perform pudendal nerve block in patients who did not receive regional anesthesia during labor. This regional block may provide adequate anesthesia for outlet operative deliveries and performance of any necessary episiotomy or repair.

Cesarean Deliveries

For most cesarean deliveries, properly administered regional or general anesthesia are both effective and have little effect on the newborn. Because of potential risks associated with airway management, intubation and the possibility of aspiration during induction of general anesthesia, regional anesthesia is usually the preferred technique and should be available in all hospitals that provide obstetric care. The advantages and disadvantages of both techniques should be discussed with the patient as completely as possible. In some circumstances, when the maternal evaluation indicates it can be safely performed, rapid induction of general anesthesia may be indicated; such circumstances might include a prolapsed umbilical cord with severe fetal bradycardia or an ominous FHR pattern from other or unknown causes.

Administration of Anesthesia Services

It is the responsibility of the director of anesthesia services to make recommendations regarding the clinical privileges of all personnel providing anesthesia services, and all anesthesia services in a given facility should be organized under a single physician director. If obstetric analgesia (other than pudendal or local techniques) is provided by obstetricians, the director of anesthesia services should participate with a representative of the obstetric department in the formulation of procedures designed to ensure the uniform quality of anesthesia services throughout the hospital. Specific recommendations regarding these procedures are provided in the *Accreditation Manual for Hospitals* published by the Joint Commission. The directors of departments providing anesthesia services are responsible for implementing processes to monitor and evaluate the quality and appropriateness of these services in their respective departments.

Regional anesthesia in obstetrics should be initiated and maintained only by health care providers who are approved through the institutional credentialing process to administer or supervise the administration of obstetric anesthesia. These individuals must be qualified to manage anesthetic complications. An obstetrician may administer the anesthesia if granted privileges for these procedures. However, having an anesthesiologist or anesthetist provide this care permits the obstetrician to give undivided attention to the delivery. Regional anesthesia should be administered only after the patient has been examined and the fetal status and progress of labor have been evaluated by a qualified individual. A physician with obstetric privileges who has knowledge of the maternal and fetal status and the progress of labor and who approves initiation of labor anesthesia should be readily available (see also "Cesarean Delivery" later in this chapter) to deal with any obstetric complications that may arise.

Risk Factors and Complications

When any of the following risk factors are present, anesthetic consultation in advance of delivery may be considered to permit formulation of a management plan:

- Marked obesity
- Severe edema or anatomic abnormalities of the face, neck, or spine, including trauma or surgery
- Abnormal dentition, small mandible, or difficulty opening the mouth
- Extremely short stature, short neck, or arthritis of the neck
- Goiter
- Serious maternal medical problems, such as cardiac, pulmonary, or neurologic diseases
- Bleeding disorders
- Severe preeclampsia
- Previous history of anesthetic complications
- Obstetric complications likely to lead to operative delivery (eg, placenta previa or high-order multiple gestation)
- Substance use disorders

When such risk factors are identified, a physician who has the credentials to provide general and regional anesthesia should be consulted in the antepartum period to allow for joint development of a plan of management, including optimal location for delivery. Strategies thereby can be developed to minimize the need for emergency induction of general anesthesia in women for whom this would be hazardous. For those women with risk factors, consideration should be given to the planned placement in early labor of an intravenous line and an epidural catheter or spinal catheter with confirmation that the catheter is functional. If a woman at unusual risk of complications from anesthesia is identified (eg, prior failed intubation), strong consideration should be given to antepartum referral of the patient to allow for delivery at a hospital that can manage such anesthesia on a 24-hour basis.

Aspiration is a significant cause of anesthetic-related maternal morbidity and mortality, and the more acidic the aspirate, the greater the harm done. Therefore, prophylactic administration of an antacid before induction of a major neuraxial or general anesthesia is often appropriate. Particulate antacids may be harmful if aspirated; a clear antacid, such as a solution of 0.3 mol/L of sodium citrate or a similar preparation, may be a safer choice.

On rare occasions, it may be impossible to intubate an obstetric patient after the induction of general anesthesia. Equipment for emergency airway management, such as the laryngeal mask airway, Combitube, and fiberoptic laryngoscope, should be available whenever general anesthesia is administered.

Delivery

Vaginal Delivery

Vaginal delivery is associated with less risk of maternal operative and postoperative complications than nonelective cesarean delivery and results in shorter hospital stays. Vaginal delivery requires consideration of factors, such as the availability of skilled personnel for the delivery (including obstetric attendants and professionals skilled in neonatal resuscitation and anesthesia administration) and the potential need to move a patient from a labor, delivery, and recovery room to an operative suite.

The risk assessment performed on the patient's admission, the course of the patient's labor, the fetal presentation, any abnormalities encountered during the labor process, and the anesthetic technique in use or anticipated for delivery will all have an effect on the need for other professionals. At least one obstetric nurse, preferably the woman's designated primary nurse for the labor, should be present in the delivery room throughout the delivery. Under no circumstances should an attempt be made to delay birth by physical restraint or anesthetic means.

The routine use of episiotomy is not necessary and may lead to an increase in the risk of third-degree and fourth-degree perineal lacerations and a delay in the patient's resumption of sexual activity. Episiotomy should only be done for a specific medical indication. Median episiotomy is associated with higher rates of injury to the anal sphincter and rectum, and mediolateral episiotomy may be preferable to median episiotomy in selected cases.

Vaginal Birth After Cesarean Delivery

The term vaginal birth after cesarean delivery (VBAC) is used to denote a vaginal delivery after a trial of labor in women who have had a previous cesarean delivery, regardless of the outcome. Trial of labor after cesarean delivery (TOLAC) provides women who desire a vaginal delivery with the possibility of achieving that goal—a vaginal birth after cesarean delivery. In addition to fulfilling a patient's preference for vaginal delivery, at an individual level VBAC is associated with decreased maternal morbidity and a decreased risk of complications in future pregnancies. At a population level, VBAC also is associated with a decrease in the overall cesarean delivery rate. Although TOLAC is appropriate for many women with a history of a cesarean delivery, several factors increase the likelihood of a failed trial of labor, which compared with VBAC, is associated with increased maternal and perinatal morbidity. Assessment of individual risks and the likelihood of VBAC is, therefore, important in determining the appropriate candidates for TOLAC (see also "Trial of Labor After Cesarean Delivery" in Chapter 5).

In addition to providing an option for those who want the experience of a vaginal birth, VBAC has several potential health advantages for women. Women who achieve VBAC avoid major abdominal surgery, which results in lower rates of hemorrhage, infection, and a shorter recovery period compared with elective repeat cesarean delivery. Additionally, for those considering larger families, VBAC may avoid potential future maternal consequences of multiple cesarean deliveries, such as hysterectomy; bowel or bladder injury; transfusion; infection; and abnormal placentation, such as placenta previa and placenta accreta.

Neither elective repeat cesarean delivery nor TOLAC is without maternal or neonatal risk. The risks of either approach include maternal hemorrhage, infection, operative injury, thromboembolism, hysterectomy, and death. Most maternal morbidity that occurs during TOLAC occurs when repeat cesarean delivery becomes necessary. Uterine rupture or dehiscence is the outcome associated with TOLAC that most significantly increases the chance of additional maternal and neonatal morbidity. One factor that markedly influences the chance of uterine rupture is the location of the prior incision on the uterus.

The preponderance of evidence suggests that most women with one previous cesarean delivery with a low transverse incision are candidates for and should be counseled about VBAC and offered TOLAC. Conversely, those at high risk of complications (eg, those with previous classical incision or T-incision, prior uterine rupture, or extensive transfundal uterine surgery) and those in whom vaginal delivery is otherwise contraindicated are not generally candidates for planned TOLAC. Individual circumstances must be considered in all cases. Some common situations that may modify the balance of risks and benefits are listed in Box 6-2.

Because of the risks associated with TOLAC and that uterine rupture and other complications may be unpredictable, it is recommended that TOLAC be undertaken in facilities with staff immediately available to provide emergency care. When resources for immediate cesarean delivery are not available, it is important that health care providers and patients considering TOLAC discuss the hospital's resources and availability of obstetric, pediatric, anesthetic, and operating room staffs. Patients should be clearly informed of potential increased

---

Box 6-2. Selected Clinical Factors Associated With
Trial of Labor After Previous Cesarean Delivery Success

Increased Probability of Success (Strong Predictors)
- Prior vaginal birth
- Spontaneous labor

Decreased Probability of Success (Other Predictors)
- Recurrent indication for initial cesarean delivery (labor dystocia)
- Increased maternal age
- Nonwhite ethnicity
- Gestational age greater than 40 weeks
- Maternal obesity
- Preeclampsia
- Short interpregnancy interval
- Increased neonatal birth weight

Vaginal birth after previous cesarean delivery. Practice Bulletin No. 115. American College of Obstetricians and Gynecologists. Obstet Gynecol 2010;116:450–63.

levels of risk and management alternatives. After counseling, the ultimate decision to undergo TOLAC or a repeat cesarean delivery should be made by the patient in consultation with her health care provider. The potential risks and benefits of both TOLAC and elective repeat cesarean delivery should be discussed. Documentation of counseling and the management plan should be included in the medical record.

Operative Vaginal Delivery

Operative vaginal deliveries are accomplished by applying direct traction on the fetal skull with forceps, or by applying traction to the fetal scalp by means of a vacuum extractor. Both forceps and vacuum extractors are acceptable and safe instruments for operative vaginal delivery. Operator experience should determine which instrument should be used in a particular situation. The vacuum extractor is associated with an increased incidence of neonatal cephalohematomata, retinal hemorrhages, and jaundice when compared with forceps delivery. Operators should attempt to minimize the duration of vacuum application, because cephalohematoma is more likely to occur as the interval increases. Forceps delivery, on the other hand, is associated with a higher rate of maternal perineal injuries. Neonatal care providers should be made aware of the mode of delivery to observe for potential complications associated with operative vaginal delivery.

Classification. In classifying forceps and vacuum extraction procedures, the station of the fetal head should be noted. Station refers to the relationship of the estimated distances, in centimeters, between the leading bony portion of the fetal head and the level of the maternal ischial spines. Engagement of the head occurs when the biparietal diameter has passed through the pelvic inlet. It is clinically diagnosed when the leading bony portion of the fetal head is at or below the level of the ischial spines (station 0 or more). The method to describe station beyond the level of the ischial spines is to estimate centimeters (+1 to +5 cm) below the spines. The following are three types of operative deliveries:

- Outlet operative vaginal delivery—Outlet operative vaginal delivery is the application of forceps or vacuum when the fetal scalp is visible at the introitus without separating the labia, the fetal skull has reached the pelvic floor, the fetal sagittal suture is in the anterior–posterior diameter or in the right or left occiput anterior or posterior position, and the fetal head is at or on the perineum. According to this definition, rotation cannot exceed 45 degrees. There is no difference in perinatal outcome when outlet operative vaginal deliveries are compared with spontaneous deliveries, and no data support the concept that rotating the head on the pelvic floor 45 degrees or less increases the rate of morbidity.

• Low operative vaginal delivery—Low operative vaginal delivery is the application of forceps or vacuum when the leading point of the fetal skull is at station +2 cm or more and is not on the pelvic floor. Low operative vaginal delivery applications have two subdivisions: 1) a rotation of 45 degrees or less (eg, left or right occipitoanterior to occiput anterior, or left or right occipitoposterior to occiput posterior) and 2) a rotation of more than 45 degrees. Although rotation of the fetal head often accompanies the use of the vacuum extractor, the vacuum never should be used to provide a direct rotational force to the fetal scalp.

• Midpelvis operative vaginal delivery—Midpelvis operative vaginal delivery is the application of forceps or vacuum when the fetal head is engaged but the leading point of the skull is above station +2 cm. Under very unusual circumstances, such as the sudden onset of severe fetal or maternal compromise, application of forceps or vacuum above station +2 cm may be attempted while simultaneously initiating preparations for a cesarean delivery in the event that the operative vaginal delivery maneuver is unsuccessful. Neither forceps nor vacuum should be applied to an unengaged fetal presenting part or when the cervix is not completely dilated.

Indications. Indications for a forceps or vacuum extraction and the position and station of the vertex at the time of application of the forceps or vacuum apparatus should be identified in a detailed operative description in the patient's medical record. No indication for operative vaginal delivery is absolute. The following indications apply when the fetal head is engaged and the cervix is fully dilated:

• Prolonged second stage

— Nulliparous women: lack of continuing progress for 3 hours with regional anesthesia, or 2 hours without regional anesthesia

— Multiparous women: lack of continuing progress for 2 hours with regional anesthesia, or 1 hour without regional anesthesia

• Suspicion of immediate or potential fetal compromise

• Shortening of the second stage for maternal benefit

The following are required for forceps or vacuum extraction operations:

- An individual with privileges for such procedures
- Assessment of maternal pelvis–fetal size relationship, including clinical pelvimetry, and an estimation of fetal weight, and the position and station of the fetal calvarium
- Adequate anesthesia
- Willingness to abandon attempted operative vaginal delivery
- Ability to perform emergency cesarean delivery (see also "Cesarean Delivery" in this chapter).

Cesarean Delivery

All hospitals offering labor and delivery services should be equipped to perform emergency cesarean delivery. The required personnel, including nurses, anesthesia personnel, neonatal resuscitation team members, and obstetric attendants, should be in the hospital or readily available. Any hospital providing an obstetric service should have the capability of responding to an obstetric emergency. Historically, the consensus has been that hospitals should have the capability of beginning a cesarean delivery within 30 minutes of the decision to operate. However, the scientific evidence to support this threshold is lacking. The decision-to-incision interval should be based on the timing that best incorporates maternal and fetal risks and benefits. For instance many of these clinical scenarios will include high-risk conditions or pregnancy complications (eg, morbid obesity, eclampsia, cardiopulmonary compromise, or hemorrhage), which may require maternal stabilization or additional surgical preparation before performance of emergent cesarean delivery. Conversely, examples of indications that may mandate more expeditious delivery include hemorrhage from placenta previa, abruptio placentae, prolapse of the umbilical cord, and uterine rupture. Therefore, it is reasonable to tailor the time to delivery to local circumstances and logistics. Sterile materials and supplies needed for emergency cesarean delivery should be kept sealed but properly arranged so that the instrument table can be made ready at once for an obstetric emergency. In-house obstetric and anesthesia coverage should be available in subspecialty care units. The anesthesia and pediatric staff responsible for covering the labor and delivery unit should be informed in advance when a complicated delivery is anticipated and upon admission of a patient with risk factors requiring a high-acuity level of care.

Before elective cesarean delivery, the maturity of the fetus should be established. For patients with an indication for an elective cesarean delivery, whether primary or repeat, fetal maturity may be assumed if one of the following criteria is met:

- Ultrasound measurement at less than 20 weeks of gestation supports gestational age of 39 weeks or greater
- Fetal heart tones have been documented as present for 30 weeks by Doppler ultrasonography
- It has been 36 weeks since a positive serum or urine hCG test

These criteria are not intended to preclude the use of menstrual dating. If any one criterion confirms gestational age assessment in a patient who has normal menstrual cycles and no immediate antecedent use of oral contraceptives, it is appropriate to schedule delivery at 39 weeks of gestation or later on the basis of menstrual dates. Another option is to await the onset of spontaneous labor.

Cesarean delivery on maternal request is defined as a primary cesarean delivery at maternal request in the absence of any medical or obstetric indication. A potential benefit of cesarean delivery on maternal request is a decreased risk of hemorrhage for the mother. Potential risks of cesarean delivery on maternal request include a longer maternal hospital stay, an increased risk of respiratory problems for the baby, and greater complications in subsequent pregnancies, including uterine rupture and placental implantation problems. Cesarean delivery on maternal request should not be performed before a gestational age of 39 weeks has been determined, utilizing the most accurate gestational dating criteria available. Maternal request for cesarean delivery should not be motivated by the unavailability of effective pain management. This form of delivery is not recommended for women desiring several children, given that the risks of placenta previa, placenta accreta, and the need for gravid hysterectomy increase with each cesarean delivery.

In women undergoing scheduled cesarean delivery, whether primary or repeat, the presence of fetal heart tones should be confirmed and documented before the surgery. There is insufficient evidence to warrant further fetal monitoring before scheduled cesarean deliveries in low-risk patients. However, in women requiring unscheduled cesarean delivery, fetal surveillance should continue until abdominal sterile preparation has begun. If internal FHR monitoring is in use, it should be continued until the abdominal sterile preparation is complete. Antimicrobial prophylaxis is recommended for all cesarean deliveries, unless the patient is already receiving appropriate antibiotics (eg, for chorio-amnionitis), and should be administered within 60 minutes of the start of the cesarean delivery. When this is not possible (eg, need for emergent delivery), prophylaxis should be administered as soon as possible. Given that cesarean delivery approximately doubles the risk of venous thromboembolism (although in the otherwise normal patient, the risk still remains low: approximately 1 per 1,000), placement of pneumatic compression devices before cesarean delivery is recommended for all women not already receiving thromboprophylaxis. However, cesarean delivery in the emergency setting should not be delayed because of the timing necessary to implement thromboprophylaxis (see also "Deep Vein Thrombosis and Pulmonary Embolism" in Chapter 7). When the cesarean delivery is performed for fetal indications, consideration should be given to sending the placenta for pathologic evaluation.

Multiple Gestation

The following factors should be considered in the delivery of multiple gestations:

- Labor and delivery—Confirmation of fetal presentations by ultrasound examination is indicated on admission. Each fetus should be monitored continuously during labor. Pediatric and anesthesia personnel should be immediately available, as well as blood bank services.

- Route of delivery—Controversy surrounds the preferred route of delivery for some multiple gestations, especially twins. Although cesarean delivery frequently is used for three or more fetuses, there are reports suggesting that vaginal delivery of triplet gestations, in appropriately monitored patients, is safe. Delivery should be based on individual needs and may depend on the physician's practice and experience. In general, twins presenting as vertex–vertex should be anticipated to deliver vaginally. If the presenting twin is nonvertex, cesarean delivery is preferred by most physicians. In vertex–nonvertex presentations, vaginal delivery of twin B in the nonvertex presentation is a reasonable option.

- Interval between deliveries—In the absence of other complications, such as bleeding or FHR abnormalities, the interval between deliveries for twins is not critical in determining the outcome of twin B. After the delivery of twin A, the FHR of twin B should be monitored.

- A physician capable of carrying out an emergent cesarean delivery should manage the labor and delivery of patients with multiple gestations.

Support Persons in the Delivery Room

Childbirth is a momentous family experience. Obstetric providers willingly should provide opportunities for those accompanying and supporting the woman giving birth to be present. These support persons must be informed about requirements for safety and must be willing to follow the directions of the obstetric staff concerning behavior in the delivery room. They also should understand the normal events and procedures in the labor and delivery area. They must conform to the dress code required of personnel in attendance in a delivery room. Both the obstetrician and the patient should consent to the presence of fathers, partners, or other support persons in the delivery room. Support persons should realize that their major function is to provide psychologic support to the mother during labor and delivery. Continuous support during labor from physicians, midwives, nurses, doulas, or lay individuals may be beneficial for women. Continuous presence of a support person appears to reduce the likelihood of medication for pain relief, operative vaginal delivery, cesarean delivery, and 5-minute Apgar scores less than 7.

The judgment of the obstetric staff, the individual obstetrician, the anesthesiologist, and pediatric support personnel, as well as the policies of the hospital, determines whether support persons may be present at a cesarean delivery. A written policy developed by all involved hospital staff is recommended.

Postpartum Maternal Care

Immediate Postpartum Maternal Care

Monitoring of maternal status postpartum is dictated in part by the events of the delivery process, the type of anesthesia or analgesia used, and the complications identified. Postanesthesia pain management should be guided by protocols established by the anesthesiologists and obstetricians in concert. Blood pressure levels and pulse should be monitored at least every 15 minutes for 2 hours, and more frequently and for longer duration if complications are encountered. The woman's temperature should be taken at least every 4 hours for the first 8 hours after delivery, then at least every 8 hours subsequently.

Nursing staff assigned to the delivery and immediate recovery of a woman should have no other obligations. Discharge from the delivery room, which may involve recovery from an anesthetic, should be at the discretion of the physician or certified nurse–midwife or the anesthesiologist in charge.

When regional or general anesthesia has been used for either vaginal or cesarean delivery, the woman should be observed in an appropriately equipped labor, delivery, and recovery room, or in an appropriately staffed and equipped postanesthesia care unit or equivalent area until she has recovered from the anesthetic. After cesarean delivery, policies for postanesthesia care should not differ from those applied to nonobstetric surgical patients receiving major anesthesia. Policy should ensure that a physician is available in the facility, or at least is nearby, to manage anesthetic complications and provide cardiopulmonary resuscitation for patients in the postanesthesia care unit. The patient should be discharged from the recovery area only at the discretion of, and after communication between, the attending physician or a certified nurse midwife, anesthesiologist, or certified registered nurse anesthetist in charge. Vital signs and additional signs or events should be monitored and recorded as they occur.

Subsequent Postpartum Care

The medical and nursing staff should cooperatively establish specific postpartum policies and procedures. In the postpartum period, staff should help the woman learn how to care for her own general needs and those of her neonate, and should identify potential problems related to her general health.

The obstetric caregiver should note postpartum orders on the patient's medical record (see also "Postpartum Form" in Appendix A). If routine postpartum orders are used, they should be printed or written in the medical record, reviewed and modified as necessary for the particular patient, and signed by the obstetric caregiver before the patient is transferred to the postpartum unit. When a labor, delivery, and recovery room is used, the same guidelines should apply.

Bed Rest, Ambulation, and Diet

It is important for the new mother to sleep, regain her strength, and recover from the effects of any analgesic or anesthetic agents that she may have received during labor. In the absence of complications, she may have a regular diet as soon as she wishes. Because early ambulation has been shown to decrease the incidence of subsequent thrombophlebitis, the mother should be encouraged to walk as soon as she feels able to do so. She should not attempt to get out of bed for the first time without assistance. She may shower as soon as she wishes. It may be necessary to administer fluids intravenously for hydration. If the patient has an intravenous line in place, her fluid and hemodynamic status should be evaluated before it is removed. If blood loss is greater than usual, the patient's hematocrit also should be assessed before discontinuing intravenous access.

Urogenital Care

Traditional teaching includes that the patient should be taught to cleanse the vulva from anterior vulva to perineum and anus rather than in the reverse direction. Application of an ice pack to the perineum during the first 24 hours after delivery may help reduce pain and swelling that have resulted from pressure of the neonate's head. Orally administered analgesics often are required and usually are sufficient for relief of discomfort from episiotomy or repaired lacerations. Pain that is not relieved by such medication suggests hematoma formation and mandates a careful examination of the vulva, vagina, and rectum. Beginning 24 hours after delivery, moist heat in the form of a warm sitz bath may reduce local discomfort and promote healing.

Women should be encouraged to void as soon as possible after delivery. Often women have difficulty voiding immediately after delivery, possibly because of trauma to the bladder during labor and delivery, regional anesthesia, or vulvar–perineal pain and swelling. In addition, the diuresis that often follows delivery can distend the bladder before the patient is aware of a sensation of a full bladder. To ensure adequate emptying of the bladder, the patient should be checked frequently during the first 24 hours after delivery, with particular attention to displacement of the uterine fundus and any indication of the presence of a fluid-filled bladder above the symphysis. Although every effort should be made to help the patient void spontaneously, catheterization may be necessary. If the patient continues to find voiding difficult, use of an indwelling catheter is preferable to repeated catheterization.

Care of the Breasts

The woman's decision about breastfeeding determines the appropriate care of the breasts. Breast care for a woman who chooses to breastfeed is outlined in Chapter 8. The woman who chooses not to breastfeed should be reassured that milk production will abate over the first few days after delivery if she does not breastfeed. During the stage of engorgement, the breasts may become painful and should be supported with a well-fitting brassiere. Ice packs and analgesics can help relieve discomfort during this period. Medications for lactation cessation are discouraged. Women who do not wish to breastfeed should be encouraged to avoid nipple stimulation and should be cautioned against continued manual expression of milk.

Postpartum Analgesia

After vaginal delivery, analgesic medication (including topical lidocaine cream) may be necessary to relieve perineal and episiotomy pain and facilitate maternal mobility. This is best addressed by administering the medications on an as-needed basis according to postpartum orders. Most mothers experience considerable pain in the first 24 hours after cesarean delivery. Although at one time pain most often was treated by intramuscular injections of narcotics, newer techniques, such as spinal or epidural opiates, patient-controlled epidural or intravenous analgesia, and potent oral analgesics, provide better pain relief and greater patient satisfaction. Regardless of the route of administration, opioids potentially can cause respiratory depression and decrease intestinal motility. Therefore, adequate supervision and monitoring should be ensured for all postpartum patients receiving these drugs.

Postpartum Immunizations

Attention should be given to maternal immunizations before hospital discharge. Regardless of a recent tetanus and diphtheria (TD) vaccination, women in the postpartum period who have not already received the tetanus toxoid, reduced diphtheria toxoid, and acellular pertussis vaccine (Tdap) should receive a dose as soon as possible after delivery to ensure pertussis immunity and reduce the risk of transmission to the newborn. Likewise, a patient who is identified as susceptible to rubella virus infection should receive the rubella vaccine in the postpartum period. In addition, women who are susceptible to varicella should be offered varicella vaccination before discharge. During the flu season, women who were not vaccinated antepartum should be offered the seasonal flu vaccine before discharge. Breastfeeding is not a contraindication to receiving any of these vaccinations.

A woman who is unsensitized and Rh D-negative and who gives birth to a neonate who is Rh D-positive or Du-positive (ie, weak Rh positive) should receive 300 micrograms of anti-D immune globulin postpartum, ideally within 72 hours, even when anti-D immune globulin has been administered in the antepartum period. No further administration of anti-D immune globulin is necessary when the infants of Rh D-negative women are also Rh D-negative. (For more information on specific vaccinations, see Chapter 10.)

Length of Hospital Stay

When no complications are present, the postpartum hospital stay usually ranges from 48 hours for vaginal delivery to 96 hours for cesarean delivery, excluding the day of delivery. A shorter hospital stay may be considered if the infant does not require continued hospitalization. When the physician and the mother want a shortened hospital stay, the following minimal criteria should be met:

- The mother is afebrile, with pulse and respirations of normal rate and quality.
- Her blood pressure level is within the normal range.
- The amount and color of lochia are appropriate for the duration of recovery.
- The uterine fundus is firm.
- Urinary output is adequate.
- Any surgical repair or wound has minimal edema and no evidence of infection and appears to be healing without complication.
- The mother is able to ambulate with ease and has adequate pain control.
- There are no abnormal physical or emotional findings.
- The mother is able to eat and drink without difficulty.
- Arrangements have been made for postpartum follow-up care.
- The mother has been instructed in caring for herself and the neonate at home, is aware of deviations from normal, and is prepared to recognize and respond to danger signs and symptoms.
- The mother demonstrates readiness to care for herself and her newborn.
- Pertinent laboratory results are available, including a postpartum measurement of hemoglobin or hematocrit, if indicated by excessive intrapartum or postpartum blood loss.
- If a perinatal drug screen was performed, the complete test results are available and the findings are negative.
- ABO blood group and Rh D type are known, and, if indicated, the appropriate amount of anti-D immune globulin has been administered.
- The mother has received instructions on postpartum activity and exercises and common postpartum discomforts and relief measures.
- Family members or other support persons are available to the mother for the first few days following discharge.
- The infant meets all criteria for discharge from the hospital (see also Chapter 8).

The medical and nursing staff should be sensitive to potential problems associated with shortened hospital stays and should develop mechanisms to address patient questions that arise after discharge. With a shortened hospital stay, a home visit or follow-up telephone conference by a health care provider, such as a lactation nurse, within 48 hours of discharge is encouraged.

When a pregnancy, labor, or delivery is complicated by medical or obstetric disorders, the mother's readiness for discharge may be based on the aforementioned criteria, as modified by the individual judgment of the obstetric care provider. The stability of the woman's medical condition, the need for continued inpatient observation, and treatment and risks of complications should be taken into consideration.

Postpartum Nutritional Guidelines

Postnatal dietary guidelines are similar to those established during pregnancy (see also Chapter 5). The minimal caloric requirement for adequate milk production in a woman of average size is 1,800 kcal per day. In general, an additional 500 kcal of energy daily is recommended throughout lactation. A balanced, nutritious diet will ensure both the quality and the quantity of the milk produced without depletion of maternal stores. Fluid intake by the mother is governed by thirst (see also "Breastfeeding" in Chapter 8).

A vitamin–mineral supplement is not needed routinely. Mothers at nutritional risk should be given a multivitamin supplement with particular emphasis on calcium and vitamin B_{12} and vitamin D (see also Chapter 5). Iron should be administered only if the mother herself needs it.

Maternal postpartum weight loss can occur at a rate of 2 lb per month without affecting lactation. On average, a woman will retain 2 lb more than her prepregnancy weight at 1 year postpartum. There is no relationship between body mass index or total weight gain and weight retention. Aging, rather than parity, is the major determinant of increases in a woman's weight over time.

Residual postpartum retention of weight gained during pregnancy that results in obesity is a concern. Special attention to lifestyle, including exercise and eating habits, will help these women return to a normal body mass index.

Postpartum Considerations

Before discharge, the mother should receive information about the following normal postpartum events:

- Changes in lochia pattern expected in the first few weeks
- Range of activities that she may reasonably undertake
- Care of the breasts, perineum, and bladder

- Dietary needs, particularly if she is breastfeeding
- Recommended amount of exercise
- Emotional responses, and risk of postpartum depression
- Signs of complications (eg, temperature elevation, chills, leg pains, episiotomy or wound drainage, or increased vaginal bleeding)

The length of convalescence that the patient can expect, based on the type of delivery, also should be discussed. For women who have had a cesarean delivery, additional precautions may be appropriate, such as wound care and temporary abstinence from lifting objects heavier than the newborn and from driving motor vehicles. It is helpful to reinforce verbal discussions with written information.

The earliest time at which coitus may be resumed safely after childbirth is unknown. Resumption of coitus should be discussed with the couple. Risks of hemorrhage and infection are minimal approximately 2 weeks postpartum. Although a common recommendation is that sexual activity should be delayed until 6 weeks postpartum, there are no data to direct this statement. Therefore, sexual activity can resume after healing of the perineum and when bleeding has decreased, depending on resolution of contraceptive management and, most importantly, on the patient's desire and comfort.

Sexual difficulties that are common in the early months after childbirth should be discussed. Healing at the episiotomy site can cause the woman some discomfort during intercourse within the first year following delivery. In the lactating woman, the vagina often is atrophic and dry. Natural lubrication during sexual excitement may be unsatisfactory. Furthermore, the demands of the newborn's care alter the couple's ability to find time for physical intimacy.

At the time of discharge, the family should be given the name of the person to contact if questions or problems arise for either the mother or the newborn. Arrangements should be made for a follow-up examination and specific instructions conveyed to the woman, including when contact is advisable.

In general, the following points should be reviewed with the mother or, preferably, with both parents; specific information to be conveyed is discussed within this section:

- Newborn care
- Immediate needs of the newborn (eg, feeding methods and environmental supports)

- Feeding techniques; skin care, including umbilical cord care; temperature assessment and measurement with a thermometer; and assessment of neonatal well-being and recognition of illness

- Roles of the obstetrician, pediatrician, and other members of the health care team concerned with the continuous medical care of the mother and the newborn

- Availability of support systems, including psychosocial support

- Instructions to follow in the event of a complication or emergency

- Importance of maintaining newborn immunization, beginning with an initial dose of the hepatitis B virus vaccine. (For more information on newborn care, see Chapter 8.)

- Importance of keeping the infant from exposure to secondhand smoke and maintaining or achieving smoking cessation if the mother smoked before or during pregnancy.

- Need for follow-up surveillance if the mother experienced gestational diabetes mellitus (GDM)

- High risk of postpartum drug overdose if the mother used opioid drugs before or during pregnancy.

Postpartum Contraception

Discussion of contraceptive options and prompt initiation of a method should be a primary focus of routine antenatal and postpartum care. The benefits of child spacing include decreases in preterm delivery and perinatal mortality, and most women wish to avoid pregnancy for at least several months, if not considerably longer, after delivering a baby. In nonbreastfeeding women, ovulation may return quickly after delivery. Lactational amenorrhea associated with exclusive breastfeeding delays ovulation for up to 6 months. However, current estimates of exclusive breastfeeding among U.S. women are low, and many women who leave the hospital intending to breastfeed never do so. Most postpartum women rapidly become fertile and should be encouraged to adopt a contraceptive method if they wish to avoid pregnancy. Important considerations in contraceptive counseling include method effectiveness and safety, continuation rates, prior success in contraceptive adherence, timing of initiation, and effect on breastfeeding. Ideally, contraceptive counseling should take place during the patient's antenatal visits, because postpartum women are typically focused on other challenges, including adapting to a new baby and breastfeeding.

The Centers for Disease Control and Prevention (CDC) have developed evidence-based medical eligibility criteria for contraceptive use that have been endorsed by the American College of Obstetricians and Gynecologists. The CDC classifies sterilization and intrauterine and implant contraception (also known as long-acting reversible contraception) as top-tier methods of contraception, based on high effectiveness, excellent continuation rates, and ease of adherence. These methods should be considered as first-line choices for postpartum women. Other methods of contraception include hormonal contraceptives and barrier methods.

Surgical Tubal Sterilization

Surgical tubal sterilization often can be safely performed in the immediate postpartum period. In the antepartum period, informed consent should be obtained, and women should receive counseling about the permanence and irreversibility of sterilization so that they can make a considered decision, review the benefits and risks of the procedure, and consider alternative reversible contraceptive methods.

If the mother is stable and has no acute medical problems after vaginal delivery, she may undergo tubal sterilization immediately or within the first few days postpartum. Tubal ligation at the time of cesarean delivery is safe and effective. In patients with medical or obstetric complications during the peripartum period—including cardiovascular, respiratory, infections, or metabolic abnormalities—the mother's stability must be ensured before proceeding with tubal sterilization. The obstetrician and anesthesiologist or certified registered nurse anesthetist should exercise medical judgment regarding the safety of the procedure. Every attempt should be made to honor the patient's wishes for a postpartum tubal ligation, particularly in women for whom a subsequent pregnancy would be dangerous or if insurance coverage may lapse. Although volume and staffing in the labor and delivery department may sometimes preclude tubal sterilization, consideration may be given to other arrangements, such as using the main operating room.

The U.S. Food and Drug Administration (FDA) has approved two devices for hysteroscopic sterilization. The first method involves placement of a metal microinsert under hysteroscopic guidance into the interstitial portion of each fallopian tube. The second technique uses bipolar radiofrequency to create a lesion in the fallopian tube, followed by deployment of a silicone matrix in the region of the tube where the lesion was formed. These minimally invasive methods can be performed without general anesthesia at 6–12 weeks after delivery, depending on the device used for tubal occlusion. Women choosing hysteroscopic sterilization must undergo hysterosalpingography 3 months after the procedure to confirm bilateral occlusion, and they must rely on a method of interim contraception until hysterosalpingography confirms occlusion.

Long-Acting Reversible Contraception

Intrauterine devices (IUDs) and contraceptive implants, or long-acting reversible contraception (LARC), are the most effective reversible contraceptives. The major advantage of LARC methods compared with other reversible contraceptive methods is that they require only a single act of motivation for long-term use. In addition, return to fertility is rapid after removal of the device. According to contraceptive use guidelines from the World Health Organization and the CDC, LARC methods have few contraindications, and almost all women, including adolescents, are eligible for implants and IUDs. Both IUD and contraceptive implant use in women with a variety of characteristics and medical conditions are addressed in the document *U.S. Medical Eligibility Criteria for Contraceptive Use* (see "Resources" in this chapter).

Intrauterine contraception is highly effective and has continuation rates approaching 80% at 1 year. Two long-acting IUDs are available in the United States. The FDA has approved use of the copper IUD for up to 10 continuous years and of the levonorgestrel IUD for up to 5 years of use. Although intrauterine contraception is typically initiated at 4–6 weeks postpartum, IUDs may be safely inserted immediately postpartum (within 10 minutes of delivery of the placenta) after either vaginal or cesarean delivery. Although a disadvantage of immediate insertion is a higher rate of expulsion, it may be outweighed by the advantage of prompt initiation. Immediate postpartum insertion is contraindicated in women in whom peripartum chorioamnionitis, endometritis, or puerperal sepsis is diagnosed. Both copper and levonorgestrel IUDs may be used by breastfeeding women.

The etonogestrel single-rod contraceptive implant is also highly effective, is FDA approved for up to 3 years of use, and has excellent continuation rates. Implants may be offered to women who are breastfeeding and more than 4 weeks postpartum. Insertion of the implant is safe at any time in nonbreastfeeding women after childbirth.

Hormonal Contraceptives

Hormonal contraceptives, including estrogen–progestin combination methods and progestin-only methods, are popular choices. Because of an increased risk of venous thromboembolism, combined hormonal contraceptives are not recommended for use by women who are less than 21 days postpartum. The risks of using combined hormonal contraceptives for women who are 21–42 days postpartum and have other risk factors for venous thromboembolism usually outweigh the benefits, and generally these methods should not be used. Benefits generally outweigh risks for those without other risk factors for venous thromboembolism, and combined hormonal contraceptives can be used by women who are more than 42 days postpartum, provided they have no other contraindications to use.

Progestin-only methods include depot medroxyprogesterone acetate injections, progestin-only pills, and the already discussed levonorgestrel IUD and etonogestrel single-rod contraceptive implant. Overall, progestin-only methods appear to have little effect on either breastfeeding success or infant growth and health, and some obstetricians routinely initiate these methods in many women before hospital discharge, including those who choose to breastfeed. The depot medroxyprogesterone acetate injection is a highly effective method that can be initiated before hospital discharge and lasts for 3 months, but continuation rates are low. Progestin-only pills may be prescribed at discharge either for immediate initiation or, as indicated above, subject to a waiting period in breastfeeding women.

Barrier Methods

Barrier methods, including the male and female condom, are particularly effective in preventing the transmission of sexually transmitted infections. These methods may be used as soon as intercourse has resumed after delivery. The diaphragm is another coital-dependent, female-controlled method. The diaphragm should not be used within 6 weeks postpartum. Barrier methods are less effective at preventing pregnancy than sterilization, intrauterine devices, and hormonal methods.

Postpartum Mood Disorders

The physical and psychosocial status of the mother and the newborn should be subject to ongoing assessment after discharge. The new mother needs personalized care during the postpartum period to hasten the development of a healthy mother–infant relationship and a sense of maternal confidence. Support and reassurance should be provided as the woman masters newborn care tasks and adapts to her maternal role. Involving the father and encouraging him to participate in the newborn's care not only can provide additional support to the woman but also can enhance the father–infant relationship.

For many women, the postpartum period can be a stressful time and may lead to the onset of mood disorders. Some patients experience *postpartum baby blues,* defined as a period of mild depressive mood and lability that typically has its onset within 2–3 days postpartum and lasts up to 2 weeks. Women who lack psychosocial support, have a history of postpartum depression or other psychiatric illnesses, or have experienced a recent stressful life event are at greater risk of postpartum depression. Screening for these risk factors is, therefore, important. Other risk factors include child care stress, low self-esteem, and low socioeconomic status. All women with postpartum baby blues should be monitored for the onset of continuing or worsening symptoms because women with the blues are at high risk of the onset of a more serious condition (see also "Clinical Depression" in Chapter 5).

The incidence of postpartum major or minor depressive disorders varies from 10% to 15%. Perinatal depression differs from general depression because of the presence of significant and debilitating anxiety. To avoid problems with maternal–infant care and bonding, depression treatment needs to be initiated quickly. An antidepressant drug generally is recommended for a major depressive disorder. Professional counseling and peer support are also effective for some women. It should be noted that a recurrence of depression might occur following discontinuation of psychotropic medication (see also "Psychiatric Disease in Pregnancy" in Chapter 7).

Postpartum psychosis is the most severe form of mental derangement and is most common in women with pre-existing disorders, such as bipolar illness or, less commonly, schizophrenia. Women with postpartum psychosis show severe symptoms, such as severe anxiety; insomnia; and delusions concerning themselves, the infant, and others. This should be considered a psychiatric emergency, and the patient should be referred for immediate, often inpatient, treatment.

The postpartum period is a time of developmental adjustment for the whole family. Family members have new roles and relationships, and an effort should be made to assess the progress of the family's adaptation. If a family member— parent or sibling—finds it difficult to assume the new role, the health care team should arrange for sensitive, supportive assistance. This is particularly important for adolescent mothers, for whom it may be necessary to mobilize multiple resources within the community.

Postpartum Visits

Approximately 4–6 weeks after delivery, the mother should visit her physician for a postpartum review and examination. This interval may be modified according to the needs of the patient with medical, obstetric, or intercurrent complications. A visit within 7–14 days of delivery may be advisable after a cesarean delivery or a complicated gestation, such as a patient requiring antihypertensives for posttreatment of severe preeclampsia or severe hypertension.

The review at the first postpartum visit should include obtaining an interval history and performing a physical examination to evaluate the patient's current status and her adaptation to the newborn. Specific inquiries regarding breastfeeding should be made. The examination should include an evaluation of weight, blood pressure levels, breasts (if not lactating or if there are specific complaints in lactating women), and abdomen as well as a pelvic examination. Episiotomy repair and uterine involution should be evaluated and a Pap test performed, if needed. Methods of birth control should be reviewed or initiated (see also "Postpartum Form" in Appendix A).

All women with GDM should be screened at 6–12 weeks postpartum and managed appropriately. The American Diabetes Association recommends repeat testing at least every 3 years for women who had a pregnancy affected by GDM and normal results of postpartum screening. Women should be encouraged to discuss their GDM history and need for screening with all of their health care providers.

Women with a history of tobacco, alcohol, or other substance use disorder should receive supportive guidance during the postpartum visit to prevent relapse to prepregnancy behaviors. If the mother used opioid drugs before or during pregnancy, she is at great risk of an overdose during the postpartum period and should be immediately referred to an addiction medicine specialist.

As already noted, many women experience some degree of emotional lability in the postpartum period. If this persists or develops into clinically significant depression, intervention may be necessary (see also "Clinical Depression" in Chapter 5). The emotional status of a woman whose pregnancy had an abnormal outcome also should be reviewed. Counseling should address specific issues regarding her future health and pregnancies. For example, it may be advantageous to discuss VBAC or the implications of diabetes mellitus, intrauterine growth restriction, preterm birth, hypertension, fetal anomalies, or other conditions that may recur in any future pregnancy. Laboratory data should be obtained as indicated. The postpartum visit is an opportune time to review adult immunizations, such as Tdap, rubella vaccination, and varicella vaccination for women who are susceptible and did not receive the vaccine immediately postpartum, and to discuss any special problems. The patient should be encouraged to return for subsequent periodic examinations.

The postpartum visit is an excellent time to begin preconception counseling for patients who may wish to have future pregnancies (see also "Preconception Care" in Chapter 5). This counseling includes risk assessment to facilitate the planning, spacing, and timing of the next pregnancy; health-promotion measures; and timely intervention to reduce medical and psychosocial risks. Such intervention may include treatment of infections; counseling regarding behaviors, such as those related to sexually transmitted infections, tobacco, alcohol, and other substance use; nutrition counseling and supplementation; and appropriate referrals for follow-up care. Although physiologic considerations indicate that a woman can return to a normal work schedule 4–6 weeks after delivery, attention also should be given to maternal–infant bonding.

Bibliography

Access to postpartum sterilization. Committee Opinion No. 530. American College of Obstetricians and Gynecologists. Obstet Gynecol 2012;120:212–15.

American Academy of Pediatrics, American College of Obstetricians and Gynecologists. Neonatal encephalopathy and cerebral palsy: defining the pathogenesis and pathophysiology. Elk Grove Village (IL): AAP; Washington, DC: ACOG; 2003.

American College of Obstetricians and Gynecologists. Operative vaginal delivery. ACOG Practice Bulletin 17. Washington, DC: ACOG; 2000.

Analgesia and cesarean delivery rates. ACOG Committee Opinion No. 339. American College of Obstetricians and Gynecologists. Obstet Gynecol 2006;107:1487–8.

Antiphospholipid syndrome. Practice Bulletin No. 118. American College of Obstetricians and Gynecologists. Obstet Gynecol 2011;117:192–9.

Batton DG, Blackmon LR, Adamkin DH, Bell EF, Denson SE, Engle WA, et al. Underwater births. American Academy of Pediatrics Committee on Fetus and Newborn, 2004-2005. Pediatrics 2005;115:1413–4.

Dystocia and augmentation of labor. ACOG Practice Bulletin No. 49. American College of Obstetricians and Gynecologists. Obstet Gynecol 2003;102:1445–54.

Episiotomy. ACOG Practice Bulletin No. 71. American College of Obstetricians and Gynecologists. Obstet Gynecol 2006;107:957–62.

Fetal monitoring prior to scheduled cesarean delivery. ACOG Committee Opinion No. 382. American College of Obstetricians and Gynecologists. Obstet Gynecol 2007: 110(4):961–2. Reaffirmed 2010.

Inappropriate use of the terms fetal distress and birth asphyxia. ACOG Committee Opinion No. 326. American College of Obstetricians and Gynecologists. Obstet Gynecol 2005;106:1469–70.

Induction of labor. ACOG Practice Bulletin No. 107. American College of Obstetricians and Gynecologists. Obstet Gynecol 2009;114:386–97.

Intrapartum fetal heart rate monitoring: nomenclature, interpretation, and general management principles. ACOG Practice Bulletin No. 106. American College of Obstetricians and Gynecologists. Obstet Gynecol 2009;114:192–202.

Long-acting reversible contraception: implants and intrauterine devices. Practice Bulletin No. 121. American College of Obstetricians and Gynecologists. Obstet Gynecol 2011;118:184–96.

Macones GA, Hankins GD, Spong CY, Hauth J, Moore T. The 2008 National Institute of Child Health and Human Development workshop report on electronic fetal monitoring: update on definitions, interpretation, and research guidelines. Obstet Gynecol 2008; 112:661–6.

Management of intrapartum fetal heart rate tracings. Practice Bulletin No. 116. American College of Obstetricians and Gynecologists. Obstet Gynecol 2010;116:1232–40.

Multiple gestation: complicated twin, triplet, and high-order multifetal pregnancy. ACOG Practice Bulletin No. 56. American College of Obstetricians and Gynecologists. Obstet Gynecol 2004;104:869–83.

Nalbuphine hydrochloride use for intrapartum analgesia. ACOG Committee Opinion No. 376. American College of Obstetricians and Gynecologists. Obstet Gynecol 2007: 110:449.

Obstetric analgesia and anesthesia. ACOG Practice Bulletin No. 36. American College of Obstetricians and Gynecologists. Obstet Gynecol 2002;100:177–91.

Optimal goals for anesthesia care in obstetrics. ACOG Committee Opinion No. 433. American College of Obstetricians and Gynecologists. Obstet Gynecol 2009;113:1197–9.

Oral intake during labor. ACOG Committee Opinion No. 441. American College of Obstetricians and Gynecologists. Obstet Gynecol 2009;114:714.

Pain relief during labor. ACOG Committee Opinion No. 295. American College of Obstetricians and Gynecologists. Obstet Gynecol 2004;104:213.

Placenta accreta. Committee Opinion No. 529. American College of Obstetricians and Gynecologists. Obstet Gynecol 2012;120:207–11.

Planned home birth. Committee Opinion No. 476. American College of Obstetricians and Gynecologists. Obstet Gynecol 2011;117:425–8.

Postpartum hemorrhage. ACOG Practice Bulletin No. 76. American College of Obstetricians and Gynecologists. Obstet Gynecol 2006;108:1039–47.

Premature rupture of membranes. ACOG Practice Bulletin No. 80. American College of Obstetricians and Gynecologists. Obstet Gynecol 2007;109:1007–19.

The Apgar score. ACOG Committee Opinion No. 333. American College of Obstetricians and Gynecologists, American Academy of Pediatrics. Obstet Gynecol 2006;107: 1209–12. Reaffirmed 2010.

Understanding and using the U.S. Medical Eligibility Criteria for Contraceptive Use, 2010. Committee Opinion No. 505. American College of Obstetricians and Gynecologists. Obstet Gynecol 2011;118:754–60.

Use of prophylactic antibiotics in labor and delivery. Practice Bulletin No. 120. American College of Obstetricians and Gynecologists. Obstet Gynecol 2011;117:1472–83.

Vaginal birth after previous cesarean delivery. Practice Bulletin No. 115. American College of Obstetricians and Gynecologists. Obstet Gynecol 2010;116:450–63.

Wong CA, Scavone BM, Peaceman AM, McCarthy RJ, Sullivan JT, Diaz NT, et al. The risk of cesarean delivery with neuraxial analgesia given early versus late in labor. N Engl J Med 2005;352:655–65.

Resources

Immunization for women. Washington, DC: American College of Obstetricians and Gynecologists; 2011. Available at: http://immunizationforwomen.org/. Retrieved December 20, 2011.

Neurological and psychiatric disorders. In: Cunningham FG, Leveno KJ, Bloom SL, Hauth JC, Rouse DJ, and Spong CY. In: Williams obstetrics. 23rd ed. New York (NY): McGraw–Hill Medical; 2010; p. 1164–84.

Shealy KR, Li R, Benton-Davis S, Grummer-Strawn LM. The CDC guide to breastfeeding interventions. Atlanta (GA): Centers for Disease Control and Prevention; 2005. Available at: http://www.cdc.gov/breastfeeding/pdf/breastfeeding_interventions.pdf. Retrieved December 22, 2011.

U.S. Medical Eligibility Criteria for Contraceptive Use, 2010. Centers for Disease Control and Prevention. MMWR Recomm Rep 2010;59(RR-4):1–86.

Update to CDC's U.S. medical eligibility criteria for contraceptive use, 2010: revised recommendations for the use of contraceptive methods during the postpartum period. Centers for Disease Control and Prevention. MMWR Morb Mortal Wkly Rep 2011;60:878–83. Available at: http://www.cdc.gov/mmwr/pdf/wk/mm6026.pdf. Retrieved July 7, 2011.

Chapter 7
Obstetric and Medical Complications

Certain complications before and during pregnancy and at the time of labor or delivery may require more intensive surveillance, monitoring, and special care of the obstetric patient (see also Appendix B and Appendix C). Often, complications can arise without warning. In some cases, early detection and timely intervention can improve outcome. When there is a high risk of complications, it may be advisable to make arrangements for such care in advance. The pediatric and anesthesia services should be made aware of such patients so that appropriate medical care can be planned in advance of the delivery.

Medical Complications Before Pregnancy

Prepregnancy medical complications that typically require special antepartum and intrapartum care include antiphospholipid syndrome, asthma, hemoglobinopathies, inherited thrombophilias, maternal phenylketonuria, obesity and bariatric surgery, pregestational diabetes, and thyroid disease.

Antiphospholipid Syndrome

Antiphospholipid antibodies are a diverse group of antibodies with specificity for binding to negatively charged phospholipids on cell surfaces. Antiphospholipid syndrome (APS) is an autoimmune disorder defined by the presence of characteristic clinical features and specified levels of circulating antiphospholipid antibodies. Antiphospholipid antibodies have been associated with a variety of medical problems, including arterial thrombosis, venous thrombosis, autoimmune thrombocytopenia, and fetal loss. In addition to fetal loss, several obstetric complications have been associated with antiphospholipid antibodies, including preeclampsia, intrauterine growth restriction, and preterm delivery (see also "Deep Vein Thrombosis and Pulmonary Embolism" later in this chapter).

Screening and Diagnosis

The three antiphospholipid antibodies that contribute to the diagnosis of antiphospholipid syndrome are 1) lupus anticoagulant, 2) anticardiolipin, and

3) anti-β_2-glycoprotein I. The diagnosis of APS requires two positive antiphospholipid antibody test results at least 12 weeks apart. Testing for antiphospholipid antibodies should be performed in women with a prior unexplained venous thromboembolism, a new venous thromboembolism during pregnancy, or in those with a history of venous thromboembolism but not tested previously. Obstetric indications for antiphospholipid antibody testing should be limited to a history of one fetal loss or three or more recurrent embryonic losses or fetal losses.

Management

The goals of treatment for APS during pregnancy are to improve maternal, fetal, and neonatal outcomes. Antepartum testing has been suggested because of the potential risk of fetal growth restriction and stillbirth in pregnancies of women with APS. Many experts recommend serial ultrasonographic assessment and antepartum testing in the third trimester. For women with APS who have had a thrombotic event, most experts recommend prophylactic anticoagulation with heparin throughout pregnancy and 6 weeks postpartum. For women with APS who have not had a thrombotic event, expert consensus suggests that clinical surveillance or prophylactic heparin (with or without low-dose aspirin) use antepartum in addition to 6 weeks of postpartum anticoagulation may be warranted.

For long-term management postpartum, patients with APS should be referred to a physician with expertise in treatment of the syndrome, such as an internist, hematologist, or rheumatologist. Women with APS should not use estrogen-containing contraceptives. (For more information, see "Deep Vein Thrombosis and Pulmonary Embolism" later in this chapter.)

Asthma

Asthma is a common, potentially serious medical condition that complicates approximately 4–8% of pregnancies. The condition is characterized by chronic airway inflammation, with increased airway responsiveness to a variety of stimuli, and airway obstruction that is partially or completely reversible. Severe and poorly controlled asthma may be associated with increased prematurity, need for cesarean delivery, preeclampsia, growth restriction, and maternal morbidity and mortality.

Diagnosis and Assessment

The diagnosis of asthma in a pregnant patient is the same as that for a nonpregnant patient. For patients who received a diagnosis of asthma and seek care, subjective assessment of disease status and pulmonary function tests should be performed. The assessment in a pregnant patient with asthma also should include the effect of any prior pregnancies on asthma severity or control because this may predict the course of the asthma during subsequent pregnancies.

Fetal surveillance should be considered in women who have moderate or severe asthma during pregnancy. Serial growth examinations should be performed (usually starting at 32 weeks of gestation) for women who have poorly controlled asthma, moderate to severe asthma, or who are recovering from a severe asthma exacerbation.

Management

The ultimate goal of asthma therapy in pregnancy is maintaining adequate oxygenation of the fetus by preventing hypoxic episodes in the mother. Optimal management of asthma during pregnancy includes objective monitoring of lung function, avoiding or controlling asthma triggers, educating patients, and individualizing pharmacologic therapy to maintain normal pulmonary function. The step-care therapeutic approach uses the lowest amount of drug intervention necessary to control a patient's severity of asthma (see Box 7-1).

Asthma medication use should not be discontinued during labor and delivery. The patient should be kept hydrated and should receive adequate analgesia in order to decrease the risk of bronchospasm. Certain medications, possibly used during labor and delivery, have the potential to worsen asthma. Nonselective β-blockers, and carboprost (15-methyl prostaglandin $F_{2\alpha}$) may trigger bronchospasm. Cesarean delivery for acute exacerbation is rarely needed. Maternal and fetal compromise usually will respond to aggressive medical management.

Hemoglobinopathies

The hemoglobinopathies are a heterogeneous group of single-gene disorders that include sickle cell disease as well as the thalassemias. The thalassemias represent a wide spectrum of hematologic disorders that are characterized by a reduced synthesis of globin chains, resulting in microcytic anemia. Thalassemias are classified according to the globin chain affected, with the most common types being α-thalassemia and β-thalassemia.

Screening and Diagnosis

Genetic screening can identify couples at risk of offspring with hemoglobinopathies and allow them to make informed decisions regarding reproduction and

---

Box 7-1. Step-Therapy Medical Management
of Asthma During Pregnancy

Mild Intermittent Asthma
- No daily medications, albutrol as needed

Mild Persistent Asthma
- Preferred—Low-dose inhaled corticosteroid
- Alternative—Cromolyn, leukotriene receptor antagonist, or throphylline (serum level 5–12 micrograms/mL)

Moderate Persistent Asthma
- Preferred—Low-dose inhaled corticosteroid and salmeterol or medium-dose inhaled corticosteroid or (if needed) medium-dose inhaled corticosteroid and salmeterol.
- Alternative—Low-dose or (if needed) medium-dose inhaled corticosteroid and either leukotriene receptor antagonist, or throphylline (serum level 5–12 micrograms/mL)

Severe Persistent Asthma
- Preferred—High-dose inhaled corticosteroid and salmeterol and (if needed) oral corticosteroid
- Alternative—High-dose inhaled corticosteroid and throphylline (serum level 5–12 micrograms/mL) and oral corticosteroid if needed

Asthma in Pregnancy. ACOG Practice Bulletin No. 90. American College of Obstetricians and Gynecologists. Obstet Gynecol 2008;112:201–7.

---

prenatal diagnosis. Individuals of African, Southeast Asian, and Mediterranean ancestry are at a higher risk of being carriers of hemoglobinopathies and should be offered carrier screening. A complete blood count and hemoglobin electrophoresis are the appropriate laboratory tests for screening for hemoglobinopathies. Solubility tests alone are inadequate for screening because they fail to identify important transmissible hemoglobin gene abnormalities affecting fetal outcome. Prenatal diagnosis of hemoglobinopathies is best accomplished by DNA analysis of cultured amniocytes or chorionic villi.

Management

Sickle Cell Disease. Regular prenatal care by or in consultation with obstetricians or maternal–fetal medicine subspecialists who are experienced in the management of sickle cell disease is recommended for pregnant women with sickle cell disease. Pregnancy in women with sickle cell disease is associated with an increased risk of maternal morbidity and mortality, spontaneous abortion, preterm labor, intrauterine growth restriction, preeclampsia, and stillbirth. Fetal surveillance with serial ultrasound examinations and antepartum fetal testing is reasonable. Because of the continual turnover of red blood cells, pregnant patients with sickle cell disease need increased prenatal folic acid supplementation (4 mg per day). Major complications (eg, worsening anemia; intrapartum complications, such as hemorrhage, septicemia, and cesarean delivery; painful crisis; and chest syndrome) may require intervention with an exchange transfusion.

Thalassemia. The course of pregnancy in women with the α-thalassemia trait usually is not significantly different from a pregnancy in women with normal hemoglobin. Hemoglobin H disease has been reported during pregnancy with favorable outcomes despite moderate anemia; however, there have been too few reported cases from which to draw definitive conclusions.

Pregnancy in women with β-thalassemia major is recommended only for those with normal cardiac function who have had prolonged hypertransfusion therapy to maintain hemoglobin levels at 10 g/dL and iron chelation therapy with deferoxamine. Fetal growth should be monitored with serial ultrasonography. In cases in which fetal growth is suboptimal, patients should have fetal surveillance. Pregnant women with β-thalassemia minor and the associated asymptomatic anemia typically have favorable pregnancy outcomes. In the absence of documented iron deficiency anemia, replacement of iron beyond prophylactic doses is not indicated.

Inherited Thrombophilias

Inherited thrombophilias are a group of disorders characterized by a propensity for blood clotting. They are caused by defects in one or more of the clotting factors and often result in potentially dangerous thrombosis. In addition to the association between thrombophilias and thrombosis, there may be an association between inherited thrombophilias and adverse pregnancy outcomes, such as fetal loss, preeclampsia, fetal growth restriction, and placental abruption; however, a definitive causal link has not been established.

Screening

Screening for thrombophilias is controversial. It is useful only when results will affect management decisions, and is not useful in situations where treatment is indicated for other risk factors. Screening may be considered in patients with a personal history of venous thromboembolism that was associated with a nonrecurrent risk factor (eg, fractures, surgery, and prolonged immobilization) or who have a first-degree relative with a history of high-risk thrombophilia or venous thromboembolism before age 50 years in the absence of other risk factors. In other situations, thrombophilia testing is not routinely recommended. Testing for inherited thrombophilias in women who have experienced a recurrence of fetal loss, placental abruption, previous intrauterine growth restriction, or previous preeclampsia is not recommended. Whenever possible, laboratory testing should be performed remote (after 6 weeks) from the thrombotic event while the patient is neither pregnant nor taking anticoagulation nor hormonal therapy.

Management

The decision to not use pharmacologic therapy or to treat with thromboprophylaxis or full anticoagulation is influenced by the venous thromboembolism history, severity of inherited thrombophilia, and additional risk factors. All patients with inherited thrombophilias should undergo individualized risk assessment, which may modify management decisions. (For information on management, see "Deep Vein Thrombosis and Pulmonary Embolism" later in this chapter.)

Obesity and Bariatric Surgery

The World Health Organization and the National Institutes of Health define obesity as a body mass index (BMI) of 30 or greater. Currently one of five women is obese at the beginning of pregnancy. As the rate of obesity increases, the number of obese women of childbearing age considering bariatric surgery also increases, which results in questions about pregnancy after these types of surgeries. It is important for obstetric care providers to counsel obese patients with specific information concerning the maternal and fetal risks of obesity in pregnancy and to address prenatal and peripartum care considerations that may be especially relevant for obese patients, including those who have undergone bariatric surgery.

Obesity

During pregnancy, obese women are at increased risk of several adverse perinatal outcomes, including anesthetic, perioperative, and other maternal and fetal complications. Compared with nonobese women, obese patients are at high risk of preeclampsia; gestational diabetes; preterm birth; cesarean delivery; and operative and postoperative complications, including prolonged operating times and increased rates of excessive blood loss, wound infection, thromboembolism, and endometritis. Obese women are less likely to have a successful vaginal delivery than nonobese patients, and the success rate of attempted vaginal birth after cesarean delivery is very low in extremely obese women. Maternal obesity can have deleterious effects on the fetus, including increased risks of congenital anomalies, growth abnormalities, miscarriage, and stillbirth. The most common types of obesity-associated birth defects are related to the neural tube, cardiac systems, and facial clefting, even after controlling for the diabetes. In addition, increased body mass impairs visualization of ultrasound images and can compromise prenatal diagnosis of fetal anomalies. Maternal obesity also may be associated with an increase risk of subsequent childhood obesity.

Antepartum Management. Height and weight should be recorded for all women at the initial prenatal visit to allow calculation of the BMI. Recommendations for prenatal weight gain should be made based on the Institute of Medicine (IOM) guidelines (see also "First-Trimester Patient Education" in Chapter 5). Nutrition consultation should be offered to all obese women and they should be encouraged to follow an exercise program. This consultation should continue postpartum and before attempting another pregnancy. Consideration should be given to screening for gestational diabetes upon presentation or during the first trimester and repeating it later in pregnancy if the initial screening result is negative. Because these patients are at increased risk of emergent cesarean delivery and anesthetic complications, anesthesiology consultation before delivery is encouraged.

Intrapartum Management. Women with a BMI of 35 or greater who have pre-existing medical conditions, such as hypertension or diabetes, may benefit from a cardiac evaluation. Because of the increased likelihood of complicated and emergent cesarean delivery, extremely obese women may require specific resources, such as additional blood products, a large operating table, and extra personnel in the delivery room. Particular attention to the type and placement of the surgical incision is needed (ie, placing the incision above the panniculus adiposus). The decision to perform a primary cesarean delivery for obese women should be based on standard maternal and fetal indications. Because of the increased risk of venous thromboembolism associated with cesarean delivery and obesity, individual risk assessment may require additional thromboprophylaxis with unfractionated heparin or low molecular weight heparin, in addition to the recommended use of pneumatic compression devices, during and after cesarean delivery in obese patients (see also "Deep Vein Thrombosis and Pulmonary Embolism" later in this chapter).

Bariatric Surgery

As the rate of obesity increases, it is becoming more common for providers of women's health care to encounter patients who are either contemplating or have had operative procedures for weight loss, also known as bariatric surgery. The types of procedures commonly performed today include the Roux-en-Y gastric bypass (a combination of restrictive and malabsorptive effect) and adjustable gastric banding (restrictive). Researchers have determined that pregnancies after bariatric surgery are less likely to be complicated by gestational diabetes, hypertension, macrosomia, and cesarean delivery than are pregnancies of obese women who have not had the surgery. Although pregnancy outcomes generally have been favorable after bariatric surgery, nutritional and surgical complications can occur and some of these complications can result in adverse perinatal outcomes. The counseling and management of patients who become pregnant after bariatric surgery can be complex.

Preconception Counseling. Contraception and preconception counseling should be a component of the overall counseling for any reproductive-aged woman undergoing bariatric surgery. Contraceptive counseling is especially important for adolescents because pregnancy rates after bariatric surgery are double the rate in the general adolescent population (12.8% versus 6.4%). Because there is an increased risk of oral contraception failure after bariatric surgery, with a significant malabsorption component, nonoral administration of hormonal contraception should be considered in these patients.

Some authorities have recommended waiting 12–24 months after bariatric surgery before conceiving so that the fetus is not exposed to a rapid maternal weight loss environment and so that the patient can achieve full weight loss goals. Should pregnancy occur before this recommended time frame, close surveillance of maternal weight and nutritional status may be beneficial.

Antepartum Management. Broad evaluation for micronutrient deficiencies (particularly, iron, vitamin B_{12}, folate, and calcium) at the beginning of pregnancy for women who have had bariatric surgery should be considered. If there is a proven deficit, then appropriate treatment should be instituted and monitored. In the absence of a deficiency, monitoring the blood count, iron, ferritin, and calcium levels in every trimester may be considered. Close nutritional surveillance should continue postpartum. Alternative testing for gestational diabetes should be considered for those patients with a malabsorptive-type surgery. All gastrointestinal problems, such as nausea, vomiting, and abdominal pain, which occur commonly during pregnancy, should be thoroughly evaluated in patients who have had bariatric surgery. Early involvement of the bariatric surgeon in evaluating abdominal pain is critical because the underlying pathology may relate to the weight loss surgery. Other concerns for patients who have had bariatric surgery relate to medication dosages. In using medications in which a therapeutic drug level is critical, testing drug levels may be necessary to ensure a therapeutic effect.

Intrapartum Management. Bariatric surgery should not alter the course of labor and delivery, and as such does not significantly affect its management. Bariatric surgery itself should not be considered an indication for a cesarean delivery. If a patient has had extensive and complicated abdominal surgery from weight loss procedures, prelabor consultation with a bariatric surgeon should be considered.

Pregestational Diabetes Mellitus

Pregestational diabetes mellitus represents one of the most challenging medical complications of pregnancy. Type 2 pregestational diabetes mellitus is most common and is characterized by onset later in life; peripheral insulin resistance; relative insulin deficiency; obesity; and the development of vascular, renal, and neuropathic complications. The rapidly increasing incidence of type 2 pregestational diabetes mellitus is caused, in part, by increasing obesity in the United States. Although 90% of cases of diabetes encountered during pregnancy are gestational diabetes mellitus (GDM), more than one half of these women eventually develop type 2 pregestational diabetes mellitus later in life (see also "Gestational Diabetes Mellitus Diagnosis and Management" later in this chapter). Type 1 diabetes mellitus tends to occur early in life. In contrast to type 2 pregestational diabetes mellitus, type 1 pregestational diabetes mellitus is characterized by an autoimmune process that destroys the pancreatic β cells, which leads to insulin deficiency and the need for insulin therapy.

Maternal Complications

Overall perinatal outcome is best when glucose control is achieved before conception and in the absence of maternal vascular disease. Pregnancy has been associated with exacerbation of many diabetes-related complications, including diabetic retinopathy, nephropathy, and ketoacidosis. Poorly controlled pregestational diabetes mellitus leads to serious end-organ damage that may eventually become life threatening. In turn, pre-existing diabetes-related end-organ disease may have deleterious effects on obstetric outcomes. The rates of spontaneous preterm labor, preeclampsia, intrauterine growth restriction, and primary cesarean delivery are all increased in women with pregestational diabetes mellitus.

Fetal and Neonatal Complications

The risk of congenital abnormalities is increased in women with pre-existing diabetes. The fetus of a woman with poorly controlled diabetes is at increased risk of intrauterine fetal death and is more likely to weigh more than 4,000 g with a disproportionate concentration of fat around the shoulders and chest, which more than doubles the risk of shoulder dystocia at vaginal delivery. The neonatal consequences of poorly controlled pregestational diabetes mellitus during pregnancy include profound hypoglycemia, a higher rate of respiratory distress syndrome, polycythemia, organomegaly, electrolyte disturbances, and hyperbilirubinemia. Long-term outcomes for neonates with type 1 diabetes mellitus include obesity and carbohydrate intolerance.

Fetal Assessment

An ultrasound examination early in gestation can be used not only to demonstrate fetal viability but also to accurately date the pregnancy. Most major anomalies can be detected at 18–20 weeks of gestation by a specialized (or targeted) ultrasound examination that includes a carefully performed assessment of fetal cardiac structure, including the great vessels. Periodic ultrasound examinations may be used to confirm appropriate fetal growth. Antepartum fetal monitoring is a valuable approach and can be used to monitor the pregnancies of women with pregestational diabetes mellitus (see also "Antepartum Tests of Fetal Well-Being" in Chapter 5).

Antepartum Management

The management of diabetes in pregnancy must focus on excellent glucose control achieved using a careful combination of diet, exercise, and insulin therapy. Patients may need to be seen every 1–2 weeks during the first two trimesters and weekly after 28–30 weeks of gestation. A registered dietitian may be of value in providing an individualized nutrition program.

Pregnancy is characterized by increased insulin resistance and reduced sensitivity to insulin action. Insulin requirements will increase throughout pregnancy, most markedly in the period between 28–32 weeks of gestation. Most insulin used in the treatment of pregestational diabetes mellitus is biosynthetic human insulin. Short-acting or rapid-acting insulins are administered before meals to reduce glucose elevations associated with eating. Longer acting insulins are used to restrain hepatic glucose production between meals and in the fasting state. Intermediate-acting insulin usually is given before breakfast with a rapid-acting or short-acting insulin and before the evening meal or at bedtime.

Frequent self-monitoring of blood glucose is essential to achieve euglycemia without significant hypoglycemia during pregnancy. Even with meticulous monitoring, hypoglycemia is more frequent in pregnancy than at other times, particularly in patients with type 1 pregestational diabetes mellitus. Patients and their families should be taught how to respond quickly and appropriately to hypoglycemia.

Intrapartum Management

Optimal timing of delivery relies on balancing the risk of intrauterine fetal death with the risks of preterm birth. Early delivery may be indicated in some patients with vasculopathy, nephropathy, poor glucose control, or a prior stillbirth. If corticosteroids are administered to accelerate lung maturation, an increased insulin requirement over the next 5 days should be anticipated, and the patient's glucose levels should be closely monitored. In contrast, patients with well-controlled diabetes may be allowed to progress to their expected date of delivery as long as antenatal testing remains reassuring. Expectant management beyond the estimated due date generally is not recommended. To prevent traumatic birth injury, cesarean delivery may be considered if the estimated fetal weight is greater than 4,500 g in women with diabetes. Induction of labor in pregnancies with a fetus with suspected macrosomia has not been found to reduce birth trauma and may increase the cesarean delivery rate.

During induction of labor, maternal glycemia can be controlled with an intravenous infusion of regular insulin titrated to maintain hourly readings of blood glucose levels less than 110 mg/dL. Avoiding intrapartum maternal hyperglycemia may prevent fetal hyperglycemia and reduce the likelihood of subsequent neonatal hypoglycemia. During active labor, insulin may not be needed. Patients who are using an insulin pump may continue their basal infusion during labor.

Insulin requirements decrease rapidly after delivery. One half of the predelivery dose may be reinstituted after starting regular food intake. Breastfeeding should be encouraged in women with pregestational diabetes mellitus.

An additional 500 kcal more than the prepregnancy caloric intake is required per day. Small snacks before breastfeeding may reduce the risks of hypoglycemia.

Thyroid Disease

Because thyroid disease is the second most common endocrine disease that affects women of reproductive age, obstetricians often care for patients in whom alterations in thyroid gland function have been previously diagnosed. In addition, both hyperthyroidism and hypothyroidism may initially manifest during pregnancy. During pregnancy, the diagnosis of thyroid abnormalities is confused by significant but reversible changes in maternal thyroid physiology that lead to alterations in thyroid function tests during gestation. However, there are gestational age-specific nomograms and thresholds for evaluating thyroid status during pregnancy. The presence of maternal thyroid disease is important information for the pediatrician to have at the time of delivery.

Thyroid Function Testing

Thyroid testing in pregnancy should be performed on symptomatic women and women with a personal history of thyroid disease or other medical conditions associated with thyroid disease (eg, type 1 diabetes mellitus). In these individuals, it is most appropriate to assess thyroid-stimulating hormone (TSH) levels first and then evaluate other thyroid functions if the TSH level is abnormal. The performance of thyroid function tests in asymptomatic pregnant women who have a mildly enlarged thyroid is not warranted. Development of a significant goiter or distinct nodules should be evaluated as in any patient. Women with established overt thyroid disease (hyperthyroidism or hypothyroidism) should be appropriately treated to maintain a euthyroid state throughout pregnancy and during the postpartum period.

Hyperthyroidism

Hyperthyroidism occurs in 0.2% of pregnancies, with Graves disease accounting for 95% of these cases. Graves disease is an autoimmune disease characterized by production of thyroid-stimulating immunoglobulin and TSH-binding inhibitory immunoglobulin to mediate thyroid stimulation or inhibition, respectively. The signs and symptoms of hyperthyroidism include nervousness, tremors, tachycardia, frequent stools, excessive sweating, heat intolerance, weight loss, goiter, insomnia, palpitations, and hypertension. Thyroid storm is a serious complication of inadequately treated Graves disease that can adversely affect both mother and fetus. Late distinctive symptoms of Graves disease are ophthalmopathy (signs including lid lag and lid retraction) and dermopathy (signs include localized or pretibial myxedema).

Compared with controlled maternal hyperthyroidism, inadequately treated maternal hyperthyroidism is associated with a greater risk of preterm delivery, severe preeclampsia, and heart failure and with an increase in medically indicated preterm deliveries, low birth weight infants, and possibly fetal loss. Hyperthyroidism in pregnancy is treated with thioamides, which decrease thyroid hormone synthesis by blocking the organification of iodide. In 2011, the U.S. Food and Drug Administration issued a black box warning for propylthiouracil because of its association with liver failure. Therefore, the preferred thioamide is methimazole. The goal of management of hyperthyroidism in pregnancy is to maintain the free thyroxine or free thyroxine index in the high normal range using the lowest possible dosage of thioamides to minimize fetal exposure to thioamides.

Hypothyroidism

The classic signs and symptoms of hypothyroidism are fatigue, constipation, intolerance to cold, muscle cramps, hair loss, dry skin, prolonged relaxation phase of deep tendon reflexes, and carpal tunnel syndrome. If left untreated, hypothyroidism will progress to myxedema and myxedema coma. It is unusual for advanced hypothyroidism to present in pregnancy. Subclinical hypothyroidism is diagnosed in asymptomatic women when the TSH level is increased and the free thyroxine level is within the reference range. However, at this time there are insufficient data characterizing perinatal risks of subclinical hypothyroidism or benefits of treatment, so routine testing is not recommended. Women with iodine-deficient hypothyroidism are at significant risk of having babies with congenital cretinism (growth failure, mental retardation, and other neuropsychologic deficits). Treatment of hypothyroidism in pregnant women is the same as for nonpregnant women and involves administering levothyroxine at sufficient dosages to normalize TSH levels.

Pregnancy-Related Complications

Anemia

The definition of *anemia* according to the Centers for Disease Control and Prevention is a hemoglobin (Hgb) or hematocrit (Hct) value less than the fifth percentile of the distribution of Hgb or Hct in a healthy reference population based on the stage of pregnancy. The two most common causes of anemia in pregnancy and the puerperium are iron deficiency and acute blood loss. Anemia may be classified according to the causative mechanism (decreased production, increased destruction, blood loss) or red blood cell morphology (microcytic, normocytic, macrocytic) or whether it is an inherited or acquired disorder. Iron deficiency anemia during pregnancy has been associated with an increased risk of low birth weight, preterm delivery, and perinatal mortality.

Screening and Diagnosis

All pregnant women should be screened for anemia during pregnancy. Measurements of serum hemoglobin (Hgb) concentration or hematocrit (Hct) are the primary screening tests for identifying anemia. Normal iron indices are listed in Table 7-1. Hemoglobin and Hct levels are lower in African American women compared with white women. Thus, for African American adults, the IOM recommends lowering the cutoff levels for Hgb and Hct by 0.8 g/dL and 2%, respectively. Asymptomatic women who meet the criteria for anemia (Hct levels less than 33% in the first trimester and third trimester and less than 32% in the second trimester) should be evaluated.

Antepartum Management

The initial evaluation of pregnant women with mild to moderate anemia may include a medical history, physical examination, and red blood cell indices, serum iron levels, and ferritin levels. Using biochemical tests, iron deficiency anemia is defined by results of abnormal values for levels of serum ferritin, transferrin saturation, and levels of free erythrocyte protoporphyrin, along with low Hgb or Hct levels. Those with iron deficiency anemia should be treated with supplemental iron, in addition to prenatal vitamins. Failure to respond to iron therapy should prompt further investigation and may suggest an incorrect diagnosis, coexisting disease, malabsorption (sometimes caused by the use of

Table 7-1. Normal Iron Indices in Pregnancy

Test	Normal Value
Plasma iron level	40–175 micrograms/dL
Plasma total iron-binding capacity	216–400 micrograms/dL
Transferrin saturation	6–60%
Serum ferritin level	More than 10 micrograms/dL
Free erythrocyte protoporphyrin level	Less than 3 micrograms/g

Anemia in pregnancy. ACOG Practice Bulletin No. 95. American College of Obstetricians and Gynecologists. Obstet Gynecol 2008;112:201–7.

enteric-coated tablets or concomitant use of antacids), nonadherence, or blood loss. Patients with anemia other than iron deficiency anemia should be further evaluated (see also "Hemoglobinopathies" in this chapter).

Intrapartum Management

Iron supplementation decreases the prevalence of maternal anemia at delivery. Transfusions of red cells seldom are indicated unless hypovolemia from blood loss coexists or an operative delivery must be performed on a patient with anemia. Severe anemia with maternal Hgb levels less than 6 g/dL has been associated with abnormal fetal oxygenation, resulting in nonreassuring fetal heart rate patterns, reduced amniotic fluid volume, fetal cerebral vasodilatation, and fetal death. Thus, maternal transfusion should be considered for fetal indications in cases of severe anemia.

Deep Vein Thrombosis and Pulmonary Embolism

Deep vein thrombosis (DVT) and pulmonary embolism (PE) are collectively referred to as venous thromboembolic events. Approximately 75–80% of cases of pregnancy-associated venous thromboembolic events are caused by DVT, and 20–25% of cases are caused by PE. Venous thromboembolism accounts for approximately 9% of all maternal deaths in the United States. Pregnant women have a fourfold to fivefold increased risk of thromboembolism compared with nonpregnant women. The most important individual risk factor for venous thromboembolism in pregnancy is a personal history of thrombosis. The next most important individual risk factor for venous thromboembolism in pregnancy is the presence of a thrombophilia (both acquired and inherited). Other risk factors for the development of pregnancy-associated venous thromboembolism include the physiologic changes that accompany pregnancy and childbirth, medical factors (such as obesity, hemoglobinopathies, hypertension, and smoking), and pregnancy complications (including operative delivery).

Evaluation and Diagnosis

Women with a history of thrombosis who have not had a complete evaluation of possible underlying etiologies should be tested for both antiphospholipid antibodies and for inherited thrombophilias. Medical records, including imaging studies, from any prior venous thromboembolic event may be helpful in evaluation. When signs or symptoms suggest new onset DVT, the recommended initial diagnostic test is compression ultrasonography of the proximal veins. Ventilation–perfusion scanning and computed tomographic angiography are used to diagnose new onset PE. Both tests are associated with relatively low radiation exposure for the fetus.

Antepartum Management

Therapeutic anticoagulation is recommended for women with acute thromboembolism during the current pregnancy or those at high risk of venous thromboembolism, such as women with mechanical heart valves. Other candidates for either prophylactic or therapeutic anticoagulation during pregnancy include women with a history of thrombosis or those who are at significant risk of venous thromboembolism during pregnancy or the postpartum period, such as those with high-risk acquired or inherited thrombophilias.

Common anticoagulation medications include unfractionated heparin, low molecular weight heparin (LMWH), and warfarin. The preferred anticoagulants in pregnancy are heparin compounds. Patients with an incidentally discovered low-risk thrombophilia without a prior venous thromboembolic event can be managed antepartum with either surveillance or prophylactic LMWH or unfractionated heparin, and in the postpartum period with either LMWH and unfractionated heparin prophylaxis or with surveillance if the patient has no additional risk factors for DVT. Guidelines recommend obtaining platelet counts when initiating therapeutic unfractionated heparin therapy in order to monitor for heparin-induced thrombocytopenia.

Intrapartum Management

Women receiving either therapeutic or prophylactic anticoagulation may be converted from LMWH to the shorter half-life unfractionated heparin in the last month of pregnancy or sooner if delivery appears imminent. An alternative option may be to stop therapeutic anticoagulation and induce labor within 24 hours, if clinically appropriate. The American Society of Regional Anesthesia and Pain Medicine guidelines recommend withholding neuraxial blockade for 10–12 hours after the most recent prophylactic dose of LMWH or 24 hours after the most recent therapeutic dose of LMWH.

Cesarean delivery approximately doubles the risk of VTE, but in the otherwise normal patient, this risk is still low (approximately 1 per 1,000 patients). Given this increased risk, and based on extrapolation from perioperative data, placement of pneumatic compression devices before cesarean delivery is recommended for all women not already receiving thromboprophylaxis. For patients with additional risk factors for thromboembolism undergoing cesarean delivery, individual risk assessment may require thromboprophylaxis with both pneumatic compression devices and unfractionated heparin or LMWH. However, cesarean delivery in the emergency setting should not be delayed because of the timing necessary to implement thromboprophylaxis.

Additional measures should be considered for certain women at particularly high risk of thrombosis at the time of delivery. Women who have antithrombin deficiency may be candidates for antithrombin concentrates peripartum. Women who have had DVT in the 2–4 weeks before delivery may be candidates for placement of a temporary vena caval filter, with removal postpartum. Other women who may be candidates for vena caval filter placement during pregnancy include women with a recurrence of a venous thromboembolic event despite therapeutic anticoagulation.

Postpartum Management

The risk of venous thromboembolic event is higher postpartum, especially during the first week postpartum, than it is during pregnancy. Most patients who receive thromboprophylaxis during pregnancy will benefit from thromboprophylaxis postpartum, but the dose and route will vary by indication. The optimal time to restart anticoagulation postpartum is unclear. A reasonable approach to minimize bleeding complications is to restart unfractionated heparin or LMWH no sooner than 4–6 hours after vaginal delivery or 6–12 hours after cesarean delivery. When reinstitution of anticoagulation is planned postpartum, pneumatic compression devices should be left in place until the patient is ambulatory and until anticoagulation is restarted. Women who require more than 6 weeks of anticoagulation may be bridged to warfarin. Because warfarin, LMWH, and unfractionated heparin do not accumulate in breast milk and do not induce an anticoagulant effect in the infant, these anticoagulants are compatible with breastfeeding.

Gestational Diabetes Mellitus Diagnosis and Management

Gestational diabetes mellitus is defined as carbohydrate intolerance that begins or is first recognized during pregnancy. This condition is associated with increased risks for the fetus and newborn, including macrosomia, shoulder dystocia, birth injuries, hyperbilirubinemia, hypoglycemia, respiratory distress syndrome, and childhood obesity. Maternal risks include preeclampsia, cesarean delivery, and an increased risk of developing type-2 diabetes later in life. The prevalence varies significantly in different populations and ethnicities, as well as with the diagnostic criteria used.

Diagnosis

The administration of a diagnostic glucose tolerance test (GTT) is advised for women whose 50-g, 1-hour glucose challenge levels meet or exceed the recommended screening test thresholds, ranging from 130 mg/dL to 140 mg/dL (see also "Routine Laboratory Testing in Pregnancy" in Chapter 5). The diagnosis of gestational diabetes can be made on the basis of the 100-g, 3-hour oral GTT, for which there is evidence that treatment improves outcome. Either the plasma or serum glucose level established by Carpenter and Coustan or the plasma level designated by the National Diabetes Data Group conversions are appropriate to use in the diagnosis of GDM (see Table 7-2). A positive diagnosis requires that two or more thresholds be met or exceeded.

Antepartum Management

Potential management strategies to prevent adverse pregnancy outcomes due to gestational diabetes include fetal surveillance, blood glucose monitoring, nutrition therapy, implementation of an exercise program, and administration of insulin.

Fetal Surveillance. Antepartum fetal testing is recommended for patients with pregestational diabetes. For women with poor glycemic control, fetal surveillance may be beneficial. There is no consensus regarding antepartum testing

Table 7-2. Diagnostic Criteria for the 100-Gram, 3-Hour Glucose Tolerance Test for Gestational Diabetes Mellitus*

Status	Plasma or Serum Glucose Level Carpenter/Coustan Conversion		Plasma Level National Diabetes Data Group Conversion	
	mg/dL	mmol/L	mg/dL	mmol/L
Fasting	95	5.3	105	5.8
One hour	180	10.0	190	10.6
Two hour	155	8.6	165	9.2
Three hour	140	7.8	145	8.0

*A positive diagnosis requires that two or more thresholds be met or exceeded.

Modified with permission of the American Diabetes Association from the Expert Committee on the Diagnosis and Classification of Diabetes Mellitus. Report of the Expert Committee on the Diagnosis and Classification of Diabetes Mellitus. Diab Care 2000;23(suppl 1):S4–S19. Copyright 2000 American Diabetes Association.

in women with well-controlled GDM. The particular antepartum test may be chosen according to local practice.

Diet. The most appropriate diet for women with GDM has yet to be established. Nutritional intervention in women with GDM should be designed to achieve normal glucose levels and avoid ketosis, while maintaining appropriate nutrition and weight gain. The American Diabetes Association recommends nutritional counseling for all patients with GDM by a registered dietician, if possible, with a personalized nutrition plan based on the individual's body mass index.

Exercise. Exercise often is recommended for individuals with diabetes, both as a way to achieve weight reduction and as a treatment to improve glucose metabolism. A regular exercise program has clear benefits for all women and may offer additional advantages for women with GDM. Women with GDM who lead an active lifestyle should be encouraged to continue a program of exercise approved for pregnancy (see also "First-Trimester Patient Education" in Chapter 5).

Blood Glucose Monitoring. Once a woman with GDM is placed on diet therapy, surveillance of blood glucose levels is required to be certain that glycemic control has been established. There is insufficient evidence concerning the optimal frequency of blood glucose testing in women with GDM.

Medical Treatment. When nutrition therapy has not resulted in fasting glucose levels less than 95 mg/dL, 1-hour postprandial values less than 130–140 mg/dL, or 2-hour postprandial values less than 120 mg/dL, insulin should be considered. The available evidence does not support a clear recommendation as to the number of times glucose values should exceed targets before insulin is added or the dosage increased. No particular insulin regimen or insulin dose has been demonstrated to be superior for GDM. Generally, it is easiest for the patient to start with the simplest regimen and work up to a more complex regimen as needed. Regardless of the starting dosage, subsequent dosage adjustments should be based on the blood glucose levels at particular times of day. Because free insulin apparently does not cross the placenta, all types of insulin have been used in patients with GDM.

Intrapartum Management

The timing of delivery in patients with GDM remains relatively open. When glucose control is good and no other complications supervene, there is no good evidence to support routine delivery before 39–40 weeks of gestation. Individuals whose metabolic control does not meet the goals described earlier, or is undocumented, or those with risk factors, such as hypertensive disorders or previous stillbirth, should be managed the same as those with pre-existing diabetes (see also "Pregestational Diabetes Mellitus" earlier in this chapter). For women with GDM and an estimated fetal weight of 4,500 g or more, cesarean delivery may be considered because it may reduce the likelihood of permanent brachial plexus injury in the infant.

Postpartum Screening

Women with a history of GDM are at increased risk of developing diabetes (generally type-2 diabetes) later in life. All women with GDM should be screened at 6–12 weeks postpartum and managed appropriately. Either a fasting plasma glucose test or the 75-g, 2-hour oral glucose tolerance test are appropriate for diagnosing diabetes. Although the fasting plasma glucose test is easier to perform, it lacks sensitivity for detecting other forms of abnormal glucose metabolism; results of the oral GTT can confirm an impaired fasting glucose level and impaired glucose tolerance. Women with abnormal testing results should be referred to the appropriate health care provider for follow-up.

The American Diabetes Association recommends repeat testing at least every 3 years for women who had a pregnancy affected by GDM and normal results of postpartum screening. For women who may have subsequent pregnancies, screening more frequently has the advantage of detecting abnormal glucose metabolism before pregnancy and provides an opportunity to ensure preconception glucose control. Women should be encouraged to discuss their GDM history and need for screening with all of their health care providers.

Hypertensive Disorders of Pregnancy

Hypertensive disease occurs in approximately 12–22% of pregnancies and accounts for approximately 18% of maternal deaths in the United States. Gestational hypertension is characterized by the onset of hypertension after the 20th week of pregnancy, with a return to prepregnancy blood pressure levels during the normal postpartum period. Other hypertensive disorders unique to pregnancy include preeclampsia (gestational hypertension with proteinuria) and eclampsia (preeclampsia with the new-onset of grand mal seizures). *Chronic hypertension* in pregnancy, however, is defined as hypertension that is present before pregnancy or before the 20th week of gestation.

Preeclampsia and Eclampsia

Preeclampsia is primarily a disorder of first pregnancies. Other risk factors include multifetal gestation, preeclampsia in a previous pregnancy, chronic hypertension, pregestational diabetes, vascular and connective tissue disease, nephropathy, antiphospholipid antibody syndrome, obesity, age of 35 years or older, and African American race. Genetic and environmental factors also play a role in the development of preeclampsia. No single screening test for preeclampsia has been found to be reliable and cost effective.

Diagnosis. Preeclampsia is a pregnancy-specific syndrome characterized by *hypertension* (defined as blood pressure of 140 mm Hg systolic or higher or 90 mm Hg diastolic or higher) that occurs after 20 weeks of gestation in a woman with previously normal blood pressure and proteinuria (defined as urinary excretion of 0.3 g protein or higher in a 24-hour urine specimen, which corresponds approximately to 1+ on a random urine dipstick). In addition to hypertension and proteinuria, preeclampsia also may be associated with a myriad of other signs and symptoms, such as edema, visual disturbances, headache, and epigastric pain. The distinction between mild and severe preeclampsia is important for decisions regarding management and timing of delivery. Hemolysis, elevated liver enzymes, low platelets (HELLP) syndrome is a constellation of laboratory abnormalities, including HELLP counts in addition to the hypertension and proteinuria typically associated with preeclampsia. Proteinuria may or may not be present in HELLP syndrome. Severe preeclampsia and HELLP syndrome are associated with an increased risk of adverse outcomes, including eclampsia, abruption, renal failure, subcapsular hepatic hematoma, a recurrence of preeclampsia, preterm delivery, and even fetal or maternal death. Superimposed preeclampsia is a diagnosis of preeclampsia made in a patient with pre-existing hypertensive disease. Diagnostic criteria include new-onset proteinuria in a woman with chronic hypertension, a sudden increase in proteinuria if already present in early gestation, a sudden increase in hypertension, or the development of HELLP syndrome.

Antepartum Management. Treatment of preeclampsia should be directed toward balancing both maternal and fetal risks. The most definitive treatment is delivery. However, other factors that may be important considerations in forming a management plan and evaluating the appropriate timing of delivery include the severity of preeclampsia, gestational age, maternal condition, fetal condition, presence of labor, and availability and capability of hospital staff and resources. Gestational hypertension and mild preeclampsia before term may be managed with careful home observation with frequent and reliable outpatient maternal and fetal assessment. Women with difficulty with adherence or other logistical barriers to frequent follow-up should be hospitalized. The management of a woman with severe preeclampsia remote from term is best accomplished in a tertiary care setting or in consultation with an obstetrician–gynecologist with training, experience, and demonstrated competence in the management of high-risk pregnancies, such as a maternal–fetal medicine subspecialist. Given the serious nature of HELLP syndrome and the possibility for severe maternal sequelae, immediate delivery is reasonable independent of gestational age for women with HELLP syndrome. When possible, the administration of antenatal corticosteroids between 24 weeks and 34 weeks of gestation should be considered for all women with preeclampsia to promote fetal lung maturity in the event of premature delivery.

Intrapartum Management. Two main goals of management of preeclampsia during labor and delivery include prevention of seizures and control of hypertension. Magnesium sulfate should be used for the prevention and treatment of seizures in women with severe preeclampsia or eclampsia. Acute antihypertensive therapy should be used for diastolic blood pressure levels of 110 mm Hg or higher or systolic blood pressure values greater than or equal to 160 mm Hg. If analgesia or anesthesia is required, regional or neuraxial analgesia or anesthesia is preferred.

Women with eclampsia require prompt intervention and should be delivered in a timely fashion. Once the patient is stabilized, the method of delivery should depend, in part, on factors, such as gestational age, fetal presentation, and the findings of the cervical examination. The decision to perform cesarean delivery should be individualized with attention to maternal stability and the anticipated time course of worsening disease.

Chronic Hypertension

Chronic hypertension in pregnancy is defined as hypertension present before pregnancy or before the 20th week of gestation. Although most women with chronic hypertension conceive when the disease is still mild and most of the pregnancies have only minor complications, chronic hypertension is associated with several adverse pregnancy outcomes, including premature birth, fetal growth restriction, fetal demise, placental abruption, and cesarean delivery.

Diagnosis. Chronic hypertension during pregnancy is most commonly classified as mild (systolic blood pressure of 140–159 mm Hg or diastolic blood pressure of 90–109 mm Hg) or as severe (systolic blood pressure of 160 mm Hg or greater or diastolic blood pressure of 110 mm Hg or greater). To establish the diagnosis of hypertension, blood pressure levels that meet the criteria should be documented on more than one occasion, at least 4–6 hours apart. Chronic hypertension can be difficult to distinguish from either gestational hypertension or preeclampsia in women who present for care with hypertension late in gestation. When hypertension develops during pregnancy, typically in the third trimester, in the absence of signs or symptoms of preeclampsia, the diagnosis of gestational hypertension is appropriate. Chronic hypertension usually can be distinguished from preeclampsia because preeclampsia typically appears after 20 weeks of gestation in a woman who was normotensive before pregnancy and most frequently includes proteinuria. The acute onset of proteinuria or a sudden increase over baseline proteinuria and baseline hypertension in women with chronic hypertension should prompt the assessment for superimposed preeclampsia.

Antepartum Management. Ideally, a woman with chronic hypertension should be evaluated before conception to identify possible end-organ involvement. Specific testing before pregnancy or early in pregnancy might include assessment of renal function, electrocardiography, echocardiography, and ophthalmologic evaluation. The choice of appropriate tests is dependent on the severity of the chronic hypertension. Evaluation of fetal growth by ultrasonography in women with chronic hypertension is warranted. If growth restriction is suspected, the fetal status should be monitored.

Antihypertensive therapy has been shown to reduce the risk of a severe maternal hypertensive crisis but has not been shown to improve overall perinatal outcome. Experts in the United States have recommended that pregnant women with hypertension in the blood pressure range of 150–160/100–110 mm Hg should be treated with antihypertensive therapy, and that their blood pressure should be kept lower than 150/100 mm Hg. It would seem reasonable to withhold antihypertensive therapy in women with mild hypertension who become pregnant unless their blood pressure is 150/100 mm Hg or greater or they have other complicating factors (eg, cardiovascular or renal disease) and to either stop or reduce medication in women who are already taking antihypertensive therapy. Based on the overall low rate of adverse effects and good efficacy, labetalol is a good option for first-line treatment of chronic hypertension in pregnancy. Calcium channel blockers or antagonists, the most commonly studied of which is nifedipine, also have been used in pregnant women with chronic hypertension. Methyldopa has been used for decades to treat hypertension in pregnancy, and it appears to be safe for this indication. However, its strong association with significant maternal sedation at therapeutic doses is a limitation to the use of this medication. Thiazide diuretic therapy used in women before pregnancy does not need to be discontinued during pregnancy. Angiotensin-converting enzyme inhibitors and angiotensin receptor blockers are contraindicated in all trimesters of pregnancy.

Intrapartum Management. Pregnant women with uncomplicated mild chronic hypertension generally are candidates for a vaginal delivery at term because most of them have good maternal and neonatal outcomes. Cesarean delivery should be reserved for obstetric indications. Women with hypertension during pregnancy and a prior adverse pregnancy outcome (eg, stillbirth) may be candidates for earlier delivery after documentation of fetal lung maturity. Women with severe chronic hypertension during pregnancy often either give birth prematurely or need premature delivery for fetal or maternal indications.

The combination of chronic hypertension and superimposed preeclampsia, particularly if it is preterm, represents a complicated situation, and the clinician should consider consultation with a subspecialist in maternal–fetal medicine. Women with severe hypertension or hypertension that is complicated by cardiovascular or renal disease may present special problems during the intrapartum period and should be collaboratively managed by the primary obstetrician and a maternal–fetal medicine subspecialist or an intensivist. Women with severe hypertension may require antihypertensive medications to treat acute elevation of blood pressure. Women with chronic hypertension complicated by significant cardiovascular or renal disease require special attention to fluid load and urine output because they may be susceptible to fluid overload with resultant pulmonary edema. General anesthesia may pose a risk in pregnant women with severe hypertension or superimposed preeclampsia. Therefore, regional analgesia and anesthesia is recommended when needed.

Intrauterine Growth Restriction

Intrauterine growth restriction is a term used to describe a fetus whose estimated weight appears to be less than expected, usually less than the 10th percentile. The term IUGR includes normal fetuses at the lower end of the growth spectrum, as well as those with specific clinical conditions in which the fetus fails to achieve its inherent growth potential as a consequence of either pathologic extrinsic influences (such as maternal smoking) or intrinsic genetic defects (such as aneuploidy). Infants with a birth weight at the lower extreme of the normal birth weight distribution are termed small for gestational age (SGA). In the United States, the most commonly used definition of SGA is a birth weight below the 10th percentile for gestational age.

Perinatal morbidity and mortality is significantly increased in the presence of low birth weight for gestational age, especially with weights below the third percentile for gestational age. Both intrapartum and neonatal complications are increased in the presence of IUGR. Long-term follow-up of infants with SGA shows that they are more prone to develop adult-onset hypertension and cardiovascular complications.

Screening

All pregnancies should be screened with serial fundal height assessments, reserving ultrasonography for those fetuses with risk factors (see Box 7-2), lagging growth, or no growth. Women who have previously given birth to an SGA infant are at an increased risk of IUGR in subsequent pregnancies. Physicians should consider an early ultrasound examination to confirm gestational age, as well as subsequent ultrasonography to evaluate sequential fetal growth, in women with significant risk factors.

Diagnosis

There are two essential steps involved in the antenatal recognition of growth restriction: 1) The elucidation of maternal risk factors associated with growth restriction (see Box 7-2) and 2) the clinical assessment of uterine size relative to gestational age. Several methods are available for clinical determination of uterine size, the most common of which is the measurement of fundal height. The second step is the ultrasonographic assessment of fetal size and growth. Ultrasonographically estimated fetal weight, head-to abdomen or femur-to-abdomen ratios, or serial observation of biometric growth patterns (growth velocity) are all acceptable and widely used methods to diagnose IUGR.

Antepartum Management

Once IUGR is suspected (ie, lagging fundal height), it should be confirmed using multiple ultrasonographic parameters, such as estimated weight percentile, amniotic fluid volume, increased head circumference, and abdominal circumference ratio. Serial ultrasound examinations to determine the rate of

---

Box 7-2. Risk Factors for Intrauterine Growth Restriction

- Maternal medical conditions
  - Hypertension
  - Renal disease
  - Restrictive lung disease
  - Diabetes (with microvascular disease)
  - Cyanotic heart disease
  - Antiphospholipid syndrome
  - Collagen-vascular disease
  - Hemoglobinopathies
- Smoking and substance use and abuse
- Severe malnutrition
- Primary placental disease
- Multiple gestation
- Infections (viral, protozoal)
- Genetic disorders
- Exposure to teratogens

American College of Obstetricians and Gynecologists. Intrauterine growth restriction. ACOG Practice Bulletin No. 12. Washington, DC: ACOG; 2000.

---

growth should be obtained approximately every 2–4 weeks, and Doppler assessment (ie, increased systolic/diastolic ratio or reversed or absent end-diastolic flow) may be useful in ongoing evaluation. If any test result is abnormal (eg, decreased amniotic fluid volume or abnormal Doppler assessments), more frequent testing, possibly daily, may be indicated.

The diagnosis of IUGR as the fetus approaches term may be an indication for delivery. If pregnancy is remote from term or if delivery is not elected, the optimal mode of monitoring has not been established. Periodic fetal assessment (approximately weekly) using Doppler velocimetry, contraction stress test, traditional biophysical profile (BPP), modified BPP, or nonstress test are all accepted monitoring techniques. The fetus should be delivered if the risk of fetal death exceeds that of neonatal death, although in many cases these risks are difficult to assess.

The timing of delivery in the growth-restricted fetus should be individualized. Early delivery may yield an infant with all the serious sequelae of prematurity, whereas delaying delivery may yield a hypoxic, acidotic infant with long-term neurologic sequelae. Gestational age and the findings of antenatal surveillance should be taken into account. The decision to deliver is based often on nonreassuring fetal assessment or a complete cessation of fetal growth assessed ultrasonographically over a 2–4-week interval. When extrauterine survival is likely despite significantly abnormal antenatal testing, delivery should be seriously considered.

Isoimmunization in Pregnancy

When any fetal blood group factor inherited from the father is not possessed by the mother, antepartum or intrapartum fetal–maternal bleeding may stimulate an immune reaction in the mother. Maternal immune reactions also can occur from blood product transfusion. The formation of maternal antibodies, or alloimmunization, may lead to various degrees of transplacental passage of these antibodies into the fetal circulation. Depending on the degree of antigenicity and the amount and type of antibodies involved, this transplacental passage may lead to hemolytic disease in the fetus and neonate. Undiagnosed and untreated, alloimmunization can lead to significant perinatal morbidity and mortality. Historically, most of the cases of Rh alloimmunization that caused transfusion reactions or serious hemolytic disease in the fetus and newborn were the result of incompatibility with respect to the D antigen. For this reason, the designation Rh positive usually indicates the presence of the D antigen and Rh negative indicates the absence of D antigen on erythrocytes. However, the use of antepartum anti-D immune globulin to prevent red cell alloimmunization has led to a relative increase in the number of cases of non–Rh-D alloimmunization, which causes fetal anemia and hemolytic disease in the newborn.

Screening

All pregnant women should be tested at the time of the first prenatal visit (or at the first presentation for obstetric care) for ABO blood group and Rh-D type and screened for the presence of erythrocyte antibodies. These laboratory assessments should be repeated in each subsequent pregnancy. Anti-D immune globulin prophylaxis is indicated only in Rh-negative women who are not previously sensitized to D. (For information on prophylaxis, see "Routine Laboratory Testing in Pregnancy" in Chapter 5.)

Maternal antibody titer levels are reported as the integer of greatest tube dilution with a positive agglutination value. If the initial antibody titer is 1:8 or less, the patient may be monitored with maternal serum antibody titer assessment every 4 weeks. Note that for a woman with a history of a previously affected fetus or neonate, serial titer assessment is inadequate for surveillance of fetal anemia. Additional evaluation is required for patients with a critical titer (ranging from 1:8 to 1:32 at most institutions), which is associated with a significant risk of severe erythroblastosis fetalis and hydrops. Similar titer levels are used to guide care for alloimmunization involving antigens other than D except in Kell-sensitized patients because Kell antibodies do not correlate with fetal status; fetal surveillance may be required even in the absence of critical antibody titers.

Antepartum Management

The initial management of a pregnancy involving an alloimmunized patient is determination of the paternal erythrocyte antigen genotype status to assess the risk of hemolytic anemia in the fetus. If the father does not carry a gene for the antigen of interest and paternity is certain, then further assessment is unnecessary. However, if the father's genotype is heterozygous or unknown, the fetal antigen type should be assessed by amniocentesis.

Measurement of the peak systolic velocity in the fetal middle cerebral artery via Doppler ultrasonography is used to assess the severity of erythroblastosis in utero. Moderate or severe anemia is predicted by values of peak systolic velocity in the fetal middle cerebral artery above 1.5 times the median for gestational age. Doppler measurements also are used to predict severe fetal anemia in patients with Kell alloimmunization. Correct technique is a critical factor when determining peak systolic velocity in the fetal middle cerebral artery with Doppler ultrasonography. This procedure should be used only by those with adequate training and clinical experience.

Intrapartum Management

It is reasonable to proceed with delivery by induction of labor at 37–38 weeks of gestation if the history and antenatal studies indicate only mild fetal hemolysis. Induction may be considered earlier if fetal pulmonary maturity is documented by amniocentesis. With severely sensitized pregnancies requiring multiple invasive procedures, the risks of continued umbilical cord blood sampling and transfusions must be considered and compared with those neonatal risks associated with early delivery. Given that the overall neonatal survival rate after 32 weeks of gestation in most neonatal intensive care nurseries is greater than 95%, it is prudent to time procedures so that the last transfusion is performed at 30–32 weeks of gestation, with delivery at 32–34 weeks of gestation after maternal steroid administration to enhance fetal pulmonary maturity.

Multifetal Pregnancy

The incidence of twin and high-order multiple gestations has increased significantly over the past 20 years primarily because of the availability and increased use of ovulation induction agents and assisted reproductive technology. There is increased fetal, neonatal, and maternal morbidity and mortality associated with multifetal gestations. The practicing obstetrician managing these high-risk patients should be familiar with their special antepartum and intrapartum problems, and consultation with maternal–fetal medicine specialists may be necessary.

Antepartum Management

Antepartum management of multifetal pregnancies requires special considerations in the areas of nutrition, prenatal diagnosis, antepartum surveillance, ultrasonography, and in the diagnosis and treatment of commonly associated pregnancy complications.

Nutritional Considerations. It is recommended that maternal dietary intake in a multiple gestation be increased by approximately 300 kcal more per day than that for a singleton pregnancy. Supplementation should include iron and folic acid. The optimal weight gain for women with multiple gestations has not been determined. However, for twin pregnancy, the IOM guidelines suggest a gestational weight gain of 37–54 pounds for women of normal weight, 31–50 pounds for overweight women, and 25–42 pounds for obese women. (For more information on nutritional guidelines, see "First-Trimester Patient Education" in Chapter 5.)

Prenatal Diagnosis. The usual indications for prenatal diagnosis and counseling in a singleton pregnancy apply to twin and high-order multiple gestations (see also "Antepartum Genetic Screening and Diagnosis" in Chapter 5). Multifetal gestations complicate prenatal genetic screening and diagnosis. Increased maternal age alone increases the risk of aneuploidy. The presence of multiple fetuses increases the mathematical probability that one or more fetuses will be affected and, thus, results in a higher risk for the pregnancy than that attributed to maternal age alone.

Amniocentesis or chorionic villous sampling may be technically difficult to accomplish in patients with multiple gestations, and only experienced physicians should perform these procedures in high-order multiple gestations. Technical problems unique to high-order multiple gestation include the need to traverse another fetus' sac to reach a different fetus for sampling, incorrect fetal karyotype caused by cross contamination with other sacs, difficulty in accurately mapping the fetuses and determining which fetus is being sampled, difficulty in accurately determining whether any of the fetuses are monochorionic twins, and difficulty in locating and reducing only the affected fetus in the event an aneuploidy is diagnosed and termination chosen.

Antepartum Fetal Surveillance. Multiple gestations are at increased risk of stillbirth. The nonstress test and the fetal biophysical profile have been shown to be effective in identifying the compromised twin or triplet gestation; however, the most effective fetal surveillance system for such pregnancies is not known. It is also not known at what gestational age testing should be initiated, whether testing should be performed once or twice per week, or whether there is a need to test normally growing dichorionic twins. At present, antepartum fetal surveillance in multiple gestations is recommended in all situations in which surveillance would ordinarily be performed in a singleton pregnancy (eg, IUGR, maternal disease, and decreased fetal movement).

Ultrasonography. Ultrasonography can be useful in both prenatal diagnosis and surveillance of multiple gestations. Early ultrasonography should be used for evaluation of chorionicity, given its importance regarding prognosis and risk of certain complications. Beginning at viability, serial estimations of fetal growth by ultrasonography (every 4–6 weeks after viability, or more closely spaced should indications arise) are a prudent measure because physical examination is less reliable.

Complications. Complications associated with multiple gestations include gestational diabetes, hypertension and preeclampsia, premature delivery, growth restriction, discordant growth, death of one fetus, and twin–twin transfusion syndrome. (For more information, see "Gestational Diabetes Mellitus Diagnosis and Management" and "Hypertensive Disorders of Pregnancy" earlier in this chapter.)

- Preterm labor and delivery—Preterm labor and preterm delivery are more common with multiple gestations, and increases with fetal number. The risks associated with tocolytic agents are amplified in multiple gestations and thus they should be used judiciously. The effect of antenatal steroid administration and the effects of steroid dose in multiple gestations have not been examined. Nonetheless, the National Institutes of Health recommends that all women in preterm labor likely to give birth between 24 weeks and 34 weeks of gestation who have no contraindications to steroid use be given one course of steroids, regardless of the number of fetuses. There currently is no evidence that prophylactic use of cerclage, hospitalization, bed rest, or home uterine monitoring improves outcome in these pregnancies. Therefore, these interventions should not be ordered prophylactically. Current evidence does not support the routine use of progesterone in women with multiple gestations (see also "Preterm Birth" later in this chapter).

- Growth restriction—Fetuses of a multiple gestation generally do not grow at the same rate as singleton fetuses. One obvious etiology is placental pathology; multiple gestations are at increased risk of having at least one fetus with a suboptimal placental implantation site or abnormal umbilical cord morphology.

- Discordant growth—Discordant fetal growth is common in multiple gestations and usually is defined by a 15–25% reduction in the estimated fetal weight of the smallest fetus when compared with the largest. The threshold at which discordant growth is most strongly associated with adverse outcomes is unclear, even in twin gestations. If both fetuses are of normal weight and are progressing appropriately on their own growth curve, then discordance may not indicate a pathologic process. Discordance can be caused by structural or genetic fetal anomalies, discordant infection, an unfavorable placental implantation or umbilical cord insertion site, placental damage (ie, partial abruption), or complications related to monochorionic placentation, such as twin–twin transfusion syndrome (discussed on the following page).

  The workup should include a review of all prenatal exposures, a specialized ultrasound examination and, depending on the gestational age, tests of fetal well-being. The ultrasound examination should be performed by someone with skill and experience in evaluating multiple gestations. Likewise, a consultation with an obstetrician–gynecologist with expertise in the management of high-risk pregnancies, such as a maternal–fetal medicine specialist, may be helpful in determining further therapy for these cases when complications arise.

- Death of one fetus—Multiple gestations, especially high-order multiple gestations, are at increased risk of losing one or more fetuses remote from delivery. No fetal monitoring protocol has been shown to predict the most losses of one fetus in a multifetal pregnancy. In addition, authorities disagree about antepartum management once a demise has occurred. Some investigators have advocated immediate delivery of the remaining fetuses. However, if the death is the result of an abnormality of the fetus itself rather than maternal or uteroplacental pathology and the pregnancy is remote from term, expectant management may be appropriate. The most difficult cases are those in which fetal demise occurs in one fetus of a monochorionic twin pair. In such cases, there may be little or no benefit in immediate delivery, especially if the surviving fetuses are very preterm; allowing the pregnancy to continue may provide the most benefit.

- Multifetal pregnancy reduction and selective fetal termination—Fetal reduction of a high-order multiple gestation has been associated with an increased risk of IUGR in the remaining twins in some studies. Monochorionicity can complicate the reduction procedure; if one fetus of a monochorionic twin pair is inadvertently reduced, sudden hypotension and thrombotic phenomena could result in death or damage of the remaining twin fetus. Whether to reduce high-order multiple gestations to twin or triplet gestations and whether to reduce triplet gestations at all are both areas of controversy. Most studies have concluded that the risks associated with a quadruplet or higher-order pregnancy clearly outweigh the risks associated with fetal reduction.

  Selective fetal termination is the application of the fetal reduction technique to the termination of an anomalous or aneuploid fetus that is part of a multiple gestation. The risks of this procedure are higher than those associated with multifetal reduction, in part because the pregnancy is often more advanced at the time of diagnosis of the anomaly. If the reduced fetus overlies the cervix or if the pregnancy is beyond 20 weeks, the risk of pregnancy loss, preterm delivery, or low birth weight of the remaining fetus may be increased.

- Twin–twin transfusion syndrome—Twin–twin transfusion syndrome is believed to occur as the result of uncompensated arteriovenous anastomoses in a monochorionic placenta, which leads to greater net blood flow going to one twin at the expense of the other. The syndrome usually becomes apparent in the second trimester and can lead rapidly to premature rupture of membranes (PROM), preterm labor, or early mortality because of heart failure in either of the fetuses. A variety of therapies have been attempted, including serial therapeutic amniocenteses of the recipient twin's amniotic sac. More aggressive therapies usually are considered only for very early, severe cases and include abolishing the placental anastomoses by endoscopic laser coagulation or selective feticide by umbilical cord occlusion. These cases should be performed in centers experienced with the procedures, monitored very closely, and managed in consultation with a maternal–fetal medicine specialist.

Intrapartum Management

Fetal and neonatal morbidity and mortality begin to increase in twin and triplet pregnancies extended beyond 37 weeks of gestation and 35 weeks of gestation, respectively. However, no prospective randomized trials have tested the hypothesis that elective delivery at these gestational ages improves outcomes in these pregnancies. If the fetuses are appropriate in size for gestational age with evidence of sustained growth and there is normal amniotic fluid volume and reassuring antepartum fetal testing in the absence of maternal complications, such as preeclampsia or gestational diabetes, the pregnancy may be continued. However, recent guidelines based on available data and expert opinion have recommended delivery at 38 weeks of gestation in uncomplicated dichorionic diamniotic twin pregnancies and at 34–37 weeks of gestation in uncomplicated monochorionic-diamniotic twin pregnancies. Alternatively, if the woman is experiencing morbidities that would improve with delivery but do not necessarily mandate delivery, delivery may be considered at these gestational ages. Determination of fetal pulmonary maturity may be necessary under certain circumstances. The route of delivery of twins should be determined by the position of the fetuses, the ease of fetal heart rate monitoring, and maternal and fetal status. Data are insufficient to determine the best route of delivery for high-order multiples.

Other Medical Complications During Pregnancy

Antepartum Hospitalization

Pregnant patients with complications who require hospitalization before the onset of labor should be admitted to a designated antepartum area, either inside or near the labor and delivery area. Obstetric patients with serious and acute complications should be assigned to an area where more intensive care and surveillance are available, such as the labor and delivery area or an intensive care unit. An obstetrician–gynecologist or a specialist in maternal–fetal medicine should be involved, either as the primary or the consulting physician, in the care of an obstetric patient with complications. When sufficiently recovered, the pregnant patient should be returned to the obstetric service, provided that her return does not jeopardize her care.

Acutely ill obstetric patients who are likely to give birth to neonates requiring intensive care should be cared for in specialty or subspecialty perinatal care centers, depending on the medical needs of the maternal–fetal dyad. When feasible, antepartum transfer to specialty or subspecialty perinatal care centers should be encouraged for these women (see also "Transfer for Critical Care" in Chapter 4).

Written policies and procedures for the management of pregnant patients seen in the emergency department or admitted to nonobstetric services should be established and approved by the medical staff and must comply with the requirements of federal and state transfer laws. When warranted by patient volume, a high-risk antepartum care unit should be developed to provide specialized nursing care and facilities for the mother and the fetus at risk. When this is not feasible, written policies are recommended that specify how the care and transfer of pregnant patients with obstetric, medical, or surgical complications will be handled and where these patients will be assigned.

Whether an obstetric patient is admitted to the antepartum unit or to a nonobstetric unit, her condition should be evaluated soon thereafter by the primary physician or appropriate consultants. The evaluation should encompass a complete review of current illnesses as well as a medical, family, and social history. The condition of the patient and the reason for admission should determine the extent of the physical examination performed and the laboratory studies obtained. A copy of the patient's current prenatal record should become part of the hospital medical record as soon as possible after admission. These policies also must comply with the requirements of federal and state transfer laws.

Critical Care in Pregnancy

Approximately 1–3% of pregnant women require critical care services in the United States each year, with the risk of death ranging from 2% to 11%. Hemorrhage and hypertension are the most common causes of intensive care unit (ICU) admission in obstetric patients. The care of any pregnant woman requiring ICU services should be managed in a facility with obstetric adult ICU and neonatal ICU capability (see also "Transfer for Critical Care" in Chapter 4). Decisions about care for a pregnant patient in the ICU should be made collaboratively with the intensivist, obstetrician, specialty nurses, and neonatologist. When a pregnant patient is transferred to the ICU, members of the care team should assess the anticipated course of her condition or disease, including possible complications, and set parameters for delivery, if appropriate. The plan should be clear to the medical team and to the patient's family, and to the patient herself if she is able to understand. Because the risk–benefit calculation for a given intervention may change as the pregnancy progresses, it is important to reevaluate the care plan on a regular basis. The plan for delivery should be made long before delivery is imminent.

Intrapartum Care

If a laboring patient requires critical care services, it is important to determine the optimal setting for her care. Factors that will affect this decision include the degree of patient instability, interventions required, staffing and expertise available, anticipated duration of ICU stay, and probability of delivery. If the fetus is previable or the maternal condition unstable, it may be appropriate to undergo vaginal delivery in the intensive care unit. Cesarean delivery in the ICU has significant disadvantages compared with procedures in a traditional operating room. Cesarean delivery in the ICU should be restricted to cases in which transport to the operating room or delivery room cannot be achieved safely or expeditiously, or to a perimortem procedure. Analgesia should still be used in the ICU setting, although assessment of pain may be more difficult in the sedated patient. Regional anesthesia is preferred but complications may preclude its use. Intravenous analgesia may be used but is less effective in treating pain (see also "Analgesia and Anesthesia" in Chapter 6).

Fetal Considerations

Fetal surveillance often is used when a patient is admitted to the ICU. Changes in fetal monitoring should prompt reassessment of maternal mean arterial pressure, acidemia, hypoxemia, or inferior vena cava compression, and every attempt should be made at intrauterine fetal resuscitation. Drugs that cross the placenta may have fetal effects; however, necessary medications should not be withheld from critically ill pregnant women because of fetal concerns. In addition, imaging studies should not be withheld out of potential concern for fetal status, although attempts should be made to limit fetal radiation exposure during diagnostic testing.

Postpartum Care

Approximately 75% of the obstetric ICU patients admitted are postpartum. Obstetric input in the care of the postpartum ICU patient may include evaluation of vaginal or intraabdominal bleeding, evaluation of obstetric sources of infection, duration of specific therapies, such as magnesium for eclampsia prophylaxis, and feasibility of breast pumping, especially compatibility of various medications with breastfeeding.

Nonobstetric Surgery in Pregnancy

Nonobstetric surgery is sometimes necessary during pregnancy, and there are no data to support specific recommendations. However, obstetric consultation to confirm gestational age, discuss pertinent aspects of maternal physiology or anatomy, and make recommendations about fetal monitoring is highly recommended. Pregnant patients who undergo nonobstetric surgery are best managed with communication between involved services, including obstetrics, anesthesia, surgery, and nursing. The decision to use fetal monitoring should be individualized, and its use should be based on gestational age, type of surgery, and facilities available.

Psychiatric Disease in Pregnancy

Approximately 500,000 pregnancies in the United States each year involve women who have psychiatric illnesses that either predate pregnancy or emerge during pregnancy and the postpartum period. The use of psychotropic medication during pregnancy requires attention to the risk of teratogenicity, perinatal syndromes, and neonatal withdrawal. Advising a pregnant or lactating woman to discontinue medication exchanges the fetal or neonatal risks of medication exposure for the risks of untreated maternal illness. Maternal psychiatric illness, if inadequately treated, or untreated can result in poor adherence to prenatal care, poor nutrition, increased alcohol or tobacco use, and disruption to mother–infant bonding. Multidisciplinary care involving the obstetrician, mental health provider, and pediatrician is recommended.

All psychotropic medications studied to date cross the placenta, are present in amniotic fluid, and enter human breast milk. The major risk of teratogenesis is during the third week through the eighth week of gestation. In general, a single medication used at a higher dose is favored over using multiple medications to obtain control of symptoms. Providing women with well-referenced patient resources for online information is a reasonable option. Electronic resources for the fetal and neonatal effects of psychotropic drug therapy during pregnancy and lactation are REPROTOX (www.reprotox.org) and TERIS (http://depts.washington.edu/terisweb/teris/). In addition, the U.S. Food and Drug Administration (FDA) web site (available at www.fda.gov) has information on the safety of individual medications during pregnancy.

Trauma During Pregnancy

Trauma is the leading cause of nonobstetric maternal death. In industrialized nations, most cases of trauma during pregnancy result from motor vehicle crashes. Other frequent causes of trauma during pregnancy are falls and direct assaults to the abdomen. The appropriate use of safety restraint systems in automobiles, compliance with traffic laws, and early identification and intervention in suspected cases of domestic violence are all preventive measures that may reduce the likelihood of both maternal and fetal morbidity and mortality. The obstetrician–gynecologist plays a central role both in the education of pregnant women on the appropriate use of seat belts while driving or riding in vehicles and in the early identification of suspected abuse.

Necessary evaluation and management of the trauma patient should not be changed because she is pregnant. Optimum management of the seriously injured pregnant woman requires an integrated effort of multiple specialties, starting with emergency medical technicians, emergency medicine physicians, trauma surgeons, and other specialists, depending on the type of injury. Obstetricians play a central role in the management of injured pregnant women. Their knowledge and expertise are vital to management decisions regarding both the woman and the fetus. The obstetrician may be consulted regarding the condition of a pregnant trauma patient and her fetus or, more commonly, may be the primary physician caring for the patient following trauma. To improve multidisciplinary management of the trauma patient who is pregnant, hospital-based guidelines for clinical management should be established with input from multiple care providers (eg, emergency medicine physicians, obstetrician–gynecologists, trauma surgeons).

Management

The primary goal and initial efforts in managing the injured pregnant woman should be evaluation and stabilization of maternal vital signs. If attention is drawn to the fetus before the woman is stabilized, serious or life-threatening maternal injuries may be overlooked, or circumstances that can compromise fetal oxygenation (eg, maternal hypoxemia, hypovolemia, or supine hypotension) may be ignored, lessening the likelihood of both maternal and fetal survival.

Fetal Assessment. The use of electronic fetal cardiac and uterine activity monitoring in pregnant trauma victims at the time of fetal viability (eg, 20–24 weeks of gestation) may be predictive of abruptio placentae. Because abruption usually becomes apparent shortly after injury, monitoring should be initiated as soon as the woman is stabilized. The duration of fetal monitoring in the viable pregnancy has been debated, with most experts recommending a minimum of 2–4 hours. Monitoring should be continued and further evaluation carried out if uterine contractions, a nonreassuring fetal heart rate pattern, vaginal bleeding, significant uterine tenderness or irritability, serious maternal injury, or rupture of the amniotic membranes is present. Upon discharge, the patient should be instructed to return if she develops vaginal bleeding, leakage of fluid, decreased fetal movement, or severe abdominal pain.

Fetal–Maternal Hemorrhage. Complications of fetal–maternal hemorrhage in trauma patients include fetal and neonatal anemia, fetal cardiac arrhythmias, and fetal death. There is no evidence that laboratory testing for fetal–maternal hemorrhage (eg, Kleihauer-Betke test) can predict or eliminate adverse immediate sequelae due to hemorrhage. Administration of D immune globulin at any time within the first 72 hours following fetal–maternal hemorrhage appears to provide protection from alloimmunization in the Rh (O) D-negative woman. Consideration should be given to administering 300 micrograms of Rh (O) D immune globulin to all unsensitized Rh (O) D-negative pregnant patients who have experienced abdominal trauma. Some experts recommend quantitative testing for fetal–maternal hemorrhage (eg, Kleihauer-Betke testing) in the Rh (O) D-negative woman to identify the unusual large-volume hemorrhage (ie, more than 30 mL of fetal–maternal hemorrhage), for which 300 micrograms of Rh(O) D immune globulin may be insufficient (see also "Isoimmunization in Pregnancy" earlier in this chapter).

Labor and Delivery Considerations and Complications

Assessment and Management of Fetal Pulmonary Maturation

The decision to deliver before 39 weeks of gestation should be based on appropriate medical (maternal or fetal) indications when the risks of continuing the pregnancy outweigh the risks of delivery. In these instances, lung maturity testing is not warranted. Because of the new appreciation of the neonatal and pediatric risks associated with delivery before 39 weeks of gestation, lung maturity is not an indication for delivery before 39 weeks of gestation. Only occasionally should the knowledge of pulmonary maturity be needed to proceed with a planned delivery before 39 weeks of gestation.

Antenatal Corticosteroid Therapy

For women at risk of preterm birth, enhancement of fetal pulmonary function with the use of antenatal steroids lessens the prevalence and severity of neonatal respiratory distress syndrome and its sequelae. A single course of corticosteroids (betamethasone or dexamethasone) is recommended for pregnant women between 24 weeks and 34 weeks of gestation who are at risk of preterm delivery within 7 days. A single course of antenatal corticosteroids should be administered to women with PROM before 32 weeks of gestation to reduce the risks of respiratory distress syndrome, perinatal mortality, and other morbidities. The efficacy of corticosteroid use at 32–33 completed weeks of gestation for preterm PROM is unclear, but treatment may be beneficial, particularly if pulmonary immaturity is documented. Sparse data exist on the efficacy of corticosteroid use before fetal age of viability, and such use is not recommended. A single rescue course of antenatal corticosteroids may be considered if the antecedent treatment was given more than 2 weeks prior, the gestational age is less than 32 6/7 weeks, and the woman is judged by the physician to be likely to give birth within the next week. However, regularly scheduled repeat courses or multiple courses (more than two) are not recommended.

Births at the Threshold of Viability

Early preterm birth or birth of an extremely low birth weight infant (less than 1,000 g), especially those weighing less than 750 g or less than 26 weeks of gestation, poses a variety of complex medical, social, and ethical considerations. The effect of such births on the infants, their families, the health care system, and society is profound. Although the prevalence of such births is less than 1%, they account for nearly one half of all cases of perinatal mortality. Information from large multicenter studies, such as those sponsored by the *Eunice Kennedy Shriver* National Institute of Child Health and Human Development (NICHD), provides sufficiently detailed data to assist the perinatal team in developing an evidence-based approach to managing the extremely preterm infant. There is now a calculator available on the NICHD web site that factors in gestational age, estimated fetal weight, fetal sex, and whether the fetus was exposed to antenatal steroids to provide a range of estimated infant outcomes (see http://www.nichd.nih.gov/about/org/cdbpm/pp/prog_epbo/epbo_case.cfm).

Family Counseling

When extremely preterm birth is anticipated, the estimated gestational age and weight should be carefully assessed, the prognosis for the fetus should be determined, and each member of the health care team should make every effort to maintain a consistent theme in their discussion with family members regarding the assessment, prognosis, and recommendations for care. Counseling from a practitioner with additional experience and expertise in extremely preterm and extremely low birth weight infants may be appropriate.

In general, parents of anticipated extremely preterm fetuses can be counseled that infants delivered before 24 weeks of gestation are less likely to survive, and those who do are not likely to survive intact. The neonatal survival rate for newborns increases from 0% at 21 weeks of gestation to 75% at 25 weeks of gestation, and from 11% at 401–500 g birth weight to 75% at 701–800 g birth weight. In addition, females generally have a better prognosis than males. Disabilities in mental and psychomotor development, neuromotor function, or sensory and communication function are present in approximately one half of extremely preterm fetuses. When the extremely preterm newborn does not survive, support should be provided to the family by physicians, nurses, and other staff after the infant's death.

Management

Retrospective studies addressing obstetric management on outcomes of extremely premature neonates have failed to document a benefit of cesarean delivery over vaginal delivery. The effect of antenatal steroid use in the extremely preterm fetus is unclear; however, it is recommended that all women at risk of preterm delivery between 24 weeks and 34 weeks of gestation be candidates for a single course of corticosteroids (see also "Assessment and Management of Fetal Pulmonary Maturation" earlier in this chapter). Maternal transport to a tertiary care center before delivery should be considered whenever possible.

Management regarding the extent of resuscitative and supportive efforts should be based on gestational age and birth weight but should be further individualized based on the newborns condition at birth and the parents' preferences. Whenever possible, data specific to the age, weight, and sex of the individual extremely preterm fetus should be used to aid management decisions made by obstetricians and parents of fetuses at risk of preterm delivery before 26 completed weeks of gestation (see NICHD calculator, available at http://www.nichd.nih.gov/about/org/cdbpm/pp/prog_epbo/epbo_case.cfm). This information may be developed by each institution and should indicate the population used in determining estimates of survivability.

Chorioamnionitis

Chorioamnionitis or intra-amniotic infection is largely a clinical diagnosis that often is made presumptively during labor if a laboring woman develops a fever for which there is no other obvious etiology. The classic signs and symptoms include maternal fever, maternal tachycardia, uterine tenderness, fetal tachycardia, and foul-smelling amniotic fluid. Common organisms that cause chorioamnionitis include gram-negative bacteria (particularly *Escherichia coli*), gram-positive bacteria (particularly group B streptococci and staphylococcus), and occasionally anaerobes. It is clear that neonates born to mothers with chorioamnionitis have less infectious outcomes if their mother is treated in utero with appropriate antibiotics. Treatment for chorioamnionitis typically is the administration of ampicillin and gentamicin; treatment with only penicillin or ampicillin is never adequate for chorioamnionitis.

Endocarditis

Most cases of endocarditis are not attributable to an invasive procedure, but rather are the result of randomly occurring bacteremia from routine daily activities. Antibiotic prophylaxis may only prevent a small number of cases of infective endocarditis in women undergoing genitourinary procedures, and the risk of antibiotic-associated adverse events exceeds the benefit, if any, from prophylactic antibiotic therapy. For these reasons, the American Heart Association and the American College of Cardiology no longer recommend infective endocarditis prophylaxis for either vaginal delivery or cesarean delivery in the absence of infection, except possibly for the small subset of patients at highest potential risk of adverse cardiac outcomes who are undergoing vaginal delivery. Only cardiac conditions associated with the highest risk of adverse outcomes from endocarditis are appropriate for infective endocarditis prophylaxis, and this is primarily for patients undergoing dental procedures that involve manipulation of gingival tissue or the periapical region of teeth, or perforation of the oral mucosa (see Box 7-3). Mitral valve prolapse is not considered a lesion that ever needs infective endocarditis prophylaxis.

In patients who have one of the high-risk conditions (see Box 7-3) and an established infection that could result in bacteremia, such as chorioamnionitis or pyelonephritis, the underlying infection should be treated to prevent infection or sepsis, but specific additional endocarditis prophylaxis is not recommended. For women not already receiving intrapartum antibiotic therapy for another indication that would also provide coverage against endocarditis, single-dose antibiotic regimens for endocarditis prophylaxis can be administered as close to 30–60 minutes before the anticipated time of delivery as is feasible. Multiple-dose combination regimens are no longer indicated or recommended for prophylaxis.

Box 7-3. Cardiac Conditions With High Risk of Endocarditis in the Presence of Bacteremia

Prophylaxis against infective endocarditis is reasonable for the following patients at highest risk of adverse outcomes from infective endocarditis who undergo dental procedures that involve manipulation of either gingival tissue or the periapical region of teeth or perforation of the oral mucosa*:

• Patients with prosthetic cardiac valve or prosthetic material used for cardiac valve repair

• Patients with previous infective endocarditis

• Patients with CHD

  —Unrepaired cyanotic CHD, including palliative shunts and conduits

  —Completely repaired congenital heart defect repaired with prosthetic material or device, whether placed by surgery or by catheter intervention, during the first 6 months after the procedure.

  —Repaired CHD with residual defects at the site or adjacent to the site of a prosthetic patch or prosthetic device (both of which inhibit endothelialization)

• Cardiac transplant recipients with valve regurgitation due to a structurally abnormal valve.

Abbreviation: CHD, congenital heart disease.

*Prophylaxis against infective endocarditis is not recommended for nondental procedures in the absence of active infection.

Data from Nishimura RA, Carabello BA, Faxon DP, Freed MD, Lytle BW, O'Gara PT, et al. ACC/AHA 2008 guideline update on valvular heart disease: focused update on infective endocarditis: a report of the American College of Cardiology/American Heart Association Task Force on Practice Guidelines: endorsed by the Society of Cardiovascular Anesthesiologists, Society for Cardiovascular Angiography and Interventions, and Society of Thoracic Surgeons. American College of Cardiology/American Heart Association Task Force. Circulation 2008;118:887–96.

Endometritis

Postpartum endometritis can be caused by a mixture of skin or vaginal flora, including organisms, such as aerobic streptococci (group B β-hemolytic streptococci and the enterococci), gram-negative aerobes (especially *Escherichia coli*), gram-negative anaerobic rods (especially *Bacteroides bivius*), and anaerobic cocci *(Peptococcus* species and *Peptostreptococcus* species). Clinically, endometritis is characterized by fever, uterine tenderness, malaise, tachycardia, abdominal pain, or foul-smelling lochia. Of these, fever is the most characteristic and may be the only sign early in the course of infection. Risk factors for postpartum endometritis include cesarean delivery, prolonged rupture of membranes, prolonged labor with multiple vaginal examinations, intrapartum fever, and lower socioeconomic status.

Prophylaxis Against Postcesarean Infection

The single most important risk factor for infection in the postpartum period is cesarean delivery. Antimicrobial prophylaxis is recommended for all cesarean deliveries unless the patient is already receiving an antibiotic regimen with appropriate coverage (eg, for chorioamnionitis), and such prophylaxis should be administered within 60 minutes before the start of the cesarean delivery. When this is not possible (eg, need for emergent delivery), prophylaxis should be administered as soon as possible after the incision is made.

A single dose of a targeted antibiotic, such as a first-generation cephalosporin, is the first-line antibiotic of choice, unless significant drug allergies are present. For women with a history of a significant penicillin or cephalosporin allergy (anaphylaxis, angioedema, respiratory distress, or urticaria), a single-dose combination of clindamycin with an aminoglycoside is a reasonable alternative choice for cesarean delivery prophylaxis. For women with a mild penicillin allergy, cefazolin is the recommended agent. After a single 1-gram intravenous dose of cefazolin, a therapeutic level is maintained for approximately 3–4 hours. A higher dose may be indicated if a woman is obese. Patients with lengthy surgeries or those who experience excessive blood loss should receive an additional intraoperative dose of the antibiotic used for preincision prophylaxis.

Management

Endometritis usually is diagnosed within a few days after delivery. A woman with postpartum fever should be evaluated by pertinent history, physical examination, blood count, and urine culture. Blood cultures rarely influence therapeutic decisions but could be indicated if septicemia is suspected. Cervical, vaginal, or endometrial cultures need not be routinely performed because the results might not indicate the infecting organism.

Principles for managing postpartum endometritis are as follows:

- Parenteral, broad-spectrum antibiotic treatment should be initiated according to a proven regimen and continued until the patient is afebrile. A combination of clindamycin and gentamicin, with the addition of ampicillin in refractory cases, is recommended for cost-effective therapy.

- Response usually is prompt. If fever persists beyond antibiotic treatment for 24–48 hours, a search for alternative etiologies, including pelvic abscess, wound infection, septic pelvic thrombophlebitis, inadequate antibiotic coverage, and retained placental tissue, should be performed.

- Because postpartum endometritis may have neonatal implications, information about the mother's condition should be provided to the neonate's health care provider.

Maternal Hemorrhage

Hemorrhage remains one of the leading causes of maternal mortality worldwide. One half of all maternal deaths occur within 24 hours of delivery and most commonly from excessive bleeding. Facilities that provide labor and delivery services should be prepared to manage maternal hemorrhage. Proper preparation and resources to manage maternal hemorrhage in a timely manner can be lifesaving. Policies to ensure the rapid availability of blood products for transfusion in the event of hemorrhage must be in place.

Postpartum Hemorrhage

There is no single definition of postpartum hemorrhage. Criteria of an estimated blood loss of greater than 500 mL after a vaginal delivery or 1,000 mL after cesarean delivery are often used, but the average volume of blood lost at delivery can approach these amounts. Symptoms of hypotension, pallor, and oliguria typically do not occur until blood loss is substantial. Risk factors for excessive bleeding include prolonged, augmented, or rapid labor; history of postpartum hemorrhage; episiotomy, especially mediolateral; preeclampsia; overdistended uterus (macrosomia, twins, or hydramnios); operative delivery; Asian or Hispanic ethnicity; and chorioamnionitis. Most cases of postpartum hemorrhage occur immediately or soon after delivery. Uterine atony is the most common cause of postpartum hemorrhage. Other etiologies include retained placenta, placenta accreta, uterine rupture, uterine inversion, obstetric lacerations, retained products of conception, maternal coagulopathy, and infection. In an effort to prevent uterine atony and associated bleeding, it is routine to administer oxytocin soon after delivery.

Management may vary greatly among patients, depending on etiology of the hemorrhage and available treatment options, and often a multidisciplinary approach is required. Less-invasive methods should be tried initially if possible, but if unsuccessful, preservation of life may require hysterectomy. Treatment options for postpartum hemorrhage due to uterine atony include administration of uterotonics and pharmacologic agents, tamponade of the uterus, surgical techniques to control the bleeding, and embolization of pelvic arteries. Treatment of hemorrhage due to uterine rupture should be tailored to the site of uterine injury, maternal condition, and her desire for future childbearing; hysterectomy may be necessary in a life-threatening situation. In the presence of previa or a history of cesarean delivery, the obstetric care provider must have a high clinical suspicion for placenta accreta and take appropriate precautions. The extent (area, depth) of the abnormal attachment will determine the response—curettage, wedge resection, medical management, or hysterectomy; abdominal hysterectomy usually is the most definitive treatment. Manual replacement with or without uterine relaxants usually is successful for management of uterine inversion. In the unusual circumstance in which it is not, laparotomy is required.

Transfusion

Transfusion therapy is used to prevent or treat hemorrhagic shock and its consequences. Transfusion of blood products is necessary when the extent of blood loss is significant and ongoing, particularly if vital signs are unstable. Clinical judgment is an important determinant, given that estimates of blood loss often are inaccurate, determination of hematocrit or hemoglobin concentrations may not accurately reflect the current hematologic status, and symptoms and signs of hemorrhage may not occur until blood loss exceeds 15%. The purpose of transfusion of blood products is to replace coagulation factors and red blood cells for oxygen-carrying capacity, not for volume replacement. To avoid dilutional coagulopathy, concurrent replacement with coagulation factors and platelets may be necessary.

Postterm Gestation

Postterm pregnancy, by definition, refers to a pregnancy that is 42 weeks of gestation or beyond (294 days, or estimated date of delivery [EDD] +14 days). Accurate pregnancy dating is critical to the diagnosis (see also "Estimated Date of Delivery" in Chapter 5). The term "postdates" is poorly defined and should be avoided. Although some cases of postterm pregnancy likely result from an inability to accurately define the EDD, many cases result from a true prolongation of gestation. Accurate assessment of gestational age and diagnosis of posterm gestation, as well as recognition and management of risk factors, may reduce the risk of adverse sequelae.

Postterm pregnancy is associated with significant fetal and maternal risks. Fetal risks include an increased perinatal mortality rate, uteroplacental insufficiency, meconium aspiration, intrauterine infection, low umbilical artery pH levels at delivery, and low 5-minute Apgar scores. Significant risks to the pregnant woman include an increase in labor dystocia, an increase in severe perineal injury related to macrosomia, and a doubling in the rate of cesarean delivery.

Management

Many authorities recommend prompt delivery in a postterm patient with a favorable cervix and no other complications. Although postterm pregnancy is defined as a pregnancy of 42 weeks or more of gestation, data suggest that routine induction at 41 weeks of gestation has fetal benefit without incurring the additional maternal risks of a higher rate of cesarean delivery.

Women with postterm gestations who have unfavorable cervices can either be managed expectantly or undergo labor induction. Despite a lack of evidence that monitoring improves perinatal outcome, it is reasonable to initiate antenatal surveillance of postterm pregnancies between 41 weeks (287 days; EDD +7 days) and 42 weeks of gestation (294 days; EDD +14 days) because of evidence that perinatal morbidity and mortality increase as gestational age advances. Many practitioners use twice-weekly testing with some evaluation of amniotic fluid volume beginning at 41 weeks of gestation. A nonstress test and amniotic fluid volume assessment (a modified BPP) are adequate. Delivery should be initiated if there is evidence of fetal compromise or oligohydramnios.

Preterm Birth

Preterm birth is defined as birth before 37 completed weeks of gestation. Spontaneous preterm birth includes preterm labor, preterm spontaneous rupture of membranes, and cervical insufficiency. It does not include indicated preterm delivery for maternal or fetal conditions. Preterm birth is the leading cause of neonatal mortality and one of the most common reasons for antenatal hospitalization. In the United States, approximately 12% of all live births occur before term, and preterm labor preceded approximately 50% of these preterm births. The pathophysiologic events that trigger preterm parturition are largely unknown but may include decidual hemorrhage (abruption), mechanical factors (uterine overdistention or cervical incompetence), hormonal changes (perhaps mediated by fetal or maternal stress), infection, and inflammation.

Risk Factor Identification and Management

A prior preterm birth is commonly reported to confer a 1.5-fold to 2-fold increased risk in a subsequent pregnancy. Other risk factors for preterm birth include African American race, age younger than 17 years or older than 35 years, low socioeconomic status, underweight prepregnancy body mass index, smoking, vaginal bleeding in more than one trimester, bacterial infections, and short cervical length.

Screening Tests. Screening for risk of preterm birth by means other than historic risk factors is not beneficial in the general obstetric population. Fetal fibronectin testing may be useful in women with symptoms of preterm labor to identify those with negative values and a reduced risk of preterm birth, thereby avoiding unnecessary intervention.

Interventions. Women with a singleton gestation and prior spontaneous preterm birth should be offered progesterone supplementation starting at 16 weeks of gestation to reduce the risk of the recurrence of preterm birth.

Diagnosis of Preterm Labor

The diagnosis of preterm labor is generally based upon clinical criteria of regular uterine contractions accompanied by cervical dilation, or effacement or presentation, or both with regular contractions and at least 2 cm dilation. Fewer than 10% of women with the clinical diagnosis of preterm labor actually deliver within 7 days of presentation. It is important to recognize that preterm labor is not the only cause of preterm birth; numerous preterm births are preceded by either rupture of membranes (see also "Premature Rupture of Membranes" later in this chapter) or other medical problems.

Patients with suspected preterm labor should be examined and observed for 1–2 hours, have their uterine activity monitored, and undergo serial cervical examinations to document the presence or absence of cervical change. The positive predictive value of a positive fetal fibronectin test result or a short cervix alone is poor and should not be used exclusively to direct management in the setting of acute symptoms. Because preterm labor often is associated with urinary tract infections, a dipstick or a microscopic examination of urine and urine culture may be helpful. Ultrasound examination also may be considered to confirm gestational age, to estimate fetal weight in order to receive appropriate counseling from pediatrics, and to assess the presence of any congenital anomalies.

Management of Preterm Labor

Interventions to reduce the likelihood of delivery should be reserved for women likely to give birth and who are at a gestational age at which delay in delivery will provide benefit to the newborn. Historically, nonpharmacologic treatments to prevent preterm births in women who have preterm labor have included bed rest, abstention from intercourse and orgasm, and hydration. Evidence for the effectiveness of these interventions is lacking, and adverse effects have been reported. Proposed pharmacologic interventions to prolong pregnancy include tocolytic drugs to inhibit uterine contractions and antibiotics to treat intrauterine bacterial infection. Therapeutics agents associated with improved neonatal outcomes include antenatal corticosteroids for fetal maturation and magnesium sulfate for neuroprotection.

Tocolytic Drugs. Evidence supports the use of first-line tocolytic treatment with beta-mimetics, calcium channel blockers, or nonsteroidal antiinflammatory drugs for short-term prolongation of pregnancy (up to 48 hours) to allow for the administration of antenatal steroids. Maintenance therapy with tocolytics has been ineffective for preventing preterm birth and improving neonatal outcomes and, therefore, is not recommended for this purpose. Tocolysis is contraindicated when the maternal and fetal risks of prolonging pregnancy or the risks associated with these drugs are greater than the risks associated with preterm birth.

Antibiotics. Antibiotic use intended only for pregnancy prolongation in women with preterm labor with intact membranes does not have short-term neonatal benefits and may be associated with long-term harm. Thus, antibiotics should not be used for this indication in women with preterm labor and intact membranes. This recommendation is distinct from recommendations for antibiotic use for preterm PROM (see also "Premature Rupture of Membranes" later in this chapter) and group B streptococci carrier status (see also "Group B Streptococci" in Chapter 10).

Antenatal Corticosteroids. The most beneficial intervention for improvement of neonatal outcome in patients who deliver preterm is the administration of antenatal corticosteroids. A single course of corticosteroids is recommended for pregnant women between 24 weeks and 34 weeks of gestation who are at risk of preterm delivery within 7 days (see also "Assessment and Management of Fetal Pulmonary Maturation" earlier in this chapter).

Magnesium Sulfate. The available evidence suggests that magnesium sulfate given before anticipated early preterm birth reduces the risk of cerebral palsy in surviving infants if administered when birth is anticipated before 32 weeks of gestation. Hospitals electing to use magnesium sulfate for fetal neuroprotection should develop uniform and specific guidelines regarding inclusion criteria, treatment regimens, concurrent tocolysis, and monitoring in accordance with one of the larger trials. The use of magnesium sulfate for inhibition of acute preterm labor has not been demonstrated to achieve significant pregnancy prolongation.

Premature Rupture of Membranes

The definition of *PROM* is rupture of membranes before the onset of labor. Membrane rupture that occurs before 37 weeks of gestation is referred to as preterm PROM. Although the term PROM results from the normal physiologic process of progressive membrane weakening, preterm PROM can result from a wide array of pathologic mechanisms acting individually or in concert. Premature rupture of membranes is a complication in approximately one third of preterm births. It typically is associated with brief latency between membrane rupture and delivery, increased potential for perinatal infection, and in utero umbilical cord compression. Because of this, both PROM at and before term can lead to significant perinatal morbidity and mortality. The gestational age and fetal status at membrane rupture have significant implications in the etiology and consequences of PROM. Management may be dictated by the presence of overt intrauterine infection, advanced labor, or fetal compromise.

Diagnosis

In most cases, PROM can be diagnosed on the basis of the patient's history and physical examination. Examination should be performed in a manner that minimizes the risk of introducing infection, particularly before term. Digital examinations should be avoided unless the patient is in active labor or imminent delivery is planned. The diagnosis of membrane rupture is confirmed by the visualization of fluid passing from the cervical canal. When the clinical history or physical examination is unclear, membrane rupture can be diagnosed unequivocally with an ultrasonographically guided transabdominal instillation of indigo carmine dye (1 mL in 9 mL of sterile normal saline), followed by observation for passage of blue fluid from the vagina.

Management

An accurate assessment of gestational age and knowledge of the maternal, fetal, and neonatal risks are essential for appropriate evaluation, counseling, and care of patients with PROM. At any gestational age, a patient with evident chorioamnionitis, abruptio placentae, or evidence of fetal compromise is best cared for by expeditious delivery. If chorioamnionitis is diagnosed, appropriate antibiotic treatment also is indicated. In the absence of an indication for immediate delivery, swabs for diagnosis of *Chlamydia trachomatis* and *Neisseria gonorrhoeae* may be obtained from the cervix, if appropriate. The need for group B streptococci intrapartum prophylaxis should be determined if preterm PROM occurs.

Term Premature Rupture of Membranes. For women with PROM at term, labor should be induced at the time of presentation, generally with oxytocin infusion, to reduce the risk chorioamnionitis. Fetal heart rate monitoring should be used to assess fetal status. Dating criteria should be reviewed to assign gestational age. When the decision to deliver is made, group B streptococci prophylaxis should be given based on prior culture results or risk factors if cultures have not been previously performed.

Preterm Premature Rupture of Membranes. Delivery is recommended when PROM occurs at or beyond 34 weeks of gestation. With PROM at 32–33 completed weeks of gestation, labor induction may be considered if fetal pulmonary maturity has been documented. The efficacy of corticosteroid use at 32–33 completed weeks is unclear based on available evidence, but treatment may be beneficial particularly if pulmonary immaturity is documented.

Patients with PROM before 32 weeks of gestation should be cared for expectantly until 33 completed weeks of gestation if no maternal or fetal contraindications exist. A 48-hour course of intravenous ampicillin and erythromycin followed by 5 days of oral amoxicillin and erythromycin is recommended during expectant management of preterm PROM remote from term to prolong pregnancy and reduce infectious and gestational age–dependent neonatal morbidity. A single course of antenatal corticosteroids should be administered to women with PROM before 32 weeks of gestation to reduce the risks of respiratory distress syndrome, perinatal mortality, and other morbidities. Tocolysis in the setting of preterm PROM has not been shown to be effective in either delaying delivery or improving neonatal outcome.

Stillbirth

Fetal death, or stillbirth (the term preferred among parent groups), is one of the most common adverse pregnancy outcomes, complicating 1 in 160 deliveries in the United States. Approximately 25,000 stillbirths at 20 weeks of gestation or greater are reported annually. In any specific case, it may be difficult to assign a definite cause to a stillbirth. A significant proportion of stillbirths remain unexplained even after a thorough evaluation.

Risk Factors and Comorbidities

In developed countries, the most prevalent risk factors associated with stillbirth are non-Hispanic black race, nulliparity, advanced maternal age, and obesity. From a public health perspective, obesity, smoking, and drug and alcohol use are common potentially modifiable risk factors for adverse pregnancy outcome. Hypertension and diabetes are two of the most common medical comorbid pregnancy conditions.

Methods of Delivery

The method and timing of delivery after a fetal death depends on the gestational age at which the death occurred, on the maternal history of a previous uterine scar, and maternal preference. Although most patients will desire prompt delivery, the timing of delivery is not critical. In the second trimester, dilation and evacuation can be offered if an experienced health care provider is available, although patients should be counseled that dilation and evacuation may limit efficacy of autopsy for the detection of macroscopic fetal abnormalities. Labor induction is appropriate at later gestational ages, if second trimester dilation and evacuation is unavailable, or based on patient preference. Induction of labor with vaginal misoprostol is safe and effective before 28 weeks of gestation in patients with a prior cesarean delivery with a low transverse uterine scar.

Evaluation of Stillbirth

After a stillbirth or neonatal death, proper management includes obtaining a complete perinatal and family history, performing a physical examination of the fetus (with documentation by description and photography, if possible), and obtaining laboratory studies. The most important tests in the evaluation of a stillbirth are fetal autopsy; examination of the placenta, cord, and membranes; and karyotype evaluation. The results of the autopsy, placental examination, laboratory tests, and cytogenetic studies should be communicated to the involved physicians and to the family of the deceased infant in a timely manner. Sensitivity is needed when discussing evaluation of a stillborn fetus with the family. Patient support should include emotional support and clear communication of test results. Referral to a bereavement counselor, religious leader, peer support group, or mental health professional may be advisable for management of grief and depression.

Recurrence Counseling

Counseling can be hampered by insufficient information regarding the etiology of the prior stillbirth. When specific risks are identified, the risk of recurrence may be quantifiable. In low-risk women with unexplained stillbirth the risk of stillbirth recurrence after 20 weeks of gestation is estimated at 7.8–10.5 per 1,000 births, with most of this risk occurring before 37 weeks of gestation. Rates of the recurrence of fetal loss are higher in women with medical complications, such as diabetes or hypertension, or in those with obstetric problems with a significant recurrence risk, such as placental abruption. Despite reassurances, the patient is likely to be anxious and to require ongoing support.

Bibliography

American College of Obstetricians and Gynecologists. Intrauterine growth restriction. ACOG Practice Bulletin 12. Washington, DC: ACOG; 2000.

American College of Obstetricians and Gynecologists. Prevention of Rh D alloimmunization. ACOG Practice Bulletin 4. Washington, DC: ACOG; 1999.

Anemia in Pregnancy. ACOG Practice Bulletin No. 95. American College of Obstetricians and Gynecologists. Obstet Gynecol 2008;112: 201–7.

Antenatal corticosteroid therapy for fetal maturation. Committee Opinion No. 475. American College of Obstetricians and Gynecologists. Obstet Gynecol 2011;117:422–4.

Antiphospholipid syndrome. Practice Bulletin No. 118. American College of Obstetricians and Gynecologists. Obstet Gynecol 2011;117:192–9.

Assessment of risk factors for preterm birth. ACOG Practice Bulletin No. 31. American College of Obstetricians and Gynecologists. Obstet Gynecol 2001;98:709–716.

Asthma in pregnancy. ACOG Practice Bulletin No. 90. American College of Obstetricians and Gynecologists. Obstet Gynecol 2008;111:457–464.

Bariatric surgery and pregnancy. ACOG Practice Bulletin No. 105. American College of Obstetricians and Gynecologists. Obstet Gynecol 2009;113:1405–13.

Chronic hypertension in pregnancy. Practice Bulletin No. 125. American College of Obstetricians and Gynecologists. Obstet Gynecol 2012;119:396–407.

Critical care in pregnancy. ACOG Practice Bulletin No. 100. American College of Obstetricians and Gynecologists. Obstet Gynecol 2009;113:443–50.

Diagnosis and management of preeclampsia and eclampsia. ACOG Practice Bulletin No. 33. American College of Obstetricians and Gynecologists. Obstet Gynecol 2002; 99:159–167.

Flegal KM, Carroll MD, Ogden CL, Curtin LR. Prevalence and Trends in Obesity Among US Adults, 1999-2008. JAMA 2010;303:235–241.

Gestational diabetes. ACOG Practice Bulletin No. 203. American College of Obstetricians and Gynecologists. Obstet Gynecol 2001;98:525–38.

Hemoglobinopathies in pregnancy. ACOG Practice Bulletin No. 78. American College of Obstetricians and Gynecologists. Obstet Gynecol 2007;109:229–37.

Inherited thrombophilias in pregnancy. Practice Bulletin No. 124. American College of Obstetricians and Gynecologists. Obstet Gynecol 2011;124:730–40.

Kim SY, Dietz PM, England L, Morrow B, Callaghan WM. Trends in pre-pregnancy obesity in nine states, 1993-2003. Obesity (Silver Spring) 2007;15:986–93.

Late-preterm infants. ACOG Committee Opinion No. 404. American College of Obstetricians and Gynecologists. Obstet Gynecol 2008;111:1029–32.

Magnesium sulfate before anticipated preterm birth for neuroprotection. Committee Opinion No. 455. American College of Obstetricians and Gynecologists. Obstet Gynecol 2010;115:669–71.

Management of alloimmunization during pregnancy. ACOG Practice Bulletin No. 75. American College of Obstetricians and Gynecologists. Obstet Gynecol 2006;108:457–64.

Management of preterm labor. Practice Bulletin No. 127. American College of Obstetricians and Gynecologists. Obstet Gynecol 2012;119:1308–17.

Management of stillbirth. ACOG Practice Bulletin No. 102. American College of Obstetricians and Gynecologists. Obstet Gynecol 2009;113:748–61.

Multifetal pregnancy reduction. ACOG Committee Opinion No. 369. American College of Obstetricians and Gynecologists. Obstet Gynecol 2007;109:1511–5.

Multiple gestation: complicated twin, triplet, and high-order multifetal pregnancy. ACOG Practice Bulletin No. 56. American College of Obstetricians and Gynecologists. Obstet Gynecol 2004;104:869–83.

Obesity in pregnancy. ACOG Committee Opinion No. 315. American College of Obstetricians and Gynecologists. Obstet Gynecol 2005;106:671–5.

Ogden CL, Carroll MD. Prevalence of overweight, obesity, and extreme obesity among adults: United States, trends 1960-1962 through 2007-2008. NCHS Health E-Stats. Hyattsville (MD): National Center for Health Statistics; 2010. p. 1-6. Available at: http://www.cdc.gov/nchs/data/hestat/obesity_adult_07_08/obesity_adult_07_08.pdf. Retrieved December 22, 2011.

Perinatal care at the threshold of viability. ACOG Practice Bulletin No. 38. American College of Obstetricians and Gynecologists. Obstet Gynecol 2002;100:617–24.

Placenta accreta. Committee Opinion No. 529. American College of Obstetricians and Gynecologists. Obstet Gynecol 2012;120:207–11.

Postpartum hemorrhage. ACOG Practice Bulletin No. 76. American College of Obstetricians and Gynecologists. Obstet Gynecol 2006;108:1039–47.

Postpartum screening for abnormal glucose tolerance in women who had gestational diabetes mellitus. ACOG Committee Opinion No. 435. American College of Obstetricians and Gynecologists. Obstet Gynecol 2009;113:1419–21.

Pregestational diabetes mellitus. ACOG Practice Bulletin No. 60. American College of Obstetricians and Gynecologists. Obstet Gynecol 2005;105:675–85.

Premature rupture of membranes. ACOG Practice Bulletin No. 80. American College of Obstetricians and Gynecologists. Obstet Gynecol 2007;109:1007–19.

Report of the Expert Committee on the Diagnosis and Classification of Diabetes Mellitus. Expert Committee on the Diagnosis and Classification of Diabetes Mellitus. Diabetes Care 2000;23 Suppl 1S4–19.

Screening and diagnosis of gestational diabetes. Committee Opinion No. 504. American College of Obstetricians and Gynecologists. Obstet Gynecol 2011;118:751–3.

Spong CY, Mercer BM, D'Alton M, Kilpatrick S, Blackwell S, Saade G. Timing of indicated late-preterm and early-term birth. Obstet Gynecol 2011;118:323–33.

Subclinical hypothyroidism in pregnancy. ACOG Committee Opinion No. 381. American College of Obstetricians and Gynecologists. Obstet Gynecol 2007;110:959–60.

Thromboembolism in pregnancy. Practice Bulletin No. 123. American College of Obstetricians and Gynecologists. Obstet Gynecol 2011;118:718–29.

Thyroid disease in pregnancy. ACOG Practice Bulletin No. 37. American College of Obstetricians and Gynecologists. Obstet Gynecol 2002;100:387–396.

Use of progesterone to reduce preterm birth. ACOG Committee Opinion No. 419. American College of Obstetricians and Gynecologists. Obstet Gynecol 2008;112: 963–5.

Use of prophylactic antibiotics in labor and delivery. Practice Bulletin No. 120. American College of Obstetricians and Gynecologists. Obstet Gynecol 2011;117:1472–83.

Use of psychiatric medications during pregnancy and lactation. ACOG Practice Bulletin No. 92. American College of Obstetricians and Gynecologists. Obstet Gynecol 2008; 111:1001–20. Reaffirmed 2009.

Resources

Food and Drug Administration. Silver Spring (MD): FDA; 2011. Available at: http://www.fda.gov. Retrieved December 22, 2011.

NICHD Neonatal Research Network (NRN):Extremely Preterm Birth Outcome Data. Bethesda (MD): NICHD; 2011. Available at: http://www.nichd.nih.gov/about/org/cdbpm/pp/prog_epbo/epbo_case.cfm. Retrieved December 22, 2011.

REPROTOX: an information system on environmental hazards to human reproduction and development. Washington, DC: The Reproductive Toxicology Center; 2011. Available at: http://www.reprotox.org/. Retrieved December 22, 2011.

Chapter 8
Care of the Newborn

All newborns should be cared for by a team of expert physicians and trained health care providers in the context of a family-centered environment. At birth, infants are quickly stabilized and assessed to determine the level of care required. Individuals trained in neonatal resuscitation are present in the delivery room and are ready to perform timely resuscitation, if needed. All infants undergo an identification process, and copies of both maternal and newborn medical records are transferred from the obstetric to the neonatal care teams.

Term (37 0/7–41 6/7 weeks of gestation) and late preterm infants (34 0/7–36 6/7 weeks of gestation) are closely observed during the transition period, the first 4–8 hours after birth. Infants who are healthy and stable should remain with their mother during this period. The infant should be kept warm and assessed by a detailed clinical examination that includes intrauterine growth status, evaluation for gestational age, and a comprehensive risk assessment for neonatal conditions that require additional monitoring or intervention. Shortly after birth, all infants are weighed; receive eye prophylaxis, parenteral vitamin K, skin care, and umbilical cord care; and are bathed and clothed.

Neonatal nutrition is ideally provided through breastfeeding. Initiation of breastfeeding should take place soon after birth, with continued monitoring of the breastfed newborn until discharge and then after by the newborn care provider. There are limited contraindications to breastfeeding. In the event breastfeeding is disrupted, breast milk may be collected and stored or pasteurized banked donor milk may serve as an alternative. Rarely, is formula feeding needed.

Preventive newborn care includes attention to hygiene and asepsis; hepatitis immunization; and screening for genetic and metabolic conditions, hearing impairment, critical congenital heart disease, risk of hyperbilirubinemia, and developmental hip dysplasia. Targeted assessment of temperature stability, glucose homeostasis, and possible sepsis are implemented on a discretionary basis, depending on individualized risk.

Delivery Room Care

Approximately 10% of newborns require some assistance to begin breathing that includes stimulation at birth, and less than 1% will need extensive resuscitative measures. Although the vast majority of newly born infants do not require intervention to make the transition from intrauterine to extrauterine life, because of the large total number of births, a sizable number will require some degree of resuscitation. Recognition and immediate resuscitation of a distressed neonate requires an organized plan of action that includes the immediate availability of proper equipment and on-site qualified personnel.

Neonatal Resuscitation Management Plan

Assessment and resuscitation of the newborn at delivery should be provided in accordance with the principles of the American Heart Association and the American Academy of Pediatrics (AAP) Neonatal Resuscitation Program™. Although the guidelines for neonatal resuscitation focus on delivery room resuscitation, most of the principles are applicable throughout the neonatal period and early infancy. Each hospital should have policies and procedures addressing the care and resuscitation of the newborn, including the qualifications of physicians and staff who provide this care. A program should be in place that ensures the competency of these individuals as well as their periodic credentialing. At every delivery, there should be at least one individual whose primary responsibility is the newborn and who is capable of initiating resuscitation, including positive pressure ventilation and chest compressions. This individual may be a physician, advanced practice neonatal nurse, nurse anesthetist, nursery nurse, physician assistant, respiratory therapist, certified nurse–midwife, or a labor and delivery nurse. Either this individual or someone else who is immediately available should have the skills required to perform a complete resuscitation, including endotracheal intubation, establishment of vascular access, and the use of medications.

The provision of services and equipment for resuscitation should be planned jointly by the medical and nursing directors of the departments involved in resuscitation of the newborn, usually the departments of obstetrics, pediatrics, and anesthesia. A physician, usually a pediatrician, should be designated to assume primary responsibility for initiating, supervising, and reviewing the plan for management of newborns requiring resuscitation in the delivery room. The following issues should be considered in this plan:

- A prioritized list should be developed of known or anticipated maternal and fetal complications that would require a routine, urgent, and an emergency delivery room presence of an individual(s) qualified in all aspects of newborn resuscitation.

- The capabilities of individuals qualified to perform neonatal resuscitation should include the following:

  — Ability to rapidly and accurately evaluate the newborn condition

  — Ability and authority to seek additional personnel and experts for immediate participation in newborn resuscitation

  — Knowledge of the pathogenesis of risk factors predisposing for the need for resuscitation (eg, hypoxia, maternal medication, hypovolemia, trauma, anomalies, infections, and preterm birth), as well as specific indications for resuscitation

  — Skills in airway management, including bag and mask ventilation, use of a laryngeal mask airway, laryngoscopy, endotracheal intubation and suctioning of the airway, chest compressions, emergency administration of drugs and fluids, establishing vascular access, and maintenance of thermal stability

  — Skill in placing an umbilical venous catheter. This is especially important because most resuscitation medications should be given by this route.

  — Although not required, skill in the recognition and decompression of a tension pneumothorax by needle aspiration is desirable.

- Procedures should be developed and policies should be in place to ensure the readiness of equipment and personnel and to provide for periodic review and evaluation of the effectiveness of the system.

- Contingency plans should be created for multiple births, unusual and life-threatening maternal complications, and other unusual circumstances.

- Guidelines should be developed for documentation of the resuscitation, including the personnel involved, interventions, medications, the time of each intervention or medication, and the response of the infant.

• Procedures should be developed and delineated for transfer of responsibility for care of the newborn.

Steps in Delivery Room Management

At birth, the neonatal care team implements a sequence of steps to quickly assess and stabilize the infant in order to institute the appropriate intensity of newborn care. With careful consideration of risk factors, most newborns who will need resuscitation can be identified before birth. If the possible need for resuscitation is anticipated, additional skilled personnel should be recruited and the necessary equipment prepared.

Assessment

Newborns who do not require resuscitation should be identified by rapid assessment of three characteristics:

1. Is the baby full term (259 days or more or 37 0/7 weeks of gestation)?
2. Is the baby breathing with a regular rhythm or crying?
3. Does the baby have good muscle tone?

If the answers to these questions are "yes," the baby does not need resuscitation and should remain with the mother. The baby should be dried, placed skin-to-skin with the mother, and covered with dry linen to maintain temperature. Observation of breathing, activity, and color should be ongoing.

If the answer to any of these questions is "no," the infant should receive one or more of the following categories of action in sequence (see Fig. 8-1 for a detailed treatment algorithm):

• Initial steps in stabilization (provide warmth, position to open the airway, clear airway if necessary, dry, stimulate breathing)

• Positive pressure ventilation, oxygen saturation monitoring, and supplemental oxygen, as needed

• Chest compressions

• Administration of epinephrine or volume expansion or both

Approximately 60 seconds ("the golden minute") are allotted for completing the initial steps, re-evaluating, and beginning ventilation if required (see Fig. 8-1). The decision to progress beyond the initial steps is determined by simultaneous assessment of two vital characteristics: 1) respirations (apnea, gasping, or

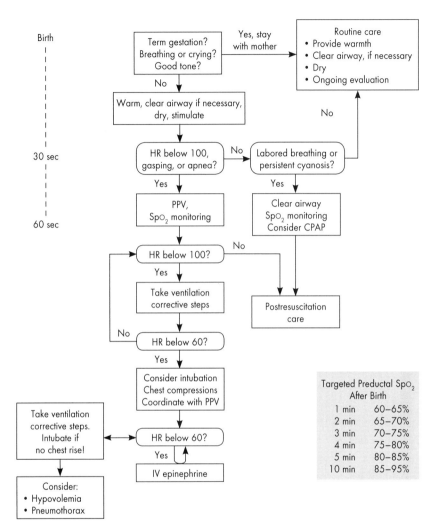

Fig. 8-1. Neonatal resuscitation algorithm. Abbreviations: CPAP, continuous positive airway pressure; HR, heart rate; IV, intravenous; PPV, positive pressure ventilation; SpO$_2$, blood oxygen saturation. Data from Kattwinkel J, Perlman JM, Aziz K, Colby C, Fairchild K, Gallagher J, et al. Neonatal resuscitation: 2010 American Heart Association Guidelines for Cardiopulmonary Resuscitation and Emergency Cardiovascular Care. American Heart Association. Pediatrics 2010;126:e1400-13 *and* Kattwinkel J, Perlman JM, Aziz K, Colby C, Fairchild K, Gallagher, et al. Part 15: neonatal resuscitation: 2010 American Heart Association Guidelines for Cardiopulmonary Resuscitation and Emergency Cardiovascular Care. Circulation. 2010;122(suppl 3):S909-S919. Reprinted with permission of the American Heart Association. Copyright 2010 American Heart Association.

labored or unlabored breathing) and 2) heart rate (whether greater than or less than 100 beats per minute). Palpation of the pulse at the base of the umbilical cord is the easiest and quickest method to determine the heart rate. If a pulse is not palpable, assessment of heart rate should be done by auscultating the precordial heart tones. Once positive pressure ventilation with or without supplemental oxygen administration is begun, assessment should consist of simultaneous evaluation of three vital characteristics: 1) heart rate, 2) respirations, and 3) the state of oxygenation (the latter optimally determined by a pulse oximeter). The most sensitive indicator of a successful response to each step is an increase in heart rate (see also "Initial Steps in Stabilization").

Initial Steps in Stabilization

Maintenance of Body Temperature. Immediately after delivery, the vigorous term infant can be dried and placed skin-to-skin with the mother—both mother and infant should be covered with a blanket. Infants who require stabilization or resuscitation should be placed under a preheated radiant warmer. The radiant warmer will reduce heat loss and allow easy access to the newborn during resuscitation procedures. For this reason, additional warming techniques are recommended (eg, prewarming the delivery room to 26°C (78.8°F), covering the baby in plastic wrapping (food or medical grade, heat-resistant plastic), placing the baby on an exothermic mattress). An infant older than 28 weeks of gestation who requires resuscitation should be dried completely with prewarmed towels and placed under a preheated radiant warmer. Very low birth weight (less than 1,500 g) preterm babies are likely to become hypothermic despite the use of traditional techniques for decreasing heat loss. Because infants younger than 28 weeks of gestation may become hypothermic while being dried, they should be immediately covered up to their necks in polyethylene wrap or a food-grade plastic bag and placed under a radiant warmer. The infant's temperature must be monitored closely because overheating has been described when plastic wrap is used in combination with an exothermic mattress. The goal should be an axillary temperature of approximately 36.5°C (97.7°F).

Clearing the Airway. When the newborn is *vigorous* (defined as having strong respiratory efforts, good muscle tone, and a heart rate greater than 100 beats per minute), there is no evidence that nasopharyngeal suctioning is necessary. It is recommended that suctioning of the airway immediately after birth (including suctioning with a bulb syringe) should be reserved for babies who have obvious airway obstruction that interferes with spontaneous breathing or who require positive pressure ventilation. The mouth should be suctioned before the nose so there is nothing to aspirate if the neonate gasps when the nose is suctioned. Vigorous suctioning of the posterior pharynx should be avoided because this may produce significant reflex bradycardia and may damage the oral mucosa, leading to interference with suckling because of pain.

When meconium is present in amniotic fluid, evidence does not support routine intrapartum oropharyngeal or nasopharyngeal suctioning, as these interventions do not prevent or alter the course of meconium aspiration syndrome. If meconium-stained amniotic fluid is present and the newborn is not vigorous, in accordance with Neonatal Resuscitation Program™ guidelines, the physician should intubate the trachea and suction to remove meconium or other aspirated material from beneath the glottis. When using suction from the wall or a pump, the suction pressure should be set so that negative pressure reads approximately 100 mm Hg when the suction tubing is blocked.

Positioning. The newborn can be positioned on either the back or the side, with the neck slightly extended. This position (known as the sniffing position) readily aligns the posterior pharynx, larynx, and trachea for optimal air entry, for both spontaneous breaths and bag and mask ventilation. The newborn's mouth and nose may be wiped with a towel or suctioned gently to remove excess mucus or blood (see also "Clearing the Airway" earlier in this section).

Stimulation. Drying and suctioning provide enough tactile stimulation for most newborns. However, if the infant does not have adequate respirations, some additional tactile stimulation may be needed. Acceptable methods of stimulation include slapping or flicking the soles of the feet, and gently rubbing the newborn's back, trunk, or extremities. If the baby does not respond to one or two slaps, flicks to the feet, or rubbing of the back, positive pressure ventilation should be initiated.

Administration of Supplemental Oxygen. Published data indicate that positive pressure ventilation should be initiated with air in the term infant; however, the data regarding the preterm infant are less clear. The goal of resuscitation is to achieve an oxygen saturation value in the interquartile range of preductal saturations for each minute after birth measured in healthy term babies after vaginal birth at sea level (see table in Fig. 8-1). In the term infant, these targets can, in most instances, be achieved by initiating resuscitation with air. The oxygen concentration may be titrated, if needed, to achieve an SpO_2 in the target range. It is recommended that oximetry be used when resuscitation can be anticipated, supplemental oxygen is administered, positive pressure is administered for more than a few breaths, or when cyanosis appears to persist. Because many babies born at less than 32 weeks of gestation will not reach target saturations when resuscitated with air, blended oxygen and air may be given judiciously and pulse oximetry should ideally be used to guide adjustments to the amount of oxygen given. Both hyperoxemia and hypoxemia should be avoided. If blended oxygen is not available, resuscitation should be initiated with air.

Ventilation. The normal newborn breathes within seconds of delivery and usually has established regular respirations within 1 minute after delivery. A newborn who is apneic or is gasping or whose heart rate is less than 100 beats per minute requires positive pressure ventilation. For most newborns, bag and mask ventilation is effective, can serve to stimulate the initiation of spontaneous respirations, and is the only resuscitation maneuver required to establish regular respirations. Effective ventilation almost always results in improved heart rate. If the heart rate does not increase with ventilation, poor ventilation due to failure to establish functional residual capacity should be suspected. In this case, corrective steps, such as opening the mouth, suctioning the oropharynx, and increasing the pressure used to deliver breaths should be considered. If resuscitation was initiated with air or blended oxygen and air, and there is no improvement in heart rate after 90 seconds of effective ventilation, the oxygen concentration should be increased to 100%.

Endotracheal intubation may be performed at various points during resuscitation, depending on the clinical circumstances. Indications for intubation include the following:

- The presence of meconium in a depressed infant
- Poor response to ventilation with mask and bag or T-piece resuscitator
- To enhance coordination of ventilation and chest compressions when chest compressions are necessary

Other possible indications for intubation include need for surfactant administration, and suspected or known congenital diaphragmatic hernia. The skill of the resuscitator also may affect the timing of intubation. Individuals not adept at intubation should obtain assistance and focus on providing effective positive pressure ventilation with a mask rather than using valuable time attempting to intubate.

Exhaled carbon dioxide detection is the recommended method to confirm endotracheal tube placement; however, critically ill infants with poor cardiac output and poor or absent pulmonary blood flow may not exhale sufficient carbon dioxide to be detected reliably and thus may give false-negative test results. As with bag and mask ventilation, effective assisted ventilation with an endotracheal tube should result in an increased heart rate. If the heart rate does not improve, esophageal intubation should be suspected.

Chest Compressions. If the heart rate does not increase promptly above 60 beats per minute after at least 30 seconds of effective ventilation with oxygen, chest compressions should be instituted while ventilation is continued. The two-thumb encircling hand technique is recommended. There should be a 3:1 ratio of compressions to ventilations with approximately 90 compressions and 30 ventilations per minute. If there is no response in the heart rate after 45–60 seconds of effective chest compressions, intubation (if not already done) and appropriate drug therapy with epinephrine, preferably by the intravenous route should be instituted.

Medications. The use of medications for resuscitation of the newborn rarely is necessary in the delivery room and should be considered only after effective ventilation and chest compressions have been established and the heart rate remains low. A list of drugs and volume expanders for resuscitation, with appropriate dosages, should be readily available, preferably in a prominent place in the resuscitation area. Neonatal Resuscitation Program™ reference charts that provide this information, as well as a flow diagram of the resuscitation procedure, are available from the AAP for use in the delivery room and on code carts.

- Epinephrine—Epinephrine is indicated when the heart rate remains less than 60 beats per minute, despite adequate ventilation and chest compressions. The recommended dose is 0.1 to 0.3 mL/kg of a 1:10,000 solution (equal to 0.01–0.03 mg/kg) given intravenously as rapidly as possible, preferably through an umbilical venous catheter placed emergently. The efficacy of endotracheal epinephrine is unproven, and use of this route results in lower and unpredictable blood levels that may not be effective. Physicians may choose to give an endotracheal tube dose while the umbilical venous catheter is being placed. If this route is used, administration of a higher dose (0.05–0.1 mg/kg, or 0.5–1 mL/kg of a 1:10,000 preparation) through the endotracheal tube may be considered, but the safety and efficacy of this practice have not been evaluated.

- Volume expanders—Volume expanders should be considered when a baby is not responding to resuscitation and blood loss is known or suspected. An isotonic crystalloid solution (normal saline or Ringer's lactate) or type O Rh-negative packed red blood cells (if fetal anemia is known or expected) is recommended for volume expansion in the delivery room. The recommended dose is 10 mL/kg given intravenously over 5–10 minutes, which may need to be repeated. It should be given by the most accessible route, which in the delivery room is usually the umbilical vein. It may be advisable to give the infusion more slowly in preterm infants because rapid infusion of large volumes may increase the risk of intraventricular hemorrhage.

- Naloxone—Administration of naloxone is not recommended as part of initial resuscitative efforts in the delivery room for newborns with respiratory depression because of concerns about the possible exposure of the infant to maternal narcotic analgesia. Adequate support of ventilation should be sufficient to restore normal heart rate and oxygenation.

Apgar Score

The Apgar score is useful for describing the status of the newborn at birth and his or her subsequent adaptation to the extrauterine environment. It should not be used to determine the need for resuscitation or the steps to be taken. If resuscitation is indicated, it is initiated before the 1-minute Apgar score is obtained. Apgar scores should be assigned at 1 minute and 5 minutes after birth, and if the 5-minute Apgar score is less than 7, additional scores should be assigned every 5 minutes for up to 20 minutes until the Apgar score is greater than 7. The AAP Committee on Fetus and Newborn has recommended the use of an assisted Apgar Scoring System (Fig. 8-2) that documents the assistance the infant is receiving at the time of assignment of the score.

Assessment of the Newborn in the Delivery Room

After delivery, the newborn must be assessed for individual needs to determine the best location for care. A healthy-appearing newborn may be kept in the mother's room or may be admitted to an observation–admission–transition nursery in preparation for rooming-in with the mother. An infant with known or anticipated medical needs may be admitted to the special care nursery or neonatal intensive care unit (NICU) either in the hospital where the infant was born or transferred to a hospital that provides the appropriate level of care (see also "Expanded Classification System for Levels of Neonatal Care" in Chapter 1 and "Transport Procedure" in Chapter 4).

Apgar Score

Gestational age: _____ weeks

Sign	0	1	2	1 min	5 min	10 min	15 min	20 min
Color	Blue or Pale	Acrocyanotic	Completely Pink					
Heart rate	Absent	Less than 100 min	Greater than 100 min					
Reflex irritability	No response	Grimace	Cry or active withdrawal					
Muscle tone	Limp	Some flexion	Active motion					
Respiration	Absent	Weak cry, hypoventilation	Good, crying					
			Total					

Comments:

		Resuscitation				
Min		1	5	10	15	20
Oxygen						
PPV/NCPAP						
ETT						
Chest compressions						
Epinephrine						

Fig. 8-2. Expanded Apgar score form. Record the score in the appropriate place at specific time intervals. The additional resuscitative measures (if appropriate) are recorded at the same time that the score is reported using a check mark in the appropriate box. Use the comment box to list other factors including maternal medications, or the response to resuscitation, or both between the recorded times of scoring. Abbreviations: PPV/NCPAP, positive-pressure ventilation/nasal continuous positive airway pressure; ETT, endotracheal tube. The Apgar Score. ACOG Committee Opinion No. 333. American College of Obstetricians and Gynecologists. Obstet Gynecol 2006;107:1209–12.

Generally, healthy newborns should remain with their mothers. If the newborn's condition is stable and the infant does not require further intervention, immediate and sustained skin-to-skin contact between the mother and her infant should be provided. If the mother has chosen to breastfeed, the newborn should be placed at the breast in the delivery room within the first hour after birth. Initial skin-to-skin contact has been associated with a longer duration of breastfeeding and improved temperature stability. Such contact maintains the infant's body temperature regulation and facilitates the opportunity for breastfeeding soon after delivery. The nursing staff in the labor, delivery, recovery, and postpartum areas should be trained in assessing and recognizing problems in the newborn.

Newborns with depressed breathing, depressed activity, or persistent cyanosis at birth who require intervention in the delivery room but respond promptly, or those with continuing symptoms, including mild respiratory distress, are at risk of developing problems and should be evaluated frequently during the immediate neonatal period. This may occur in an observation–admission–transition nursery, where frequent vital signs can be obtained and the nursing staff is familiar with the signs and symptoms of an infant who is in distress. If the vital signs stabilize and the infant has no other risk factors, the newborn can then room-in with the mother.

Infants who require more extensive resuscitation are at risk of developing subsequent complications and may require ongoing support. These infants should be managed in an area where ongoing evaluation and monitoring are available. This may take place in the birth hospital, if it is an appropriate facility, or may require transport to another hospital for a higher level of care.

Immediate plans for the newborn should be discussed with the parents or other support person(s), preferably before leaving the delivery room. Whenever possible, the parents should have the opportunity to see, touch, and hold the newborn before transfer to a nursery or before transfer to another facility. The physician or other responsible individual delivering the newborn should also be advised of the status and plans for the newborn, including potential transfer or admission to a special care nursery or NICU.

Noninitiation or Withdrawal of Intensive Care for High-Risk Infants

Parents should be active participants in the decision-making process concerning the treatment of severely ill infants. This approach requires honest and open communication. Ongoing evaluation of the condition and prognosis of the high-risk infant is essential, and the physician, as the spokesperson for the health care team, must convey this information accurately and openly to the parents of the infant.

Compassionate and Comfort Care

Compassionate care to ensure comfort must be provided to all infants, including those for whom intensive care is not being provided. The decision to initiate or continue intensive care should be based only on the judgment that the infant will benefit from the intensive care. It is inappropriate for life-prolonging treatment to be continued when the condition is incompatible with life or when the treatment is judged to be harmful, of no benefit, or futile.

Whenever nonresuscitation is considered an option, a qualified individual should be involved and present in the delivery room to manage this complex situation. Whenever possible, this individual should be a neonatologist. Comfort care should be provided for all infants for whom resuscitation is not initiated or is not successful.

Parent Counseling Regarding Resuscitation of Extremely Low Gestational Age Infants

Whether to initiate resuscitation of an infant born at an extremely low gestational age is a difficult decision because the consequences of this decision are either the inevitable death of the infant or the uncertainties of providing intensive care for an unknown length of time with an uncertain outcome. Each hospital that provides obstetric care should have a comprehensive and consistent approach to counseling parents and decision making. Parents should be provided the most accurate prognostic data available to help them make decisions. These predictions should not be based on gestational age alone but should include all relevant information affecting the prognosis. It is not possible to develop specific criteria for when the initiation of resuscitation should or should not be offered. Rather, the following general guidelines are suggested when discussing this situation with parents. If the physicians involved believe that there is no chance of survival, resuscitation is not indicated and should not be initiated. If the physicians consider a good outcome to be very unlikely, then parents should be given the choice of whether resuscitation should be initiated, and physicians should respect their preference. When the physicians' judgment is that a good outcome is reasonably likely, physicians should initiate resuscitation and, together with the parents, continually re-evaluate whether intensive care should be continued.

Identification

The possibility of newborns being switched in the hospital requires strict guidelines to prevent these events. Human error continues to be the major cause of infants being accidentally switched, and establishing procedures with multiple checks or electronic matching systems minimizes this risk. Infant identification procedures should begin in the delivery room with matching bands for the infant and the mother. The nurse in the delivery room should be responsible for preparing and securely fastening these identification bands on the newborn and the mother while the newborn is still in the delivery room. These identical bands should indicate the mother's admission number, the infant's sex, the date and time of birth, and other information specified in hospital policy. Footprinting and fingerprinting alone are not adequate methods of patient identification. The birth records and identification bands should be checked and verified for accuracy before the newborn leaves the delivery room. Policies and procedures requiring personnel to match identification bands each time the infant is taken to the mother while in the hospital and at discharge will minimize errors. If the condition of the newborn does not allow placement of identification bands (eg, extreme preterm birth), the identification bands should accompany the infant and should be placed on the incubator or warmer. In these instances, the identification bands should be attached to the infant as soon as is practical.

With multiple births, each of the newborns should be identified according to birth order (eg, A, B, C or 1, 2, 3), and the corresponding umbilical cords should be identified according to hospital policy (eg, use of different number of clamps). This will ensure that umbilical cord blood specimens will be labeled correctly and can be correlated with the correct newborn. All umbilical cord blood samples must be labeled with an indication that these are samples of the newborn's umbilical cord blood and not that of the mother. The birth order may or may not correlate with the number assigned to the fetus in utero (see also "Infant Safety" later in this chapter).

Communication of Information

Care of the newborn is aided by effective communication of information about the mother and her fetus to the pediatrician or other health care provider.

With an uncomplicated pregnancy, labor, and delivery, the information on the medical record accompanying the newborn, if complete, may be sufficient. The obstetric staff should record the following information, which also should be available on a medical record that accompanies the newborn during any transfer of responsibility for care:

- The mother's name, medical record number, blood type, serologic test result, rubella status, hepatitis B test result, and human immunodeficiency virus (HIV) status

- Other maternal test results, if obtained, that are relevant to neonatal care, such as colonization with group B streptococci or intrapartum maternal antibiotic therapy (including type and number of doses of antibiotics)

- Maternal illness potentially affecting the fetus, evidence of chorioamnionitis, and maternal medications (including tocolytics and corticosteroids)

- Any history of illicit substance use or any other known socially high-risk circumstances, such as unstable housing, adolescent mother, maternal psychiatric disease, domestic violence, or history of previous child abuse or neglect

- Complications of pregnancy associated with abnormal fetal growth, fetal anomalies, or abnormal results from tests of fetal well-being and the corresponding interpretation

- Information regarding the labor (eg, duration) and delivery (eg, method), complications of labor (eg, deviations in fetal heart rate patterns), duration of rupture of amniotic membranes, presence or absence of meconium in amniotic fluid, and need for resuscitation

- Situations in which lactation may be compromised, such as history of breast surgery, trauma, or previous lactation failure

The obstetric staff should communicate problems before and after delivery in a timely manner to the physician or other health care provider who will be caring for the newborn. For some high-risk pregnancies, a neonatal consultation during the antepartum period may be helpful in obstetric management and can assist the parents in understanding what to expect for their newborn. This is of particular importance when fetal anomalies are significant or the delivery of a very preterm infant is expected.

Assessment of the Newborn Infant

Initial Assessment

A detailed clinical examination and assessment of the infant is performed by nursery personnel soon after birth and includes the following: evaluation of airway patency and skin color; auscultation of the heart and lungs; assessment of muscle tone, level of consciousness, response to handling; measurement of vital signs (ie, body temperature, heart rate, and respiratory rate); and measurement of head circumference, body length, and body weight. Each newborn should be weighed shortly after birth or after the first breastfeeding, and daily thereafter. The newborn must be kept warm during weighing. The scale pan should be covered with clean paper before each newborn is weighed. Additional targeted evaluations may include assessment of capillary refill, blood pressure, oxygen saturation, and need for supplemental oxygen.

Assessment of Intrauterine Growth

The newborn's gestational age can be estimated from the results of an ultrasound examination before 20 weeks of gestation or the mother's menstrual history (see also "Estimated Date of Delivery" in Chapter 5) and from the nursery assessment of gestational age (Fig. 8-3). Gestational age should be assigned after all nursing, pediatric, and obstetric data have been assessed. Any marked discrepancy between the presumed duration of pregnancy by obstetric assessment and the physical and neurologic findings in the newborn should be documented on the medical record. Growth parameters should be plotted on a birth weight–gestational age record appropriate for the community. Determination of gestational age and its relationship to weight should be used to identify newborns at risk of postnatal complications. For example, newborns who are either large or small for their gestational ages are at increased risk of alterations of glucose homeostasis, and appropriate tests (eg, serum glucose screen) are indicated.

Assessment of Late-Preterm Status

Infants born at 34 0/7–36 6/7 weeks of gestation (239–259 days since the first day of the last menstrual period) are referred to as late preterm. Late preterm infants are physiologically immature and have limited compensatory responses to the extrauterine environment compared with term infants. Late preterm infants are at a greater risk of acute as well as long-term morbidity and mortality than are term infants. During the birth hospitalization, temperature instability, hypoglycemia, respiratory distress, apnea, hyperbilirubinemia, and feeding difficulties are more likely to be diagnosed in late preterm infants than term infants. During the first month after birth, late preterm infants are more likely than term infants to be rehospitalized for phototherapy, severe hyperbilirubinemia, feeding difficulties, dehydration, suspected sepsis, parenteral antibiotic treatment, apneic events, and poor weight gain.

Risk factors that have been identified for rehospitalization or neonatal morbidity in late preterm infants include being the first born, being suboptimally breastfed at discharge, having a mother who had labor and delivery complications, being a recipient of public insurance at delivery, and being of Asian or Pacific Island descent. Collaborative counseling before delivery by both obstetric and neonatal physicians about the outcomes of late preterm births is warranted unless precluded by emergent conditions.

Risk Assessment for Neonatal Conditions

No later than 2 hours after birth, nursery personnel should evaluate the newborn's status and assess risk of neonatal illness and complications (see also "Initial Assessment" earlier in this section). Risks can be assessed through the history as documented on the antepartum and intrapartum records, as well as from the gestational age assessment and growth parameter determination. If the newborn's physician (or other health care provider) is not present at the delivery, he or she should be notified of the admission and of the status of the newborn within a time frame established by institutional policy.

Nursery policies should delineate those conditions (eg, low birth weight or small for gestational age) that require specific actions by nurses or immediate notification of the infant's physician or other health care provider, as defined by institutional policy. Clinical conditions, such as suspected maternal infection or low Apgar scores at 5 minutes or more, are associated with increased risk of neonatal illness and should prompt immediate notification of the infant's health care provider. The obstetrician should be notified of the newborn's status in a timely manner, particularly if problems or complications arise.

If immediate attention is not indicated, the newborn's physician or other health care provider should examine the apparently normal newborn within 24 hours after birth and within 24 hours before discharge from the hospital. This may be accomplished with at least one physical examination. The results of the examination should be recorded on the newborn's medical record and discussed with the parents. The health care provider should be made aware of any deviation or variance in the newborn's transition, postpartum stabilization, or risk status.

Neuromuscular maturity

	-1	0	1	2	3	4	5
Posture							
Square window (wrist)	>90°	90°	60°	45°	30°	0°	
Arm recoil		180°	140–180°	110–140°	90–110°	<90°	
Popliteal angle	180°	160°	140°	120°	100°	90°	<90°
Scarf sign							
Heel to ear							

Physical maturity

Skin	Sticky, friable, transparent	Gelatinous, red, translucent	Smooth, pink, visible veins	Superficial peeling or rash or both, few veins	Cracking, pale areas, rare veins	Parchment, deep cracking, no vessels	Leathery, cracked, wrinkled
Lanugo	None	Sparse	Abundant	Thinning	Bald areas	Mostly bald	
Plantar surface	Heel–toe 40–50 mm:-1 <40 mm:-2	<50 mm, no crease	Faint red marks	Anterior transverse crease only	Creases on anterior 2/3	Creases over entire sole	
Breast	Impercep-tible	Barely perceptible	Flat areola– no bud	Stripped areola 1–2 mm bud	Raised areola 3–4 mm bud	Full areola 5–10 mm bud	
Eye/ear	Lids fused loosely (-1), tightly (-2)	Lids open, pinna flat, stays folded	Slightly curved pinna; soft; slow recoil	Well-curved pinna, soft but ready recoil	Formed and firm, instant recoil	Thick cartilage, ear stiff	
Genitals male	Scrotum flat, smooth	Scrotum empty, faint rugae	Testes in upper canal rare rugae	Testes descending, few rugae	Testes down, good rugae	Testes pendulous, deep rugae	
Genitals female	Clitoris prominent, labia flat	Prominent clitoris, small labia minora	Prominent clitoris, enlarging minora	Majora & minora equally prominent	Majora large, minora small	Majora cover clitoris & minora	

Maturity rating	
Score	Weeks
-10	20
-5	22
0	24
5	26
10	28
15	30
20	32
25	34
30	36
35	38
40	40
45	42
50	44

Fig. 8-3. The expanded new Ballard Score includes extremely preterm infants and has been refined to improve accuracy in more mature infants. Reprinted with permission from Ballard JL, Khoury JC, Wedig K, Wang L, Eilers-Walsman BL, Lipp R. New Ballard Score, expanded to include extremely premature infants. J Pediatr 1991;119:417–23.

Transitional Care

After the initial evaluation of the newborn's condition, a care plan should be established, and the newborn should be carefully observed during the subsequent stabilization–transition period (the first 2–24 hours after birth). If the infant is healthy and stable, the care plan should facilitate ongoing contact between the mother and the infant (eg, rooming-in together) during this period. Temperature, heart and respiratory rates, skin color, peripheral circulation, respiration, level of consciousness, tone, and activity should be monitored and recorded at least once every 30 minutes until the newborn's condition has remained stable for 2 hours. Rooming-in for the mother and her infant is optimal because it allows unrestricted contact and feeding.

Clinical care includes the following: conjunctival (eye) care, administration of vitamin K, care of the skin, care of the umbilical cord, male circumcision (if chosen by the parents) and care of the circumcision site, and provision for appropriate clothing. Hospital staff can easily assess the infant's status in the mother's room. The newborn should be observed for any signs of illness or variations from normal behavior (as listed in Box 8-1). Knowledge and understanding of the processes of newborn transition allows for early detection of newborn disorders. For example, meconium is typically passed within the first 24 hours after birth. If a term newborn has not passed meconium by 48 hours after birth, the lower gastrointestinal tract may be obstructed. Urine is normally passed within the first 12 hours after birth. Failure to void within the first 24 hours may indicate genitourinary obstruction or abnormality. The newborn's physician or other health care provider should be informed to determine if the clinical event requires immediate medical attention.

Box 8-1. Potential Signs of Neonatal Illness

- Temperature instability
- Change in activity, including refusal of feedings
- Unusual skin color (pallor, jaundice, plethora, mottling)
- Abnormal cardiac or respiratory rate and rhythm
- Abdominal distention or bilious vomiting and gastric aspirate
- Excessive lethargy, sleepiness, or hypotonicity
- Jitteriness, irritability, or abnormal movements
- Delayed (more than 24 hours) or abnormal stools
- Delayed voiding (more than 12 hours)
- Weight change that is greater than expected

Conjunctival (Eye) Care

Prophylaxis against gonococcal ophthalmia neonatorum is mandatory for all newborns, including those born by cesarean delivery. Antimicrobial ophthalmic prophylaxis soon after delivery is recommended for all neonates but may be delayed until after the initial breastfeeding in the delivery room. A variety of topical agents appear to be equally efficacious. Acceptable prophylactic regimens are an application of a 1-cm ribbon of sterile ophthalmic ointment containing erythromycin (0.5%) or tetracycline (1%) in each lower conjunctival sac. Care should be taken to ensure that the agent reaches all parts of the conjunctival sac. The eyes should not be irrigated with saline or distilled water after application of any of these agents; however, after 1 minute, excess solution or ointment can be wiped away with sterile cotton. A 1% solution of silver nitrate is an effective alternative for prevention of gonococcal ophthalmia, but is associated with a 10-20% incidence of transient chemical conjunctivitis. Of these agents, only erythromycin ointment is commercially available in the United States. None of the topical agents are effective against *Chlamydia trachomatis* (see also "Chlamydial Infection" in Chapter 10).

Gonococcal ophthalmia or disseminated gonococcal infection can occur in neonates born to women with gonococcal disease. Single-dose systemic antibiotic therapy is an effective treatment for gonococcal ophthalmia and prophylaxis for disseminated disease (see also "Gonorrhea" in Chapter 10).

Administration of Vitamin K

Every newborn should receive a single parenteral dose of natural vitamin K_1 oxide (phytonadione) (0.5–1 mg) to prevent vitamin K-dependent hemorrhagic disease of the newborn. This dose should be administered shortly after birth but may be delayed until after the first breastfeeding in the delivery room. Oral administration of vitamin K has not been shown to be as efficacious as parenteral administration for the prevention of late hemorrhagic disease.

Skin Care

Skin care, including bathing, may be important for the health and appearance of the individual newborn and for infection control within the nursery. Removal of blood and secretions from the skin after delivery may minimize the risk of infection with potentially contaminating microorganisms, such as hepatitis B virus, herpes simplex virus, and HIV. Because bathing can be associated with significant heat loss, the first bath should be postponed until the newborn's thermal stability is ensured unless indicated by maternal infection risk factors, particularly HIV. The medical and nursing services of each hospital should develop guidelines regarding the time of the first bath, measures to protect against excessive heat loss, circumstances and methods of skin cleansing, and the roles of personnel and parents. The effects on the newborn's skin should be considered in selecting skin care techniques. Whole-body bathing of the newborn may not be necessary. Sterile cotton sponges (not gauze) soaked with warm water may be used to remove blood and meconium from the newborn's face, head, and body. Alternatively, the newborn can be cleansed with a mild, nonmedicated soap and then rinsed with water. After washing by either method, the infant should be dried well, with particular attention to the head to minimize heat loss.

For the remainder of the newborn's stay in the hospital, local skin care of the buttocks and perianal regions with warm water and cotton, a mild soap and water, or baby wipes at diaper changes should be adequate. Ideally, agents used on the newborn's skin should be dispensed in single-use containers, or each newborn should have a personal dispenser.

Umbilical Cord Care

The umbilical cord should be kept clean and dry. The application of antiseptics, including alcohol, triple dye, and chlorhexidine, has no advantage over dry umbilical cord care in reducing the incidence of omphalitis in developed countries, although these agents may reduce neonatal morbidity and mortality in low-resource settings.

Circumcision

Existing scientific evidence demonstrates that the preventive health benefits of elective circumcision of newborn males outweigh the risks of this procedure. Benefits include significant reductions in the risk of urinary tract infection in the first year of life and, subsequently, in the risk of heterosexual acquisition of HIV and other sexually transmitted infections. Although health benefits are not great enough to recommend routine circumcision for all newborn males, the benefits of circumcision are sufficient to justify access to this procedure for families choosing it and to warrant third-party payment for circumcision of newborn males. There are no data indicating that the circumcision of male newborn infants who may have been exposed to herpes simplex virus at birth should be postponed. It may be prudent, however, to delay circumcision for approximately 1 month in neonates at the highest risk of disease (eg, neonates delivered vaginally to women with active genital lesions).

The exact incidence of complications after circumcision is not known, but data indicate that the rate is low and that the most common complications are local infection and bleeding. To make an informed choice, the parents of all male newborns should be given accurate and unbiased information on circumcision and be given an opportunity to discuss this decision. Parents will need to weigh medical information in the context of their own religious, ethical, and cultural beliefs and practices, as it is the parents who must ultimately decide whether circumcision is in the best interests of their male child. Information sheets for parents about circumcision are available through AAP.

Analgesia should be provided if circumcision is performed. Swaddling, sucrose by mouth, and acetaminophen administration may reduce the stress response but are not sufficient for the operative pain and cannot be recommended as the sole method of analgesia. Although local anesthesia and combination preparations of lidocaine and prilocaine provide some anesthesia benefit, both ring blocks and dorsal penile blocks have been proved to be more effective.

Postprocedure care of the circumcised neonate should include cleaning and protecting the site from infection and irritation. With each diaper change, the penis should be cleaned and petroleum jelly can be placed over the surgical site. The jelly can be placed on a bandage or clean gauze pad and applied directly on the penis or placed on the diaper in the area with which the penis comes into contact. The petroleum jelly is not necessary for healing, but it keeps the surgical site from sticking to the diaper and causing irritation and bleeding when the diaper is removed. This will be necessary for approximately 4–7 days after circumcision.

If the family decides against circumcision, gentle washing of the genital area while bathing is sufficient for normal hygiene of the uncircumcised penis. Because of physiologic adhesions, the foreskin usually does not retract fully for several years and should not be forcibly retracted.

Clothing

Once thermal stability has been established, most newborns require only a cotton shirt or gown without buttons in addition to a soft diaper. A supply of soft, clean cotton clothing; bed pads; sheets, and blankets should be kept at the bedside. Nontoxic dyes should be used to mark clothing, blankets, or other items used in the care of newborns. A cap prevents excessive heat loss from the head.

Neonatal Nutrition

Breastfeeding

There are diverse and important advantages to infants, mothers, families, and society for breastfeeding and the use of human milk for infant feeding. These include health, nutritional, immunologic, developmental, psychological, social, economic, and environmental benefits. Human milk feeding supports optimal growth and development of the infant while decreasing the risk of a variety of acute and chronic diseases. Prenatal counseling and education regarding methods of newborn feeding may allow correction of misperceptions about feeding methods. Virtually all mothers who are initially undecided or hesitant to breastfeed can do so successfully with appropriate counseling, education, and knowledgeable support. Formula feeding should not be portrayed as equivalent to human milk feeding. If the mother chooses not to breastfeed after these interventions have been implemented, she should be supported in her decision.

Initiation of Breastfeeding

Successful breastfeeding begins during pregnancy. Prenatal care should include discussion of prior breastfeeding experience, feeding plans, and breast care. Ascertainment of history of breast surgery, trauma, or prior lactation failure is important because these situations may present special challenges to successful breastfeeding. The integration of breastfeeding into the total care of the newborn in the first months of life should be discussed. The mother should be offered the opportunity and be encouraged to breastfeed her newborn as soon as possible after delivery. A healthy newborn is capable of latching on to a breast without specific assistance within the first hour after birth, and breastfeeding should be initiated within the first hour unless medically contraindicated. Infants should be placed in direct skin-to skin contact with their mothers immediately after delivery and should remain there until the first breastfeeding is completed.

Rooming-in with the mother facilitates breastfeeding. From the time of delivery to discharge from the hospital, the mother and her healthy infant should be together continuously. The mother should be encouraged to offer the breast whenever the infant shows early signs of hunger, such as increased alertness, increased physical activity, mouthing, or rooting, and not to wait until the infant cries.

When awake, the newborn should be encouraged to feed frequently (8–12 times per day) until satiety (usually 10–15 minutes on each breast) to help stimulate milk production. In the early weeks after birth, an infant may need to be aroused to feed if 4 hours have elapsed since the last nursing. Usually, it is practical to alternate the breast used to initiate the feeding and to equalize the time spent at each breast over the day. When satisfied, the newborn will fall asleep or unlatch, although some infants may fall asleep before consuming sufficient nutrition.

Supplemental feedings including water, glucose water, formula, and other fluids should not be given to the breastfeeding infant unless ordered by the health care provider after documentation of a medical indication. Supplementation of the breastfed infant is best accomplished with expressed human milk or formula. Intermittent bottle-feeding of a breastfed newborn may lessen the success of breastfeeding and, if the newborn's appetite is partially satisfied by water or formula supplements, the newborn will take less from the breast, and milk production will be diminished.

Monitoring the Breastfed Newborn

During the newborn hospitalization, trained caregivers should use a standardized evaluation tool, such as the LATCH score to assess breastfeeding. The mother should be encouraged to record the time and duration of each feeding, as well as the infant's urine and stool output, during the early days of breastfeeding to facilitate assessment of her infant's milk intake.

A pediatrician or other knowledgeable and experienced health care professional should see the newborn infant at 3–5 days of age or within 48 hours of discharge. A second ambulatory visit should be scheduled when the infant is 2–3 weeks of age, unless indicated earlier, to monitor progress. The initial visit should include measurement of the infant's weight, a physical examination (especially for jaundice and hydration), questions about maternal history of breast problems (including pain or engorgement), assessment of the infant's elimination patterns (expect three to five urine eliminations and three to four stool eliminations per day by 3–5 days of age, and four to six urine eliminations and three to six stool eliminations per day by 5–7 days of age), and documentation of the transition in stools from meconium to yellow around 3–4 days after birth. A formal observation of breastfeeding, including position, latch, and milk transfer should be documented using a standardized evaluation tool.

Tracking an infant's weight provides a useful assessment of adequacy of breast milk intake. Weight loss beyond 3 days of age, weight loss of more than 7% of birth weight, or failure to regain birth weight by 10 days of age in the term infant requires a careful evaluation of the feeding techniques being used and the adequacy of breastfeeding (Table 8-1). Infants with impaired tongue mobility resulting in poor latch and maternal nipple pain should be evaluated

Table 8-1. Weight Change in Breastfed Infants

	Median (95% CI)	95th Percentile (95% CI)
Weight Loss (%)		
Breast	6.6 (6.3–6.9)	11.8 (11.2–12.9)
Formula	3.5 (3.0–3.9)	8.4 (7.8–8.9)
Mixed	5.9 (4.8–6.9)	11.5 (10.6–12.8)
Timing of Loss (d)		
Breast	2.7 (2.5–2.8)	9.1 (7.7–10.2)
Formula	2.7 (2.5–2.9)	7.1 (6.7–9.2)
Mixed	2.5 (2.2–2.8)	9.3 (6.5–12.0)
Regain Birth Weight (d)		
Breast	8.3 (7.7–8.9)	18.7 (16.7–20.8)
Formula	6.5 (6.2–7.1)	14.5 (13.8–16.7)
Mixed	7.9 (7.0–8.5)	19.0 (15.7–20.3)

Abbreviation: CI, confidence interval; d; days.

Adapted with permission from BMJ Publishing Group Limited. Macdonald PD, Ross SR, Grant L, Young D. Neonatal weight loss in breast and formula fed infants. Arch Dis Child Fetal Neonatal Ed 2003;88:F472–6.

for ankyloglossia (tongue tie). Although most infants with this condition breastfeed successfully, some may benefit from frenotomy. Some mothers may experience a delay in lactogenesis, such as that associated with retained placental fragments. If unrecognized, this failure of lactation may lead to significant dehydration in the infant, hypernatremia, and hyperbilirubinemia. First-time breastfeeding mothers are most likely to have difficulty in recognizing failure of lactation and its associated signs and consequences. Exclusive breastfeeding is the ideal nutrition and sufficient to support optimal growth and development for the healthy term infant for approximately 6 months after delivery. In families with a strong history of allergy, breastfeeding is likely to be especially beneficial. Infants weaned before the age of 12 months should not receive cow's milk feedings; instead, they should receive iron-fortified infant formula.

Contraindications to Breastfeeding

Contraindications to breastfeeding include certain maternal infectious diseases and medications. A mother with active herpes simplex virus infection may breastfeed her infant if she has no vesicular lesions in the breast area, as long as the she observes careful hand hygiene. A mother who has herpes simplex lesions on a breast should not breastfeed her infant on that breast until the lesions are cleared. Endometritis or mastitis that is being treated with antibiotics is not a contraindication to breastfeeding.

Despite the demonstrated benefits of breastfeeding, there are some situations in which breastfeeding is not in the best interest of the newborn. These include the newborn with galactosemia, who must be fed nonlactose based formula, the newborn whose mother uses illicit drugs, or the newborn whose mother is positive for human T-cell lymphotrophic virus type I or II. In the United States and other developed countries where formula is safe and readily available, women infected with HIV should not breastfeed their infants. Mothers who have received radioactive materials should not breastfeed as long as there is radioactivity in the milk, and mothers who are receiving antimetabolites or chemotherapy should not breastfeed until the medication has cleared from the milk.

Conditions That Are Not Contraindications to Breastfeeding

Certain maternal conditions have been shown to be compatible with breastfeeding, including: positive test results for hepatitis B surface antigen (HBsAg), if the infant receives both hepatitis B vaccine and hepatitis B immune globulin (breastfeeding need not be delayed while waiting for the administration of hepatitis B vaccine and hepatitis B immune globulin); positive test results for hepatitis C (either hepatitis C virus antibody or hepatitis C virus-RNA-positive blood) because there have been no reported cases of transmission via human milk; uncomplicated maternal fever or chorioamnionitis; and seropositivity (not recent conversions) for cytomegalovirus (CMV), if the infant is term. Preterm infants born to women who become seropositive for CMV during lactation can develop a sepsis–like syndrome from CMV excretion in human milk (and all maternal mucosal surfaces). Pasteurization of milk inactivates CMV, and freezing milk at -20°C (-4°F) decreases viral titers but does not eliminate CMV reliably. However, the benefits of human milk for preterm infants outweigh the risk of acquiring the CMV sepsis-like syndrome.

The effects on the newborn of medications taken by a nursing mother have been closely studied. The AAP Committee on Drugs reviewed the current data on the transfer of drugs and other chemicals into human milk. There are few drugs that are absolute contraindications to breastfeeding. Physicians are encouraged to review available data and recommendations from reputable sources before advising against breastfeeding when mothers are taking medications. (LactMed is a peer-reviewed, referenced, and frequently updated database of drugs to which breastfeeding mothers may be exposed and is available at http://toxnet.nlm.nih.gov/cgi-bin/sis/htmlgen?LACT.) The mother should discuss the use of these medications with her obstetrician and infant's health care provider if she wishes to continue breastfeeding. It must be determined whether the drug therapy is needed, whether a safer drug is available, and whether an infant's drug exposure can be minimized by having the woman take the medication after feedings. If the drug presents a risk to the infant, the infant should be carefully monitored to detect any adverse effects, and consideration should be given to measuring blood concentrations. Breastfeeding mothers may use oral contraceptives once lactation has been established but it is preferred that these be low-dose estrogen or progestin-only pills to limit the effect on milk production (see also "Postpartum Contraception" in Chapter 6).

Human Milk Storage

There are many situations in which a mother might be separated from her infant, necessitating her to express and store her milk. A mother who is in school or employed outside of the home can maintain exclusive human milk feeding by providing expressed milk to be given in her absence. Therefore, it is important to encourage and support mothers in providing their infants with expressed milk. All mothers who provide milk for their infants should be instructed in the proper techniques of milk collection to minimize bacterial contamination. Careful hand hygiene is critical before handling the breast, the equipment, or the milk. Previous practices of washing the breast and discarding the first expressed milk did not result in a decrease in colonization of the milk. Although manual expression, when performed correctly, yields relatively uncontaminated milk, many women prefer to use a breast pump. All parts of the pump that are in contact with the milk should be washed carefully with hot, soapy water, and rinsed and dried thoroughly after each use.

Mothers who are HBsAg positive may breastfeed their infants after the infants have received hepatitis B immune globulin vaccine and hepatitis B vaccine. However, they should not store milk for their infants while in the nursery because of the risk of infection to other newborns from milk that is potentially contaminated with hepatitis B virus.

The Academy of Breastfeeding Medicine recommends that fresh expressed milk be stored in sterile glass, plastic containers, or plastic bags that are free of bisphenol A and made specifically for human milk storage. According to the Academy of Breastfeeding Medicine, milk that is refrigerated (at or below 4°C [39°F]) should optimally be used within 72 hours (Table 8-2), although recommendations vary widely and use up to 96 hours appears to be safe. Frozen milk should be thawed quickly—usually by holding the container under warm running water or setting it in a container of warm water—using precautions to avoid contamination from the water, or thawed gradually in the refrigerator at or below 4°C (39°F). Human milk should not be defrosted by extremely hot

Table 8-2. Breast Milk Storage Guidelines

Location of Storage	Temperature	Maximum Recommended Storage Duration
Room Temperature	16–29°C (60–85°F)	3–4 hours optimal 6–8 hours acceptable under very clean conditions
Refrigerator	4°C (39°F) or below	72 hours optimal 5–8 days under very clean conditions
Freezer	below –17°C (0°F)	6 months optimal 12 months acceptable

Reprinted with permission from ABM clinical protocol #8: human milk storage information for home use for full-term infants (original protocol March 2004; revision #1 March 2010). Academy of Breastfeeding Medicine Protocol Committee. Breastfeed Med 2010;5:127–30.

water or in a microwave oven. The very high temperatures that may be reached with these methods can destroy valuable components of the milk and may result in thermal injury to the infant. Previously frozen milk thawed for 24 hours should not be left at room temperatures for more than a few hours because of its reduced ability to inhibit bacterial growth. Whether thawed breast milk can be safely refrozen is uncertain. When using human milk in neonatal care units, it is essential to have policies and procedures for storing the milk, appropriately identifying the milk, and checking the milk before giving it to an infant (see also "Milk and Formula Preparation Areas" in Chapter 2).

Banked Donor Milk

Banked human milk may be a suitable alternative for infants whose mothers are unable or unwilling to provide their own milk. Human milk banks in North America follow national guidelines for quality control of screening and testing of donors and pasteurize all milk before distribution. Fresh human milk from unscreened donors is not recommended because of concerns about infectious disease transmission. Women who donate milk for other newborns should be interviewed carefully regarding past and current infectious diseases, use of drugs and medications, and other factors that may impair the quality or safety of the milk that they provide. Before women are accepted as milk donors, they should be tested for HIV, HBsAg, hepatitis C, tuberculosis, syphilis, medications, and illicit drug use. Women with positive test results should not be accepted as donors. These tests should be repeated periodically for donors who continue to provide milk or who seek reinstatement as a donor. The potential risks should be explained to mothers whose newborns are to receive donated milk.

Use of Formula Milk Preparations

If a mother chooses not to breastfeed or is medically unable to breastfeed her infant, the infant may be prescribed a standard infant formula. Fresh cow's milk should not be given for the first 12 months. The health care provider caring for the infant should direct the selection of milk formula. Appropriate hospital committees and the director of the newborn nursery should review the components and reported benefits of marketed formula-milk preparations before their use. For mothers who intend to breastfeed their newborns, direct marketing and distribution of formula packages on discharge should be discouraged. For mothers who intend to feed their newborns with a milk formula, the distribution of formula marketing packages on discharge should be consistent with the written discharge orders.

Many hospitals use prepared formula units with separate nipples that allow for ready attachment to the bottles just before use. These need not be refrigerated and may be stored in a convenient, clean, cool area. The sterile cap should be kept on the nipple until the infant is ready to be fed. If there is a special area where nipples are uncapped and placed on the bottle, it should be kept very clean and should be used only for formula preparation, donor human milk, or expressed milk handling. Alternatively, nipples may be uncapped and attached to bottles at the mother's bedside just before feeding. The formula and nipple unit should be used as soon as possible, certainly within 4 hours after the bottle is uncapped, and then discarded. Particular attention is needed to maintain hygiene and safety, prevent cross-contamination of oral feeding units, and ensure correct identification of the infant.

Vitamin and Mineral Supplementation

Vitamin D

The vitamin D content of human milk is low, and rickets can occur in deeply pigmented breastfed infants or in those with inadequate exposure to sunlight. Adequate exposure to sunlight is difficult to guarantee and supplementation at the recommended dose is safe. To prevent rickets and vitamin D deficiency in healthy infants, a vitamin D intake of at least 400 international units per day has been recommended. Breastfed and partially breastfed infants should be supplemented with 400 international units per day of vitamin D beginning in the first several days after birth. Formula fed infants do not need vitamin D supplementation unless they are consistently ingesting less than 1 liter per day of vitamin D fortified formula. Fluoride supplementation for both breastfed and bottle-fed infants can begin at age 6 months.

Iron

The iron content of human milk is low; however, the bioavailability is high. Approximately 50% of the iron in breast milk is absorbed by newborns who are breastfed exclusively. Breastfed and partially breastfed infants who receive human milk as more than half their daily feedings should be given supplemental elemental iron (1 mg/kg/day) starting at 4 months of age. Formula-fed newborns should be placed on iron-containing milk formulas that contain 12 mg of elemental iron per liter. Term newborns consuming commercial milk formulas do not need vitamin and mineral supplementation for the first 6 months of life.

Preventive Care

Immunization

Hepatitis B

Each hospital should establish procedures to assess the newborn's status regarding hepatitis exposure and timely, appropriate intervention and immunization (see also "Hepatitis B Virus" in Chapter 10). Early hepatitis B immunization is recommended for all medically stable infants with birth weights greater than 2 kg, irrespective of maternal hepatitis B status. For infants born to mothers with negative hepatitis B serology, it is preferable that the initial dose is administered before discharge from the nursery.

If the mother is HBsAg positive, both hepatitis B immune globulin vaccine and hepatitis B vaccine should be administered at different sites within 12 hours of birth. Infants born to women with unknown HBsAg status should receive the hepatitis B vaccine and if the mother's HBsAg status cannot be determined within the first 12 hours after delivery, the hepatitis B immune globulin vaccine should be administered as well. The initial dose of hepatitis B vaccine given to preterm infants born to HBsAg-positive women should not be counted as part of the required three-dose hepatitis B immunization series. (For more information, see also "Hepatitis B Virus" in Chapter 10.)

Other Vaccines

Neonatal intensive care units should implement guidelines for immunization of term and preterm infants who require prolonged hospital stays. Preterm infants should begin the immunization series at the usual chronologic age of 2 months, unless otherwise indicated for a specific vaccine or disease process (see also "Immunization of Hospitalized Infants" in Chapter 9). Palivizumab should be administered for respiratory syncytial virus prophylaxis when indicated (see also "Respiratory Syncytial Virus" in Chapter 10). Maternal immunity is the only effective strategy for influenza protection in newborns because the vaccine is not approved for use in infants younger than 6 months.

Newborn Screening

Newborn screening programs are mandated, state-based public health programs that provide newborns in the United States with presymptomatic testing and necessary follow-up care for a variety of medical conditions. The goal of these essential public health programs is to decrease morbidity and mortality by screening for disorders for which early intervention will improve neonatal and long-term health outcomes for the individual. Newborn screening programs test infants for various congenital disorders, including metabolic conditions, endocrinopathies, hemoglobinopathies, cystic fibrosis, hearing loss, and, more recently, severe combined immunodeficiency and related T-cell lymphocyte deficiencies, and critical congenital heart disease. Most of the disorders screened through these programs have no clinical findings at birth.

Newborn Blood Spot Screening

Almost all states have adopted the 2010 Recommended Uniform Screening Panel suggested by the U.S. Secretary of Health and Human Services' Advisory Committee on Heritable Disorders in Newborns and Children. The list of recommended conditions for newborn screening is continually being evaluated; for an updated list, see the Secretary's Advisory Committee on Heritable Disorders in Newborns and Children web site, available at (http://www.hrsa. gov/advisorycommittees/mchbadvisory/heritabledisorders/). Although the newborn screening program in most states includes the Recommended Uniform Screening Panel, there is some variability from state to state. The selection of an individual state's screening panel is influenced by the disease prevalence within the state, detection rates, and cost considerations. The National Newborn Screening and Genetic Resource Center maintains a current list of conditions screened for in each state, available at http://genes-r-us.uthscsa.edu/resources/ consumer/statemap.htm.

Newborn blood spot screening programs are developed and managed on the state level and operate through collaborations between public health programs, laboratories, hospitals, pediatricians, subspecialists, and specialty diagnostic centers.

A comprehensive screening program includes the following components:

- Education of parents and practitioners about newborn screening and their participation in the activity

- Reliable acquisition and transportation of adequate specimens

- Reliable and prompt performance of screening tests

- Prompt retrieval and follow-up of individuals with test results that are out of range. Appropriate further testing of individuals with out-of-range test results to establish accurate diagnoses

- Appropriate intervention, treatment, and follow-up of affected individuals

- Education, genetic counseling, and psychosocial support for families with affected newborns

Every birthing facility should establish routines to ensure that all newborns are screened in accordance with state law. States test newborns primarily through blood samples collected from heel pricks that are placed on a special filter paper. Umbilical cord blood is never an appropriate specimen because it will be inaccurate for detection of disorders in which metabolite accumulation occurs after birth and after the initiation of feeding. Newborn screening blood specimens are ideally collected between 24 hours and 48 hours of age and sent to the designated state newborn screening laboratory as soon as possible. In most states if the initial specimen is obtained before the infant is 24 hours old, it is recommended that a second specimen be obtained to decrease the probability that disorders with metabolite accumulation (eg, phenylketonuria) will be missed as a consequence of early testing. Some states also mandate, or strongly recommend, that an additional newborn screening blood specimen be collected on all infants at 10–14 days of age in order to reduce the chance of missed identification of infants with clinically significant disorders because of early testing. Diagnostic testing should be performed if clinically indicated, regardless of the initial screening results. Some newborns with disorders included in the newborn screening panel will not be identified even with a properly conducted screening test because of individual or biologic variations, very early discharge, or administrative or laboratory error.

An adequate dried blood specimen must be provided to the laboratory for accurate testing. Limitations for obtaining an adequate specimen include newborns who require a transfusion or total parenteral nutrition, are sick, or are preterm. The Clinical and Laboratory Standards Institute recommends that screening of preterm and sick neonates be performed on admission to the NICU, at 48–72 hours of age, and again either at 28 days of age or discharge (whichever is sooner). For these infants, nurseries should develop protocols that comply with state regulations.

The responsibility for transmitting the screening test results to the physician or other health care providers should rest with the authority or agency that performed the test. However, primary care providers must develop policies and procedures to ensure that newborn screening is conducted, that results are transmitted to them in a timely fashion, and that the information is carefully documented in the medical record of each infant. Primary care providers also must develop strategies to employ should these systems fail.

In order to respond appropriately, primary care providers require immediate access to clinical and diagnostic information and guidance. The American College of Medical Genetics and Genomics ACT sheets and confirmatory algorithms for the various disorders included in newborn screening panels are a valuable source of such guidance. The ACT sheets describe the short-term actions a health professional should consider in communicating with the family and determining the appropriate steps in the follow-up of the infant that has screened positive for a particular disorder. The ACT sheets are available online at http://www.acmg.net/AM/Template.cfm?Section=ACT_ Sheets_and_Confirmatory_Algorithms&Template=/CM/HTMLDisplay. cfm&ContentID=5127.

Hearing Screening

The prevalence of newborn hearing loss is approximately 1–2 per 1,000 live births, with an incidence of 1 per 1,000 in the normal newborn nursery population and 20–40 per 1,000 in the newborn intensive care unit population. In accordance with the recommendations of the AAP Task Force on Improving the Effectiveness of Newborn Hearing Screening, Diagnosis, and Intervention and the Joint Committee on Infant Hearing, the hearing of all infants should be screened by 1 month of age. Every hospital with an obstetric service and children's hospitals that accept newborns transferred for care should develop and implement a universal newborn hearing screening protocol to ensure that all newborns are screened in accordance with jurisdictional guidelines. Screening should be performed with a physiologic measure, using an automated auditory brainstem response device, an otoacoustic emission device, or a combination of the two. Every effort should be made to complete screening before discharge from the hospital. Many programs use a two-step screening protocol, in which all infants have an initial screening test. If they pass the screening test, no further testing is done; if they fail the first screening test, a repeat screening test is performed before discharge. Other screening protocols include a return visit after hospital discharge for outpatient hearing screening. For infants who are admitted to the NICU for more than 5 days, a separate screening protocol that includes auditory brainstem response is recommended to identify infants with neural hearing loss.

All infants who fail the newborn hearing screening test should receive complete diagnostic testing by a qualified pediatric audiologist no later than 3 months of age, with intervention provided no later than 6 months of age from health care and education professionals with expertise in hearing loss and deafness in infants and young children. Tracking and close follow-up by the state Early Hearing Detection and Intervention programs are essential to ensure that children receive appropriate and necessary evaluation and intervention.

Regardless of previous hearing-screening outcomes, all infants with or without risk factors should receive ongoing surveillance of communicative development beginning at 2 months of age during well-child visits in the medical home and should be re-evaluated periodically throughout childhood with objective measures of hearing (see the AAP Recommendations for Preventive Pediatric Health Care [Periodicity Schedule], available at http://practice.aap.org/content.aspx?aid=1599). A number of infants may develop progressive or late-onset hearing loss, and continued surveillance is essential to identify these children in a timely manner.

Glucose Homeostasis Screening

Blood glucose concentrations as low as 30 mg/dL are common in healthy neonates by 1–2 hours after birth; these low concentrations usually are transient, asymptomatic, and considered to be part of normal adaptation to postnatal life. Clinically significant neonatal hypoglycemia reflects an imbalance between supply and use of glucose and alternative fuels and may result from a multitude of disturbed regulatory mechanisms. Current evidence does not support a specific concentration of glucose that can discriminate normal from abnormal or can potentially result in acute or chronic irreversible neurologic damage. Early identification of the at-risk infant and institution of prophylactic measures to prevent neonatal hypoglycemia are recommended as a pragmatic approach despite the absence of a consistent definition of hypoglycemia in the literature. The following section describes the screening of neonatal hypoglycemia in at-risk late preterm (born between 34 0/7 weeks and 36 6/7 weeks of gestation) and term infants. Management of neonatal hypoglycemia is discussed in Chapter 9.

Risk Factors and Clinical Signs. Routine screening and monitoring of blood glucose concentration is not needed in healthy term newborns after an entirely normal pregnancy and delivery. Blood glucose concentration should only be measured in term infants who are known to be at risk or who have clinical manifestations. Neonatal hypoglycemia occurs most commonly in infants who are small for gestational age, infants born to mothers who have diabetes, and late preterm infants; whether otherwise healthy infants who are large for gestational age are at increased risk is uncertain, although this is assumed for practical reasons because it is difficult to exclude maternal hyperglycemia or diabetes. The clinical signs of neonatal hypoglycemia are not specific and include a wide range of local or generalized manifestations that are common in sick neonates, including jitteriness, cyanosis, seizures, apneic episodes, tachypnea, weak or high-pitched cry, floppiness or lethargy, poor feeding, and eye rolling. It is important to screen for other possible underlying disorders (eg, infection) as well as hypoglycemia. Coma and seizures may occur with prolonged neonatal hypoglycemia (plasma or blood glucose concentrations lower than 10 mg/dL range) and repetitive hypoglycemia. Because avoidance and treatment of cerebral energy deficiency is the principal concern, greatest attention should be paid to neurologic signs.

When to Screen. Plasma or blood glucose concentration should be measured as soon as possible (minutes, not hours) in any infant who manifests clinical signs compatible with a low blood glucose concentration. At-risk infants should be fed by 1 hour of age and screened 30 minutes after the feeding. Glucose screening should continue until 12 hours of age for infants born to mothers with diabetes and those who are large for gestational age, and until 24 hours of age for late preterm and small for gestational age infants. At-risk asymptomatic infants should be fed every 2–3 hours and screened before each feeding. The target plasma glucose concentration is greater than or equal to 45 mg/dL before feedings. Management of infants who do not achieve target glucose levels is discussed in Chapter 9.

Screening Methods. When neonatal hypoglycemia is suspected, the plasma or blood glucose concentration must be determined immediately by using one of the laboratory enzymatic methods (eg, glucose oxidase, hexokinase, or dehydrogenase method). Although a laboratory determination is the most accurate method of measuring the glucose concentration, the results may not be available quickly enough for rapid diagnosis of neonatal hypoglycemia, which thereby delays the initiation of treatment. Bedside reagent test-strip glucose analyzers can be used if the test is performed carefully and the physician is aware of the limited accuracy of these devices. Because of limitations with rapid bedside methods, the blood or plasma glucose concentration must be confirmed by laboratory testing ordered stat. Treatment of suspected neonatal hypoglycemia should not be postponed while waiting for laboratory confirmation. (For information on management, see also "Hypoglycemia" in Chapter 9.)

Hyperbilirubinemia Screening

Jaundice occurs in most newborns. Most jaundice is benign, but because of the potential toxicity of bilirubin, newborns must be monitored to identify those who might develop severe hyperbilirubinemia and, in rare cases, acute or chronic bilirubin encephalopathy. Based on a consensus of expert opinion and review of available evidence, universal predischarge bilirubin screening is recommended and can be performed by measuring total serum bilirubin levels at the time of routine metabolic screening or measuring transcutaneous bilirubin levels and plotting the result on an hour-specific nomogram to determine the risk of subsequent hyperbilirubinemia that will require treatment.

Before discharge it is recommended that a systematic assessment for the risk of severe hyperbilirubinemia be made, a plan for treatment be developed (when indicated), and early follow-up after discharge be arranged based on the risk assessment (see also "Hyperbilirubinemia" in Chapter 9). Each nursery should develop policies and procedures for hyperbilirubinemia screening. These policies should consider the following elements:

- Promotion and support of successful breastfeeding
- Protocols for identification and evaluation of hyperbilirubinemia
- Provision for measurement of the total serum bilirubin or transcutaneous bilirubin concentration in infants who are jaundiced in the first 24 hours
- Recognition that visual estimation of the degree of jaundice can lead to errors, especially in darkly pigmented infants
- Interpretation of all bilirubin levels according to the infant's age in hours (Fig. 8-4)
- Recognition that infants born at less than 38 weeks of gestation, especially those who are breastfed, are at higher risk of developing hyperbilirubinemia and require closer surveillance and monitoring
- Performance of a systematic assessment on all infants before discharge for the risk of severe hyperbilirubinemia (Box 8-2)
- Provision of both written and verbal information to parents about newborn jaundice
- Provision of appropriate follow-up based on the time of discharge and the risk assessment
- Treatment of newborns, when indicated, with phototherapy or exchange transfusion (see also "Hyperbilirubinemia" in Chapter 9).

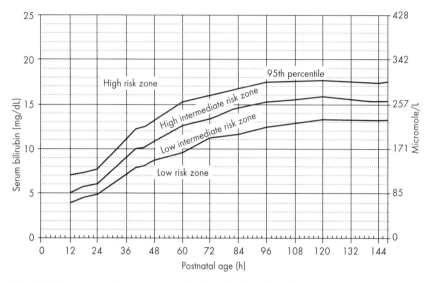

Fig. 8-4. Nomogram for designation of risk in 2,840 well newborns at 36 or more weeks of gestational age with birth weight of 2,000 g or more or 35 or more weeks of gestational age and birth weight of 2,500 g or more based on the hour-specific serum bilirubin values. Management of hyperbilirubinemia in the newborn infant 35 or more weeks of gestation. American Academy of Pediatrics Subcommittee on Hyperbilirubinemia. Pediatrics 2004; 114:297–316.

Developmental Dysplasia of the Hip Screening

Developmental dysplasia of the hip (DDH) refers to the condition in which the femoral head has an abnormal relationship to the acetabulum. Developmental dysplasia of the hip includes frank dislocation (luxation), partial dislocation (subluxation), instability wherein the femoral head comes in and out of the socket, and an array of radiographic abnormalities that reflect inadequate formation of the acetabulum. The term developmental more accurately reflects the biologic features of hip dysplasia than does the term congenital, because not every dislocated hip is detectable at birth and hips continue to dislocate throughout the first year of life.

Physicians should screen all newborns for DDH by physical examination and identification of risk factors. The two maneuvers for assessing hip stability in the newborn are the 1) Ortolani test and 2) Barlow test. The Ortolani test elicits the sensation of the dislocated hip reducing, and the Barlow test detects the unstable hip dislocating from the acetabulum. Universal newborn screening by ultrasonography is not recommended. Risk factors for DDH are female

---

Box 8-2. Major Risk Factors for Development of Severe
Hyperbilirubinemia in Infants of 35 or More Weeks of Gestation
(in Approximate Order of Importance)

- Predischarge TSB or TcB level in the high-risk zone
- Jaundice observed in the first 24 hours
- Blood group incompatibility with positive direct antiglobulin test, other known hemolytic disease (eg, G6PD deficiency), elevated ETCOc
- Gestational age 35–36 weeks
- Previous sibling received phototherapy
- Cephalohematoma or significant bruising
- Exclusive breastfeeding, particularly if nursing is not going well and weight loss is excessive
- East Asian race*

Abbreviations: ETCOc, end-tidal carbon monoxide corrected for ambient carbon monoxide; G6PD, glucose-6-phosphate dehydrogenase; TcB, transcutaneous bilirubin; TSB, total serum bilirubin.

*Race as defined by mother's description.

Modified from Management of hyperbilirubinemia in the newborn infant 35 or more weeks of gestation. American Academy of Pediatrics Subcommittee on Hyperbilirubinemia. Pediatrics 2004;114:297–316.

---

gender, breech birth, or having a positive family history. Physicians should follow a process of care that will minimize the likelihood of late diagnosis of hip dislocation. In the newborn, this includes the following:

- Examine the hips of all newborns using the Ortolani and Barlow tests.

- Determine the presence of risk factors: breech birth, positive family history, and female gender.

- If there are no risk factors and the physical examination is negative, examine the infant's hips according to the AAP periodicity schedule and follow up until the child is walking.

- If the Ortolani or Barlow test results are positive, refer the newborn to an orthopedist.

- If the Ortolani or Barlow test results are equivocal, repeat the examination in 2 weeks; depending on the findings at 2 weeks, follow up, refer to an orthopedist, or obtain ultrasonography.

- If the Ortolani or Barlow test results are negative or equivocal and risk factors are present, consider repeat examination in 2 weeks, referral to an orthopedist, or age-appropriate imaging.

Cyanotic Congenital Heart Disease Screening

In 2011, the U.S. Secretary of Health and Human Services recommended that screening with pulse oximetry for critical congenital heart disease be added to the Recommended Uniform Screening Panel. A detailed description of issues related to implementing screening has been published by AAP. The publication includes a detailed screening algorithm developed by the Secretary's Advisory Committee on Heritable Disorders in Newborns and Children and also provides detailed recommendation regarding necessary equipment, personnel and training, and appropriate management of a positive screening result (see "Bibliography" at the end of this chapter).

Infant Safety

Visiting Policies

The father or support person should be encouraged to remain with the mother throughout the intrapartum and postpartum periods. Flexible and liberal visiting policies for families are encouraged. Some institutions offer sibling classes to prepare other children in the family for the event of childbirth. Contact with the mother and newborn in the hospital helps prepare siblings for the new family member and is reassuring for younger children. The presence of siblings may be appropriate in labor, at delivery, or in the postpartum period, as local policy permits. The children must be accompanied by an adult to help them understand what is occurring and to remove them if circumstances demand.

Physical contact of siblings with infants is a topic of ongoing concern because of the possible transmission of viral infectious diseases. If siblings are allowed to have direct contact with the newborn, the visit may take place in the mother's private room or, if the mother is not in a private room, in a special sibling visitation area. Thorough hand hygiene, as practiced at the institution, should be required before physical contact with the infant. Parents should share the responsibility of preventing the exposure of their newborn to a sibling with a contagious illness by providing accurate information about illness or exposures. Contact of the newborn with children other than siblings should be avoided.

An institution that allows sibling visitation should have clearly defined, written policies and procedures that are based on currently available information. Basic guidelines for sibling visits that may serve as the basis for policy formulation are listed as follows:

- Sibling visits should be encouraged for both healthy and ill newborns.

- Before the visit, a member of the hospital staff should interview the parents to assess the current health of each sibling visitor. Children with fever or symptoms of an acute illness, such as upper respiratory infection or gastroenteritis, should not be allowed to visit. Children who have been exposed recently to a known communicable disease (eg, chickenpox) should not be allowed to visit.

- Children should be prepared in advance for their visit.

- Children should only visit their siblings.

- Children should practice hand hygiene according to the unit guidelines before patient contact.

- Throughout the visit, parents or a responsible adult should supervise sibling activity.

Because available data on the risks and benefits of sibling visitation are limited, continued evaluation and reporting are needed. Evaluation should include both psychologic and infectious-disease factors. Institutions offering controlled sibling visitation in NICUs have noted no adverse effects, although chickenpox exposures have occurred, but more study is needed before a general recommendation can be made.

Infant Security

The threat of infant abduction requires that hospitals have active programs to prevent such an event. Prevention of infant abduction is minimized by policies that include educating staff about the risk factors for abduction, educating families about safe procedures for handing over their infant, and controlling access to the postpartum area. Each institution should develop a newborn security system to protect the physical safety of newborns, families, and staff, which may include the use of electronic sensor devices. When the newborn is rooming-in, the families should be instructed to hand over their infants only to an individual with a picture identification badge, and they should question why and where their infants are being taken. Access to the labor and delivery area as well as the postpartum area should be controlled. All neonatal care units should be designed to minimize the risk of newborn abduction while maintaining a family-friendly atmosphere. Policies and procedures for visitation, transfer, and discharge of neonates should include identification and verification of the neonate and designated attendants and visitors.

Hospital Discharge and Parent Education

Discharge of Healthy Newborns

The hospital stay of a mother and her newborn should be long enough to allow identification of problems and to ensure that the mother is sufficiently recovered and prepared to care for herself and her newborn at home. Many neonatal cardiopulmonary problems related to the transition from the intrauterine to the extrauterine environment usually become apparent during the first 12 hours after birth. Other neonatal problems, such as jaundice, ductal-dependent cardiac lesions, and gastrointestinal obstruction, may require a longer period of observation by skilled and experienced personnel. Likewise, significant maternal complications, such as endometritis, may not become apparent during the first day after delivery. The length of stay, therefore, should be based on the unique characteristics of each mother–infant dyad, including the health of the mother, the health and stability of the newborn, the ability and confidence of the mother to care for herself and her newborn, the adequacy of support systems at home, and access to appropriate follow-up care. All efforts should be made to keep a mother and her newborn together to encourage on-demand breastfeeding and to ensure simultaneous discharge.

The timing of discharge from the hospital should be the decision of the health care provider caring for the mother and her newborn. This decision should be made in consultation with the family and should not be based on arbitrary policies established by third-party payers. A shortened hospital stay (less than 48 hours after delivery) for healthy, term newborns can be accomplished but is not appropriate for every mother and newborn. Institutions should develop guidelines through their professional staff in collaboration with appropriate community agencies, including third-party payers, to establish hospital-stay programs for mothers and their healthy, term newborns. State and local public health agencies also should be involved in the oversight of existing hospital-stay programs for quality assurance and monitoring.

The following minimum criteria should be met before a newborn is discharged from the hospital after an uncomplicated pregnancy, labor, and delivery.

- The infant's vital signs are documented to be normal and stable for the 12 hours before discharge, including a respiratory rate of less than 60 breaths per minute, a heart rate of 100–160 beats per minute, and an axillary temperature of 36.5–37.4°C (97.7–99.3°F) in an open crib with appropriate clothing.

- The infant has urinated and has passed at least one stool spontaneously.
- The infant has completed at least two successful feedings.
- If the infant is bottle-feeding, it is documented that the newborn is able to coordinate sucking, swallowing, and breathing while feeding.
- If the infant is breastfeeding, a caregiver knowledgeable in breastfeeding, latch, swallowing, and infant satiety should observe an actual feeding and document the observation in the medical record.
- Physical examination reveals no abnormalities that require continued hospitalization.
- There is no evidence of excessive bleeding at the circumcision site for at least 2 hours.
- The clinical significance of jaundice, if present before discharge, has been determined, and appropriate management or follow-up plans have been put in place.
- The mother's knowledge, ability, and confidence to provide adequate care for the infant are documented by the fact that training and information has been received in the following areas:
  - Appropriate urination and stooling frequency for the infant
  - Umbilical cord, skin, and newborn genital care, as well as temperature assessment and measurement with a thermometer
  - Signs of illness and common newborn problems, particularly jaundice
  - Infant safety, such as use of an appropriate car safety seat, supine positioning for sleeping, maintaining a smoke-free environment, and sleeping in proximity but not bed sharing
  - Hand hygiene, especially as a way to reduce infection
- A car safety seat appropriate for the infant's maturity and medical condition that meets Federal Motor Vehicle Safety Standard 213 has been obtained and is available at hospital discharge.
- Family members or other support persons, including health care providers who are familiar with newborn care and are knowledgeable about lactation and the recognition of jaundice and dehydration, are available to the mother and the infant after discharge.
- Instructions to follow in the event of a complication or emergency have been provided.

- Maternal and infant laboratory tests are available and have been reviewed, including the following:
  - Maternal syphilis, HBsAg, and HIV status
  - Umbilical cord or newborn blood type and direct Coombs test result, if clinically indicated.
  - Screening tests, in accordance with state requirements. If a test was performed before 24 hours of milk feeding, a system for repeating the test during the follow-up visit must be in place in accordance with local or state policy.

- Initial hepatitis B vaccine has been administered or an appointment scheduled for its administration as indicated by the infant's risk status and according to the current immunization schedule.

- Hearing screening has been completed per hospital protocol.

- Family, environmental, and social risk factors have been assessed. When these or other risk factors are present, the discharge should be delayed until they are resolved or a plan to safeguard the newborn is in place. Such factors may include, but are not limited to the following:
  - Untreated parental use of illicit substances or positive urine toxicology test results in the mother or the newborn
  - History of child abuse or neglect
  - Mental illness in a parent who is in the home
  - Lack of social support, particularly for single, first-time mothers
  - No fixed home
  - History of domestic violence, particularly during this pregnancy
  - Adolescent mother, particularly if other risk factors are present
  - Barriers to adequate follow-up, such as lack of transportation, lack of access to telephone communication, and non-English speaking parents

- A physician-directed source of continuing medical care (medical home) for both the mother and the infant has been identified. For newborns discharged before 48 hours after delivery, an appointment has been made for the infant to be examined within 48 hours of discharge. If this cannot be ensured, discharge should be deferred until a mechanism for follow-up is identified.

Discharge of Late Preterm Infants

The timing of discharge for late preterm infants is individualized and depends on the infant's competency in thermoregulation and feeding, as well as absence of medical illness and social risk factors similar to term infants. Late preterm infants are not expected to achieve these competencies before at least 48 hours of birth. In addition to meeting the aforementioned criteria outlined for term infants, late preterm infants should not be discharged until there has been

- accurate determination of gestational age.

- demonstration of 24 hours of successful feeding by breast or bottle, and the ability to coordinate sucking, swallowing, and breathing with feeding. An infant with weight loss greater than 2–3% of birth weight per day or a maximum of 7% of birthweight during the birth hospitalization should be assessed for dehydration before discharge.

- if breastfeeding, a formal evaluation with observation of position, latch, and milk transfer should be documented by a trained caregiver at least twice daily after birth.

- a follow-up visit scheduled for 24–48 hours after discharge; additional visits may be needed to ensure a pattern of appropriate weight gain.

- documentation that the infant has passed the car safety seat study to observe for apnea, bradycardia, or oxygen desaturation (see also "Safe Transportation of Late Preterm and Low Birth Weight Infants" later in this chapter and "Hospital Discharge of High-Risk Infants" in Chapter 9).

Parent Education and Psychosocial Factors

The short duration of a newborn's hospital stay compromises the opportunity for parent education. Traditional methods of individual teaching of parents by nurses cannot be accomplished within a short hospital stay. This requires that other methods of education be developed, including prenatal classes, audiovisual materials, printed materials at appropriate literacy levels, and online education programs. Audiovisual materials that have been reviewed and approved by the obstetric and pediatric staff, printed materials, and education by a variety of hospital personnel (eg, postpartum and nursery nurses, registered dietitians and nutritionists, lactation specialists, and physical and occupational therapists) can be helpful to parents. Many educational resources can be made available via the Internet. There is a parent-education site on the AAP web site (www.aap.org), and many individual hospitals have their own web sites with appropriate information. Other beneficial activities are group or individual educational sessions held regularly during the postpartum period to teach and discuss patient self-care, including exercises and self-examination of the breasts; parent–infant relationships; care of the newborn, including bathing and feeding; and child growth and development. Family-planning techniques appropriate to the patient's needs and desires also should be explained in detail (see also "Postpartum Considerations" in Chapter 6).

The educational activities should include information explaining the rapid changes in physiology that occur in the newborn. Parents should be familiar with normal and abnormal changes in wake–sleep patterns, temperature, respiration, voiding, stooling, and the appearance of the skin, including jaundice. They also should observe and become familiar with the behavior, temperament, and neurologic capabilities of the newborn. Awareness of newborn cardiopulmonary resuscitation techniques also may be helpful.

Parent education should include instruction on breastfeeding. Mothers often seek breastfeeding assistance from their health care professional, who should be able to provide advice that is correct and up-to-date. Before discharge, mothers should be provided with sources for outpatient lactation support.

During the postpartum hospital stay, health care personnel can provide the mother with professional assistance when she is most likely to be uncomfortable and can help her to anticipate how she may feel once she is home. The mother may be unsure of the normal physical changes that occur after delivery and of her ability to care for the newborn. The mother should be evaluated when she is with her newborn to identify any problems she is having so that appropriate instructions can be provided before and after discharge. Prenatal instructions given to prepare the family for the newborn's care at home also should be reinforced.

Both in-hospital and community agencies often are available to assist the family. Information on public and private groups that provide services to families with newborns, and the circumstances under which these organizations may be asked for such assistance, should be available in the hospital. Information may be obtained from the following sources:

- The in-hospital social services department, as an integral part of the interdisciplinary effort to coordinate hospital and discharge activities, to obtain public or private assistance, and to render psychosocial support

- Members of the home care service, for home visits to assess the parents' child-rearing skills, the home environment, the mother's emotional stability, and the infant's status and development (under the physician's direction, home care nurses may administer drugs or provide other types of therapy)

- Groups that lend support and provide education on special activities (eg, breastfeeding)

Safe Sleep Position and Sudden Infant Death Syndrome

In the United States, sudden infant death syndrome (SIDS) is a leading cause of mortality for infants between 1 month and 12 months of age. Several modifiable risk factors have been identified, including prone sleeping position, soft sleep surfaces, loose bedding, second-hand smoke exposure, overheating the infant, and bed sharing. Investigations on the hazards of prone sleeping and reviews of the epidemiology of SIDS with attention to sleep position have resulted in the recommendation that healthy infants not be placed in the prone position for sleeping. Supine positioning (lying wholly on the back) carries the lowest risk of SIDS and is preferred; although the side position is safer than the prone position, there remains a significantly higher risk of SIDS in the side position and it should not be used. Infants should be placed supine when resting, sleeping, or when left alone, and all caregivers, baby sitters, and child-care centers should have this emphasized to them by the parent. Parents can reduce their babies' risk of SIDS by not smoking when pregnant and not smoking in the home or around the baby after the baby is born. Hence, mothers must be educated about this during their hospital stay. Additionally, parents should be instructed to avoid excessively loose or soft bedding materials by which the infant's airway may become occluded. Overheating may be an independent risk factor or may be associated with the use of additional clothing or blankets. The use of a pacifier during sleep may be protective; however, pacifier use in breastfeeding infants should be delayed until approximately 1 month of age to ensure that breastfeeding is well established.

Bed sharing or co-sleeping is of concern because of the risk of suffocation through overlaying, as well as the risk of entrapment, wedging, falling, or strangulation on an adult bed. Proponents of bed sharing propose that breastfeeding, especially nocturnal breastfeeding, is enhanced, and some mothers will choose to co-sleep. Co-sleeping is associated with an increased risk of SIDS, although the risk is greater when the infant co-sleeps with children or other adults rather than with the mother. The Task Force on Sudden Infant Death Syndrome recommends a separate but proximate sleeping environment because the risk of SIDS has been shown to decrease when the infant sleeps in the same room as the mother.

For infants with gastroesophageal reflux disease, obstructive sleep apnea, or certain congenital malformations, the physician should recommend specific sleep positioning. Preterm infants in the newborn intensive care unit should be placed supine as determined by physician judgment as far in advance of discharge as possible.

Decreases in deaths caused by SIDS have been documented in countries where parents have changed from placing infants in prone positions to back positions for sleeping. Cardiorespiratory monitoring has not been demonstrated to decrease the incidence of SIDS, and home cardiorespiratory monitoring should not be prescribed to prevent SIDS. Serious adverse effects to the newborn because of supine positioning have not been reported. There has been an increase in the diagnosis of cranial asymmetry or positional plagiocephaly temporally related to the Back to Sleep national campaign positioning recommendation. This can be minimized by alternating the supine head position during sleep and by encouraging "tummy time" for awake playtime and when under direct observation by the caregiver. Upright "cuddle time" should be encouraged, and spending excessive time in car-seat carriers and rockers or bouncers in which pressure is applied to the occiput, should be avoided.

Safe Transportation of Late Preterm and Low Birth Weight Infants

Proper selection and use of car safety seats or car beds are important for ensuring that preterm and low birth weight infants are transported as safely as possible. The increased frequency of oxygen desaturation or episodes of apnea or bradycardia experienced by preterm and low birth weight infants positioned semireclined in car safety seats may expose them to an increased risk of cardiorespiratory events and adverse neurodevelopmental outcomes. It is suggested that preterm infants should have a period of observation of 90–120 minutes (or longer, if time for travel home will exceed this amount) in a car safety seat before hospital discharge to detect complications such as apnea, bradycardia, and oxygen desaturation. Educating parents about the proper positioning of preterm and low birth weight infants in car safety seats is important for minimizing the risk of respiratory compromise. Providing observation and avoiding extended periods in car safety seats for vulnerable infants and using car seats only for travel should also minimize risk of adverse events.

Follow-up Care

The physical and psychosocial status of the mother and her infant should be subject to ongoing assessment after discharge. The mother needs personalized care during the postpartum period to facilitate the development of a healthy mother–infant relationship and a sense of maternal confidence. Support and reassurance should be provided as the mother masters and adapts to her maternal role. Involving the other parent or other close support person and encouraging participation in the infant's care not only can provide additional support to the mother but also enhance the relationship between the newborn and the family.

The follow-up visit can take place in a home or clinic setting, as long as the personnel examining the infant are competent in newborn assessment and the results of the follow-up visit are reported to the infant's health care provider on the day of the visit. The follow-up visit should be considered an independent service to be reimbursed as a separate package and not part of a global fee for labor, delivery, and routine neonatal care. The follow-up visit is designed to fulfill the following functions:

- Weigh the infant; assess the infant's general health, hydration, and degree of jaundice; and identify any new problems
- Review feeding patterns and technique, including observation of breast-feeding for adequacy of position, latch, and swallowing, and obtain historical evidence of adequate stool and urine patterns
- Assess quality of mother–infant interaction and details of newborn behavior
- Reinforce maternal or family education in infant care, particularly regarding feeding and sleep position
- Review results of laboratory tests performed at discharge
- Perform screenings accordance with state regulations and other tests that are clinically indicated, such as serum bilirubin
- Verify the plan for health care maintenance, including a method for obtaining emergency services, preventive care and immunizations, periodic evaluations and physical examinations, and necessary screening

The postpartum period is a time of developmental adjustment for the whole family. Family members have new roles and relationships, and an effort should be made to assess the progress of the family's adaptation. If a family member finds it difficult to assume the new role, the health care team should arrange for sensitive, supportive assistance. This is particularly important for adolescent mothers, for whom it may be necessary to mobilize multiple resources within the community. The frequency of follow-up visits for the well infant varies with patient, locale, and community practices. The intervals should be consistent with the AAP's guidelines on preventive health care. Regular follow-up visits and good records of development should be maintained. Physicians and other professionals who provide follow-up care to women and infants should be aware of and look for the following physical, social, and psychological factors associated with child abuse:

- Preterm birth
- Neonatal illness with long periods of hospitalization, especially in neonatal intensive care units
- Single parenthood
- Adolescent motherhood
- Closely spaced pregnancies
- Infrequent family visits to hospitalized infants
- Substance use

Infants and parents with such a history or with other factors associated with child abuse require closer follow-up than does the average family. The interaction of the parents, especially the mother with the infant, should be evaluated periodically. The infant or child who fails to thrive may be a victim of neglect, if not outright abuse, and a causal relationship between neglect and failure to thrive should be suspected always. In every state, providers of health care to children are legally obligated to report suspected child abuse by calling statewide hotlines, local child protective services, or law enforcement agencies.

Adoption

Health care for infants who are to be adopted should focus on the needs of the child, the adoptive family, and the birth parents. These infants may have acute and long-term medical, psychological, and developmental problems because of their genetic, emotional, cultural, psychosocial, or medical backgrounds. The pediatrician should perform a careful medical assessment of the infant and should counsel the adopting family appropriately. Just as a birth family cannot be certain that its biologic child will be healthy, an adoptive family cannot be guaranteed that an adopted child will not have future health problems. Most adopted children, even those from high-risk backgrounds, are healthy. Those with certain disorders and special problems, however, also can be adopted successfully. The risks should be defined and explained carefully to the family so that problems can be anticipated and addressed expediently.

The pediatrician's role is not to judge the advisability of a proposed adoption but to apprise the prospective parents clearly and honestly of any special health needs detected at examination or anticipated in the future. Physicians evaluating a newborn for adoption should obtain as an extensive history as possible from the birth parents and enter these data into the formal medical record. There may never again be a comparable opportunity to obtain this information. If the pediatrician is unable to interview the parents personally, an adoption agency social worker who is trained to do a skilled genetic and medical interview should obtain a complete prenatal and postpartum history. The prenatal history should include information on the birth parents' lifestyle that may affect the fetus at birth or later in development. Physicians and adoption agency social workers should be trained to obtain lifestyle information in a manner that is sensitive to psychological and cultural issues. Such information includes parental use of alcohol or other drugs and history of sexual practices that increase the risk of sexually transmitted diseases in both birth parents. After reviewing whatever history is available, the pediatrician should examine the adopted child carefully and perform metabolic, genetic, and other assessments as indicated.

Physicians must be careful with semantics when dealing with the adoptive family. This is an adoptive family, not only an adopted child. The term parents applies to the parents in the adoptive family; the birth parents are those who conceived the child. Real or natural parent(s) are confusing terms that should be eliminated because they may reflect negatively on adoptive families and imply a temporary or less-than-genuine relationship between adoptive families and their children. The physician should be aware of state laws regarding adoption procedures. Hospital nurseries should have policies regarding the handling of adoptions in accordance with these laws. Policies should reflect sensitivity toward both the adoptive family as well as the birth parents. Although adoption is generally an elective decision initiated by the birth parents, the birth parents often need support adjusting to the separation from their infant.

Bibliography

ABM clinical protocol #8: human milk storage information for home use for full-term infants (original protocol March 2004; revision #1 March 2010). Academy of Breastfeeding Medicine Protocol Committee. Breastfeed Med 2010;5:127–30.

Adamkin DH. Postnatal glucose homeostasis in late-preterm and term infants. American Academy of Pediatrics Committee on Fetus and Newborn. Pediatrics 2011;127:575–9.

American Academy of Pediatrics, American Heart Association. Textbook of neonatal resuscitation. 6th. Elk Grove Village (IL): Dallas (TX): AAP; AHA; 2011.

Apnea, sudden infant death syndrome, and home monitoring. American Academy of Pediatrics Committee on Fetus and Newborn. Pediatrics 2003;111:914–7.

Ballard JL, Khoury JC, Wedig K, Wang L, Eilers–Walsman BL, Lipp R. New Ballard Score, expanded to include extremely premature infants. J Pediatr 1991;119:417–23.

Barfield WD. Standard terminology for fetal, infant, and perinatal deaths. American Academy of Pediatrics. Committee on Fetus and Newborn. Pediatrics 2011;128:177–181.

Batton DG. Clinical report—Antenatal counseling regarding resuscitation at an extremely low gestational age. American Academy of Pediatrics Committee on Fetus and Newborn. Pediatrics 2009;124:422–7.

Batton DG, Barrington KJ, Wallman C. Prevention and management of pain in the neonate: an update. American Academy of Pediatrics Committee on Fetus and Newborn; American Academy of Pediatrics Section on Surgery; Canadian Paediatric Society Fetus and Newborn Committee. Pediatrics 2006;118:2231–41.

Bell EF. Noninitiation or withdrawal of intensive care for high-risk newborns. American Academy of Pediatrics Committee on Fetus and Newborn. Pediatrics 2007;119:401–3.

Best D. Technical report—Secondhand and prenatal tobacco smoke exposure. The American Academy of Pediatrics Committee on Environmental Health; Committee on Native American Child Health; Committee on Adolescence. Pediatrics 2009;124:e1017–44.

Bhutani VK, Committee on Fetus and Newborn, American Academy of Pediatrics. Phototherapy to prevent severe neonatal hyperbilirubinemia in the newborn infant 35 or more weeks of gestation. Pediatrics 2011;128:e1046–52.

Breastfeeding and the use of human milk. American Academy of Pediatrics. Section on Breastfeeding. Pediatrics 2012;129:e827–41.

Bull M, Agran P, Laraque D, Pollack SH, Smith GA, Spivak HR, et al. Safe transportation of newborns at hospital discharge. American Academy of Pediatrics. Committee on Injury and Poison Prevention. Pediatrics 1999;104:986–7.

Bull MJ, Engle WA. Safe transportation of preterm and low birth weight infants at hospital discharge. American Academy of Pediatrics Committee on Injury, Violence, and Poison Prevention and Committee on Fetus and Newborn. Pediatrics 2009;123:1424–9.

Circumcision policy statement. American Academy of Pediatrics. Task Force on Circumcision. Pediatrics 2012;130:585–6.

Clinical practice guideline: early detection of developmental dysplasia of the hip. Committee on Quality Improvement, Subcommittee on Developmental Dysplasia of the Hip. American Academy of Pediatrics. Pediatrics 2000;105:896–905.

Cohen GJ. The prenatal visit. Committee on Psychosocial Aspects of Child and Family Health. Pediatrics 2009;124:1227–32.

Controversies concerning vitamin K and the newborn. American Academy of Pediatrics Committee on Fetus and Newborn. Pediatrics 2003;112:191–2.

Endorsement of health and human services recommendation for pulse oximetry screening for critical congenital heart disease. American Academy of Pediatrics. Section on Cardiology and Cardiac Surgery Executive Committee. Pediatrics 2012;129:190–192.

Engle WA, Tomashek KM, Wallman C. "Late-preterm" infants: a population at risk. American Academy of Pediatrics Committee on Fetus and Newborn. Pediatrics 2007;120: 1390–401.

Families and adoption: the pediatrician's role in supporting communication. American Academy of Pediatrics Committee on Early Childhood, Adoption, and Dependent Care. Pediatrics 2003;112:1437–41.

Family-centered care and the pediatrician's role. American Academy of Pediatrics Committee on Hospital Care. Pediatrics 2003;112:691–7.

Havens PL, Mofenson LM. Evaluation and management of the infant exposed to HIV-1 in the United States. American Academy of Pediatrics Committee on Pediatric AIDS. Pediatrics 2009;123:175–87.

HIV testing and prophylaxis to prevent mother-to-child transmission in the United States. American Academy of Pediatrics Committee on Pediatric AIDS. Pediatrics 2008;122: 1127–34.

Hospital stay for healthy term newborns. American Academy of Pediatrics. Committee on Fetus and Newborn. Pediatrics 2010;125:405–9.

Ip S, Chung M, Kulig J, O'Brien R, Sege R, Glicken S, et al. An evidence-based review of important issues concerning neonatal hyperbilirubinemia. American Academy of Pediatrics Subcommittee on Hyperbilirubinemia. Pediatrics 2004;114:e130–53.

Kattwinkel J, Perlman JM, Aziz K, Colby C, Fairchild K, Gallagher J, et al. Neonatal resuscitation: 2010 American Heart Association Guidelines for Cardiopulmonary Resuscitation and Emergency Cardiovascular Care. American Heart Association. Pediatrics 2010;126:e1400–13.

Kaye CI, Accurso F, La Franchi S, Lane PA, Hope N, Sonya P, et al. Newborn screening fact sheets. American Academy of Pediatrics Committee on Genetics. Pediatrics 2006; 118:e934–63.

Lee PA, Houk CP, Ahmed SF, Hughes IA. Consensus statement on management of intersex disorders. International Consensus Conference on Intersex. International Consensus Conference on Intersex organized by the Lawson Wilkins Pediatric Endocrine Society and the European Society for Paediatric Endocrinology. Pediatrics 2006; 118:e488–500.

Levels of neonatal care. Policy statement. American Academy of Pediatrics. Committee on Fetus and Newborn. Pediatrics 2012;130:587–97.

Macdonald PD, Ross SR, Grant L, Young D. Neonatal weight loss in breast and formula fed infants. Arch Dis Child Fetal Neonatal Ed 2003;88:F472–6.

Management of hyperbilirubinemia in the newborn infant 35 or more weeks of gestation. American Academy of Pediatrics Subcommittee on Hyperbilirubinemia. Pediatrics 2004;114:297–316.

Markenson D, Reynolds S. The pediatrician and disaster preparedness. American Academy of Pediatrics Committee on Pediatric Emergency Medicine, Task Force on Terrorism. Pediatrics 2006;117:e340–62.

Moon RY. SIDS and other sleep-related infant deaths: expansion of recommendations for a safe infant sleeping environment. American Academy of Pediatrics. Task Force on Sudden Infant Death Syndrome. Pediatrics 2011;128:1030–9.

Neonatal drug withdrawal. American Academy of Pediatrics Committee on Drugs, Committee on Fetus and Newborn. Pediatrics 2012;129:1–21.

Newborn screening expands: recommendations for pediatricians and medical home—implications for the system. American Academy of Pediatrics Newborn Screening Authoring Committee. Pediatrics 2008;121:192–217.

Policy statement—Tobacco use: a pediatric disease. The American Academy of Pediatrics Committee on Environmental Health; Committee on Substance Abuse; Committee on Adolescence; Committee on Native American Child. Pediatrics 2009;124:1474–87.

Principles and guidelines for early hearing detection and intervention programs. American Academy of Pediatrics, Joint Committee on Infant Hearing. Pediatrics 2007;120: 898–921.

Recommendations for preventive pediatric health care (periodicity schedule). Elk Grove Village (IL): AAP; 2008. Available at: http://practice.aap.org/content.aspx?aid=1599. Retrieved December 22, 2011.

Slutzah M, Codipilly C, Potak D, Clark RM, Schanler RJ. Refrigerator storage of expressed human milk in the neonatal intensive care unit. J Pediatr 2010; 156:26–28.

The Apgar score. ACOG Committee Opinion No. 333. American College of Obstetricians and Gynecologists. Obstet Gynecol 2006;107:1209–12.

The Apgar score. American Academy of Pediatrics, Committee on Fetus and Newborn. Pediatrics 2006;117:1444–7.

Verani JR, McGee L, Schrag SJ. Prevention of perinatal group B streptococcal disease—revised guidelines from CDC, 2010. Centers for Disease Control and Prevention. MMWR Recomm Rep 2010;59(RR-10):1–36.

Wagner CL, Greer FR. Prevention of rickets and vitamin D deficiency in infants, children, and adolescents. American Academy of Pediatrics Section on Breastfeeding; American Academy of Pediatrics Committee on Nutrition. Pediatrics 2008;122:1142–52.

Wallman C. Advanced practice in neonatal nursing. American Academy of Pediatrics Committee on Fetus and Newborn. Pediatrics 2009;123:1606–7.

Resources

American Academy of Pediatrics. Safe and healthy beginnings: a resource toolkit for hospitals and physicians offices. Elk Grove Village (IL): AAP; 2011.

Breastfeeding initiatives: health professionals resource guide. Elk Grove Village (IL): AAP; 2011. Available at: https://www2.aap.org/breastfeeding/healthProfessionals ResourceGuide.html. Retrieved December 22, 2011.

Drugs and Lactation Database (LactMed). Bethesda (MD): NIH; 2012. Available at http://toxnet.nlm.nih.gov/cgi-bin/sis/htmlgen?LACT. Retrieved January 25, 2012.

Newborn screening act sheets and confirmatory algorithms. Bethesda (MD): ACMG; 2011. Available at: http://www.acmg.net/AM/Template.cfm?Section=ACT_Sheets_and_ Confirmatory_Algorithms&Template=/CM/HTMLDisplay.cfm&ContentID=5127. Retrieved May 16, 2012.

Newborn screening: state map page. Austin (TX): NNSGRC; 2011. Available at: http://genes-r-us.uthscsa.edu/resources/consumer/statemap.htm. Retrieved December 22, 2011.

Shipman SA, Helfand M, Moyer VA, Yawn BP. Screening for developmental dysplasia of the hip: a systematic literature review for the US Preventive Services Task Force. Pediatrics 2006;117:e557–76.

Secretary's Advisory Committee on Heritable Disorders in Newborns and Children. Washington, DC: DHHS; 2011. Available at: http://www.hrsa.gov/advisorycommittees/ mchbadvisory/heritabledisorders/. Retrieved December 22, 2011.

Chapter 9

Neonatal Complications and Management of High-Risk Infants

This chapter highlights some of the common complications encountered in the care of high-risk infants and, whenever possible, provides an evidence-based approach to management.

Neonatal Complications

Anemia

Anemia of prematurity results from multiple factors and varies with the degree of immaturity, illness, postnatal age, and nutrition. Current evidence indicates that most cases of anemia that occur in the first 2–3 weeks after delivery mainly result from the volume of blood sampling obtained for clinical management. During growth, the balance of oxidative substrate (polyunsaturated free fatty acids), antioxidants (eg, vitamin E), and pro-oxidants (eg, iron) in the diet may play a role in red blood cell survival. As growth accelerates with advancing postnatal age, depletion of iron stores begins to affect erythropoiesis. Adding to these factors is the very low birth weight infant's limited capacity to increase erythropoietin production in response to anemia, which further decreases red blood cell production and increases the likelihood of dilutional anemia from an expanding blood volume.

A multipronged approach to decreasing red blood cell transfusion is recommended, particularly in very low birth weight infants, to address both causation and correction of anemia of prematurity. This approach includes limiting blood sampling when possible, extensive use of noninvasive oxygen monitoring, optimal nutritional intake, adherence to a protocol with strict indications for transfusion of packed red blood cells, and establishment of a system of blood banking that limits donor exposure. Emerging evidence suggests that delayed cord clamping in preterm infants reduces the need for blood transfusion.

Controlled clinical trials have shown that adherence to protocols with strict indications for transfusion reduces both the volume of blood transfused and donor exposure; however, an appropriate threshold for transfusion remains uncertain. Two studies have suggested that restrictive transfusion guidelines could be associated with adverse neurodevelopmental effects. However, this must be balanced with risks associated with transfusion. Recombinant human erythropoietin, whether administered early in the neonatal course or initiated after several weeks, has demonstrated little utility in reducing the number of transfusions or the volume of transfused blood in clinical trials. Thus, routine use of human recombinant erythropoietin in preterm infants is not supported by current evidence. In some circumstances, such as an infant born to parents who are Jehovah's Witnesses, the physician may choose to administer erythropoietin to derive any possible benefit.

Apnea

Apnea of prematurity can persist beyond 36 weeks postmenstrual age in very low birth weight infants, particularly in extremely preterm infants and in those with bronchopulmonary dysplasia (BPD). Neurologic immaturity of respiratory control is hypothesized to be a common underlying mechanism. Persistent apnea often is associated with inadequate oral feeding, which may be the only remaining issue to be resolved before discharge from the hospital. In the absence of objective measurements that clearly identify infants at risk of significant cardiorespiratory instability, physicians have used an empiric approach of requiring an event-free interval of some days before discharge. The precise number of days without apnea or bradycardia episodes that defines full maturation and diminished risk after discharge has not been determined. Home cardiorespiratory monitors are rarely indicated for detection of apnea solely because of immature respiratory control and should not be used to justify discharge of infants who are still at risk of apnea.

Although preterm infants have been found to have a higher incidence of sudden infant death syndrome (SIDS), no correlation between apnea of prematurity and SIDS has been established. In addition, formal analyses of breathing patterns (ie, pneumograms) are of no value in predicting SIDS and are not helpful in identifying patients who should be discharged with home monitors. Home cardiorespiratory monitoring may be useful for some infants who are technology dependent (see also "Hospital Discharge of High-Risk Infants" later in this chapter).

Brain Injury

Hemorrhagic and Periventricular White Matter Brain Injury

Infants born at 32 weeks of gestation or less or who have birth weights of 1,500 g or less are at highest risk of hemorrhagic and other brain injuries. Both the incidence and severity increase with decreasing gestational age. The vulnerability of the preterm infant arises from the vascular and cellular immaturity of the developing brain and may be compounded by inadequate cerebral autoregulation of blood flow during the frequent periods of physiologic instability characteristic of this group of newborns. Periventricular–intraventricular hemorrhage, the most frequent hemorrhagic lesion, ranges from a small germinal matrix hemorrhage to varying amounts of intraventricular blood to massive intraparenchymal hemorrhage or hemorrhagic infarction. Most periventricular–intraventricular hemorrhage occurs in the first 72 hours after birth. Posthemorrhagic hydrocephalus secondary to intraventricular hemorrhage often is apparent within 2–4 weeks after delivery, but can develop later. Periventricular leukomalacia is the most frequent white matter lesion identified. Residual lesions after brain injury include minimal to extensive cystic lesions in the periventricular white matter and ventriculomegaly secondary to diffuse cerebral atrophy. Porencephaly may develop after severe, localized ischemic or hemorrhagic infarction. These lesions evolve over the course of several weeks after the precipitating insult.

Screening and Follow-up. Portable bedside cranial ultrasonography is the most frequent imaging modality used to diagnose and monitor the evolution of brain injury. There can be great variability in interpretation. The quality of the images is affected by the choice of equipment and the expertise of the ultrasonographer in obtaining consistent positioning of the sensor. It is recommended that each center establish a protocol for screening cranial ultrasound examinations in infants who are at risk. The initial screening study can be performed between 7 and 14 postnatal days. Follow-up studies to monitor for the evolution of severity or emergence of a complication may be based on the clinical course and the initial findings. Although cranial ultrasonography is useful in diagnosing and monitoring the development of posthemorrhagic hydrocephalus, this modality is poorly predictive of neurodevelopmental sequelae. Studies of the predictive value of magnetic resonance imaging (MRI) are ongoing; however, to date there has been no recommendation for routine MRI for all preterm infants who are at risk.

Prevention. Prenatal corticosteroids given to accelerate fetal lung maturation decreases the incidence and severity of periventricular–intraventricular hemorrhage. Postnatally, only prophylactic indomethacin has been documented to decrease severe periventricular–intraventricular hemorrhage in a large randomized controlled trial; however, this decrease did not result in improved neurodevelopmental outcome at 18–21 months corrected age. No other postnatal intervention has been found to consistently prevent either periventricular–intraventricular hemorrhage or other lesions, although many approaches have been tried. Hypocapnia has been associated with cystic periventricular leukomalacia and should be avoided.

Hypoxic–Ischemic Encephalopathy

Hypoxic–ischemic encephalopathy can be a neurologically devastating or fatal condition. Previous therapeutic interventions to ameliorate hypoxic–ischemic encephalopathy have failed to provide benefit; however, randomized trials of selective head cooling and whole-body cooling have demonstrated that mild hypothermia consistently results in a significant improvement in survival without major neurodevelopmental impairment. The components of a hypothermia regimen include the criteria for inclusion, the timing of initiation, the length of cooling, the depth of hypothermia, and the type of cooling method. Thus far, infants with moderate to severe hypoxic–ischemic encephalopathy, as judged by the Sarnat criteria, and who are greater than 35 weeks of gestational age have been enrolled. Both selective head cooling and total body cooling have been successfully employed when instituted before 6 hours of postnatal age, with a target core temperature of 33–34°C (91.4–93.2°F) for 72 hours. The usefulness of amplitude-integrated electroencephalography as an entry criterion is not yet clear.

Although inducing hypothermia may seem technologically straightforward, the critically ill nature of the patient requires a full range of specialty and subspecialty support available only at a level III or level IV neonatal intensive care unit (NICU) with experience in instituting and monitoring this therapy. In addition, at this time, the unknown risks of overshooting the desired temperature and other adverse events under uncontrolled circumstances outweigh the possible benefits of instituting cooling prior to arrival at a level III or level IV NICU. A recent randomized controlled trial (RCT) demonstrated the feasibility of instituting cooling at the birth hospital with application of cold packs; importantly, however, the study design included continuous monitoring of core temperature.

Although hospitals without level III NICUs are not advised to institute therapeutic hypothermia at this time, data from the *Eunice Kennedy Shriver National Institute of Child Health and Development* whole-body hypothermia trial demonstrated that hyperthermia was clearly associated with worsened outcomes in these patients. It is not known whether hyperthermia itself causes worse outcomes or whether infants destined to have worse outcomes also have hyperthermia as a manifestation of their disease. However, it seems prudent to take steps to avoid abnormally high temperatures in infants with hypoxic–ischemic encephalopathy. Such steps may include turning off the radiant warmer if the infant's temperature is greater than 37.5°C (99.5°F) and giving a tepid bath for a persistent temperature above 38°C (100.4°F).

Ongoing and proposed trials of hypothermia may clarify issues, such as whether delayed institution of hypothermia is beneficial, whether deeper or longer hypothermia regimens can further improve outcomes, and whether amplitude-integrated electroencephalography is a useful and generalizable tool for decision making and outcome prediction. Until those results are available, practitioners should take care to institute therapeutic hypothermia only in a regimen similar to those used in published trials and only at institutions with practitioners who are trained in its use.

Hyperbilirubinemia

Although bilirubin is toxic to the central nervous system, the factors that determine its toxicity in the infant are many, complex, and incompletely understood. They include factors affecting the serum albumin concentration, the binding of bilirubin to albumin and the penetration of bilirubin into the brain, as well as comorbidities, gestational age, postnatal age, and the vulnerability of brain cells to the toxic effects of bilirubin. The relationship of specific serum bilirubin concentrations to bilirubin encephalopathy (the clinical neurologic findings caused by bilirubin toxicity to the basal ganglia and various brainstem nuclei), either in the first weeks after birth (acute bilirubin encephalopathy) or as the chronic and permanent neurologic condition (kernicterus), is not clear. In addition, it is not known whether hyperbilirubinemia can result in chronic neurologic impairment less severe than that caused by kernicterus. Because of limited evidence and individual variations, it is difficult to provide recommendations suitable to all situations. However, adherence to recommended practices is likely to reduce the risk of severe hyperbilirubinemia and associated adverse neurologic outcomes.

Term and Late Preterm Infants With Hemolytic Disease

A direct association between severe and increasing unconjugated hyperbilirubinemia, bilirubin encephalopathy, and kernicterus has been demonstrated in infants with erythroblastosis fetalis. Survivors may manifest serious sequelae, including athetoid cerebral palsy, hearing loss, paralysis of upward gaze, and dentoalveolar dysplasia. Although no specific total serum bilirubin threshold for neurotoxicity has been established, clinical observations of term infants with hemolytic disease indicate that clinical kernicterus is highly unlikely at unconjugated bilirubin concentrations of less than 20 mg/dL (342 micromoles per liter).

Term and Late Preterm Infants Without Hemolytic Disease

There are no properly designed studies, or even observational data, on term or late preterm infants without hemolytic disease on which to base clinical guidelines for the treatment of serum bilirubin concentrations of less than 20 mg/dL (342 micromoles per liter). Follow-up data for apparently healthy term infants with bilirubin concentrations as high as 25 mg/dL (428 micromoles per liter) show no apparent neurologic sequelae. However, historical data and subsequent studies have shown that a total serum bilirubin greater than 30 mg/dL (513 micromoles per liter) carries a decidedly higher risk of kernicterus. The current American Academy of Pediatrics (AAP) guidelines for phototherapy and exchange transfusion in infants born at 35 weeks of gestation or greater are based on this limited evidence (see Figure 9-1 and Figure 9-2).

Preterm Infants

Kernicterus is rare in preterm infants, and it is controversial whether modest increases of total serum bilirubin result in encephalopathy. Although some observational studies have suggested that bilirubin levels less than or equal to 5 mg/dL (86 micromoles per liter) may cause neurodevelopmental impairments, others have suggested that modest increases have no such effects. Some published guidelines for the management of jaundice in extremely preterm infants have suggested early phototherapy and exchange transfusion for bilirubin concentrations as low as 10 mg/dL (171 micromoles per liter); however, several studies have failed to confirm a relationship between serum bilirubin concentrations and later neurodevelopmental handicap at concentrations of less than 20 mg/dL (342 micromoles per liter). In a recent multicenter trial, the neurodevelopmental effects of aggressive phototherapy versus conservative phototherapy were compared in almost 2,000 extremely low birth weight infants.

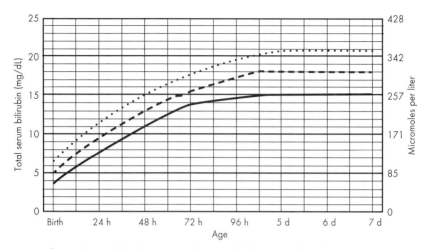

• • • Infants at lower risk (equal to or greater than 38 wk of gestation and well)
— — Infants at medium risk (equal to or greater than 38 wk of gestation with risk factors or
        35–37% wk of gestation and well)
——— Infants at higher risk (35–37% wk of gestation with risk factors)

Fig. 9-1. Guidelines for phototherapy in hospitalized infants at 35 weeks of gestation or older. These guidelines are based on limited evidence, and the levels shown are approximations. The guidelines refer to the use of intensive phototherapy, which should be used when the total serum bilirubin level exceeds the line indicated for each category. Infants are designated as "higher risk" because of the potential negative effects of the conditions listed on albumin binding of bilirubin, the blood-brain barrier, and the susceptibility of the brain cells to damage by bilirubin. Use total bilirubin. Do not subtract direct reacting or conjugated bilirubin. Risk factors are isoimmune hemolytic disease, G6PD deficiency, asphyxia, significant lethargy, temperature instability, sepsis, acidosis, or albumin less than 3 g/dL (if measured). For well infants 35-37 6/7 wk of gestation, total serum bilirubin levels can be adjusted for intervention around the medium risk line. It is an option to intervene at lower total serum bilirubin levels for infants closer to 35 wk of gestation and at higher total serum bilirubin levels for those closer to 37 6/7 wk of gestation. It is an option to provide conventional phototherapy in the hospital or at home with total serum bilirubin levels 2-3 mg/dL (35-50 micromoles per liter) below those shown, but home phototherapy should not be used in any infant with risk factors. Management of hyperbilirubinemia in the newborn infant 35 or more weeks of gestation. American Academy of Pediatrics. Subcommittee on Hyperbilirubinemia [published erratum appears in Pediatrics 2004;114:1138]. Pediatrics 2004;114:297-316.

Aggressive phototherapy was started at study entry and continued for total bilirubin values exceeding 5 mg/dL during the first week and values greater than 7 mg/dL during the second week, whereas conservative phototherapy was started at 8 mg/dL for infants with birth weights of 501–750 g and at 10 mg/dL for infants with birth weights of 751–1,000 g. Exchange transfusion was performed if intensive phototherapy failed to bring the bilirubin below 13 mg/dL for the lower weight group and 15 mg/dL for the higher weight group. In this

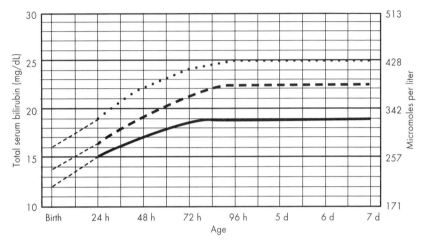

• • • Infants at lower risk (equal to or greater than 38 wk of gestation and well)
━ ━ Infants at medium risk (equal to or greater than 38 wk of gestation with risk factors or
       35–37% wk of gestation and well)
━━━ Infants at higher risk (35–37% wk of gestation with risk factors)

Fig. 9-2. Guidelines for exchange transfusion in infants at 35 weeks of gestation or older. These suggested levels represent a consensus of most of the committee but are based on limited evidence, and the levels shown are approximations. During birth hospitalization, exchange transfusion is recommended if the total serum bilirubin level increases to these levels despite intensive phototherapy. For readmitted infants, if the total serum bilirubin level is above the exchange level, repeat total serum bilirubin measurement every 2–3 hours and consider exchange if the total serum bilirubin level remains above the levels indicated after intensive phototherapy for 6 hours. The dashed lines for the first 24 hours indicate uncertainty because of a wide range of clinical circumstances and a range of responses to phototherapy. Immediate exchange transfusion is recommended if the infant shows signs of acute bilirubin encephalopathy (hypertonia, arching, retrocollis, opisthotonos, fever, or high pitched cry) or if the total serum bilirubin level is equal to or greater than 5 mg/dL (85 micromoles per liter) above these lines. Risk factors are isoimmune hemolytic disease, G6PD deficiency, asphyxia, significant lethargy, temperature instability, sepsis, and acidosis. Measure serum albumin level and calculate bilirubin/albumin ratio. Use total bilirubin. Do not subtract direct reacting or conjugated bilirubin. If the infant is well and at 35-37 6/7 wk of gestation (medium risk), total serum bilirubin levels for exchange can be individualized based on actual gestational age. Management of hyperbilirubinemia in the newborn infant 35 or more weeks of gestation. American Academy of Pediatrics. Subcommittee on Hyperbilirubinemia [published erratum appears in Pediatrics 2004;114:1138]. Pediatrics 2004;114:297-316.

study, aggressive phototherapy did not significantly reduce the rate of death or neurodevelopmental impairment at 18–22 months of corrected age (52% versus 55%). Aggressive phototherapy did significantly reduce neurodevelopmental impairment in survivors (26% versus 30%), but this reduction was offset by an increase in mortality in infants weighing 501–750 g at birth (39% versus 34%). Thus, best practice for instituting phototherapy in the extremely LBW infant remains uncertain.

Breastfeeding and Jaundice

Some evidence indicates that frequent breastfeeding (8–12 times per 24 hours) may reduce the incidence of hyperbilirubinemia in infants. Supplementing nursing with water or dextrose-water is not necessary and will not decrease serum bilirubin concentrations in healthy, breastfeeding infants. Breastfeeding significantly affects the level and duration of unconjugated hyperbilirubinemia compared with formula feeding, primarily in two ways:

1. Inadequate fluid intake—This condition most often occurs in the setting of a primiparous or first-time breastfeeding mother with a late preterm infant. Early hospital discharge is an additional risk factor. Inadequate milk production can result in weight loss of as much as 30% of birth weight over the initial 7–14 days of life, marked hyperbilirubinemia, and, rarely, kernicterus or death. It is likely that caloric deprivation and its effect on the enterohepatic circulation of bilirubin is more responsible for this result than dehydration itself. Proper education and support of the mother, together with early and close follow-up after hospital discharge to evaluate the feeding process and the health of the infant, are essential to prevent adverse outcomes. With such support, successful breastfeeding usually is achievable. If failure of milk production persists, infants should be evaluated, rehydrated as needed, and changed to infant formula.

2. Breast milk jaundice—This condition is characterized by a persistence of physiologic jaundice beyond the first week of age. Breastfed infants commonly have serum bilirubin concentrations greater than 5 mg/dL (85.5 micromoles per liter) for several weeks after delivery. This persistent, mild unconjugated hyperbilirubinemia is caused by a factor in human milk, which is yet unidentified, that promotes an increase in intestinal absorption of bilirubin. Infants with jaundice that persists beyond the first week of life should be monitored to ensure that it is unconjugated hyperbilirubinemia, that the concentration of bilirubin is not increasing, and that other pathologic causes for jaundice are not present.

If the serum unconjugated bilirubin level in a breastfed, term, healthy infant is increasing and is higher than 20 mg/dL (171 micromoles per liter), the physician has several options:

- Breastfeeding may be continued and the infant may be treated with phototherapy while the infant and mother undergo thorough evaluation and assistance with the feeding process.
- Breastfeeding may continue while the infant is supplemented with infant formula and treated with phototherapy.
- Infant formula may be substituted for breast milk for 24–48 hours. This can be combined with phototherapy and will almost always result in a rapid decrease in serum bilirubin concentrations. The mother should be strongly encouraged to maintain lactation and should be provided a breast pump during the period of interrupted nursing.

Dehydration and Hyperbilirubinemia

Some infants who are admitted to the hospital with high bilirubin concentrations also may be dehydrated and may need supplemental enteral formula or pumped breast milk, or intravenous fluid, or both. Enteral supplementation with dextrose-water is not indicated. Sick very low birth weight infants receiving phototherapy may have increased evaporative water loss and require increased intravenous fluid intake, or environmental humidity, or both to compensate for ongoing losses. Routine increases in fluid intake are probably not warranted; however, the state of hydration should be carefully monitored.

Clinical Assessment

Physicians should ensure that all infants are routinely monitored for the development of jaundice, and nurseries should have established protocols for the assessment of jaundice (see also "Hyperbilirubinemia Screening" in Chapter 8). In most infants with total serum bilirubin levels of less than 15 mg/dL (257 micromoles per liter), noninvasive transcutaneous bilirubin measurement devices can provide a valid estimate of the total serum bilirubin level.

Laboratory Evaluation

A noninvasive transcutaneous bilirubin measurement, or total serum bilirubin measurement, or both should be performed on every infant who is jaundiced in the first 24 hours after birth. The need for and timing of a repeat noninvasive transcutaneous bilirubin measurement or total serum bilirubin measurement will depend on the age of the infant and the evolution of the hyperbilirubinemia. A noninvasive transcutaneous bilirubin measurement, or total serum bilirubin measurement, or both should be performed if the jaundice appears excessive for the infant's age. If there is any doubt about the degree of jaundice, the noninvasive transcutaneous bilirubin or total serum bilirubin should be measured. Visual estimation of bilirubin levels from the degree of jaundice can lead to errors, particularly in darkly pigmented infants. All bilirubin levels and the need for treatment should be interpreted according to the infant's age in hours (see Fig. 8-4).

Risk Assessment

Universal predischarge bilirubin screening using total serum bilirubin or transcutaneous bilirubin measurements is recommended to assess the risk of subsequent severe hyperbilirubinemia. In addition, a structured approach to management and follow-up is recommended according to the predischarge total serum bilirubin or transcutaneous bilirubin measurements, gestational age, and other risk factors for hyperbilirubinemia. In addition to predischarge total serum bilirubin or transcutaneous bilirubin measurements in the high risk or high intermediate risk zone, the important risk factors most frequently associated with severe hyperbilirubinemia are exclusive breastfeeding, gestational age less than 38 weeks, jaundice in the first 24 hours of age, isoimmune or other hemolytic disease (eg, G6PD deficiency), previous sibling with jaundice, cephalohematoma or other significant bruising, or East Asian race. Appropriate follow-up after discharge is essential.

Follow-up

All hospitals should provide written and verbal information for parents at the time of discharge, which should include an explanation of jaundice, the need to monitor infants for jaundice, and advice on how monitoring should be done. (An example of a parent-information handout is available in English and Spanish at http://www.healthychildren.org/English/news/pages/Jaundice-in-Newborns.aspx.) All infants should be examined by a qualified health care professional in the first few days after discharge to assess the infant's well-being and the presence or absence of jaundice. The timing and location of this assessment will be determined by the length of stay in the nursery, risk zone assessed on the appropriate nomogram by plotting the predischarge noninvasive transcutaneous bilirubin level or total serum bilirubin level according to the baby's age in hours (see Fig. 8-4), presence or absence of risk factors for hyperbilirubinemia, and risk of other neonatal problems.

The follow-up assessment should include the infant's weight and percent change from birth weight, adequacy of intake, the pattern of voiding and stooling, and the presence or absence of jaundice. Clinical judgment that incorporates an assessment of the risk of hyperbilirubinemia needing treatment (predischarge risk zone and clinical risk factors) should be used to determine the need for a bilirubin measurement. Jaundice that persists beyond 2 weeks requires further investigation, including measurement of total and direct serum bilirubin concentrations. An increase of the direct serum bilirubin concentration always requires further investigation.

Treatment

There are two commonly used treatment options for neonatal hyperbilirubinemia. These options are phototherapy and exchange transfusion.

Phototherapy. There is no standardized method for delivering phototherapy. However, detailed recommendations regarding the use of phototherapy can be found in the AAP hyperbilirubinemia clinical practice guideline and the technical report on phototherapy (see "Bibliography" at the end of this chapter). Commonly used phototherapy units contain daylight, cool white, blue, or special blue fluorescent tubes. Other units use tungsten-halogen lamps in different configurations, either freestanding or as part of a radiant-warming device. Fiber optic systems have been developed that deliver high-intensity light via a fiber optic blanket.

The efficacy of phototherapy is influenced by the energy output (irradiance) in the blue spectrum (measured in microwatts per centimeter squared), the spectrum of light source, and the surface area of the infant exposed to the light source. The irradiance of a unit should be monitored and bulbs changed as needed to maintain maximum energy output. It is acceptable to interrupt phototherapy during feeding or brief parental visits. Intensive phototherapy can be achieved by using blue lights, decreasing the distance of the source from the infant, and increasing the surface area exposed to the lights. The infant's temperature should be monitored frequently while phototherapy is being applied.

Although phototherapy has many biologic effects, it has no known lasting toxic effects in the human infant. Because experiments in animals have documented retinal damage from phototherapy, the infant's eyes should be covered with opaque patches during exposure to phototherapy light. Complications from improper monitoring of eye-patch placement include exposure to high-energy light, obstruction of the nares, lid opening and resultant corneal abrasion, and conjunctivitis from use without intermittent removal to assess the condition of the covered tissues.

Some infants with uncomplicated nonhemolytic jaundice may be treated with phototherapy at home. With proper instruction of the parents or guardians, home phototherapy using a freestanding device or a fiber optic blanket can be provided. Guidelines should be developed by each institution to define criteria for infants who are eligible for home phototherapy. Home care requires appropriate follow-up and supervision by a health care professional who is capable of obtaining blood samples for the measurement of serum bilirubin when clinically indicated. If serum bilirubin concentrations do not decrease in response to home phototherapy, admission to the hospital may be indicated for more intensive phototherapy or and for further investigation for an underlying cause (Fig. 9-1 and Fig. 9-2).

Exchange Transfusion. Guidelines for exchange transfusion in infants 35 weeks of gestation or older are shown in Figure 9-2. The figure legend provides guidance for the clinical approach for the management of such infants.

Hypoglycemia

Neonatal hypoglycemia occurs most commonly in infants who are small for gestational age, infants born to mothers who have diabetes, and late preterm infants (see also "Glucose Homeostasis Screening" in Chapter 8). Routine screening and monitoring of blood glucose concentration is not needed in healthy term newborns after an entirely normal pregnancy and delivery. Blood glucose concentration should only be measured in term infants who are known to be at risk or who have clinical manifestations.

The definition of a plasma glucose concentration at which intervention is indicated needs to be tailored to the clinical situation and the particular characteristics of a given infant. Because severe, prolonged, symptomatic hypoglycemia may result in neuronal injury, prompt intervention is necessary for infants who manifest clinical signs and symptoms. A reasonable (although arbitrary) cutoff for treating symptomatic infants is 40 mg/dL. A plasma sample for a laboratory glucose determination needs to be obtained just before giving an intravenous minibolus of glucose (200 mg of glucose per kg, 2 mL/kg dextrose 10% in water [$D_{10}W$], intravenously), or starting a continuous infusion of glucose ($D_{10}W$ at 80–100 mL/kg per day), or both. A reasonable goal is to maintain plasma glucose concentrations in symptomatic infants between 40 mg/dL and 50 mg/dL.

Figure 9-3 is a guideline for the screening and management of neonatal hypoglycemia in asymptomatic late preterm infants and term infants who are born to mothers with diabetes, small for gestational age, or large for gestational age. The figure is divided into two time periods (birth to 4 hours and 4–12 hours) and accounts for the changing values of glucose that occur over the first 12 hours after birth. The recommended values for intervention are intended to provide a margin of safety over concentrations of glucose associated with clinical signs. The recommendations also provide a range of values over which the physician can decide to re-feed or provide intravenous glucose. The target glucose concentration is greater than 45 mg/dL before each feeding. At-risk infants should be fed by 1 hour of age and screened 30 minutes after the feeding. Gavage feeding may be considered in infants who are not suckling well. Glucose screening should continue until 12 hours of age for infants born to mothers with diabetes and those who are large for gestational age.

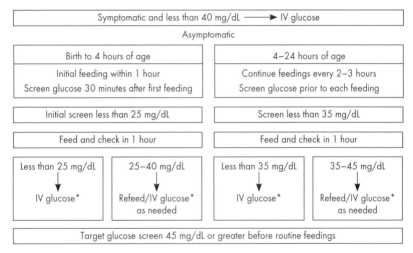

Fig. 9-3. Screening and management of postnatal glucose homeostasis in late-preterm (34-36 6/7 weeks of gestation) infants, small-for-gestational age infants, infants who were born to mothers with diabetes, and large-for-gestational age infants. Screen late-preterm and small-for-gestational age infants every 0-24 hours and infants born to mothers with diabetes and large-for-gestational age infants who are 34 or more weeks of gestation, every 0 -12 hours. Abbreviation: IV, intravenous. *Glucose dose is 200 mg/kg (D$_{10}$W at 2 mL/kg) and/or IV infusion at 5-8 mg/kg per min (80-100 mL/kg per d). Achieve plasma glucose level of 40-50 mg/dL. Adamkin DH. Postnatal glucose homeostasis in late-preterm and term infants. American Academy of Pediatrics Committee on Fetus and Newborn. Pediatrics 2011;127:575-9.

Late-preterm infants and infants who are small for gestational age require glucose monitoring for at least 24 hours after birth, especially if regular feedings are not yet established. It is recommended that the at-risk asymptomatic infant who has glucose concentrations of less than 25 mg/dL (birth to 4 hours of age) or less than 35 mg/dL (4–24 hours of age) be re-fed and that the glucose value be rechecked 1 hour after refeeding. Subsequent concentrations lower than 25 mg/dL, or lower than 35 mg/dL, respectively, after attempts to re-feed, necessitate treatment with a minibolus of 2 mL/kg $D_{10}W$ (200 mg/kg), or intravenous infusion of $D_{10}W$ at 5–8 mg/kg per minute, 80–100 mL/kg per day, or both; the goal is to achieve a plasma glucose concentration of 40–50 mg/dL (higher concentrations will only stimulate further insulin secretion). If it is not possible to maintain blood glucose concentrations of greater than 45 mg/dL after 24 hours of using this rate of glucose infusion, consideration should be given to the possibility of hyperinsulinemic hypoglycemia. A blood sample should be sent for measurement of insulin along with a glucose concentration at the time when a bedside blood glucose concentration is less than 40 mg/dL, and an endocrinologist should be consulted.

Neonatal Drug Withdrawal

Maternal use of certain drugs during pregnancy can result in transient neonatal signs consistent with withdrawal or acute toxicity, or may cause sustained signs consistent with a lasting drug effect. In addition, hospitalized infants who are treated with opioids or benzodiazepines to provide analgesia or sedation may be at risk of manifesting signs of withdrawal. Signs characteristic of neonatal withdrawal have been attributed to intrauterine exposure to a variety of drugs (Table 9-1). Other drugs cause signs in infants because of acute toxicity. Chronic in utero exposure to a drug (eg, alcohol) can lead to permanent phenotypical, or neurodevelopmental behavioral abnormalities, or both consistent with drug effect. Signs and symptoms of withdrawal worsen as drug levels decrease, whereas signs and symptoms of acute toxicity abate with drug elimination. Clinically important neonatal withdrawal most commonly results from intrauterine opioid exposure. The constellation of clinical findings associated with opioid withdrawal has been termed neonatal narcotic abstinence syndrome. Withdrawal signs will develop in 55–94% of infants exposed to opioids in utero. Neonatal withdrawal signs also have been described in infants exposed antenatally to benzodiazepines, barbiturates, and alcohol.

Because fetal drug exposure often is unrecognized in the immediate newborn period, affected infants may be discharged to homes where they are at

Table 9-1. Maternal Nonnarcotic Drugs That Cause Neonatal Psychomotor Behavior Consistent With Withdrawal

Drug	Signs	Onset of Signs
Alcohol[1,2]	Hyperactivity, crying, irritability, poor suck, tremors, seizures; poor sleeping pattern, hyperphagia, diaphoresis; onset of signs at birth	3–12 hours
Barbiturates[3,4]	Irritability, severe tremors, hyperacusis, excessive crying, vasomotor instability, diarrhea, restlessness, increased tone, hyperphagia, vomiting, disturbed sleep; onset first 24 hours of life or as late as 10–14 days of age	1–14 days
Caffeine[5]	Jitteriness, vomiting, bradycardia, tachypnea	At birth
Chlordiazepoxide[6]	Irritability, tremors; signs may start at 21 days	Days–weeks
Clomipramine[7]	Hypothermia, cyanosis, tremors; onset 12 hours of age	
Diazepam[8]	Hypotonia, poor suck, hypothermia, apnea, hypertonia, hyperreflexia, tremors, vomiting, hyperactivity, tachypnea (mother receiving multiple drug therapy)	Hours–weeks
Ethchlorvynol[9]	Lethargy, jitteriness, hyperphagia, irritability, poor suck, hypotonia (mother receiving multiple drug therapy)	
Glutethimide[10]	Increased tone, tremors, opisthotonos, high-pitched cry, hyperactivity, irritability, colic	
Hydroxyzine[11]	Tremors, irritability, hyperactivity, jitteriness, shrill cry, myoclonic jerks, hypotonia, increased respiratory and heart rates, feeding problems, clonic movements (mother receiving multiple drug therapy)	
Meprobamate[12]	Irritability, tremors, poor sleep patterns, abdominal pain	
SSRIs[13–16]	Crying, irritability, tremors, poor suck, feeding difficulty, hypertonia, tachypnea, sleep disturbance, hypoglycemia, seizures	Hours–days

Abbreviation: SSRIs, selective serotonin reuptake inhibitors.

1. Pierog S, Chandavasu O, Wexler I. Withdrawal symptoms in infants with the fetal alcohol syndrome. J Pediatr. 1977;90(4):630–3.

2. Nichols MM. Acute alcohol withdrawal syndrome in a newborn. Am J Dis Child. 1967;113(6):714–5.

3. Bleyer WA, Marshall RE. Barbiturate withdrawal syndrome in a passively addicted infant. JAMA. 1972;221(2):185–6.

4. Desmond MM, Schwanecke RP, Wilson GS, Yasunaga S, Burgdorff I. Maternal barbiturate utilization and neonatal withdrawal symptomatology. J Pediatr. 1972;80(2):190–7.

(continued)

Table 9-1. Maternal Nonnarcotic Drugs That Cause Neonatal Psychomotor Behavior Consistent With Withdrawal *(continued)*

5. McGowan JD, Altman RE, Kanto WP Jr. Neonatal withdrawal symptoms after chronic maternal ingestion of caffeine.South Med J. 1988;81(9):1092-4.

6. Athinarayanan P, Pierog SH, Nigam SK, Glass L. Chloriazepoxide withdrawal in the neonate. Am J Obstet Gynecol. 1976;124(2):212-3.

7. Musa AB, Smith CS. Neonatal effects of maternal clomipramine therapy. Arch Dis Child. 1979;54(5): 405.

8. Rementería JL, Bhatt K. Withdrawal symptoms in neonates from intrauterine exposure to diazepam. J Pediatr. 1977;90(1):123-6.

9. Rumack BH, Walravens PA. Neonatal withdrawal following maternal ingestion of ethchlorvynol (Placidyl). Pediatrics. 1973;52(5):714-6.

10. Reveri M, Pyati SP, Pildes RS. Neonatal withdrawal symptoms associated with glutethimide (Doriden) addiction in the mother during pregnancy. Clin Pediatr (Phila). 1977;16(5):424-5.

11. van Baar AL, Fleury P, Soepatmi S, Ultee CA, Wesselman PJ. Neonatal behavior after drug dependent pregnancy. Arch Dis Child. 1989;64(2):235-40.

12. Desmond MM, Rudolph AJ, Hill RM, Claghorn JL, Dreesen PR, Burgdorff I. Behavioral alterations in infants born to mothers on psychoactive medication during pregnancy. In: Farrell G, ed. Congenital Mental Retardation. Austin, TX: University of Texas Press; 1969:235-44.

13. Dahl ML, Olhager E, Ahlner J. Paroxetine withdrawal syndrome in a neonate. Br J Psychiatry. 1997; 171:391-2.

14. Sanz EJ, De-las-Cuevas C, Kiuru A, Bate A, Edwards R. Selective serotonin reuptake inhibitors in pregnant women and neonatal withdrawal syndrome: a database analysis. Lancet. 2005;365(9458): 482-7.

15. Chambers CD, Johnson KA, Dick LM, Felix RJ, Jones KL. Birth outcomes in pregnant women taking fluoxetine. N Engl J Med.1996;335(14):1010-5.

16. Haddad PM, Pal BR, Clarke P, Wieck A, Sridhiran S. Neonatal symptoms following maternal paroxetine treatment: serotonin toxicity or paroxetine discontinuation syndrome? J Psychopharmacol. 2005;19 (5):554-7.

Modified from Neonatal drug withdrawal. American Academy of Pediatrics Committee on Drugs, Committee on Fetus and Newborn. Pediatrics 2012;129:e540-60.

increased risk of a variety of medical and social problems, including abuse and neglect. Women who use illicit substances are at risk of human immunodeficiency virus (HIV), acquired immunodeficiency syndrome (AIDS), herpes, hepatitis, and syphilis, each of which can have significant adverse effects on the fetus and newborn. In addition, these women may have received little or no prenatal care, further increasing risks for the infant.

The specific effect of drug exposure on the fetus and newborn varies widely with the substance ingested, the amount received, and individual susceptibility. Illicit drugs that have been reported to have adverse effects on nursing infants include cocaine, methamphetamine, heroin, marijuana, and phencyclidine. (Note that methadone is not a contraindication to breastfeeding and is included in the AAP "approved" category for breastfeeding women.)

Breastfeeding women should be counseled about the adverse effects of substance use. However, breastfeeding should be encouraged for most substance-using women, as long as it poses no risk to the infant.

Screening

Before the onset of withdrawal signs, the presence of maternal or infant characteristics known to be associated with drug use in pregnancy can be considered indications to screen for intrauterine drug exposure, by using meconium or urine samples. Maternal characteristics that suggest a need for screening include no prenatal care, previous unexplained fetal demise, precipitous labor, abruptio placentae, hypertensive episodes, severe mood swings, cerebrovascular accidents, myocardial infarction, and repeated spontaneous abortions. Infant characteristics that may be associated with maternal drug use include prematurity; unexplained intrauterine growth restriction; neurobehavioral abnormalities; urogenital anomalies; and atypical vascular incidents, such as cerebrovascular accidents, myocardial infarction, and necrotizing enterocolitis in otherwise healthy full-term infants. The legal implications of testing and the need for consent from the mother may vary among the states; therefore, pediatricians should be aware of local laws and legislative changes that may influence regional practice.

The duration of urinary excretion of most drugs is relatively short, and maternal or neonatal urinary screening only addresses drug exposure in the hours immediately before urine collection. Thus, false-negative urine test results may occur in the presence of significant intrauterine drug exposure. Meconium analysis provides a more accurate indication of exposure over a longer gestational period than does urine analysis. Although newborn meconium screening also may yield false-negative test results, the likelihood is lower than with urinary screening. Additional assessment of infants of drug-abusing mothers includes screening for hepatitis B, hepatitis C, HIV, and other sexually transmitted infections.

Treatment

Drug withdrawal should be considered as a diagnosis in infants in whom compatible signs develop. Physicians and nursery staff should be trained to recognize signs of neonatal withdrawal (Box 9-1). Physicians should also be aware of other potential diagnoses that should be evaluated and treated, if confirmed. Drug withdrawal should be scored using an appropriate scoring tool, such as the modified Neonatal Abstinence Scoring System (Fig. 9-4). Consistent scoring of

---

Box 9-1. Clinical Features of Neonatal Narcotic Abstinence Syndrome

Neurologic Excitability
- Tremors
- Irritability
- Increased wakefulness
- High-pitched crying
- Increased muscle tone
- Hyperactive deep tendon reflexes
- Exaggerated Moro reflex
- Seizures
- Frequent yawning and sneezing

Gastrointestinal Dysfunction
- Poor feeding
- Uncoordinated and constant sucking
- Vomiting
- Diarrhea
- Dehydration
- Poor weight gain

Autonomic Signs
- Increased sweating
- Nasal stuffiness
- Fever
- Mottling
- Temperature instability

Neonatal drug withdrawal. American Academy of Pediatrics Committee on Drugs, Committee on Fetus and Newborn. Pediatrics 2012;129:e540–60.

---

signs of withdrawal enables decisions about the institution of pharmacologic therapy to be more objective and allows a quantitative approach to increasing or decreasing dosing. Each nursery should have a written policy for implementation of a standard scoring system for neonatal withdrawal and appropriate treatment of the withdrawing infant.

System	Signs and Symptoms	Score	AM			
Central nervous system disturbnces	Excessive high pitched (or other) cry	2				
	Continuous high pitched (or other) cry	3				
	Sleeps less than 1 hour after feeding	3				
	Sleeps less than 2 hours after feeding	2				
	Sleeps less than 3 hours after feeding	1				
	Hyperactive moro reflex	2				
	Markedly hyperactive moro reflex	3				
	Mild tremors disturbed	1				
	Moderate-severe tremors disturbed	2				
	Mild tremors undisturbed	3				
	Moderate-severe tremors undisturbed	4				
	Increased muscle tone	2				
	Excoriation (specific area)	1				
	Myoclonic jerks	3				
	Generalized convulsions	5				
Metabolic/vasomotor/respiratory disturbances	Sweating	1				
	Fever 100.4°-101°F (38°-38.3°C)	1				
	Fever more than 101°F (38.3°C)	2				
	Frequent yawning (more than 3-4 times/interval)	1				
	Mottling	1				
	Nasal stuffiness	1				
	Sneezing (more than 3-4 times/interval)	1				
	Nasal flaring	2				
	Respiratory rate more than 60/min	1				
	Respiratory rate more than 60/min with retractions	2				
Gastrointestinal disturbances	Excessive sucking	1				
	Poor feeding	2				
	Regurgitation	2				
	Projectile vomiting	3				
	Loose stools	2				
	Watery stools	3				
	Total score					
	Initials of scorer					

Fig. 9-4. Modified Finnegan's Neonatal Abstinence Scoring Tool. Adapted from Finnegan LP. Neonatal abstinence. In: Nelson NM, ed. Current Therapy in Neonatal-Perinatal Medicine. 2nd ed. Toronto,Ontario: BC Decker Inc; 1990. Neonatal drug withdrawal. American Academy of Pediatrics Committee on Drugs, Committee on Fetus and Newborn. Pediatrics 2012;129:e540-60.

		PM					Comments
							Daily Weight

Infants with confirmed drug exposure who have no signs or minimal signs of withdrawal do not require pharmacologic therapy. Initial treatment of the infants experiencing drug withdrawal should be primarily supportive, because pharmacologic therapy may prolong hospitalization and subject the infant to exposure to drugs that may not be indicated. Supportive care includes swaddling to decrease sensory stimulation; frequent small feedings of hypercaloric (24 cal/oz) formula to supply the additional caloric requirements; and observation of sleeping habits, temperature stability, weight gain or weight loss, or change in clinical status that might suggest another disease process.

Withdrawal-associated seizures should be treated with pharmacologic therapy. Other causes of neonatal seizures also must be evaluated. Vomiting, diarrhea, or both, associated with dehydration and poor weight gain, in the absence of other diagnoses, are relative indications for treatment, even in the absence of high total withdrawal scores. Drug selection should match the type of agent causing withdrawal. Physicians should be aware that the severity of withdrawal signs, including seizures, has not been proven to be associated with differences in long-term outcome after intrauterine drug exposure. Furthermore, treatment of drug withdrawal may not alter the long-term outcome.

Discharge and Follow-up Care

Documentation of in utero illicit substance exposure and alcohol use by the mother should preclude early discharge after birth. Appropriate planning for discharge and subsequent follow-up care requires social work assessment and may include referral for child protective services if there is a concern about the future well-being of the infant.

Long-term effects on learning and school performance, behavioral problems, and emotional instability of infants exposed to illicit drugs, alcohol, and tobacco in utero remain major concerns. Drug exposure during development may have long-lasting effects on behavioral and cognitive outcomes. These effects also may result from environmental factors that place drug-exposed infants at high risk of physical, sexual, and emotional abuse, neglect, and developmental delay. Multidisciplinary long-term follow-up should include medical, developmental, and social support. In general, a coordinated multidisciplinary approach without criminal sanctions has the best chance of helping infants and families.

Management of Acquired Opioid and Benzodiazepine Dependency

One of the cornerstones in caring for critically ill infants is to provide adequate and safe analgesia, sedation, amnesia, and anxiolysis using both pharmacologic and nonpharmacologic measures. Pharmacologic treatment typically includes medications in the opioid and benzodiazepine drug classes. If these drugs cannot safely be discontinued within a few days, physical dependence on one or both of these classes of medication can develop, and infants often manifest signs and symptoms of withdrawal upon acute dosage reduction or cessation of therapy. Infants who undergo complex surgery, who require prolonged medical intensive care for conditions such as respiratory failure or persistent pulmonary hypertension, or who are supported with extracorporeal membrane oxygenation (ECMO) therapy are among those at greatest risk of acquired drug dependency. Infants cared for in intensive care units who have developed tolerance to opioids and benzodiazepines due to an extended duration of treatment can be converted to an equivalent regimen of oral methadone and lorazepam. Doses may be increased as necessary to achieve patient comfort. These medications can then be reduced by 10–20% every 1–2 days based on the clinical response and the serial assessments using a standardized abstinence instrument.

Respiratory Complications

Oxygen Therapy

The hazards associated with administration of supplemental oxygen to preterm infants have been recognized for many years. Studies conducted in the 1950s indicated that prolonged unmonitored oxygen therapy was associated with increased rates of retinopathy of prematurity (ROP), formerly called retrolental fibroplasia. This discovery led to widespread restriction of oxygen therapy, which caused a marked decrease in ROP but an increase in cerebral palsy and mortality. Current practice recommends supplemental oxygen as needed, based on objective monitoring of oxygenation. Clinical assessment of physical signs to determine the amount of supplemental oxygen needed may be useful for short periods, emergencies, or abrupt clinical changes, but should not be the basis for ongoing supplemental oxygen therapy.

Supplemental oxygen can be delivered via endotracheal tube, mask, oxygen hood, nasal prongs, or cannula. Except in emergency situations, supplemental oxygen should be warmed and humidified, and the concentration or flow should be monitored and regulated. Orders for oxygen therapy should include desired ambient concentration, flow, or both. The concentration or flow rate of oxygen should be checked routinely. Orders should be written to adjust fraction of inspired oxygen (FIO_2) or flow within a stated range to maintain oxygen saturation within specific limits. There should be an institutional guideline for ordering, delivering, and documenting oxygen therapy and monitoring. Oxygen analyzers should be calibrated in accordance with manufacturers' recommendations.

An important development in the care of infants who require oxygen therapy is the ability to monitor oxygenation continuously with noninvasive techniques. The pulse oximeter measures the percentage of hemoglobin saturated with oxygen. Throughout most of the oxygen-hemoglobin dissociation curve, pulse oximetry will closely predict PaO_2 when adjustments are made for the presence of fetal hemoglobin, and it is an excellent continuous monitor of oxygenation; however, at saturations greater than 96%, the PaO_2 may be extremely high. The transcutaneous oxygen analyzer provides an indirect measurement of PaO_2. This device has the potential advantage of monitoring for high PaO_2; however, the heated membrane may cause burns, and the membrane may not read accurately because of poor perfusion or skin thickness, and it has been largely replaced by oximetry.

Continuous measurement of pulse oximetry combined with periodic measurement of PaO_2 in samples from an umbilical or peripheral artery catheter is the most complete method of monitoring oxygen therapy. In infants whose condition is unstable, noninvasive measurements should be correlated with PaO_2 as often as every 8–24 hours. More frequent analyses of arterial blood gas may be indicated for the assessment of pH and $PaCO_2$. In infants whose condition is stable, correlation with arterial blood gas samples may be performed when clinically indicated.

In the absence of an indwelling arterial catheter, arterialized capillary sampling provides reasonable estimates of arterial pH and $PaCO_2$ if perfusion to the extremity is not compromised. Although PaO_2 is not accurately estimated in arterialized capillary samples, the combined use of continuous oxygen saturation monitoring and intermittent capillary arterialized blood gases can guide oxygen therapy. In this circumstance, oxygen saturation should not be allowed to remain above 95%, as previously described, particularly in preterm infants at risk of ROP.

The use of either pulse oximetry or transcutaneous oxygen measurement may shorten the time required to determine optimum inspired oxygen concentration and ventilator settings in the acute care setting. Both measurements are also useful in monitoring oxygen therapy in infants who are recovering from respiratory distress or who require long-term supplemental oxygen. Pulse oximetry is particularly advantageous for long-term monitoring of oxygen therapy because transcutaneous oxygen measurements underestimate oxygenation in older infants with BPD and may cause burns.

In consideration of the current, but incomplete, understanding of the effects of oxygen administration, the following recommendations are offered:

- Supplemental oxygen should be used for specific indications, such as cyanosis, low PaO_2, or low oxygen saturation.

- For infants who require oxygen therapy for acute care, measurements of blood pH and $PaCO_2$ should accompany measurements of PaO_2. In addition, a record of blood gas measurements, noninvasive measurements of oxygenation, details of the oxygen delivery system (eg, ventilator, continuous positive airway pressure, nasal cannula, hood, mask, settings), and ambient oxygen concentrations (FIO_2, liter of flow per minute, or both) should be maintained.

- The optimal range for oxygen saturation and PaO_2 that balances tissue metabolism, growth and development, and toxicity has not been elucidated for preterm infants receiving supplemental oxygen. Data from cohort studies initially suggested that lower saturation ranges may decrease ROP. However, three RCTs demonstrated that although a target saturation range of 85–89% was associated with a decrease in severe ROP, it also was associated with an increase in mortality, compared with a target saturation range of 91–95%. These findings resulted in early study closure of two of these three studies, and a recommendation to target a saturation range higher than 85–89%. Of note, even with careful monitoring, oxygen saturation and PaO_2 often fluctuate outside specified ranges, particularly in infants with cardiopulmonary disease.

- Regular and periodic (every 1–4 hours) measurement and recording of the concentration of oxygen delivered to the infant receiving supplemental oxygen is recommended.

- Except for an emergency situation, air–oxygen mixtures should be warmed and humidified before being administered to infants.

Respiratory Distress Syndrome

Respiratory distress syndrome (RDS) is associated with surfactant deficiency and typically occurs in preterm infants, but may occasionally be seen in term infants, particularly in the setting of maternal diabetes. Multiple randomized controlled trials have demonstrated the benefits of surfactant replacement therapy, including reduction in the severity of RDS, decrease in pulmonary complications (eg, air leak), and improvement in survival. Surfactant therapy does not change the incidence of BPD in infants born at less than 30 weeks of gestation, but does reduce the incidence of BPD in infants born at or beyond 30 weeks of gestation. Surfactant therapy has no effect on coexisting morbidities, such as necrotizing enterocolitis, nosocomial infection, patent ductus arteriosus, and intraventricular hemorrhage. Long-term outcome of treated infants has shown possible improvement in pulmonary function studies, but has not shown beneficial or adverse effects on growth and neurodevelopment.

Antenatal corticosteroid administration stimulates structural and functional maturation of the fetal lung and, like postnatal surfactant replacement, improves survival and reduces the incidence of RDS. Antenatal corticosteroids and postnatal surfactant replacement have additive effects. Therefore, both antenatal steroid administration to women at risk of preterm delivery and postnatal surfactant administration to infants at high risk of RDS are important treatments to optimize outcomes for preterm infants.

Surfactant replacement has proved clearly efficacious for infants with respiratory distress associated with primary surfactant deficiency and should be administered to these infants as soon as possible after intubation. Preterm infants born at less than 30 weeks of gestation are at high risk of primary surfactant deficiency. Prophylactic surfactant given soon after birth may reduce mortality and morbidity in such infants, particularly for those without exposure to antenatal steroids; however, RCTs that compared early continuous positive airway pressure administration and early surfactant therapy have shown similar rates of death or BPD. Thus, early continuous positive airway pressure appears to be a reasonable alternative to prophylactic surfactant therapy. Rescue surfactant also may be efficacious in, and should be considered for, infants with hypoxic respiratory failure attributable to secondary surfactant deficiency (eg, meconium aspiration, sepsis or pneumonia, pulmonary hemorrhage).

Surfactant replacement with either animal-derived (natural) or synthetic surfactant preparations has shown efficacy for respiratory distress due to surfactant deficiency. Animal-derived products from bovine and porcine sources are similar in efficacy, and have not been associated with long-term immunologic or infectious complications. First-generation synthetic surfactant preparations are less effective than animal-derived surfactants, in part because of their inability to mimic the spreading and recycling functions of surfactant-associated proteins. Second-generation synthetic surfactant preparations contain recombinant surfactant proteins or peptides that mimic the function of surfactant-associated proteins. Clinical studies comparing animal-derived and second-generation synthetic surfactants are progressing.

Infants receiving surfactant replacement therapy often have associated multisystem organ dysfunction that requires specialized care. Caring for these infants in nurseries that do not have the full range of required capabilities may affect overall outcome adversely. Therefore, infants with respiratory failure requiring surfactant therapy should be managed in NICUs that have the expertise to provide comprehensive care for sick newborns.

In view of the documented efficacy of surfactant replacement therapy, the following recommendations should be incorporated into neonatal care systems:

• Surfactant should be administered by physicians with the technical and clinical expertise to respond to rapid changes in lung volume and lung compliance and complications of surfactant instillation into the airway.

• Surfactant therapy should be provided by experienced personnel who are capable of managing multisystem disorders in sick newborns.

• Surfactant replacement therapy should be directed by physicians who are trained in the respiratory management of sick newborns and have knowledge and experience in mechanical ventilation.

• Nursing and respiratory therapy personnel who are experienced in the management of sick newborns, including the use of mechanical ventilation, should be available when surfactant therapy is administered.

• The equipment necessary for managing and monitoring the condition of sick newborns, including that needed for mechanical ventilation, should be available when surfactant therapy is administered.

• The radiology and laboratory support necessary to manage a broad range of needs of sick newborns should be immediately available in facilities where surfactant therapy is prescribed.

• At institutions that do not meet these requirements, when timely transfer of a high-risk newborn to an appropriate institution cannot be achieved, surfactant therapy may be given by physicians who are skilled in endotracheal intubation and surfactant administration. Newborns who have received surfactant should be transferred from such institutions as soon as feasible to a center with appropriate facilities and trained staff to care for multisystem morbidity in sick newborns.

Hypoxic Cardiorespiratory Failure

Hypoxic cardiorespiratory failure in term or late preterm infants may result from diverse conditions, such as primary persistent pulmonary hypertension, RDS, aspiration of meconium, pneumonia, sepsis, or congenital diaphragmatic hernia. Hypoxemia, hypercarbia, and acidosis generally are reversible with conventional therapies, such as administration of oxygen, mechanical ventilation, and supportive care. Additionally, inotropic agents, intravascular volume expansion, and antibiotics may be indicated.

Term and late preterm infants who fail to respond to conventional interventions may benefit from rescue therapies targeting specific physiologic abnormalities that may accompany hypoxic respiratory failure, such as surfactant replacement for primary or secondary surfactant deficiency or inhaled nitric oxide for pulmonary hypertension. In small, randomized trials involving infants with meconium aspiration syndrome, persistent pulmonary hypertension, and sepsis, surfactant replacement reduced mortality and the need for ECMO without an increase in morbidity. Randomized clinical trials have demonstrated that inhaled nitric oxide, a selective pulmonary vasodilator, improves oxygenation and reduces the need for ECMO in term and late preterm infants. Response to inhaled nitric oxide is optimized when the lungs are adequately recruited; if conventional mechanical ventilation is not successful in this regard, high frequency ventilation may be useful.

It is essential that newborns with hypoxic cardiorespiratory failure receive care in institutions that have appropriately skilled personnel—including physicians, nurses, and respiratory therapists who are qualified to use multiple modes of ventilation—and readily accessible radiologic and laboratory support. Newborns who are not responding to conventional therapies should be transferred in a timely manner to the appropriate level NICU capable of providing rescue therapies, such as inhaled nitric oxide or ECMO.

Nitric Oxide. The use of inhaled nitric oxide in preterm infants with acute hypoxic respiratory failure appears to be of little clinical benefit in the large randomized controlled trials thus far reported. Until new trials report significant beneficial results, preterm infants should receive inhaled nitric oxide for acute hypoxic respiratory failure only within the context of clinical research protocols. Individual preterm infants with documented pulmonary hypertension may respond to inhaled nitric oxide.

Extracorporeal Membrane Oxygenation. Extracorporeal membrane oxygenation refers to prolonged (days to weeks) cardiopulmonary bypass for infants with hypoxic respiratory or cardiac failure who are unresponsive to less invasive therapies. Lung rest during ECMO allows pulmonary and cardiac recovery with reduced risk of secondary injury from exposure to high oxygen and ventilator support. Extracorporeal membrane oxygenation is highly invasive and accompanied by risks associated with systemic anticoagulation, mechanical complications, and the cannulation procedures.

Criteria for initiating or transferring for ECMO are complex because numerous factors, including gestational age, weight, diagnosis, severity of cardio-respiratory failure, clinical course, presence of complications, postnatal age, proximity of an ECMO center, risk of transport, and parental preferences all must be considered. In general, however, a late preterm or term infant with respiratory failure who is deteriorating and has an oxygenation index greater than 25 on conventional mechanical ventilation (oxygenation index=[mean airway pressure/PaO_2]×FIO_2×100) has a moderately high risk of requiring ECMO. Consultation and possible transfer to an ECMO center is advised when the oxygenation index reaches 25. Newborns with oxygenation index calculations greater than 35–45 on conventional mechanical ventilation are at high risk of death without ECMO. Contraindications to ECMO may include gestational age less than 34–35 weeks, birth weight less than 2,000 g, profound hypoxic–ischemic encephalopathy, large intracranial hemorrhage, congenital anomalies associated with grave prognosis, or irreversible pulmonary or cardiac disorder.

Improved survival without an increase in morbidity has been demonstrated in clinical trials for infants receiving ECMO. Medical complications may include BPD, feeding problems, gastroesophageal reflux, and slow growth. Significant neurologic abnormality, developmental delay, or neurocognitive disability occurred in approximately 15% of ECMO survivors evaluated at 5 years of age. Complications, such as seizures; hearing loss; visual disturbances; learning disability; and social, attention, and behavioral problems are seen in many neonatal patients with complex medical courses, including those treated with inhaled nitric oxide and ECMO. Because of the risk of these adverse outcomes and the emergence of subtle disabilities during the school age and adolescent years, it is recommended that infants who have been critically ill, especially those who survive with the use of rescue therapies, such as ECMO, be monitored by developmental specialists throughout childhood.

Bronchopulmonary Dysplasia/Chronic Lung Disease

Bronchopulmonary dysplasia, or chronic lung disease, complicates the recovery of many preterm infants with RDS and infants of any gestational age with severe pulmonary insufficiency or hypoplasia. Classic BPD is characterized pathologically by alveolar and airway destruction, inflammation, and fibrosis, which results in emphysema, atelectasis, bronchial and bronchiolar mucosal hyperplasia and metaplasia, interstitial fibrosis, narrowed airways, excess mucus accumulation, interstitial edema, lymphatic dilation, pulmonary vascular smooth muscle hypertrophy, and reduction in capillary bed size. With advances in care, such as antenatal corticosteroids and postnatal surfactant, many extremely preterm infants have mild initial lung disease but still develop BPD. This new BPD is characterized by alveolar and capillary simplification, and likely results from a complex interaction of antenatal and postnatal factors superimposed on an arrest of lung development due to extremely preterm birth. Infants with severe BPD may develop pulmonary hypertension or cor pulmonale, or may die from acute bronchospasm or infection.

Bronchopulmonary dysplasia has been variably defined as the need for oxygen at 28 days postnatal age or at 36 weeks of postmenstrual age, with or without clinical and radiographic abnormalities. Because oxygen often is administered according to inconsistent, subjective criteria, it is a challenge to compare outcomes across NICUs. To reduce variability in reporting, improve comparability among different NICUs, and develop research priorities, specific diagnostic definitions were created at a consensus workshop sponsored by the National Heart, Lung, and Blood Institute (Table 9-2). In conjunction with this set of definitions, a physiologic definition of BPD also has been introduced; that is, the diagnosis of BPD can be established if infants require supplemental oxygen to maintain an oxygen saturation level at or above 90%. Infants receiving supplemental oxygen of 0.30 FIO_2 or less at 36 weeks of postmenstrual age, and are not on positive pressure ventilation, should have an oxygen reduction test performed to determine whether supplemental oxygen is necessary to maintain the saturation level at or above 90%. Infants who are receiving positive pressure ventilation, continuous positive airway pressure, or oxygen supplementation greater that 0.30 FIO_2 at 36 weeks of postmenstrual age (or 56 days postnatal age for infants born at or beyond 32 weeks of gestation) are considered to have BPD without verification by an oxygen reduction test.

Therapeutic Approaches. Multiple pharmacologic interventions and respiratory support strategies have been proposed to decrease development of BPD in sick infants, but few are supported by controlled clinical trials of appropriate size and design:

- Antenatal administration of corticosteroids decreases the incidence of RDS and, thereby, decreases the population at risk.
- Surfactant replacement has decreased the incidence of BPD in infants born at or beyond 30 weeks of gestation but not in infants born at less than 30 weeks of gestation.

Table 9-2. Definition of Bronchopulmonary Dysplasia

Assessment	Gestational Age	
	Less Than 32 wk	**32 wk or Older**
Time point of assessment	36 wk PMA or discharge to home, whichever comes first Treatment with oxygen greater than 21% for at least 28 d plus:	28 d but less than 56 d postnatal age or discharge to home, whichever comes first Treatment with oxygen more than 21% for at least 28 d plus:
Mild BPD	• Breathing room air at 36 wk PMA or discharge, whichever comes first	• Breathing room air by 56 d postnatal age or discharge, whichever comes first
Moderate BPD	• Need for less than 30% oxygen at 36 wk PMA or discharge, whichever comes first	• Need for less than 30% oxygen at 56 d postnatal age or discharge, whichever comes first
Severe BPD	• Need for 30% or greater oxygen or positive pressure (PPV or NCPAP), or both, at 36 wk PMA or discharge, whichever comes first	• Need for 30% or greater oxygen or positive pressure (PPV or NCPAP), or both, at 56 d postnatal age or discharge, whichever comes first

Abbreviations: BPD, bronchopulmonary dysplasia; NCPAP, nasal continuous positive airway pressure; PMA, postmenstrual age; PPV, positive-pressure ventilation.
Jobe AH, Bancalari E. Bronchopulmonary dysplasia. Am J Respir Crit Care Med 2001;163:1723–9.

- Caffeine supplementation started within the first 10 days of life has been associated with a significantly decreased incidence of BPD and improved neurodevelopmental outcomes at 18–21 months of corrected age in babies weighing 500–1,250 g at birth.

- Vitamin A supplementation has been shown to significantly decrease the risk of BPD in mechanically ventilated, extremely low birth weight infants.

- Postnatal corticosteroids:

  — Postnatal dexamethasone given in the first week of life to very low birth weight infants facilitates extubation and decreases BPD; however, its benefits are outweighed by numerous documented adverse effects, particularly possible compromise of neurodevelopment. Therefore, the routine use of systemic dexamethasone for the prevention and treatment of chronic lung disease in very low birth weight infants is not recommended.

  — After the first week of life, dexamethasone may be beneficial, but also carries risks. Given the limitations of current evidence, dexamethasone should be reserved for infants who cannot be weaned from mechanical ventilation, and the dose and duration of treatment should be minimized. Parents should be fully informed about the known short-term risks and long-term risks and consent to treatment.

— Hydrocortisone given in the first postnatal week may result in a decrease in BPD, but the evidence is not clear, and this therapy cannot be recommended at this time. To date, there are no randomized controlled trials of its use in infants after the first week of life.

— Inhaled corticosteroids have not been shown to decrease BPD.

• Early use of inhaled nitric oxide appears to be of little clinical benefit; however, one large randomized trial of nitric oxide treatment initiated between 7–21 days and continued for 24 days was reported to increase survival without BPD and without adverse effects on growth or neurodevelopment at 2 years of age.

• Assisted ventilation strategies that avoid hyperinflation are desirable, but strong supportive evidence for most specific, individual ventilation strategies are lacking; however, a meta-analysis of five studies, including 413 infants, suggested that volume-targeted ventilation may reduce BPD compared with pressure-limited ventilation.

• Continuous positive airway pressure beginning in the delivery room has not been proven to reduce the incidence of BPD.

• Permissive hypercapnia (ie, accepting higher $PaCO_2$ levels than previously was customary) has been suggested, but controlled studies in neonates have not demonstrated a reduction in risk of BPD.

• High-frequency ventilation using various modalities and strategies has not been found to be consistently efficacious.

• The use of synchronized ventilation and short inspiratory times seems reasonable but the effects on BPD have not been demonstrated in large randomized trials.

Other modalities directed at specific antecedents of inflammatory injury have included antioxidants (vitamin E and superoxide dismutase) and erythromycin (prophylaxis or treatment for *Ureaplasma* colonization). None of these can be recommended at this time either because of safety issues (erythromycin) or unconfirmed efficacy (vitamin E supplementation beyond that required to prevent vitamin E deficiency is not beneficial); superoxide dismutase and other antioxidant medications have not been studied adequately. High volumes of fluid intake in the first week are associated with persistence of a patent ductus arteriosus and the development of BPD. Diuretics may acutely improve pulmonary function and decrease oxygen requirement, but their effectiveness in decreasing BPD is unsubstantiated in clinical trials.

Treatment. Treatment of developing or established BPD is primarily pragmatic, and includes oxygen supplementation, careful attention to optimize nutrition and growth, and appropriate immunizations. The optimal oxygen saturation range is unknown, but oxygen supplementation has been shown to improve growth and decrease the likelihood of progression to pulmonary hypertension. Growth failure is well recognized to accompany severe BPD, and energy expenditure has been shown to be significantly higher in these infants. In addition, inadequate nutrition impairs lung healing. Therefore, although not supported by controlled trials, provision of calories, minerals, and protein to sustain a growth rate comparable with non-BPD gestational age peers seems a logical approach. Immunoprophylaxis for respiratory syncytial virus and influenza has reduced the posthospitalization morbidity of infants with BPD. Infants born to mothers who have received the influenza vaccine during pregnancy have been shown to have less influenza disease during their first months of life. Infants should receive all immunizations in accordance with AAP recommendations (see also "Immunization" in Chapter 8).

Retinopathy of Prematurity

A myriad of factors, including but not limited to hyperoxia, may contribute to the pathogenesis of ROP. Prematurity; low birth weight; multiple gestation; severity of illness; prolonged ventilatory support (especially when accompanied by episodes of hypoxia and hypercapnia); and clinical conditions, including acidosis, shock, sepsis, apnea, anemia, chronic lung disease, intraventricular hemorrhage, patent ductus arteriosus, and vitamin E deficiency also have been associated with retinopathy of prematurity.

To date, a safe level of PaO_2 in relation to retinopathy of prematurity has not been established, perhaps because multiple other factors, such as those listed previously play a part in its pathogenesis. Retinopathy of prematurity has occurred in preterm infants who have never received supplemental oxygen therapy and in infants with cyanotic congenital heart disease in whom PaO_2 levels never exceeded 50 mm Hg. Conversely, ROP has not developed in some preterm infants after prolonged periods of hyperoxemia. Data have demonstrated no additional progression of active prethreshold retinopathy of prematurity when supplemental oxygen was administered at pulse oximetry saturations between 96% and 99%. Further, continuous, close monitoring of transcutaneous oxygen tension has not resulted in a decrease in the incidence of ROP when compared with intermittent transcutaneous monitoring. On the basis of published data, the following statements regarding ROP and oxygen use are warranted:

- Retinopathy of prematurity is not preventable in some infants, especially extremely premature infants.
- Many factors other than hyperoxia contribute to the pathogenesis of retinopathy of prematurity.
- Transient hyperoxemia alone cannot be considered sufficient to cause retinopathy of prematurity.
- Strict adherence to existing guidelines for supplemental oxygen therapy will not completely prevent complications or adverse effects.

Screening and Initial Examination

An ophthalmologist with sufficient knowledge and experience in retinopathy of prematurity and the use of binocular indirect ophthalmoscopy should examine the retinas of all preterm infants born at 30 weeks of gestation or less or weighing less than 1,500 g at birth, as well as selected infants weighing 1,500–2,000 g at birth with an unstable clinical course and who are thought to be at risk by their attending pediatrician or neonatologist. Sterile instruments should be used to examine each infant in order to avoid possible cross contamination of infectious agents. Pretreatment of the eyes with a topical anesthetic agent, such as proparacaine may minimize the discomfort and systemic effect of this examination. Consideration also may be given to the use of nonpharmacologic pain management interventions, such as pacifiers and oral sucrose.

Table 9-3 presents a suggested schedule for timing of initial eye examinations based on postmenstrual age and chronologic (postnatal) age. This schedule was designed to detect retinopathy of prematurity before it progresses to retinal detachment and to allow for earlier intervention, while minimizing the number of potentially traumatic examinations. The timing of follow-up examinations is best determined from the findings of the first examination, using the International Classification of Retinopathy of Prematurity (see also "Treatment and Follow-up Care" later in this section). One examination is sufficient only if it unequivocally shows the retina to be fully vascularized in each eye.

Table 9-3. Timing of First Eye Examination Based on Gestational Age at Birth*

Gestational Age at Birth (wk)	Age at Initial Examination (wk)	
	Postmenstrual	Chronologic
22[†]	31	9
23[†]	31	8
24	31	7
25	31	6
26	31	5
27	31	4
28	32	4
29	33	4
30	34	4
31[‡]	35	4
32[‡]	36	4

*Shown is a schedule for detecting prethreshold retinopathy of prematurity with 99% confidence, usually well before any required treatment.

[†]This guideline should be considered tentative rather than evidence-based for infants with a gestational age of 22–23 weeks because of the small number of survivors in these gestational-age categories.

[‡]If necessary

Screening examination of premature infants for retinopathy of prematurity. Section on Ophthalmology, American Academy of Pediatrics; American Academy of Ophthalmology; American Association for Pediatric Ophthalmology and Strabismus. Pediatrics 2006;117:572–6.

Digital photographic retinal image capture with remote interpretation is a developing approach to ROP screening. However, outcome trial data comparing large-scale operational photoscreening systems with remote interpretation to binocular indirect ophthalmoscopy have not been published. Off-site photo interpretation requires close collaboration among neonatologists, imaging staff, and ophthalmologists. Specific responsibilities of each individual must be carefully delineated in a written protocol in advance so that repeat imaging, confirmatory examinations, and required treatments can be performed without delay.

Treatment and Follow-up Care

If intervention is considered necessary, it generally should be performed within 72 hours of the diagnosis, if possible, to minimize the risk of retinal detachment. The retinal findings requiring strong consideration of ablative treatment are as follows:

- Zone I retinopathy of prematurity: any stage with plus disease
- Zone I retinopathy of prematurity: stage 3, no plus disease
- Zone II: stage 2 or 3 with plus disease

Published data indicate that intravitreal bevacizumab monotherapy, as compared with conventional laser therapy, in infants with stage 3+ retinopathy of prematurity showed a significant benefit for zone I disease but not zone II disease. However, the number of infants treated was small and there remain unanswered questions involving dosage, timing, safety, visual outcomes, and other long-term effects.

If hospital discharge or transfer to another neonatal unit or hospital is contemplated before retinal maturation into zone III has taken place or if the infant has been treated by ablation for ROP and is not yet fully healed, the availability of an appropriate follow-up ophthalmologic examination by an experienced ophthalmologist must be ensured, and specific arrangement for that examination must be made before such discharge or transfer occurs. Responsibility for examination and follow-up of infants at risk of ROP must be carefully defined by each NICU. Unit-specific criteria for screening and follow-up examinations should be established by consultation and agreement between neonatology and ophthalmology services. These criteria should be recorded and should automatically trigger ophthalmologic examinations.

Management of High-Risk Infants

Nutritional Needs of Preterm Infants

Optimal nutrition is critical in the management of preterm infants. There is no standard for the precise nutritional needs of preterm infants comparable with the human milk standard for term infants. Present recommendations are designed to provide nutrients to approximate the rate of growth and composition of weight gain for a normal fetus of the same postmenstrual age and to maintain normal concentrations of blood and tissue nutrients. Acute illness and organ system immaturity can make provision of optimal nutrition challenging, particularly for the sickest and most immature infants, yet inadequate nutrition during this period may have life-long consequences.

Parenteral Nutrition

Parenteral administration of amino acids, glucose, and fat is an important aspect of the nutritional care of preterm infants, particularly those who weigh

Table 9-4. Comparison of Parenteral Intake Recommendations for Growing Preterm Infants in Stable Clinical Condition

Element	Consensus Recommendations		Consensus Recommendations	
	Less than 1,000 g/kg per day	Less than 1,000 g/ 100 kcal	1,000– 1,500 g/kg per day	1,000– 1,500 g/ 100 kcal
Water/fluids, mL	140–180	122–171	120–160	120–178
Energy, kcal	105–115	100	90–100	100
Protein, g	3.5–4.0	3.0–3.8	3.2–3.8	3.2–4.2
Carbohydrate, g	13–17	11.3–16.2	9.7–15	9.7–16.7
Fat, g	3–4	2.6–3.8	3–4	3.0–4.4
Linoleic acid, mg	340–800	296–762	340–800	
Linoleate: linolenate (C18:2–C18:3)	5–15	5–15	5–15	5–15
Vitamin A, IU	700–1500	609–1,429	700–1,500	700–1,667
Vitamin D, IU	40–160		40–160	
Vitamin E, IU	2.8–3.5	2.4–3.3	2.8–3.5	2.8–3.9
Vitamin K_1 µg	10	8.7–9.5	10	10.0–11.1
Ascorbate, mg	15–25	13.0–23.8	15–25	15.0–27.8
Thiamine, µg	200–350	174–333	200–350	200–389
Riboflavin, µg	150–200	130–190	150–200	150–222
Pyridoxine, µg	150–200	130–190	150–200	150–222
Niacin, mg	4–6.8	3.5–6.5	4–6.8	4.0–7.6
Pantothenate, mg	1–2	0.9–1.9	1.2	1.0–2.2
Biotin, µg	5–8	1.3–7.6	5–8	5.0–8.9
Folate, µg	56	49–53	56	56–62
Vitamin B_{12}, µg	0.3	0.26–0.29	0.3	0.30–0.33
Sodium, mg	69–115	60–110	69–115	69–128
Potassium, mg	78–117	68–111	78–117	78–130
Chloride, mg	107–249	93–237	107–249	107–277
Calcium, mg	60–80	52–76	60–80	60–89
Phosphorus, mg	45–60	39–57	45–60	45–67
Magnesium, mg	4.3–7.2	3.7–6.9	4.3–7.2	4.3–8.0
Iron, µg	100–200	87–190	100–200	100–222
Zinc, µg	400	348–381	400	400–444
Copper, µg	20	17–19	20	20–22
Selenium, µg	1.5–4.5	1.3–4.3	1.5–4.5	1.5–5.0
Chromium, µg	0.05–0.3	0.04–0.29	0.05–0.3	0.05–0.33

(continued)

Table 9-4. Comparison of Parenteral Intake Recommendations for Growing Preterm Infants in Stable Clinical Condition *(continued)*

Element	Consensus Recommendations		Consensus Recommendations	
	Less than 1,000 g/kg per day	Less than 1,000 g/ 100 kcal	1,000– 1,500 g/kg per day	1,000– 1,500 g/ 100 kcal
Manganese, µg	1	0.87–0.95	1	1.00–1.11
Molybdenum, µg	0.25	0.22–0.24	0.25	0.25–0.28
Iodine, µg	1	0.87–0.95	1	1.00–1.11
Taurine, mg	1.88–3.75	1.6–3.6	1.88–3.75	1.9–4.2
Carnitine, mg	~2.9	~2.5–2.8	~2.9	~2.9–3.2
Inositol, mg	54	47–51	54	54–60
Choline, mg	14.4–28	12.5–26.7	14.4–28	14.4–31.1

Data from Tsang RC, Uauy R, Koletzko B, Zlotkin SH. Nutrition of the preterm infant: scientific basis and practical guidelines. Cincinnati, OH: Digital Education Publishing Inc; 2005:417–8.

American Academy of Pediatrics. Pediatric Nutrition Handbook. 6th ed. Elk Grove Village (IL): American Academy of Pediatrics; 2009.

less than 1,500 g (Table 9-4). The high incidence of respiratory and other morbidities, combined with intestinal immaturity, may necessitate slow advancement of the volume of enteral feedings. Parenteral nutrition can supplement the gradually increasing enteral feedings so that total intake by both routes meets the infant's nutritional needs.

Current evidence indicates that parenteral administration of amino acid and glucose may be safely initiated within hours of birth. Positive nitrogen balance, indicating an anabolic state, can occur with amino acid intakes of 1.5–2.0 g/kg per day and with parenteral lipid and glucose energy intakes of 60 kcal/kg per day. Growth generally requires nonprotein energy intake of at least 70 kcal/kg per day; nitrogen retention may occur at the fetal rate with nonprotein energy intake of 80–85 kcal/kg per day and amino acid intakes of 2.7–3.5 g/kg per day. At a minimum, amino acids should be provided to very low birth weight infants at 1.5–2.0 g/kg per day as soon as possible after birth to prevent negative nitrogen balance; amino acid intake at this level is well tolerated in even the most immature infants. As nonprotein energy and amino acid intake is increased, a balanced supply of glucose and intravenous lipid generally is recommended to prevent some of the metabolic complications of parenteral nutrition.

Enteral Nutrition

The method of enteral feeding chosen for each infant should be based on gestational age, birth weight, and clinical condition. Historically, enteral feedings have been delayed in the small, preterm infant because of extreme immaturity, perceived increased risk of necrotizing enterocolitis, or significant respiratory or other morbidity. However, evidence indicates that early introduction of trophic feeding or priming feeding is safe, well tolerated, and associated with significant benefits. The actual route of enteral feeding (eg, nasogastric, orogastric, gastrostomy, transpyloric, or nipple) again is determined on the basis of gestational age, clinical condition, and oromotor integrity (ability to coordinate sucking, swallowing, and breathing).

Human milk has a number of special features that make its use desirable in feeding preterm infants. Fresh or properly stored refrigerated human milk contains immunologic and antimicrobial factors that are protective against infection. Fat digestion is facilitated by the lipase and the triglycerides found in human milk. However, human milk does not provide adequate protein, calcium, phosphorus, sodium, trace metals, and some vitamins to meet the tissue and bone growth needs of the very low birth weight infant. Human milk fortifiers that are nutritionally balanced to correct these deficiencies when added to human milk are available commercially and can enhance growth and bone mineralization in very low birth weight infants.

Preterm infants who weigh more than 2,000 g at birth generally achieve adequate growth when fed their mother's milk, postdischarge formula, or a regular term infant formula of 67 kcal/dL. However, calcium and phosphorus retention rates are slower than fetal accretion rates. These infants may require vitamin supplementation during the period when the volume of formula or human milk ingested does not provide the recommended daily vitamin intake, particularly of vitamin D (see Table 9-5 and "Breastfeeding" in Chapter 8).

Special formulas for very low birth weight infants (preterm formulas) contain additional protein, easily absorbed carbohydrates (glucose polymers and lactose), and easily digested and absorbed lipids (15–50% medium-chain triglycerides). The calcium and phosphorus contents are high to achieve a bone mineralization rate equivalent to the fetal rate. The sodium content also is high, reflecting the increased sodium requirement of preterm infants. Trace metals and vitamins have been added to meet the increased needs of the very low birth weight infant. The use of formulas for preterm infants, compared with the

Table 9-5. Comparison of Enteral Intake Recommendations for Growing Preterm Infants in Stable Clinical Condition

Element	Consensus Recommendations		Consensus Recommendations	
	Less than 1,000 g/kg per day	Less than 1,000 g/ 100 kcal	1,000– 1,500 g/kg per day	1,000– 1,500 g/ 100 kcal
Water/fluids, mL	160–220	107–169	135–190	104–173
Energy, kcal	130–150	100	110–130	100
Protein, g	3.8–4.4	2.5–3.4	3.4–4.2	2.6–3.8
Carbohydrate, g	9–20	6.0–15.4	7–17	5.4–15.5
Fat, g	6.2–8.4	4.1–6.5	5.3–7.2	4.1–6.5
Linoleic acid, mg	700–1,680	467–1,292	600–1,440	462–1,309
Linoleate: linolenate (C18:2–C18:3)	5–15	5–15	5–15	5–15
Docosahexaenoic acid, mg	≥21	≥16	≥18	≥16
Arachidonic acid, mg	≥28	≥22	≥24	≥22
Vitamin A, IU	700–1,500	467–1,154	700–1,500	538–1,364
Vitamin D, IU	150–400	100–308	150–400	115–364
Vitamin E, IU	6–12	4.0–9.2	6–12	4.6–10.9
Vitamin K_1 µg	8–10	5.3–7.7	8–10	6.2–9.1
Ascorbate, mg	18–24	12.0–18.5	18–24	13.8–21.8
Thiamine, µg	180–240	120–185	180–240	138–218
Riboflavin, µg	250–360	167–277	25–3600	192–327
Pyridoxine, µg	150–210	100–162	150–210	115–191
Niacin, mg	3.6–4.8	2.4–3.7	3.6–4.8	2.8–4.4
Pantothenate, mg	1.2–1.7	0.8–1.3	1.2–1.7	0.9–1.5
Biotin, µg	3.6–6	2.4–4.6	3.6–6	2.8–5.5
Folate, µg	25–50	17–38	25–50	19–45
Vitamin B_{12}, µg	0.3	0.2–0.23	0.3	0.23–0.27
Sodium, mg	69–115	46–88	69–115	53–105
Potassium, mg	78–117	52–90	78–117	60–106
Chloride, mg	107–249	71–192	107–249	82–226
Calcium, mg	100–220	67–169	100–220	77–200
Phosphorus, mg	60–140	40–108	60–140	46–127
Magnesium, mg	7.9–15	5.3–11.5	7.9–15	6.1–13.6
Iron, mg	2–4	1.33–3.08	2–4	1.54–3.64
Zinc, µg	1,000–3,000	337–2,308	1,000–3,000	769–2,727

(continued)

Table 9-5. Comparison of Enteral Intake Recommendations for Growing Preterm Infants in Stable Clinical Condition *(continued)*

Element	Consensus Recommendations		Consensus Recommendations	
	Less than 1,000 g/kg per day	Less than 1,000 g/ 100 kcal	1,000– 1,500 g/kg per day	1,000– 1,500 g/ 100 kcal
Copper, µg	120–150	80–115	120–150	92–136
Selenium, µg	1.3–4.5	0.9–3.5	1.3–4.5	1.0–4.1
Chromium, µg	0.1–2.25	0.07–1.73	0.1–2.25	0.08–2.05
Manganese, µg	0.7–7.75	0.5–5.8	0.7–7.75	0.5–6.8
Molybdenum, µg	0.3	0.20–0.23	0.3	0.23–0.27
Iodine, µg	10–60	6.7–46.2	10–60	7.7–54.5
Taurine, mg	4.5–9.0	3.0–6.9	4.5–9.0	3.5–8.2
Carnitine, mg	˜2.9	˜1.9–2.2	˜2.9	˜2.2–2.6
Inositol, mg	32–81	21–62	32–81	25–74
Choline, mg	14.4–28	9.6–21.5	14.4–28	11.1–25.2

Data from Tsang RC, Uauy R, Koletzko B, Zlotkin SH. Nutrition of the preterm infant: scientific basis and practical guidelines. Cincinnati, OH: Digital Education Publishing Inc; 2005:417–8.
American Academy of Pediatrics. Pediatric Nutrition Handbook. 6th ed. Elk Grove Village (IL): American Academy of Pediatrics; 2009.

use of formulas intended for term infants, has been shown to contribute to weight gain and a bone mineralization rate closer to that of the reference fetus and improved long-term growth and development. Also, improved neurodevelopmental outcome is seen in preterm infants fed preterm formulas or human milk versus term formula. Formulas containing long-chain polyunsaturated fatty acids may confer visual and neurodevelopmental benefits, although study results are conflicting. Formulas supplemented with docosahexaenoic acid and arachidonic acid are now available and appear safe.

Nutrient Enhancement for Preterm Infants After Discharge
Specialized formulas that provide increased protein, energy, and mineral intake to meet the continuing growth needs of the small, preterm infant after hospital discharge are available at a cost slightly higher than that of standard formulas. Some studies have shown their use to result in improved growth, bone mineralization, and accrual of lean body mass when compared with the use of

standard formulas; however, current data do not provide strong evidence that feeding a nutrient-enriched formula to preterm infants after hospital discharge affects growth rates or development up to 18 months postterm. In the face of a continuing paucity of data on what to feed the preterm infants after hospital discharge, it may be reasonable to provide small, preterm infants (born at or before 34 weeks of gestation, with a birth weight less than or equal to 1,800 g) and infants with other morbidities (eg, BPD) specialized formulas after hospital discharge to promote catch-up growth, acquisition of lean body mass, and improved bone mineralization.

Pain Prevention and Management

Pain consists of the perception of painful stimuli (nociception) and the psychological response to painful stimuli (anxiety). Studies measuring a variety of physiologic factors, including oxygen saturation, β-endorphin, glucose, cortisol, and epinephrine concentrations, confirm that infants of all gestational ages have a nociceptive response to pain stimuli. Observations of infant behavior suggest that anxiety also is a component of the infantile pain response, but its character, intensity, and duration remain undetermined. Therefore, the significance of anxiety in the newborn remains unknown.

The prevention of pain is important not only because it is an ethical expectation, but also because repeated painful exposures can have long-term deleterious consequences, including altered pain sensitivity and permanent neuroanatomic and behavioral abnormalities. Measures for assessing pain in the newborn have been developed and validated. Every health care facility caring for newborns should implement an effective pain-prevention and stress-reduction program that includes strategies to achieve the following goals:

- Assess pain
- Minimize the number of painful procedures performed
- Effectively use nonpharmacologic and pharmacologic therapies for the prevention of pain associated with routine minor procedures
- Eliminate pain associated with surgery and other major procedures

Validated pain assessment tools must be used in a consistent manner, and caregivers should be trained to assess newborns for pain. Any unnecessary noxious stimuli (including acoustic, visual, tactile, and vestibular) should be avoided. Simple comfort measures, such as swaddling, nonnutritive sucking, kangaroo care or breastfeeding, and developmentally appropriate positioning (eg, facilitated tuck position), should be used whenever possible for minor procedures. Oral administration of sucrose reduces pain associated with painful procedures. These environmental and nonpharmacologic interventions should be provided as baseline measures to prevent, reduce, or eliminate stress and pain.

The risks and benefits of pharmacologic pain management techniques must be considered on an individualized basis. Pharmacokinetic and pharmacodynamic properties and efficacy of these drugs vary in the newborn; to the extent possible, agents whose properties have been studied in the newborn should be used. It is important to remember that sedatives and anxiolytics do not provide analgesia. Agents known to compromise cardiorespiratory function should be administered only by individuals experienced in airway management and in settings with the capacity for continuous cardiorespiratory monitoring.

Intraoperative and Postoperative Pain Management

Pain is an inevitable consequence of surgery at any age. A health care facility providing surgery for infants should have an established protocol for pain management, based on a coordinated, multidimensional strategy. Although it is now considered unethical to perform surgery in the newborn without anesthesia, the appropriate levels of anesthesia for various surgical procedures have not been well investigated. The use of paralytic agents without analgesia during surgery is unacceptable. For major surgical procedures, general anesthesia by inhalation of anesthetic gases, intravenous administration of narcotic agents, or regional techniques can be safe and effective. Anesthesia for surgical procedures for all newborns should be administered by specially trained physicians, and the choice of technique and agent should be based on a comprehensive assessment of the infant, efficacy and safety of the drug, and the technical requirements of the procedure.

The use of analgesic agents is important in the immediate postoperative period and should be continued as required. Continuous or bolus infusions of opioids and continuous caudal or epidural blockade can be used to provide a steady course of pain relief, but both require careful management and continuous monitoring of cardiorespiratory and hemodynamic status. Acetaminophen can be used as an adjunct to regional anesthetics or opioids, but there are inadequate data on pharmacokinetics at gestational ages less than 28 weeks to permit calculation of appropriate doses.

Pain Management for Other Invasive Procedures

Intercostal Drain Placement and Removal. Insertion of a chest drain is a painful procedure. Because there have been no prospective trials of analgesia for this procedure to date, recommendations based on general principles include slow infiltration of the skin with a local anesthetic and systemic analgesia with a rapidly acting opioid. Removal of the chest drain can also be very painful, and a short-acting, rapid-onset systemic analgesic agent should be considered for this procedure.

Retinal Examination. These examinations are painful. Although there are insufficient data to make specific recommendations, a reasonable approach would be administration of oral sucrose and a topical anesthetic. Nonpharmacologic measures, such as swaddling or nonnutritive sucking, should be used in conjunction with these agents.

Circumcision. For information on pain management during circumcision, see "Circumcision" in Chapter 8.

Intubation. The experience of being intubated is unpleasant and painful. Except for emergent intubation during resuscitation, and perhaps for infants with upper airway anomalies, premedication should be used for all endotracheal intubations in newborns. Medications with rapid onset and short duration of action are preferable, and the following principles should be observed:

- Analgesics should be given
- Vagolytic agents and rapid-onset muscle relaxants should be considered
- Use of hypnotics or sedatives without analgesics should be avoided
- A muscle relaxant without an analgesic should not be used
- In circumstances when intravenous access is not available, alternative routes, including intramuscular or intranasal administration, can be considered

Topical Anesthetics for Minor Invasive Procedures

Topical anesthetics, such as a mixture of lidocaine and prilocaine, can effectively reduce pain associated with minor invasive procedures, such as venipuncture, lumbar puncture, and intravenous catheter insertion, if the agent is applied for a sufficient length of time before the procedure (at least 30 minutes). Repeated use should be limited to avoid the risk of methemoglobinemia. These agents are not effective for heel-stick blood draws because the pain from heel sticks is primarily from squeezing the heel rather than from the lancet.

Medication for Infants Receiving Mechanical Ventilation

The routine use of continuous analgesic or sedative agents for mechanically ventilated infants has not been shown to be helpful and may be harmful; therefore, this practice cannot be recommended. Use of analgesic and anxiolytic agents for amelioration of the discomfort associated with prolonged endotracheal intubation in newborns should be undertaken only after careful consideration of the observed response of the individual infant and the adverse effects of the commonly used agents. A recent Cochrane review concluded that if sedation is required, morphine sulfate is safer than midazolam.

Concepts that must be remembered when considering medication for intubated infants include the following:

- Chronic use of many sedatives or hypnotics may lead to tolerance, dependency, and withdrawal.

- Effects of chronic sedation on neurodevelopmental outcome are unknown.

- Sedatives or hypnotics may cause respiratory and cardiovascular depression.

- Combined treatment with a sedative or hypnotic and an opioid requires a decreased dosage of each.

- Agitation in the chronically ventilated infant may indicate the need to confirm airway patency and position, adjust ventilatory settings, or reduce noxious environmental stimuli.

Radiation Risk

Computed tomography (CT) is a valuable imaging modality; however, it entails an obligatory radiation exposure far in excess of many other common radiographic procedures. Compared with adults, infants have an increased risk of cancer from radiation exposure for the following three reasons: 1) growing and developing tissues are more sensitive to radiation effects, 2) the oncogenic effect of radiation has a long latent period, and 3) the radiation exposure from a fixed set of CT parameters results in a dose that is relatively higher for an infant's smaller cross-sectional area compared with an adult.

The amount of radiation that CT provides depends on many factors, especially the protocols used and the equipment settings. The radiologist has the responsibility to create protocols and adjust scanning techniques on the basis of special considerations of neonatal patients. If the same settings are used for both newborns and adults, newborns will receive an unnecessary and excessive amount of radiation. The radiologist can assist the pediatrician by suggesting alternative imaging techniques, such as MRI or ultrasonography when suitable, by using a low-dose technique, and by limiting the number of times (phases) the infant is scanned for an individual examination.

Surgical Procedures in the Neonatal Intensive Care Unit

Infants in the NICU often require surgical procedures during hospitalization. The transport of an acutely ill infant to the operating room may be associated with a number of risks, including hypothermia, changes in blood pressure, and dislodging of an intravenous catheter or endotracheal tube. For this reason, many centers perform selected surgical procedures (eg, laser ablation) within the NICU. Studies have suggested that this approach can be safe and effective and may result in improved outcomes.

If surgical procedures are performed within the NICU, there must be adequate lighting and work space, as well as ongoing monitoring and anesthetic management. Personnel should wear appropriate operating room attire, and strict sterile techniques must be used. Hospitals should develop policies governing all surgical procedures performed within the NICU, including management of anesthesia. Such policies should be developed in conjunction with the institutional operating room committee to ensure that all appropriate guidelines are met.

Immunization of Hospitalized Infants

Guidelines for immunization of both preterm and term infants who require prolonged hospital stays should be implemented in each NICU. Medically stable preterm infants should begin the immunization series at the usual chronological age of 6–8 weeks, unless otherwise indicated. Some very low birth weight infants have been found to have a reduced immune response when the usual timing of immunizations is followed. Additional studies are needed to define the optimal immunization schedule for this group of infants. Vaccine doses should not be reduced for very low birth weight infants or preterm infants. Term infants who remain in the hospital at 6–8 weeks of age should receive vaccines according to the schedule recommended by the Centers for Disease Control and Prevention Advisory Committee on Immunization Practices and included in the AAP Redbook. Rotavirus vaccine, which is a live virus vaccine, should not be administered until discharge. Immunization recommendations and vaccine safety information are frequently updated and can be verified from the Centers for Disease Control and Prevention Advisory Committee on Immunization Practices web page at http://www.cdc.gov/vaccines/recs/acip/. (See also "Immunization" in Chapter 8.)

Death of a Newborn

Loss of a pregnancy or death of a newborn touches every aspect of a family's life. The intense emotions of grieving can be confusing and overwhelming. Every effort should be made to determine the cause of the loss, to understand the family's grief responses, and to facilitate healthy coping and adjustment. Efforts to obtain organs for donation are strongly encouraged.

In-Hospital Support and Counseling

Bereavement counseling support is important to family members' abilities to adjust to their loss and to continue with their lives. Counseling should be tailored to the specific circumstances surrounding the death; should be sensitive to specific ethical, cultural, religious, and family considerations; and should be provided by specific staff within the hospital. The period after a neonatal death always has an element of confusion because of the continuing grief, the tasks of informing relatives and friends, and the need to make final arrangements.

The time in the hospital before and after the newborn has died is the parents' only opportunity to create memories of the newborn and experience being the newborn's parent. Therefore, involvement of the parents in as much of the bedside care of even critically ill infants as is commensurate with safety and their needs is of major importance. Whether a neonatal death is expected or unexpected, specific management procedures can be useful in facilitating parental adjustment to the loss:

- Offer the parents, and extended family if desired, an opportunity to see, hold, and spend time with the infant both before and immediately after the death.

- Facilitate involvement with the clergy or spiritual adviser of the family's choice in preparing the family for the death and supporting them afterward.

- Encourage the family to name the infant, if they have not done so previously, as it is easier to connect memories to a name.

- Obtain pictures and remembrances (eg, identification tags, footprints, a lock of hair, birth and death certificates, height and weight records, a receiving blanket for the infant, plaster molds of the hands and feet). Even if the parents initially say that they do not want these mementos, they frequently ask for them days, weeks, or months later.

• Provide information about options for burial, cremation, funerals, or memorial services. Encourage both parents to take an active part in making these arrangements.

• Visit the parents daily while the mother is in the hospital; listen to them sympathetically, and give them information as it becomes available.

• Provide reliable preliminary information from the appropriate medical professionals concerning the cause and circumstances of death.

• Be aware that the staff's potential reactions—a sense of guilt, failure, and uncertainty—may cause them to avoid the parents, thereby impeding discussion of the deceased infant with the family. The grief of caregivers, like that of parents and family, should be addressed and supported by appropriate hospital personnel.

• Ensure that the parents have access to support from their families and friends. Anticipate with parents the difficulties they may have in sharing information about the loss with other children, family, and friends. Provide information and suggestions on how they might handle difficult situations or times and information on the availability of support groups.

• Explain the grieving process so that the parents understand the usual reactions. Parents frequently demonstrate reactions of acute grief, such as somatic disturbances, a preoccupation with the newborn's appearance or probable future appearance, guilt, hostility, and loss of ability to function. Mourning should be allowed and encouraged to proceed.

• Encourage the parents to communicate their thoughts and feelings openly with one another. Help them understand and accept the differences in how each of them grieves.

• Provide written materials for the parents to read in the hospital and after discharge. Although there is no substitute for a multidisciplinary group of professionals carefully organized to provide support, written materials can provide concrete information about specific procedures, such as autopsy and funeral arrangements, as well as guidance on long-term issues, such as grief, marital stress, explanations for young children, and consideration of another pregnancy. These materials can be designed by the individual hospital or obtained through various associations.

Because families may come from a distance and may not be well acquainted with the attending physicians, it is especially important that referral centers that provide neonatal care designate a member of the team to be an advocate for the family during the hospital stay and after discharge. The designated individual also should be responsible for documenting the management and follow-up of each death. Too often families are lost to follow-up when physicians, nurses, and families avoid sharing the sadness of bereavement.

Determining Cause of Death

When a neonatal death occurs, a special effort should be made to determine the cause of death. This process is helpful for several reasons:

- It helps the family to understand the medical reasons for the death.

- It provides a basis for counseling the family about future pregnancies, including family planning, genetic counseling, and obstetric and neonatal management.

- It provides correct diagnoses for statistical reporting and analysis of perinatal care outcomes.

Requesting an autopsy after the death of a newborn must be handled with sensitivity and gentleness. Selecting the right time to introduce the idea is critical. It can be helpful when it is apparent that a newborn is dying, particularly when the underlying cause is uncertain, to introduce the idea of a postmortem examination to the parents. Its value as a means of gaining information that will be helpful in answering their future questions often is perceived as a compelling reason for consent. Involvement of the primary care physician and the mother's obstetrician in the request for autopsy consent also may facilitate the family's acceptance of the idea.

If there is reluctance for consent for a complete examination of the body, consideration should be given to a limited one, to obtaining specimens of body fluids for microbial culture or other analyses as indicated, and to obtaining postmortem imaging studies if such information could further elucidate the cause of death. In all neonatal deaths, every effort should be made to obtain histopathologic examination of the placenta, membranes, and umbilical cord. When an underlying genetic disorder is suspected and premortem testing is incomplete, advance planning for appropriate specimen retrieval with or without a full autopsy should occur. In every instance, the family should receive the final written results of the autopsy and other examinations in person, if possible, in conjunction with a verbal explanation of the findings.

Each unit should have a formal process for periodic review of all neonatal deaths. In addition, when there has been an unexpected clinical deterioration leading to a death, a contemporaneous review of the specific clinical events and decisions with all the involved staff participating can be helpful to resolve interpersonal conflicts, relieve feelings of guilt or failure, and improve both understanding and team interaction. Such sessions usually are best led by the attending neonatologist, although, on occasion, employment of an uninvolved facilitator can be useful.

Bereavement Follow-up

The responsibility for ongoing bereavement counseling depends on the specific circumstances of the death and on the family's relationship with the physician. Usually a multidisciplinary approach is best. In general, such counseling should include the following:

- An initial session 4–6 weeks after the death
- Assessment of the grieving process
- Additional genetic services, if indicated
- Review of preliminary autopsy data, if available
- Answers for parents' specific questions
- Education and reassurance regarding the normal grieving process
- Follow-up visits as indicated by the individual family needs
- Referral of family members to bereavement support groups or bereavement counselors

Hospital Discharge of High-Risk Infants

Discharge Planning

Discharge planning for high-risk infants should begin early in hospitalization and includes six critical elements:

1. Parental education
2. Completion of appropriate elements of primary care in the hospital
3. Development of a management plan for unresolved medical problems
4. Development of the comprehensive home-care plan
5. Identification and involvement of support services
6. Determination and designation of follow-up care

Discharge planning for infants who have been transported back to community hospitals for convalescent care should follow the same principles, and the care plan should be coordinated between the two units before the transfer of the infant occurs.

Readiness for Hospital Discharge

The decision of when to discharge an infant from the hospital after a stay in the NICU is complex and includes assessment of the infant's physiologic stability, the family's readiness to care for their infant, and the mobilization of appropriate community resources to ensure continuing care and follow-up, including identification of a primary care physician experienced in the care of such infants. The following recommendations are offered as a framework for guiding decisions about the timing of discharge. It is prudent for each institution to establish guidelines that ensure a consistent approach yet allow some flexibility on the basis of physician and family judgment. It is of foremost importance that the infant, family, and community be prepared for the infant to be safely cared for outside the hospital.

Infant Readiness

The infant is considered ready for discharge if, in the judgment of the responsible physician, the following have been accomplished:

- A sustained pattern of weight gain of sufficient duration has been demonstrated.

- The infant has demonstrated adequate maintenance of normal body temperature when fully clothed in an open bed with normal ambient temperature (20–25°C [68–77°F]).

- The infant has established competent feeding by breast or bottle without cardiorespiratory compromise.

- Physiologically mature and stable cardiorespiratory function has been documented for a sufficient duration.

- Appropriate immunizations have been administered.

- Appropriate metabolic screening has been performed.

- Hematologic status has been assessed and appropriate therapy has been instituted, if indicated.

- Nutritional risks have been assessed and therapy and dietary modification have been instituted, if indicated.

- Hearing evaluation has been completed.
- Funduscopic examinations for red reflux and retinopathy of prematurity have been completed, as indicated.
- Neurodevelopmental and neurobehavioral status has been assessed and demonstrated to the parents.
- Car seat evaluation has been completed (see also "Safe Transportation of Late Preterm and Low Birth Weight Infants" in Chapter 8).
- Review of the hospital course has been completed, unresolved medical problems have been identified, and plans for follow-up monitoring and treatment have been instituted.
- An individualized home-care plan has been developed with input from all appropriate disciplines.

Family and Home Environmental Readiness

Assessment of the family's caregiving capabilities, resource availability, and home physical facilities has been completed as follows:

- Identification of at least two family caregivers, and assessment of their ability, availability, and commitment
- Psychosocial assessment for parenting strengths and risks
- Home environmental assessment that may include an on-site evaluation
- Review of available financial resources and identification of adequate financial support

In preparation for home care of the technology-dependent infant, it is essential to complete an assessment documenting availability of 24-hour telephone access, electricity, safe in-house water supply, and adequate heating. Specific modification of home facilities must have been completed, if needed, to accommodate home-care systems. Plans must be in place for responding to loss of electrical power, heat, or water, and for emergency relocation mandated by natural disaster. Detailed financial assessment and planning are also essential. Caregivers should have demonstrated the necessary capabilities to provide all components of care, including the following:

- Feeding, whether breast, bottle, or alternative technique, including formula preparation if required
- Basic infant care, including bathing; skin, and genital care; temperature measurement; dressing and comforting

- Infant cardiopulmonary resuscitation and emergency intervention
- Assessment of clinical status, including understanding and detection of the general early signs and symptoms of illness, as well as the signs and symptoms specific to the infant's condition
- Infant safety precautions, including proper positioning during sleep and proper use of car seats (see also "Parent Education and Psychosocial Factors" in Chapter 8)
- Specific safety precautions for the artificial airway, if any; feeding tube; intestinal stoma; infusion pump; and other mechanical and prosthetic devices, as indicated
- Administration of medications, specifically proper storage, dosage, timing, and administration; and recognition of signs of potential toxicity
- Equipment operation, maintenance, and problem solving for each mechanical support device required
- Appropriate technique for each special care procedure required, including special dressings for infusion entry sites, intestinal stomas, or healing wounds; maintenance of an artificial airway; oropharyngeal and tracheal suctioning; and physical therapy, as indicated.

Community and Health Care System Readiness

An emergency intervention and transportation plan must be developed, and emergency medical service providers identified and notified, if indicated. Follow-up care needs must be determined, appropriate physicians identified, and appropriate information exchanged, including the following:

- A primary care physician has been identified, and has accepted responsibility for care of the infant.
- Surgical specialty and pediatric medical subspecialty follow-up care requirements have been identified and appropriate arrangements have been made.
- Neurodevelopmental follow-up requirements have been identified and appropriate referrals have been made.
- Home nursing visits for assessment and parent support have been arranged as indicated, and the home care plan has been transmitted to the home health agency.
- For breastfeeding mothers, information on breastfeeding support and availability of lactation counselors has been provided.

Special Considerations

The final decision for discharge, which is the responsibility of the attending physician, must be tailored to the unique constellation of issues posed by each infant's situation. Within this framework, there are four broad categories of high-risk infants that require individual consideration: 1) preterm infants, 2) infants with special health care needs or dependence on technology, 3) infants at risk because of family issues, and 4) infants with anticipated early death.

Preterm Infants

Criteria for hospital discharge of preterm infants should include physiologic stability rather than attainment of a specific weight. The three physiologic competencies generally recognized as essential before discharge are 1) oral feeding sufficient to sustain appropriate growth, 2) the ability to maintain normal body temperature in a home environment, and 3) sufficiently mature respiratory control. These competencies usually are achieved by 36–37 weeks of postmenstrual age; infants born earlier in gestation and with more complicated medical courses tend to take longer to achieve these physiologic competencies. Home monitors are rarely indicated (see also "Apnea" earlier in this chapter). Preterm infants should be placed supine for sleeping, and hospitals should model this behavior for parents by positioning infants supine after approximately 32 weeks of postmenstrual age. Late preterm infants (34–37 weeks of gestation) are at increased risk of feeding problems and hyperbilirubinemia after discharge. These infants require close follow-up after discharge to monitor bilirubin concentrations and weight gain (see also "Discharge of Late Preterm Infants" in Chapter 8).

Infants With Special Health Care Needs or Dependence on Technology

Increasing numbers of infants are being discharged from the hospital with continuing medical problems requiring specialized technologic support. For infants discharged from the NICU, these supports are primarily nutritional and respiratory, although additional special services may be necessary.

When infants are unable to achieve adequate oral feedings to sustain growth, alternatives include gavage or gastrostomy feedings, parenteral nutrition, or both. Gavage feeding has a limited role and should be considered only when feeding is the last issue requiring continued hospitalization and the parents or caregivers have demonstrated competence and comfort with this procedure. When little to no progress is being made with oral feedings, gastrostomy tube placement can make hospital discharge feasible and allow the infant to develop competent oral feeding skills if possible. Home parenteral nutrition requires thorough education of caregivers and the availability of a home-care company that is well versed in infant nutritional support and monitoring.

Respiratory support can include supplemental oxygen, tracheostomy, or home ventilation. Home oxygen therapy for infants with BPD has become a fairly common practice, allowing earlier hospital discharge for an otherwise stable infant. Oxygen saturation levels should be assessed intermittently at home to ensure sufficient oxygen is being delivered during a range of activities and sleep. Some infants who are discharged on supplemental oxygen also are discharged on a cardiorespiratory monitor or pulse oximeter in case the oxygen supply is interrupted. Reducing or stopping supplemental oxygen should be supervised by the physician or other health care professional and attempted only when the infant demonstrates acceptable oxygen saturations (greater than 90%) with good growth velocity and sufficient stamina for usual activity. Home care of the infant with a tracheostomy requires extensive parental teaching and coordinated multidisciplinary follow-up care. Infants with tracheostomy should be discharged on a cardiorespiratory monitor in case the airway should become obstructed. If the infant also requires continuing assisted ventilation, home nursing support will be needed for at least part of each day and the ventilator must have a disconnect alarm.

Infants at Risk Because of Family Issues

Preterm birth, prolonged hospitalization, birth defects, and disabling conditions are known family stressors and risk factors for subsequent family dysfunction and child abuse. An organized approach to planning for discharge may help identify infants who require extra support or whose home environments present unacceptable risks. Adverse social conditions, including lower maternal education, lack of social support or stability, fewer prenatal visits, or concern for parental substance abuse should prompt awareness of the need for increased support after discharge. Most interventions have focused on multidisciplinary teams that provide follow-up monitoring, including home visits, although the efficacy of these interventions has been difficult to demonstrate.

Infants With Anticipated Early Death

For many infants with terminal conditions, the best place to spend the last days or weeks is at home. If the family wishes, assisted ventilation can even be withdrawn at home, rather than in the hospital. Preparation to discharge an infant for home hospice care should include arrangements for medical follow-up and home nursing, necessary equipment and supplies, management of pain, and bereavement support for the family. The parents should be given a letter to confirm to health care personnel that the infant should not be resuscitated (see also "Noninitiation or Withdrawal of Intensive Care for High-Risk Infants" in Chapter 8). Involvement of a multidisciplinary hospice or palliative care team before and after discharge can be very helpful to both the health care team and the family.

Hospice care may be chosen by families whose infant has an irreversible, fatal disease. The site for such care may vary with local community resources and family wishes. Enhancing the quality of the remaining life for the neonate and family is more important than the site of care delivery. Although less well studied than for older children, the components of neonatal hospice care are not unlike those established for pediatric hospice care. These components include the following elements:

- Involvement of skilled professionals
- Control of distressing conditions and provision of physical comfort
- Coordinated, multidisciplinary service delivery
- Social support of the family
- Follow-up and bereavement care

Follow-up Care of High-Risk Infants

The designation "high-risk" encompasses the broad spectrum of medical, neurologic, developmental, and psychosocial outcomes experienced by vulnerable neonatal subgroups described in the previous section. The organization of follow-up care will vary with the neonatal subgroup being monitored, potential adverse outcomes frequently associated with individual subgroups, and the purpose for ongoing evaluation. Specific requirements for follow-up care of high-risk neonatal subgroups include the following components:

- Primary care—monitoring of growth and development, preventive care, and guidance
- Management of unresolved medical problems
- Early detection of abnormality or delayed developmental progress
- Early intervention and habilitation

- Infant safety
- Parent education
- Evaluation of treatment benefit and complications
- Documentation of outcomes
- Neurosensory follow-up
- Environmental and psychosocial concerns
- Referral to other community resources

Role of the Primary Care Provider

The infant's primary care physician should provide a medical home and share in the responsibility for providing continuity of care with the level II, level III, or level IV care center. Frequently, the more detailed developmental and psychological evaluations and the initial management of complex unresolved medical problems are primarily the responsibility of the level III or level IV care center. As recovery progresses, medical care is increasingly assumed by the primary care physician. The primary care physician likely will assume the responsibility for referral to subspecialty consultation and care. Within any format of shared patient care delivery, it is imperative that all professionals communicate information in a timely manner and share in the planning and execution of the long-term care for infants with multidisciplinary service needs.

Surveillance and Assessment

The timing of follow-up visits for high-risk infants will vary with the needs of the individual infant and family. It may be necessary to examine some of these infants weekly or semimonthly at first. Neurologic, developmental, behavioral, and sensory status should be assessed more than once during the first year in high-risk infants to ensure early identification of problems and referral for appropriate interventions. A multidisciplinary perinatal follow-up program is especially valuable in providing these assessments.

Many infants who are born preterm have increased difficulty with emotional and attentional regulation, resulting in irritability, dependency, and other attentional problems. These factors as well as prolonged hospitalization inevitably disrupt family relationships, particularly the parent–child relationship. Infants with such a history may be at higher risk of child abuse, and these families benefit from close follow-up and support. (For more information on child abuse risk factors, see "Follow-up Care" in Chapter 8.)

Growth should be assessed at each follow-up visit—including weight gain, linear growth, and head growth—and plotted on standardized, birth-weight-appropriate growth curves with the appropriate-age correction for gestational age at birth. Review of nutritional intake and calculation of caloric intake are helpful in case management.

Physical examination should assess neuromotor, cardiac, pulmonary, gastrointestinal, and nutritional status, as well as the presence of any hernias, anomalies, or orthopedic deformities. Residual scars from invasive procedures during the neonatal course should be monitored for satisfactory healing. On occasion, referral for reconstructive procedures may be necessary.

Medication dosage should be re-evaluated, doses increased with weight gain and age, and blood concentrations monitored as indicated. Immunization status should be reviewed, and age-appropriate administration should be maintained. Follow-up audiology and visual assessments should be obtained when indicated.

Neurologic assessment should include an appraisal of muscle tone, development, protective and deep-tendon reflexes, and visual and auditory responses. In addition, developmental progress should be monitored both by parental report of milestone acquisition and by assessment using a standard developmental screening tool. When neurologic findings are suspect or developmental delays are suspected, children should be referred to either a neonatal follow-up program or an appropriate community program for more in-depth assessment.

Infants at greatest risk of adverse neurodevelopmental outcome (eg, those with a birth weight of 1,500 g or less; hypoxic–ischemic encephalopathy or neonatal seizures; hypoxic cardiorespiratory failure; or complex, multiple congenital anomalies) should have formal neurodevelopmental testing with a battery of standardized tests at least at 1 year and 2 years corrected age to monitor development in all domains (gross motor; fine motor and adaptive; visual perceptive and problem solving; hearing, language, and speech; and socialization). Primary care physicians should ensure that such testing is completed, irrespective of the results of developmental screening.

Early Intervention

Intervention programs for high-risk infants have been established under federal legislation to provide early detection of developmental delay and other disabilities. Intervention services may be provided up to 3 years of age for individual infants with confirmed neurodevelopmental delay or other disability. Programs also offer therapeutic guidelines for families, parent support groups, and respite care programs. Although no definitive data confirm the beneficial effects of infant-stimulation programs, early intervention may improve social adaptation, limit residual functional disability, and provide valuable family support.

Bibliography

Adamkin DH. Postnatal glucose homeostasis in late-preterm and term infants. American Academy of Pediatrics Committee on Fetus and Newborn. Pediatrics 2011;127:575–9.

Aher SM, Ohlsson A. Early versus late erythropoietin for preventing red blood cell transfusion in preterm and/or low birth weight infants. Cochrane Database of Systematic Reviews 2006, Issue 3. Art. No.: CD004865. DOI: 10.1002/14651858.CD004865. pub2; 10.1002/14651858.CD004865.pub2.

Aher SM, Ohlsson A. Late erythropoietin for preventing red blood cell transfusion in preterm and/or low birth weight infants. Cochrane Database of Systematic Reviews 2006, Issue 3. Art. No.: CD004868. DOI: 10.1002/14651858.CD004868.pub2; 10.1002/14651858.CD004868.pub2.

American Academy of Pediatrics. Pediatric nutrition handbook. 6th. Elk Grove Village (IL): American Academy of Pediatrics; 2009.

American Academy of Pediatrics. Red book: report of the Committee on Infectious Diseases. 29th. Elk Grove Village (IL): American Academy of Pediatrics; 2012.

American Academy of Pediatrics, American Heart Association. Textbook of neonatal resuscitation. 6th. Elk Grove Village (IL): Dallas (TX): AAP; AHA; 2011.

American Association of Blood Banks. Standards for blood banks and transfusion services. 27th. Bethesda (MD): AABB; 2011.

Antenatal corticosteroid therapy for fetal maturation. ACOG Committee Opinion No. 475. American College of Obstetricians and Gynecologists. Obstet Gynecol 2011; 117:422–4.

At-risk drinking and illicit drug use: ethical issues in obstetric and gynecologic practice. ACOG Committee Opinion No. 422. American College of Obstetricians and Gynecologists. Obstet Gynecol 2008;112:1449–60.

Ballard RA, Truog WE, Cnaan A, Martin RJ, Ballard PL, Merrill JD, et al. Inhaled nitric oxide in preterm infants undergoing mechanical ventilation. NO CLD Study Group. N Engl J Med 2006;355:343–53.

Barrington KJ, Finer N. Inhaled nitric oxide for respiratory failure in preterm infants. Cochrane Database of Systematic Reviews 2010, Issue 12. Art. No.: CD000509. DOI: 10.1002/14651858.CD000509.pub4; 10.1002/14651858.CD000509.pub4.

Batton DG, Barrington KJ, Wallman C. Prevention and management of pain in the neonate: an update. American Academy of Pediatrics Committee on Fetus and Newborn;

American Academy of Pediatrics Section on Surgery; Canadian Paediatric Society Fetus and Newborn Committee. Pediatrics 2006;118:2231–41.

Bellù R, de Waal KA, Zanini R. Opioids for neonates receiving mechanical ventilation. Cochrane Database of Systematic Reviews 2008, Issue 1. Art. No.: CD004212. DOI: 10.1002/14651858.CD004212.pub3; 10.1002/14651858.CD004212.pub3.

Brody AS, Frush DP, Huda W, Brent RL. Radiation risk to children from computed tomography. American Academy of Pediatrics Section on Radiology. Pediatrics 2007;120:677–82.

Cools F, Henderson-Smart DJ, Offringa M, Askie LM. Elective high frequency oscillatory ventilation versus conventional ventilation for acute pulmonary dysfunction in preterm infants. Cochrane Database of Systematic Reviews 2009, Issue 3. Art. No.: CD000104. DOI: 10.1002/14651858.CD000104.pub3; 10.1002/14651858.CD000104.pub3.

El Shahed AI, Dargaville PA, Ohlsson A, Soll R. Surfactant for meconium aspiration syndrome in full term/near term infants. Cochrane Database of Systematic Reviews 2007, Issue 3. Art. No.: CD002054. DOI: 10.1002/14651858.CD002054.pub2; 10. 1002/14651858.CD002054.pub2.

Engle WA. Surfactant-replacement therapy for respiratory distress in the preterm and term neonate. American Academy of Pediatrics Committee on Fetus and Newborn. Pediatrics 2008;121:419–32.

Finer N, Barrington KJ. Nitric oxide for respiratory failure in infants born at or near term. Cochrane Database of Systematic Reviews 2006, Issue 4. Art. No.: CD000399. DOI: 10.1002/14651858.CD000399.pub2; 10.1002/14651858.CD000399.pub2.

Glass P, Brown J. Outcome and follow-up of neonates treated with ECMO. In: Van Meurs K, Lally KP, Peek G and Zwischenberger JB, editors. In: ECMO: extracorporeal cardiopulmonary support in critical care. 3rd ed. Ann Arbor (MI): Extracorporeal Life Support Organization; 2005. p. 319–28.

Halliday HL, Ehrenkranz RA, Doyle LW. Early (<8 days) postnatal corticosteroids for preventing chronic lung disease in preterm infants. Cochrane Database of Systematic Reviews 2010, Issue 1. Art. No.: CD001146. DOI: 10.1002/14651858.CD001146. pub3; 10.1002/14651858.CD001146.pub3.

Halliday HL, Ehrenkranz RA, Doyle LW. Late (>7 days) postnatal corticosteroids for chronic lung disease in preterm infants. Cochrane Database of Systematic Reviews 2009, Issue 1. Art. No.: CD001145. DOI: 10.1002/14651858.CD001145.pub2; 10. 1002/14651858.CD001145.pub2.

Henderson-Smart DJ, De Paoli AG, Clark RH, Bhuta T. High frequency oscillatory ventilation versus conventional ventilation for infants with severe pulmonary dysfunction born at or near term. Cochrane Database of Systematic Reviews 2009, Issue 3. Art. No.: CD002974. DOI: 10.1002/14651858.CD002974.pub2; 10.1002/14651858. CD002974.pub2.

Higgins RD, Raju T, Edwards D, Azzopardi DV, Bose CL, Clark RH, et al. Hypothermia and other treatment options for neonatal encephalopathy: an executive summary of the Eunice Kennedy Shriver NICHD Workshop. J Pediatr 2011;159:851–8.e1.

Hospital discharge of the high-risk neonate. American Academy of Pediatrics Committee on Fetus and Newborn. Pediatrics 2008;122:1119–26.

Jacobs SE, Hunt R, Tarnow–Mordi WO, Inder TE, Davis PG. Cooling for newborns with hypoxic ischaemic encephalopathy. Cochrane Database of Systematic Reviews 2007, Issue 4. Art. No.: CD003311. DOI: 10.1002/14651858.CD003311.pub2; 10.1002/ 14651858.CD003311.pub2.

Jobe AH, Bancalari E. Bronchopulmonary dysplasia. Am J Respir Crit Care Med 2001; 163:1723–9.

Kumar P, Denson SE, Mancuso TJ. Premedication for nonemergency endotracheal intubation in the neonate. American Academy of Pediatrics Committee on Fetus and Newborn, Section on Anesthesiology and Pain Medicine. Pediatrics 2010;125:608–15.

Maisels MJ, Bhutani VK, Bogen D, Newman TB, Stark AR, Watchko JF. Hyperbilirubinemia in the newborn ≥ 35 weeks' gestation: an update with clarifications. Pediatrics 2009; 124:1193-8.

Management of hyperbilirubinemia in the newborn infant 35 or more weeks of gestation. American Academy of Pediatrics Subcommittee on Hyperbilirubinemia. Pediatrics 2004;114:297–316.

Moon RY. SIDS and other sleep-related infant deaths: expansion of recommendations for a safe infant sleeping environment. American Academy of Pediatrics. Task Force on Sudden Infant Death Syndrome. Pediatrics 2011;128:1030–9.

Morley CJ, Davis PG, Doyle LW, Brion LP, Hascoet JM, Carlin JB. Nasal CPAP or intubation at birth for very preterm infants. COIN Trial Investigators. N Engl J Med 2008;358:700–8.

Morris BH, Oh W, Tyson JE, Stevenson DK, Phelps DL, O'Shea TM, et al. Aggressive vs. conservative phototherapy for infants with extremely low birth weight. NICHD Neonatal Research Network. N Engl J Med 2008;359(18):1885–96.

Neonatal drug withdrawal. American Academy of Pediatrics Committee on Drugs, Committee on Fetus and Newborn. Pediatrics 2012;129:e540–60.

Ohlsson A, Aher SM. Early erythropoietin for preventing red blood cell transfusion in preterm and/or low birth weight infants. Cochrane Database of Systematic Reviews 2006, Issue 3. Art. No.: CD004863. DOI: 10.1002/14651858.CD004863.pub2; 10. 1002/14651858.CD004863.pub2.

Policy statements—Modified recommendations for use of palivizumab for prevention of respiratory syncytial virus infections. American Academy of Pediatrics Committee on Infectious Diseases. Pediatrics 2009;124:1694–701.

Prevention of rotavirus disease: updated guidelines for use of rotavirus vaccine. American Academy of Pediatrics Committee on Infectious Diseases. Pediatrics 2009;123:1412–20.

Screening examination of premature infants for retinopathy of prematurity. American Academy of Pediatrics Section on Ophthalmology; American Academy of Ophthalmology; American Association for Pediatric Ophthalmology and Strabismus. Pediatrics 2006;117:572–6.

Substance abuse reporting and pregnancy: the role of the obstetrician-gynecologist. AGOG Committee Opinion No. 473. American College of Obstetricians and Gynecologists. Obstet Gynecol 2011;117:200–1.

Supplemental Therapeutic Oxygen for Prethreshold Retinopathy Of Prematurity (STOP-ROP), a randomized, controlled trial. I: primary outcomes. Pediatrics 2000;105: 295–310.

Walsh MC, Wilson-Costello D, Zadell A, Newman N, Fanaroff A. Safety, reliability, and validity of a physiologic definition of bronchopulmonary dysplasia. J Perinatol 2003;23:451–6.

Watterberg KL. Policy statement—postnatal corticosteroids to prevent or treat bronchopulmonary dysplasia. American Academy of Pediatrics Committee on Fetus and Newborn. Pediatrics 2010;126:800–8.

Whyte RK, Kirpalani H, Asztalos EV, Andersen C, Blajchman M, Heddle N, et al. Neurodevelopmental outcome of extremely low birth weight infants randomly assigned to restrictive or liberal hemoglobin thresholds for blood transfusion. PINTOS Study Group. Pediatrics 2009;123:207–13.

Resources

Advisory Committee on Immunization Practices (ACIP). Atlanta (GA): CDC; 2011. Available at: http://www.cdc.gov/vaccines/recs/acip/. Retrieved January 3, 2012.

Jaundice in newborns—Q&A. Elk Grove Village (IL): AAP; 2009. Available at: http://www.healthychildren.org/English/news/pages/Jaundice-in-Newborns.aspx. Retrieved January 3, 2012.

Chapter 10
Perinatal Infections

Certain infections that occur in the antepartum or intrapartum period may have a significant effect on the fetus and newborn. Appropriate antepartum and intrapartum care of the mother and subsequent care of the newborn soon after birth can reduce the frequency of or ameliorate many serious problems and can minimize the risk of subsequent transmission in the nursery. In addition, some infections, such as influenza and varicella, may have more severe outcomes in pregnant women than in other adults. Communication and cooperation among all perinatal care personnel are essential to obtain the best results. The infections discussed in this chapter have been selected on the basis of new and evolving information that affects management.

Viral Infections

Cytomegalovirus

Cytomegalovirus (CMV), a member of the herpesvirus group, is the most common congenital viral infection. Approximately 1% of newborns are infected with CMV in utero and excrete CMV after birth. Approximately 10% of infants with congenital CMV infection have signs of infection at birth, with manifestations including intrauterine growth restriction, jaundice, purpura, hepatosplenomegaly, microcephaly, intracerebral calcifications, and retinitis; developmental delays in early childhood are common. Sensorineural hearing loss is the most common sequela of congenital CMV infection, which makes CMV the leading nongenetic cause of sensorineural hearing loss in children in the United States, accounting for one third of all cases.

Transmission

Transmission occurs via transplacental passage of the virus, contact of the infant with infectious secretions at the time of birth, ingestion of infected breast milk, or transfusion of blood from seropositive donors. Infection acquired intrapartum from maternal cervical secretions or postpartum from human milk usually is not associated with clinical illness in term infants. In preterm infants, infection resulting from human milk or from transfusion from CMV-seropositive donors has been associated with systemic infections, including lower respiratory tract disease and disseminated disease. Both primary CMV infection and reactivation of a latent infection can occur during pregnancy and result in congenital CMV infection. CMV-associated illness in a congenitally infected infant is more likely to occur in an infant born to a mother with primary CMV infection, especially among pregnant women infected before the third trimester.

Breastfeeding is not contraindicated for term infants of mothers who are seropositive carriers of CMV and have a past history of CMV infection. Transmission of CMV to newborns who receive milk from human milk banks can be minimized by limiting donor milk to CMV-negative donors or by ensuring appropriate pasteurization. (For breastfeeding guidelines, see Chapter 8.) Transmission via transfusion has been virtually eliminated by the use of blood from CMV-negative donors, the use of frozen deglycerolized red blood cells, and filtration to remove white blood cells.

Screening

Because there is neither a vaccine for prevention of infection nor an established, effective therapy for acute CMV infection, routine serologic screening of women or neonates is of no proven benefit. Testing generally is limited to pregnant women and neonates in whom CMV exposure is suspected. Routine serologic testing of personnel in newborn nurseries is not recommended.

Diagnosis

Active infection with CMV in pregnant women can be diagnosed by polymerase chain reaction (PCR) or viral culture of CMV from urine, saliva, throat swab specimens, or other body tissues. Serologic tests that detect CMV antibodies (immunoglobulins M and G) are widely available and can be used to document susceptibility to CMV or primary infection. Congenital CMV infection can be diagnosed if an infant has the virus detected in his or her urine, saliva, blood or other tissues within 2–3 weeks after birth. Later in infancy, differentiation between intrauterine and perinatal infection is difficult to determine. Isolation of the virus or detection of CMV genome by PCR from amniotic fluid is the most sensitive test for detecting fetal infection. Fetal blood obtained by cordocentesis may be tested for CMV-specific immunoglobulin M (IgM), but this test is less sensitive than culture or PCR of amniotic fluid.

Treatment

No treatment is currently indicated for CMV infection in healthy individuals. Antiviral treatment is used for immunocompromised patients who have either sight-related or life-threatening illnesses due to CMV infection. There are limited data suggesting the possible benefits of parenteral administration of the antiviral medication ganciclovir in neonates ill with congenital CMV involving the central nervous system to protect against hearing deterioration and to decrease the risk of neurodevelopmental impairment. However, intravenous treatment with ganciclovir requires prolonged (42-day) hospitalization, has significant adverse effects (eg, neutropenia) that may force discontinuation of treatment, and places the infant at increased risk of an adverse event associated with prolonged intravenous therapy. There are little data regarding the efficacy of ganciclovir therapy in preterm infants with perinatally acquired CMV infection.

There is limited evidence that administration of CMV hyperimmune globulin to pregnant women with a primary CMV infection can lower the risk of congenital CMV disease. However, there are insufficient efficacy data to recommend its use at this time.

Enteroviruses

The enteroviruses comprise a group of viruses that includes the polioviruses, Coxsackie viruses, echoviruses, and other enteroviruses. Through the widespread use of vaccines, wild-type poliovirus infection has been eliminated from the Western Hemisphere as well as the Western Pacific and European regions. Nonpolio enteroviral infections are common and are spread by fecal–oral and respiratory routes. Enteroviruses are common and pregnant women are frequently exposed to them, especially during summer and fall months. Most enterovirus infections during pregnancy cause mild or no illness in the mother. However, infection in the third trimester can trigger labor.

Enteroviruses rarely cross the placenta and cause disease in the fetus. Vertical transmission of enteroviruses can occur at birth after exposure to virus-containing maternal blood or cervical secretions. Signs of an enterovirus infection in the neonate generally begin 3–7 days after birth. Neonates who acquire infection perinatally or within days of birth are at risk of severe disease. Manifestations can include pneumonia, exanthems, aseptic meningitis, encephalitis, paralysis, hepatitis, conjunctivitis, myocarditis, and pericarditis.

Diagnosis is confirmed by recovery of the virus from swabs of the throat or rectum and samples of stool, cerebrospinal fluid, or blood. Polymerase chain reaction testing of spinal fluid is more sensitive than a culture.

No specific therapy is available. Immune globulin given intravenously has been used in life-threatening neonatal infections, suspected viral myocarditis, and enterovirus 71 neurologic disease, but efficacy data are lacking. Hospitalized newborns should be managed with standard as well as contact precautions.

Hepatitis A Virus

The hepatitis A virus (HAV) is a small RNA virus that can produce either asymptomatic infection or acute illness. Serious effects of HAV infection are uncommon. Hepatitis A virus has little effect on pregnancy and rarely is transmitted perinatally. The risk of transplacental transmission to the fetus is negligible, and there is no evidence that the virus is a teratogen. The most common mode of transmission is by the fecal–oral route. Diagnosis is confirmed by the demonstration of anti-HAV IgM antibodies in infant serum.

Vaccines for hepatitis A are highly effective and approved for use during pregnancy, if indicated. Although vaccine safety in pregnancy has not been established, the theoretical risk to the developing fetus is negligible because the vaccine contains inactivated, purified viral proteins. Pregnant women with the following risk factors are candidates for hepatitis A vaccination: history of or current intravenous drug use, travel to endemic regions, residence in communities with a high prevalence of hepatitis A, working or having close contact with HAV-infected primates, diagnosis of chronic liver disease or receipt of a liver transplant, or receiving clotting factor concentrate for treatment of a clotting disorder. Immunoglobulin is effective for both pre-exposure and postexposure prophylaxis, does not pose a risk to either a pregnant woman or her fetus, and should be administered during pregnancy if indicated.

Nosocomial outbreaks have been reported in neonatal intensive care units, but these are rare. Prevention of virus spread is based on contact precautions. With appropriate hygienic precautions, breastfeeding by a mother with HAV infection is permissible. Although immunoglobulin has been administered to newborns if the mother's symptoms began 2 weeks before delivery through 1 week after delivery, the efficacy of this practice has not been established.

Hepatitis B Virus

Hepatitis B virus (HBV) is a small DNA virus that contains three principal antigens: 1) hepatitis B surface antigen (HBsAg), 2) hepatitis B core antigen, and 3) hepatitis B e antigen (HBeAg). People acutely infected with HBV may be asymptomatic or symptomatic. Among people with symptomatic HBV infection, the spectrum of signs and symptoms is varied and includes subacute illness with nonspecific symptoms (eg, anorexia, nausea, or malaise), clinical hepatitis with jaundice, or fulminant hepatitis. Transmission of HBV occurs through contact with infected blood or bodily fluids (ie, semen, cervical secretions, and saliva).

Perinatal transmission of HBV infection is highly efficient and generally occurs from exposure to maternal blood during labor and delivery. If appropriate and timely treatment is not instituted, perinatal infection occurs in 70–90% of infants born to mothers who are both HBsAG positive and HBeAg positive. Transplacental passage of HBV is rare. More than 90% of infants who are infected perinatally will develop chronic HBV infection.

Antepartum Screening and Immunization

Because historical information about risk factors identifies less than one half of chronic carriers, serologic testing for HBsAg is recommended for all pregnant women as part of routine prenatal care. A copy of the original laboratory report should be entered into the patient's medical record at the delivery hospital. Women who have not been screened prenatally, those who are at high risk of infection (eg, intravenous drug users and women with a recurrence of sexually transmitted infections [STIs]), and those with clinical hepatitis should be tested at admission for delivery. Pregnant women with chronic HBV should be informed about transmission risks and ways to prevent newborn infection. Although recent studies have demonstrated potential benefit from antiviral treatment in decreasing the risk of in utero HBV infection in women with high viral loads late in pregnancy, this approach is not yet recommended.

Women who are HBsAg negative but who have risk factors for HBV infection should be offered vaccination during pregnancy. The recommended adult dose of HBV vaccine is 10–20 micrograms (1 mL) injected into the deltoid muscle. A series of three doses is required; the second and third doses are given 1 month and 6 months after the first dose. A two-dose schedule, administered at time zero and again 4–6 months later, is available for adolescents aged 11–15 years using the adult dose of a hepatitis B recombinant vaccine.

Hepatitis B vaccine also is recommended for household contacts and sexual partners of chronic carriers of HBV (ie, those who are positive for HBsAg) unless immunity has previously been demonstrated. Nonimmunized sexual partners of individuals with acute HBV infection should receive a single dose of hepatitis B immune globulin (HBIG) and should begin an HBV vaccine series if their test results are serologically negative.

Neonatal Immunization

Universal HBV immunization is recommended for all neonates. Delivery hospitals should develop policies and procedures that ensure administration of the vaccine as part of the routine care of all medically stable infants weighing at least 2,000 g at birth, unless there is a physician's order to defer immunization and the serologic status of the mother is documented in the infant's medical record. Three intramuscular doses are required to provide effective protection (Table 10-1).

Hepatitis B Surface Antigen-Negative Mother. For neonates born to women who are known to be HBsAg negative, the first 0.5 mL dose of monovalent vaccine should be administered preferably before discharge from the hospital or by 2 months of age. The second dose is given 1–2 months later; and the

Table 10-1. Hepatitis B Immunoprophylaxis Scheme by Infant Birth Weight*

Maternal Status	Infant Birth Weight 2,000 g or More	Infant Birth Weight Less than 2,000 g
HBsAg positive	Hepatitis B vaccine + HBIG (within 12 hours of birth)	Hepatitis B vaccine + HBIG (within 12 hours of birth)
	Continue vaccine series beginning at 1–2 months of age according to recommended schedule for infants born to HBsAg-positive mothers	Continue vaccine series beginning at 1–2 months of age according to recommended schedule for infants born to HBsAg-positive mothers
		Immunize with four vaccine doses; do not count birth dose as part of vaccine series
	Check anti-HBs and HBsAg after completion of vaccine series†	Check anti-HBs and HBsAg after completion of vaccine series†
	HBsAg-negative infants with anti-HBs levels ≥10 mIU/mL are protected and need no further medical management	HBsAg-negative infants with anti-HBs levels ≥10 mIU/mL are protected and need no further medical management
	HBsAg-negative infants with anti-HBs levels <10 mIU/mL should be reimmunized with a second three-dose vaccine series and retested	HBsAg-negative infants with anti-HBs levels <10 mIU/mL should be reimmunized with a second three-dose series and retested
	Infants who are HBsAg positive should receive appropriate follow-up, including medical evaluation for chronic liver disease	Infants who are HBsAg positive should receive appropriate follow-up, including medical evaluation for chronic liver disease

(continued)

Table 10-1. Hepatitis B Immunoprophylaxis Scheme by Infant Birth Weight*
(continued)

Maternal Status	Infant Birth Weight 2,000 g or More	Infant Birth Weight Less than 2,000 g
HBsAg status unknown	Test mother for HBsAg immediately after admission for delivery	Test mother for HBsAg immediately after admission for delivery
	Hepatitis B vaccine (within 12 hours of birth)	Hepatitis B vaccine (within 12 hours of birth)
	Administer HBIG (within 7 days) if mother tests HBsAg positive; if mother's HBsAg status remains unknown, some experts would administer HBIG (within 7 days)	Administer HBIG if mother tests HBsAg positive or if mother's HBsAg result is not available within 12 hours of birth
	Continue the three-dose vaccine series beginning at 1–2 months of age according to recommended schedule based on mother's HBsAg result	Continue vaccine series beginning at 1–2 months of age according to recommended schedule based on mother's HBsAg result
		Immunize with four vaccine doses; do not count birth dose as part of the three-dose vaccine series
HBsAg negative	Hepatitis B vaccine at birth[‡]	Delay first dose of hepatitis B vaccine until 1 month of age or hospital discharge, whichever is first
	Continue vaccine series beginning at 1–2 months of age	Continue the three-dose vaccine series beginning at 2 months of age
	Follow-up anti-HBs and HBsAg testing not needed	Follow-up anti-HBs and HBsAg testing not needed

Abbreviations: HBsAg, hepatitis B surface antigen; HBIG, hepatitis B immune globulin; anti-HBs, antibody to HBsAg.

*Extremes of gestational age and birth weight no longer are a consideration for timing of hepatitis B vaccine doses.

[†]Test at 9–18 months of age, generally at the next well-child visit after completion of the primary series. Use testing method that allows determination of a protective concentration of anti-HBs (10 mIU/mL or greater).

[‡]The first dose may be delayed until after hospital discharge for an infant who weighs 2,000 g or greater and whose mother is HBsAg negative, but only if a physician's order to withhold the birth dose and a copy of the mother's original HBsAg-negative laboratory report are documented in the infant's medical record.

American Academy of Pediatrics. Red book: report of the Committee on Infectious Diseases, 29th. Elk Grove Village (IL): American Academy of Pediatrics; 2012.

third dose, by 6–18 months of age. Alternatively, vaccines can be administered at 2-month intervals, concurrent with other childhood vaccines, at 2, 4, and 6 months of age.

Because of suboptimal immune response in some preterm infants, the current American Academy of Pediatrics recommendation is to delay the start of hepatitis B immunization in low-risk preterm infants (whose mothers are HBsAg negative) who weigh less than 2,000 g at birth until they reach the chronologic age of 30 days, regardless of initial birth weight or gestational age. Preterm infants weighing 2,000 g or more and low birth weight infants who are medically stable and showing consistent weight gain when discharged from the hospital before 30 days of age can receive the first dose of vaccine at the time of discharge. The appropriate dose (Table 10-2) can be given into the anterolateral thigh muscle of neonates.

Hepatitis B Surface Antigen-Positive Mother. Newborns of HBsAg-positive women should receive timely postexposure prophylaxis and follow-up. Both term and preterm infants born to women known to be HBsAg positive should receive one 0.5 mL dose of HBIG within 12 hours of birth and monovalent hepatitis B vaccine. Prophylaxis for exposed newborns can prevent perinatal HBV infection in approximately 95% of neonates when HBIG is given within 12 hours after birth and the three-dose immunization series is completed. The initial dose of HBV vaccine can be administered concurrently with HBIG but should be given at a different site. No special care of the infant is indicated other than removal of maternal blood to avoid the virus contaminating the skin. The second dose of vaccine should be administered at 1–2 months of chronologic age, regardless of the infant's gestational age or birth weight. The third dose should be given at 6 months of age. For preterm infants who weigh less than 2,000 g at birth, the initial vaccine dose is given at birth but is not counted in the required three-dose schedule; therefore, these infants receive four doses: 1) at birth, 2) when their weight reaches 2,000 g or at 2 months of age, 3) 1–2 months later, and 4) at 6 months of age.

At 1–3 months after completion of the immunization schedule for newborns of HBsAg-positive women, testing is indicated to ensure immune response or to identify neonates who have become chronically infected. Breastfeeding of newborns by HBsAg-positive women poses no additional risk for the transmission of HBV.

HBsAg Status Unknown. Newborns of women whose HBsAg status is unknown should receive HBV vaccine within 12 hours of birth in a dose appropriate for neonates born to HBsAg-positive women. The woman's blood should be obtained for testing at hospital admission for delivery. If the woman subsequently is found to be HBsAg positive, the neonate should receive HBIG

Table 10-2. Recommended Dosages of Hepatitis B Vaccines

Patients	Vaccine*		Combination Vaccine
	Recombivax HB† Dose, μg (mL)	Engerix-B‡ Dose, μg (mL)	Twinrix§
Infants of mothers who are HBsAg-negative and children and adolescents younger than 20 years	5 (0.5)	10 (0.5)	Not applicable
Infants of mothers who are HBsAg-positive (HBIG [0.5 mL] also is recommended)	5 (0.5)	10(0.5)	Not applicable
Adults 20 years or older	10 (1.0)	20 (1.0)	20 (1.0)
Adults undergoing dialysis and other immunosuppressed adults	40 (1.0)‖	40 (2.0)¶	Not applicable

Abbreviations: HBsAg, hepatitis B surface antigen; HBIG, hepatitis B immune globulin.

*Both vaccines are administered in a three-dose schedule at 0, 1, and 6 months; four doses may be administered if a birth dose is given and a combination vaccine is used (at 2, 4, and 6 months) to complete the series. Only single-antigen hepatitis B vaccine can be used for the birth dose. Single-antigen or combination vaccine containing hepatitis B vaccine may be used to complete the series.

†Available from Merck & Co Inc.

  • A two-dose schedule, administered at 0 months and then 4 to 6 months later, is licensed for adolescents 11–15 years of age using the adult formulation of Recombivax HB (10 micrograms).

  • A combination of hepatitis B (Recombivax, 5 micrograms) and Haemophilus influenzae type b (PRP-OMP) vaccine is recommended for use at 2, 4, and 12–15 months of age (Comvax). This vaccine should not be administered at birth (before 6 weeks of age) or after 71 months of age.

‡Available from GlaxoSmithKline Biologicals. The U.S. Food and Drug Administration also has licensed this vaccine for use in an optional four-dose schedule at 0, 1, 2, and 12 months for all age groups. A 0-, 12-, and 24-month schedule is licensed for children 5–16 years of age, and a 0-, 1-, and 6-month schedule is licensed for adolescents 11–16 years of age.

  • A combination of diphtheria and tetanus toxoids and acellular pertussis (DTaP), inactivated poliovirus (IPV), and hepatitis B (Engerix-B, 10 micrograms) is recommended for use at 2, 4, and 6 months of age (Pediarix). This vaccine should not be administered at birth (before 6 weeks of age) or at 7 years of age or older.

§A combination of hepatitis B (Engerix-B, 20 micrograms) and hepatitis A (Havrix, 720 enzyme-linked immunosorbent assay units [ELU]) vaccine (Twinrix) is licensed for use in people 18 years of age and older in a three-dose schedule administered at 0 months,1 month, and 6 or more months later. Alternately, a four-dose schedule at days 0, 7, and 21–30 followed by a booster dose at 12 months may be used.

‖Special formulation for adult dialysis patients given at 0, 1, and 6 months.

¶Two 1.0-mL doses given in one or two injections in a four-dose schedule at 0, 1, 2, and 6 months of age.

American Academy of Pediatrics. Red book: report of the Committee on Infectious Diseases, 29th. Elk Grove Village (IL): American Academy of Pediatrics; 2012.

as soon as possible (within 7 days of birth) and should receive the second and third doses of vaccine as recommended for infants of HBsAg-positive women. Both maternal HBsAg test results and the infant's hepatitis vaccine administration should be documented in the infant's medical record.

Hepatitis C Virus

Hepatitis C virus (HCV) is a small RNA virus that has at least six identified, distinct genotypes, with broad geographic variation and widely ranging prognoses for both disease progression and response to therapy. The prevalence of HCV infection in the general population of the United States is estimated to be approximately 1.8% but varies in different populations in proportion to risk factors. The primary known route of transmission is parenteral exposure to blood and blood products from individuals who are infected with HCV. Sexual transmission among monogamous couples is uncommon, as is transmission among family contacts. In most cases, no source can be identified. The risk of maternal–fetal (vertical) transmission of HCV ranges from 2% to 12%. The risk of transmission, which correlates with maternal HCV RNA levels, appears to be increased for women also infected with human immunodeficiency virus (HIV). Neonates infected with HCV usually appear healthy. Of infants perinatally infected, approximately 20% will clear their infection. Maternal HCV infection is not a contraindication to breastfeeding.

Infection with HCV is diagnosed serologically by the presence of HCV antibodies via a third-generation enzyme immunoassay, which has a sensitivity of 97% and specificity of 99%. Positive antibody test results should be confirmed with a more specific anti-HCV assay (ie, recombinant immunoblot assay) or HCV-specific RNA testing and genotyping. Liver enzyme and function tests should be performed in patients with positive test results for the antibodies, because as many as 70% of patients with HCV infection develop chronic liver disease, with cirrhosis ultimately developing in 20–25% of these patients. However, data suggest that liver function tests are not helpful in assessing the development of aggressive hepatitis and cirrhosis.

Children born to HCV-positive women should be tested for HCV infection. However, antibody testing should be deferred until at least 18 months of age, when passively transferred maternal HCV antibodies have decreased below detectable levels. If earlier diagnosis of HCV infection is desired, testing for HCV RNA could be performed at age 1–2 months. Hepatitis C virus RNA testing should then be repeated at a subsequent visit, independent of the initial HCV RNA test result.

Currently, no preventive measures are available to lower the risk of vertical HCV infection in infants. Routine serologic testing during pregnancy for HCV infection is not recommended. Testing should be reserved for women seeking evaluation or care for an STI, including HIV, or whose histories suggest an increased risk of infection, such as blood transfusions before 1990, intravenous drug use, occupational or recreational percutaneous exposure, or mucosal surface blood exposure. The natural history of perinatally acquired hepatitis C infection is the subject of ongoing studies. Immune globulin manufactured in the United States does not contain antibodies to HCV and has no role in postexposure prophylaxis. Immunoglobulin G and antiviral agents are not recommended for postexposure prophylaxis of infants born to women with HCV. Recently, benefits have been demonstrated in nonpregnant adults infected with HCV when treated with pegylated interferon. Benefits in pregnant women or to the fetus and newborn by potentially decreasing vertical transmission await further study.

Herpes Simplex Virus

Herpes simplex virus (HSV) is a DNA virus with two distinct species: HSV type 1 (HSV-1) and HSV type 2 (HSV-2). Most genital infections with HSV are caused by HSV-2. However, genital HSV-1 infections are increasingly recognized as the cause of genital herpes infection. Genital herpes infection is classified as primary when it occurs in a woman with no evidence of prior HSV infection (ie, seronegative for both HSV-1 and HSV-2), as a nonprimary first episode when it occurs in a woman with a history of heterologous infection (eg, first HSV-2 infection in a woman with prior HSV-1 infection or vice versa), and as recurrent when it occurs in a woman with clinical or serologic evidence of prior genital herpes (of the same serotype). In most adults with unequivocal serologic evidence of HSV-2 infection, the infection has not been diagnosed clinically, indicating that most primary infections are asymptomatic.

Antepartum Management

Women who have primary genital HSV infection in late pregnancy (whether symptomatic or asymptomatic) and who give birth vaginally have a high risk (30–50%) of transmitting the virus to their infants. Similarly, nonprimary first-episode HSV infection occurring late in pregnancy also has a high risk of vertical transmission. The risk of transmission during a vaginal delivery is much lower with recurrent infection (less than 2–5%). Currently, most newborns infected with HSV are delivered to women who have asymptomatic or unrecognized infections.

Diagnosis. Although routine antepartum genital cultures for HSV screening are not recommended, all suspected herpes virus infections should be evaluated and confirmed through viral detection techniques (viral culture or PCR viral antigen detection) or by type-specific serologic antibody testing. For patients who do not present with active lesions or whose lesions have negative culture or PCR test results, type-specific serologic assays that accurately distinguish between HSV-1 and HSV-2 antibodies can be useful in confirming a clinical diagnosis of genital herpes. Valid type-specific assays for HSV antibodies must be based upon HSV-specific glycoprotein G. The U.S. Food and Drug Administration has approved several such assays (refer to www.fda.gov for a current list). Routine antepartum genital HSV cultures in asymptomatic patients with a recurrence of disease are not recommended.

Antiviral Therapy. At the time of the outbreak of a primary herpes infection, antiviral treatment may be administered orally to pregnant women to reduce the duration and the severity of the symptoms as well as reduce the duration of viral shedding. The efficacy of suppressive therapy during pregnancy to prevent recurrences near term has been evaluated in numerous studies. In pregnant women near term, acyclovir use has been found to reduce the risk of clinical HSV recurrence at delivery and decrease both HSV shedding at delivery and the rate of cesarean delivery for a recurrence of genital herpes. Women with a history of a recurrence of genital herpes should be offered suppressive viral therapy at or beyond 36 weeks of gestation. Acyclovir can be administered orally to pregnant women with first-episode genital herpes or a severe recurrence of herpes, and intravenous administration is indicated for pregnant women with severe genital HSV infection or with disseminated herpetic infections.

Patient Counseling on Prevention. All pregnant women and their partners should be asked about a history of genital HSV infection. Couples should be educated about the natural history of genital HSV infection and should be advised that, if either partner is infected, they should abstain from sexual contact while lesions or prodromes are present. To minimize the risk of sexual transmission, use of condoms is recommended for HSV-infected individuals when asymptomatic. However, protection provided by condoms is incomplete (estimated to be approximately 50% effective). Susceptible pregnant women should avoid sexual contact during the last 6–8 weeks of gestation if their partners have active genital HSV infections. In addition, oral–genital sexual contact should be avoided in the latter weeks of pregnancy to avoid acquisition of HSV-1 in susceptible individuals.

Intrapartum Management

Women with a history of genital HSV infection should be questioned about recent symptoms and should undergo careful examination of the perineum before delivery. If no lesions are observed, infants can be delivered vaginally. A detailed examination of the cervix is not required because recurrent infections rarely cause isolated cervical lesions.

Cesarean delivery is indicated for all women with active genital HSV lesions or with a typical herpetic prodrome at the time of delivery. In patients with active HSV infection and ruptured membranes at or near term, a cesarean delivery should be performed as soon as the necessary personnel and equipment can be readied. In active HSV infection and premature rupture of membranes remote from term, there is no consensus on the gestational age at which the risks of prematurity outweigh the risks of HSV. When expectant management is elected, treatment with an antiviral drug may be considered. Local neonatal infection can result from the use of fetal scalp electrode monitoring in patients with a history of herpes, even when maternal lesions are not present. However, if there are indications for fetal scalp monitoring, it may be appropriate in a woman who has a history of HSV recurrence and no active lesions.

Contact precautions, use of gown or gloves, and covering of all lesions (in addition to standard precautions), should be used for women with clinically evident or serologically confirmed primary genital HSV infection or nongenital HSV infection in the labor, delivery, recovery, and postpartum care areas. For a recurrence of mucocutaneous lesions, standard precautions are sufficient. Infected family members and others in contact with the infant also should use contact precautions. Health care personnel and the woman herself should use gloves for direct contact with the infected area or with contaminated dressings, and meticulous handwashing is essential. Labor, delivery, recovery rooms require only routine, careful cleaning and disinfection before using the rooms for other patients.

Neonatal Diagnosis

Most neonatal infections are caused by HSV-2, although infection with HSV-1 also can occur. Most infants who develop HSV infection acquire the infection during passage through the infected maternal lower genital tract or by ascending infection to the fetus, sometimes even though membranes apparently are intact. Less common sources of neonatal infection include postnatal transmission from the parents, hospital personnel, or other close contact, most often from a nongenital infection (eg, mouth, hands, or around the breasts).

Uncommonly, intrauterine transmission occurs, and signs of infection appear within 48 hours of birth.

Infants Born to Women With Active Lesions at Delivery. Infants born vaginally to women with active lesions require close observation. Specimens for HSV cultures should be obtained at 24 hours after birth from skin lesions, conjunctiva, nasopharynx, mouth, and rectum in healthy appearing newborns exposed to HSV. If skin lesions are present, blood buffy coat and cerebrospinal fluid HSV cultures should be obtained. Cerebrospinal fluid also should be studied by PCR, which is a sensitive method for detecting HSV DNA. Acyclovir therapy should be initiated if the infant has clinical signs of infection, the cultures or PCR test results are positive, or if HSV infection is otherwise strongly suspected.

Some experts recommend empiric treatment with acyclovir for infants born vaginally to a mother with symptomatic primary herpes infection, pending results of cultures, although no data exist to support the efficacy of this approach. Other experts recommend awaiting positive culture results or clinical manifestations of infection before starting acyclovir therapy if the mother has a prior history of genital herpes infection. Parents and physicians should be educated about the signs and symptoms of neonatal HSV infection, which include vesicular lesions of the skin, respiratory distress, seizures, or signs of sepsis. A newborn with any of these manifestations should be evaluated immediately for possible HSV infection and treated pending results of the evaluation.

Infants born vaginally (or by cesarean delivery if membranes have ruptured) to women with active HSV lesions should be physically separated from other infants and managed with contact precautions if they remain in the nursery during the incubation period; an isolation room is not essential. Alternatively, the infant may stay with the mother in a private room after the mother has been instructed on proper preventive care to reduce postpartum transmission.

Infants Born to Asymptomatic Women With History of Genital Herpes. The risk of HSV infection is extremely low in infants born vaginally to asymptomatic women with a history of a recurrence of genital herpes and in those born to symptomatic women by cesarean delivery before rupture of membranes. Infants born by cesarean delivery to women with herpetic lesions with intact membranes should be cultured for HSV, as recommended previously for infants exposed by vaginal delivery, and should also be observed. The length of in-hospital observation is empirical and is based on risk factors, local resources, and access to adequate follow-up. Special isolation precautions are not needed for these infants. Parents should be instructed to report early signs of infection. Antiviral therapy should be initiated if culture results from the infant are positive or if HSV infection is strongly suspected for other reasons.

Neonatal Treatment

Cultures obtained from the eye, mouth, or rectum of infants born to women who are known or who are strongly suspected of being infected with HSV can assist in management decisions. A positive culture obtained 24 hours or more after delivery suggests HSV infection and is an indication for immediate institution of acyclovir therapy, even in the absence of symptoms. The dosage of acyclovir is 60 mg/kg per day in three divided doses, given intravenously for 14 days for disease of the skin, eyes, and mouth and for 21 days in central nervous system disease or disseminated disease. Of treated infants, 5–10% will develop recurrent disease requiring retreatment in the first month of life. Six months of oral acyclovir suppressive therapy for infants with clinical HSV infection (skin, eyes, mouth, or CNS) has been demonstrated to reduce the risk of a recurrence of HSV infection.

Infants with HSV disease should be managed in a facility that provides neonatal intensive care and consultation with an infectious diseases specialist. The infant should be physically segregated and managed with contact precautions for the duration of the illness; an isolation room is desirable.

Although HSV infection is more likely to occur at a site of skin trauma, no data indicate that the circumcision of male infants who may have been exposed to HSV at birth should be postponed. It may be prudent, however, to delay circumcision for approximately 1 month in infants at the highest risk of disease (eg, infants delivered vaginally to women with active genital lesions).

Contact of Infants With Infected Mothers

A woman with active HSV infection should be taught about her infection and about hygienic measures to prevent postpartum transmission of herpes to her infant. Before touching her newborn, the woman should wash her hands carefully and use a clean barrier to ensure that the infant does not come into contact with lesions or potentially infectious material. If the woman has genital HSV infection, her infant can room with her after she has been instructed in protective measures. Breastfeeding is permissible if the woman has no vesicular herpetic lesions in the breast area and other active cutaneous lesions are covered.

A woman with herpes labialis (cold sore) or stomatitis should not kiss or nuzzle her infant until the lesions have cleared. Careful hand hygiene is important. She should wear a disposable surgical mask when she touches her infant until the lesions have crusted and dried. Herpetic lesions on other skin sites should be covered. Direct contact of an infant with other family members or friends who have active HSV infection should be avoided.

Human Immunodeficiency Virus

Acquired immunodeficiency syndrome (AIDS) is caused by HIV type 1 (HIV-1) and, less commonly, HIV type 2 (HIV-2), a related virus. Human immunodeficiency virus type 2 is extremely uncommon in the United States but is more common in West Africa and South America.

Transmission

Human immunodeficiency virus has been isolated from blood (including lymphocytes, macrophages, and plasma), cerebrospinal fluid, pleural fluid, human milk, semen, cervical secretions, saliva, urine, and tears. However, only blood, semen, cervical secretions, and human milk have been implicated epidemiologically in the transmission of infection. Well-documented modes of HIV transmission in the United States are sexual contact (both heterosexual and homosexual), skin penetration by contaminated needles or other sharp instruments, transfusion of contaminated blood products, and mother-to-infant transmission during pregnancy, around the time of labor and delivery, and postnatally through breastfeeding. Cases of probable HIV transmission from HIV-infected caregivers to their infants through feeding blood-tinged premasticated food have been reported in the United States.

Before effective perinatal HIV interventions, the risk of infection for a neonate born to an HIV seropositive mother was approximately 25% (range, 13–39%). All pregnant women who are infected with HIV should be offered antiretroviral drug regimens, which will likely decrease the HIV viral load to undetectable levels.

The exact timing of transmission from an infected mother to her infant is uncertain. Evidence suggests that in the absence of breastfeeding, 30% of transmission occurs before birth and 70% occurs around the time of delivery.

Antepartum Management

Clear medical benefits are derived from pregnant women knowing their HIV serostatus. Demonstrated benefits include early diagnosis and treatment to delay active disease in women and significant reduction in perinatal transmission through early treatment.

Prenatal Screening. All pregnant women should be told that HIV screening is recommended during pregnancy and that an HIV test is part of the routine panel of prenatal tests unless it is declined (opt-out screening). If a woman declines HIV testing, this should be documented in the medical record. Repeat testing in the third trimester (preferably before 36 weeks of gestation) is recommended for women in areas with a high HIV prevalence, women known to be at high risk of acquiring HIV infection, and women who declined testing earlier in pregnancy. In some states, it is necessary to obtain the woman's written authorization before disclosing her HIV status to health care providers who are not members of her health care team. Obstetrician–gynecologists should be aware of and comply with their states' legal requirements for perinatal HIV screening.

The conventional HIV testing algorithm, which may take up to 2 weeks to complete if a result is positive, begins with a screening test, the enzyme-linked immunosorbent assay (ELISA) that detects antibodies to HIV; if the test results are positive, a confirmatory test (either a Western blot or an immunofluorescence assay) is performed. If the ELISA test result is positive and the Western blot or immunofluorescence assay test result is negative, the woman is not infected and repeat testing is not indicated.

If the screening and confirmatory test results are both positive, the patient should be given her results in person. The implications of HIV infection and vertical transmission should be discussed with the patient. Additional laboratory evaluation, including CD4 count, HIV viral load, HIV antiretroviral resistance testing, hepatitis C virus antibody, HBsAg, complete blood count with platelet count, and baseline chemistries with liver function tests, will be useful before prescribing antiretroviral prophylaxis. Coordination of care of the mother and fetus should be done in consultation with an infectious disease or obstetric infectious disease specialist.

Maternal Antiretroviral Therapy. Combination antiretroviral drug regimens that maximally suppress viral replication are recommended for HIV-1 infected adults. Pregnancy does not preclude the use of these standard antiretroviral regimens. Offering antiretroviral therapy to infected women during pregnancy, either to treat HIV-1 infection or to reduce perinatal transmission or both, should be accompanied by discussion of the known and unknown short-term and long-term benefits and risks of such therapy for affected women and their infants. It is recommended that zidovudine chemoprophylaxis be included in the antiretroviral combination regimen, except in cases of known intolerance. No significant short-term adverse effects have been observed from zidovudine use other than mild, self-limited anemia in the infants. In addition, infants have been monitored for several years and no untoward effects of zidovudine have been observed.

Current recommendations for adults are that plasma viral load determinations be done at baseline and every 3 months or after changes in therapy. Additionally, CD4+ T-lymphocyte counts should be monitored during pregnancy. Because of the rapid advances in this area, refer to the Centers for Disease Control and Prevention (CDC) (www.cdc.gov) and the U.S. Department of Health and Human Services AIDSinfo web sites (http://www.aidsinfo.nih.gov/) for treatment recommendations.

Intrapartum Management

As noted, a substantial proportion of neonatal HIV cases occur as a result of exposure to the virus during labor and delivery. Intrapartum strategies to prevent mother-to-child transmission include rapid HIV antibody testing for women with unknown HIV status during labor and delivery; administration of antepartum, intrapartum, and neonatal antiretroviral prophylaxis; and cesarean delivery performed before the onset of labor and before rupture of membranes in women with viral loads of more than 1,000 copies per milliliter.

Rapid HIV Testing. Any woman whose HIV status is unknown during labor and delivery should be given a rapid HIV test, unless she declines (opt-out screening), in order to provide an opportunity to begin prophylaxis before delivery. A negative rapid HIV test result is definitive. A positive HIV test result is not definitive and must be confirmed with a supplemental test, such as a Western blot test or immunofluorescence assay.

If the rapid HIV test result at labor and delivery is positive, the obstetric provider should take the following seven steps:

1. Tell the woman she may have HIV infection and that her infant also may be exposed.

2. Explain that the rapid test result is preliminary and that false-positive test results are possible.

3. Assure the woman that a second test is being done right away to confirm the positive rapid test result.

4. Immediate initiation of antiretroviral prophylaxis should be recommended without waiting for the results of the confirmatory test to reduce the risk of transmission to the infant.

5. Once the woman gives birth, discontinue maternal antiretroviral therapy until the result of the confirmatory test is known.

6. Tell the woman that she should postpone breastfeeding until the confirmatory result is available because she should not breastfeed if she is infected with HIV.

7. Inform pediatric care providers (depending on state requirements) of positive maternal test results so that they may institute the appropriate neonatal prophylaxis.

Route of Delivery. A viral load obtained late in the third trimester is useful to guide the decision concerning mode of delivery. Consistent results indicating a significant relationship between route of delivery, viral load, and vertical transmission of HIV have been published. This body of evidence indicates that when care includes scheduled cesarean delivery (performed before the onset of labor and before the rupture of membranes) and zidovudine therapy, the likelihood of vertical transmission of HIV is reduced to approximately 2%. There are insufficient data to demonstrate a benefit of cesarean delivery performed after the onset of labor or rupture of membranes. Thus, a scheduled cesarean delivery at 38 weeks of gestation without an amniocentesis for lung maturity is recommended for all HIV-1 infected pregnant women with viral loads greater than 1,000 copies per milliliter near the time of delivery (or who have an unknown viral load), whether or not they are receiving antiretroviral prophylaxis. It is clear that the rate of maternal morbidity is higher with cesarean delivery than with vaginal delivery. However, the benefit to the infant outweighs the increased maternal morbidity associated with cesarean delivery (see also "Cesarean Delivery" in Chapter 6).

Women with plasma viral loads less than 1,000 copies per milliliter have a low risk of vertical transmission (less than 2%), even without routine use of scheduled cesarean delivery. There are not enough data to demonstrate a benefit of scheduled cesarean delivery for women with plasma viral loads of less than 1,000 copies per milliliter. The decision regarding route of delivery in these circumstances must be individualized. The patient's autonomy in making the decision regarding route of delivery must be respected.

Because HIV may be present in blood, vaginal secretions, amniotic fluid, and other fluids, standard precautions should be followed strictly during all vaginal and cesarean deliveries. Gloves should be used when handling the infant until blood and amniotic fluid have been removed from the infant's skin.

Postpartum Management

After delivery, HIV infected women can receive care in the postpartum care unit, with the use of standard precautions. Human immunodeficiency virus RNA has been detected in both the cellular and cell-free fractions of human breast milk, and breastfeeding has been implicated in the transmission of HIV infection. Women in developed countries who are infected with HIV should be counseled not to breastfeed their babies, and they should not donate to milk banks. Obstetric providers may need to refer women who are infected with HIV to another health care provider with special expertise in HIV infection for continuing medical care after pregnancy. Few infants with HIV infection show clinical evidence of infection in the first weeks after delivery.

To minimize risk to health care personnel, routine standard precautions should be used when caring for the infant. Prompt and careful removal of blood from the infant's skin is important. There is no need for other special precautions or for isolation of the infant from an HIV-infected mother; rooming-in is acceptable. Gloves should be worn for contact with blood or blood-containing fluids, for procedures that entail exposure to blood and for diaper changes.

Evaluation and Management of Exposed Newborns

Screening and Antiretroviral Prophylaxis. Newborn infants born to women who are HIV-infected or whose HIV status is unknown should have a rapid antibody test performed as soon as possible after birth and receive postpartum antiretroviral drugs within 12 hours of birth to reduce the risk of perinatal HIV-1 transmission. Because of possible contamination with maternal blood (and a high incidence of false-positive test results), umbilical cord blood should not be used for this determination. If the result is positive, a confirmatory test should be performed. If the confirmatory test result is negative, antiretroviral drugs should be stopped. For infants with a positive confirmatory test result, a 6-week course of zidovudine is recommended. Infants born to HIV-infected women who did not receive antiretroviral therapy before the onset of labor should receive a 2-drug prophylaxis regimen.

Maternal health information should be reviewed to determine if the infant may have been exposed to maternal coinfections (such as tuberculosis, syphilis, toxoplasmosis, hepatitis B or hepatitis C, cytomegalovirus, or HSV), and diagnostic testing and treatment of coinfections in the infant should be based on maternal findings and evaluation of the infant. Immunizations and tuberculosis screening should be given in accordance with current published guidelines. Both mother and infant should have prescriptions for HIV drugs when they leave the hospital, and the infant should have an appointment for a postnatal visit at 2–4 weeks of age to monitor medication adherence and to screen the infant for anemia from zidovudine therapy. Pediatricians should provide counseling to parents and caregivers of HIV-1 exposed infants about HIV-1 infection, including anticipatory guidance on the course of illness, infection-control measures, care of the infant, diagnostic tests, and potential drug toxicities.

Diagnostic Testing. Because passively transferred maternal HIV-1 antibodies may be detectable in an exposed but uninfected infant's bloodstream until 18 months of age, assays that directly detect HIV-1 DNA or RNA (generically referred to as HIV-1 nucleic acid amplification tests [NAATs]) represent the preferred method of diagnostic testing of infants and young children younger than 18 months. Approximately 30–40% of HIV-infected infants will have a positive HIV DNA PCR assay result in samples obtained before 48 hours of age. A positive result by 48 hours of age suggests in utero transmission. Approximately 93% of infected infants have detectable HIV DNA by 2 weeks of age, and approximately 95% of HIV-infected infants have a positive HIV DNA PCR assay result by 1 month of age.

All HIV-1 exposed infants should undergo virologic testing with HIV-1 DNA or RNA assays at 14–21 days of life, and if results are negative, the tests should be repeated at 1–2 months of age and again at 4–6 months of age. An infant is considered infected if two separate samples test positive. For infants with negative virologic test results, many experts confirm the absence of HIV-1 infection with HIV-1 antibody assay testing at 12–18 months of age. If infection is confirmed, a pediatric HIV specialist should be consulted for advice regarding antiretroviral therapy and care.

Pneumocystis jiroveci pneumonia prophylaxis. *Pneumocystis jiroveci* pneumonia is the most common opportunistic infection in HIV-1 infected infants and children. All HIV-1 exposed infants should be considered for prophylaxis beginning at 4–6 weeks of age. Infants in whom HIV-1 is diagnosed should be given prophylaxis until 1 year of age, at which time reassessment is made on the basis of age-specific CD4+ T-lymphocyte count and percentage thresholds. Infants with indeterminate HIV-1 infection status should receive prophylaxis starting at 4–6 weeks of age until they are deemed to be presumptively or definitively uninfected.

Human Papillomavirus

Infections caused by the human papillomavirus (HPV) are common. More than 100 types of HPV exist, more than 40 of which can infect the genital area. Infection with certain HPV types can cause genital warts and a recurrence of respiratory papillomatosis (eg, HPV-6 and HPV-11) as well as cervical and anogenital carcinomas (eg, HPV-16 and HPV-18). Most cervical HPV infections are transient. Persistent infection is more likely with oncogenic types. Cervical or vaginal HPV infections usually are asymptomatic. Pap tests are less useful for the diagnosis of subclinical cervical infection. Most genital HPV infections are sexually transmitted.

Genital HPV infections may be exacerbated during pregnancy. Papillary lesions (condylomata acuminata) may proliferate on the vulva and in the vagina, and lesions can become increasingly friable during pregnancy. Cryotherapy, laser therapy, and trichloroacetic acid can be used safely to treat genital HPV infection in pregnancy. Imiquimod, sinecatechins, podophyllin, and podofilox should not be used during pregnancy because they may be toxic to the fetus. Fetal death has been reported after treating the mother with large topical doses of podophyllin. Currently, there are two FDA-approved vaccines shown to be effective in preventing HPV infection in adolescents and young adults. HPV vaccines have not been shown to have a harmful effect on pregnancy when inadvertent administration occurs, but pregnant women should not be vaccinated. If a woman discovers she is pregnant during the vaccine schedule, she should delay completing the three-dose series until after she gives birth. Women who are breastfeeding can receive the vaccine.

The risk that an infant born to a mother who has a genital HPV infection will develop subsequent respiratory papillomatosis is very small. These lesions are thought to result from aspiration of infectious secretions during passage through the birth canal. Because the risk of respiratory papillomatosis is so low, cesarean delivery is not recommended for the sole purpose of protecting the infant from HPV infection. In women with extensive condylomata, however, cesarean delivery may be necessary because of poor vaginal or vulvar distensibility and the related increased likelihood of extensive vulvovaginal lacerations. Infants born to mothers with HPV infection should receive routine care in the nursery.

Influenza Virus

Influenza A and influenza B viruses are the main types of human influenza virus that are responsible for seasonal influenza epidemics each year. During the course of influenza season, different types and subtypes of influenza viruses can circulate and cause illness. Influenza viruses are spread from person to person primarily through hand-to-hand contact and large-particle respiratory droplet transmission. Contact with respiratory-droplet contaminated surfaces is another possible source of transmission. Uncomplicated influenza illness is characterized by the abrupt onset of constitutional and respiratory signs and symptoms (eg, fever, myalgia, headache, malaise, nonproductive cough, sore throat, and rhinitis) and typically resolves after 3–7 days, but malaise can persist for up to 14 days.

Pregnant women and young children are at greater risk of serious influenza complications, which can include influenza or secondary bacterial pneumonia, ear infections, sinus infections, dehydration, and worsening of chronic medical conditions, such as congestive heart failure, asthma, or diabetes. Pregnant women also have higher mortality and hospitalization rates than nonpregnant women. Preventing influenza during pregnancy is an essential element of prenatal care, and the most effective strategy for preventing influenza is annual immunization. Immunizing pregnant women against seasonal influenza can protect the mother and is associated with reduced febrile respiratory viral illness in her infant. Obstetrician–gynecologists are an important source of information and advice on immunization for pregnant women and play a crucial role in recommending influenza vaccine to every pregnant woman.

The seasonal trivalent inactivated influenza vaccine is safe for pregnant women and their unborn infants and can be given during any trimester. The CDC Advisory Committee on Immunization Practices recommends that all women who are pregnant during influenza season (October through May in the United States) receive the trivalent inactivated influenza vaccine at any point in gestation. Regardless of gestational age, vaccination early in the season is optimal. Live attenuated influenza vaccine is contraindicated for pregnant women.

No study to date has shown an adverse consequence of the inactivated influenza vaccine in pregnant women or their offspring. Thimerosal, a mercury-containing preservative used in multidose vials of influenza vaccine, has not been shown to cause any adverse effects except for occasional local skin reactions. There is no scientific evidence that thimerosal-containing vaccines cause adverse effects in children born to women who received vaccines with thimerosal. Hence, the Advisory Committee on Immunization Practices does not indicate a preference for thimerosal-containing or thimerosal-free vaccines for any group, including pregnant women. In addition to the benefits of immunization for pregnant women, a prospective, controlled, randomized trial demonstrated fewer cases of laboratory-confirmed influenza in infants whose mothers had been immunized compared with women in the control group, as well as fewer cases of respiratory illness with fever. Maternal immunity is the only effective strategy in newborns because the vaccine is not approved for use in infants younger than 6 months.

Infants born to mothers with a suspected influenza infection should room in with their mothers. Those requiring hospitalization in the neonatal intensive care units should be placed in an isolation room and given routine supportive care. All health care professionals who care for high-risk newborns should receive seasonal influenza vaccine annually as soon as the vaccine becomes available. Antiviral chemoprophylaxis can be used in infected family members or health care providers who are unimmunized and who are likely to have ongoing close exposure to infants who are younger than 12 months. Because antiviral resistance patterns can change over time, antiviral drug recommendations are updated regularly. Physicians are advised to monitor local antiviral resistance surveillance data and visit the CDC's "Vaccines & Immunizations" web page (http://www.cdc.gov/vaccines/) for current immunization information and recommendations. Additional health care provider and patient immunization information and resources are available on the American College of Obstetrician and Gynecologists' "Immunization for Women" web site, which can be accessed at http://www.immunizationforwomen.org.

Human Parvovirus

Parvovirus B19 is a DNA virus that causes childhood exanthem erythema infectiosum, also known as fifth disease. Transmission most commonly occurs through respiratory secretions and hand-to-mouth contact. In immunocompetent adults, the most common symptoms of parvovirus B19 infection are a reticular rash on the trunk and peripheral arthropathy, although approximately 33% of infections are asymptomatic. Most individuals experience mild infection and have a complete recovery.

Perinatal Transmission

Parvovirus B19 infects fetal erythroid precursors and causes anemia, which can lead to nonimmune hydrops, isolated pleural and pericardial effusions, intrauterine growth restriction, and death. Parents should be reassured that although the rate of intrauterine transmission is high (approximately 50%), the risk of fetal death is between 2% and 6%, and most infected infants are healthy at birth. More than one half of pregnant women are immune to parvovirus B19. In most cases of B19 infection during pregnancy, the fetus is not affected. Most reported maternal infections that have resulted in fetal death occur between the 10th week and 20th week of pregnancy, and fetal death and spontaneous abortion usually have occurred 4–6 weeks after infection. Congenital anomalies caused by parvovirus have been reported in small series and rare case reports. However, the determination that parvovirus is a teratogen remains unproven at this time.

Diagnosis and Management

Because of widespread asymptomatic parvovirus infection in adults and children, all women are at some risk of exposure, particularly those exposed to school-aged children. Pregnant women who learn that they have been exposed to parvovirus B19 should be counseled about the potential risk to the fetus and have serologic testing (ELISA, and Western blot tests) to determine if they are immune. If they are nonimmune, the test should be repeated in 3–4 weeks and paired samples tested to document whether the woman becomes seropositive for parvovirus.

If seroconversion does occur, the fetus should be monitored for 10 weeks by serial ultrasound examination to evaluate for the presence of hydrops fetalis, placentomegaly, and growth disturbances. If hydrops fetalis develops, percutaneous umbilical blood sampling should be performed to determine the fetal hematocrit, leukocyte and platelet count, and viral DNA in preparation for supportive care.

Prevention

In view of the high prevalence of parvovirus B19 seropositive women, the low risk of ill effects to the fetus, and the fact that avoidance of childcare or teaching can reduce but not eliminate the risk of infection, pregnant women should not be excluded from workplaces where B19 is present. Pregnant health care workers should be aware that otherwise healthy patients with erythema infectiosum are contagious the week before, but not after the onset of rash. In contrast, patients who are immunocompromised or who have a hemoglobinopathy remain contagious from before the onset of symptoms through the time of the rash. Routine infection control practices, such as standard precautions and droplet precautions, reduce transmission.

Respiratory Syncytial Virus

Respiratory syncytial virus (RSV), an RNA virus of the family Paramyxoviridae, is a common cause of respiratory infection in infancy and the most common cause of hospitalization for lower respiratory illness in infants. Characteristics that increase the risk of severe RSV lower respiratory tract illness are preterm birth; cyanotic or complicated congenital heart disease, especially conditions causing pulmonary hypertension; chronic lung disease; and immunodeficiency disease or therapy causing immunosuppression at any age.

Transmission

Respiratory syncytial virus usually occurs in annual fall and winter epidemics and during early spring in temperate climates. Spread among household and child care contacts, including adults, is common. Transmission usually is by direct or close contact with contaminated secretions, which may occur from exposure to large-particle droplets at short distances (less than 3 feet) or fomites. Enforcement of infection-control policies is important to decrease the risk of health care-related transmission of RSV.

Diagnosis and Treatment

Rapid diagnostic assays, including immunofluorescent and enzyme immunoassay techniques for detection of viral antigen in nasopharyngeal specimens, are available commercially and generally are reliable in infants and young children. Primary treatment is supportive and should include hydration, careful clinical assessment of respiratory status, including measurement of oxygen saturation, use of supplemental oxygen, suction of the upper airway, and if necessary, intubation and mechanical ventilation.

Prophylaxis

Prophylaxis to prevent RSV in infants at increased risk of severe disease, particularly those with chronic lung disease receiving medical management on a long-term basis, is available using an intramuscular monoclonal antibody—palivizumab. Prophylaxis with palivizumab decreases the risk of severe RSV disease and hospitalization by approximately 50%. Palivizumab is administered as a maximum of three to five monthly intramuscular injections (15 mg/kg per dose) during RSV season, with the first dose typically administered in November in North America. The current American Academy of Pediatrics' recommendations for RSV prophylaxis are listed here and summarized in Table 10-3:

- Infants with chronic lung disease. In order to be considered a candidate for RSV prophylaxis, infants with chronic lung disease require ongoing medical management (eg, supplemental oxygen, diuretics, corticosteroids, bronchodilator therapy) within 6 months before the onset of RSV season. Those with more severe chronic lung disease may benefit from prophylaxis for two RSV seasons.

- Infants without chronic lung disease who were less than 32 weeks of gestation at birth. Infants born at 29–32 weeks of gestation may benefit from prophylaxis up to 6 months of age, whereas those born at 28 weeks of gestation or younger may benefit from prophylaxis up to 12 months of age.

- Infants without chronic lung disease who were 32 0/7–34 6/7 weeks of gestation at birth. Respiratory syncytial virus prophylaxis should be limited to infants who are at greatest risk of hospitalization due to RSV, namely infants younger than 3 months of age at the onset of the RSV season or born during the RSV season and who are likely to have an increased risk of exposure to RSV. Epidemiologic data suggest that RSV infection is more likely to occur and more likely to lead to hospitalization for infants in this gestational age group when either of the following two risk factors is present: 1) infant attends child care or 2) has a sibling or child living in the home who is younger than 5 years of age. Infants in this gestational age category should receive prophylaxis until they reach the age of 3 months. Palivizumab should not be given beyond 90 days of age in these infants. Therefore, this group should receive a maximum of three monthly injections.

- Infants with congenital heart disease. Infants with hemodynamically significant congenital heart disease should receive palivizumab throughout RSV season and may benefit from prophylaxis for two RSV seasons.

Respiratory syncytial virus can be transmitted in the hospital setting and may cause serious disease in high-risk newborns. The major means to prevent RSV disease in the hospital is strict observance of infection control practices, including identifying and cohorting RSV-infected patients. Palivizumab is not indicated as a control measure for hospital outbreaks of RSV infection.

A critical aspect of RSV prevention is parent education about the importance of avoiding exposure to and transmission of the virus. Preventive measures include limiting, when feasible, exposure to contagious settings, such as child care centers. The importance of hand hygiene should be emphasized in all settings, including the home.

Rubella

Rubella virus is an RNA virus that can manifest clinically as postnatal rubella or congenital rubella syndrome. Before widespread use of rubella vaccine, rubella

Table 10-3. Maximum Number of Monthly Doses of Palivizumab for Respiratory Syncytial Virus Prophylaxis

Infants Eligible for a Maximum of Five Doses	Infants Eligible for a Maximum of Three Doses
Infants younger than 24 months with chronic lung disease and requiring medical therapy	Preterm infants with gestational age of 32 weeks, 0 days to 34 weeks, 6 days with at least one risk factor, and born 3 months before or during RSV season
Infants younger than 24 months and requiring medical therapy for congenital heart disease	
Preterm infants born at 31 weeks, 6 days of gestation or less	
Certain infants with neuromuscular disease or congenital abnormalities of the airways	

Abbreviation: RSV, respiratory syncytial virus.

Policy statements—Modified recommendations for use of palivizumab for prevention of respiratory syncytial virus infections. American Academy of Pediatrics Committee on Infectious Diseases. Pediatrics 2009;124: 1694-701.

was an epidemic disease. More recently, infection has occurred in foreign-born or underimmunized people, because endemic rubella has been eliminated from the United States. Clinical disease usually is mild and characterized by a generalized erythematous maculopapular rash, lymphadenopathy, and slight fever.

Maternal rubella during pregnancy can result in miscarriage, fetal death, or congenital rubella syndrome. The most common manifestations associated with congenital rubella syndrome are ophthalmologic (cataracts, pigmentary retinopathy, microphthalmos, and congenital glaucoma), cardiac (patent ductus arteriosus, peripheral pulmonary artery stenosis), auditory (sensorineural hearing impairment), and neurologic (behavioral disorders, meningoencephalitis, and mental retardation). Mild forms of congenital rubella syndrome can be associated with few or no obvious clinical manifestations at birth.

Antepartum Management

Surveillance for susceptibility to rubella infection is essential in prenatal care. Each patient should have serologic screening for rubella immunity at the first prenatal visit unless she is known to be immune by previous serologic testing. Seropositive women do not need further testing, regardless of their subsequent history of exposure. If a seronegative pregnant woman is exposed to rubella or develops symptoms that suggest infection, she should be retested for rubella-specific antibody. Specimens should be obtained as soon as possible after exposure, again 2 weeks later, and, if necessary, 4 weeks after exposure. Acute and chronic serum specimens should be tested on the same day in the same laboratory. Detection of rubella-specific IgM antibodies usually indicates recent infection, but false-positive test results occur. Isolation of the virus from throat swabs establishes a diagnosis of acute rubella.

If rubella is diagnosed in a pregnant woman, she should be advised of the risks of fetal infection; the choice of pregnancy termination should be discussed. Structural malformation may be caused by infection during embryogenesis, and although fetal infection may occur throughout pregnancy, defects are rare when infection occurs after the 20th week of gestation.

The rubella vaccine is a live-attenuated virus and is highly effective with few adverse effects. However, rubella vaccination is not recommended during pregnancy. Women found to be susceptible during pregnancy should be offered vaccination postpartum and before discharge from the hospital. Breastfeeding is not a contradiction to receiving the rubella vaccine. After immunization, women should be advised to avoid conception for 1 month. However, a woman who conceives within 1 month of rubella vaccination or who is inadvertently vaccinated in early pregnancy should be counseled that the teratogenic risk to the fetus is theoretic. Although asymptomatic fetal infection can occur, no case of congenital rubella syndrome has arisen from a woman given the current rubella vaccine (human diploid vaccine RA 27/3) during pregnancy. Therefore, receipt of the rubella vaccine during pregnancy is not an indication for termination of pregnancy. All suspected cases of congenital rubella syndrome, whether caused by wild-type virus or vaccine virus infection, should be reported to local and state health departments. A pregnant household member is not a contraindication to vaccination of a child.

Neonatal Management

Infants who show signs of congenital rubella infection or who were born to women with a history of rubella during pregnancy should be managed with contact isolation. Care of the infant should be restricted to personnel who are immune to rubella. Efforts should be made to obtain viral cultures from the infant to document the infection. Affected infants should be considered contagious until 1 year of age unless nasopharyngeal and urine cultures (after 3 months of age) are repeatedly negative for the rubella virus.

Varicella Zoster Virus

Varicella zoster virus (VZV) is a highly contagious DNA herpesvirus that is transmitted by respiratory droplets or close contact. The primary infection causes chickenpox, which is characterized by fever, malaise, and a maculopapular pruritic rash that becomes vesicular. The disease usually is a benign and self-limited illness in children; severe complications, such as encephalitis and pneumonia, are more common in adults than in children. After the primary infection, VZV remains dormant in sensory ganglia and can be reactivated to cause a vesicular erythematous skin rash known as herpes zoster. The antibody to VZV develops within a few days after the onset of infection, and prior infection with VZV confers lifelong immunity.

Varicella in pregnant women can result in VZV transmission to the fetus or newborn. Intrauterine VZV infection can cause congenital varicella syndrome or neonatal varicella. Congenital varicella syndrome is manifested by low birth weight, cutaneous scarring, limb hypoplasia, microcephaly, chorioretinitis, and cataracts. It occurs in 1.5% of infants born to women who contract VZV in the first 28 weeks of gestation. Fetuses infected by VZV during the second half of gestation can develop zoster early in life without having had extrauterine chickenpox. The onset of varicella in pregnant women 5 days before to 2 days after delivery may result in severe varicella in newborns, which, if untreated, has a high mortality rate.

Antepartum Management

Diagnosis of maternal VZV infection usually is based on clinical findings, and laboratory testing is not needed, especially if a rash occurs after known exposure. The VZV antigen can be demonstrated within skin lesions or vesicular fluid by immunofluorescence. Varicella infection also can be documented by the detection of the fluorescence antibody to the membrane antigen or of the VZV antibody by ELISA. Pregnant women who are seronegative for VZV (per expeditious determination of the VZV membrane antigen or equivalent anti-VZV antibody status) can receive varicella immune globulin up until 10 days postexposure, but it is not known whether this will prevent or ameliorate fetal infection.

Varicella during pregnancy can be treated with oral acyclovir to minimize maternal symptoms. Maternal treatment with acyclovir has not been shown to ameliorate or prevent the fetal effects of congenital varicella syndrome. Pregnant women with VZV infection should be advised of pulmonary complications and to seek medical care immediately if any pulmonary symptoms develop. Although women with VZV infection during pregnancy are no more likely to develop varicella pneumonia than are other adults, varicella pneumonia is more severe during pregnancy. Maternal varicella complicated by pneumonia should be treated with intravenous acyclovir, because intravenous acyclovir may reduce maternal morbidity and mortality associated with varicella pneumonia.

Neonatal Management

Neonatal VZV infection is associated with a high neonatal death rate when maternal disease develops from 5 days before delivery up to 48 hours postpartum as a result of the relative immaturity of the neonatal immune system and the lack of protective maternal antibody. Varicella zoster immune globulin should be given to infants born to women who develop varicella during this interval, although this does not universally prevent neonatal varicella. Infants who develop varicella within the first 2 weeks of life should be treated with intravenous acyclovir.

Infants born at less than 28 weeks of gestation or less than 1,000 g who are exposed to VZV postnatally are at increased risk of severe varicella, regardless of maternal history. These infants should receive varicella zoster immune globulin regardless of the maternal history of varicella or varicella zoster serostatus. Hospitalized, preterm infants born at 28 weeks of gestation or later who are exposed postnatally to chickenpox and whose mothers have no history of chickenpox also should receive varicella zoster immune globulin.

Infection Control

Hospitalized women with VZV infection must be kept under airborne and contact precautions. Similar precautions are recommended for infants born to mothers with varicella and, if still hospitalized, should continue during the incubation period (21 days or 28 days). Infants with VZV infection should be isolated in a private room for the duration of the illness. Infants with congenital VZV infection acquired earlier in gestation do not require special precautions or isolation unless vesicular lesions are present. Hospitalized infants who are exposed postnatally should be isolated from 8 days to 21 days after onset of the rash in the index case.

Immunization

Pregnant women should not be vaccinated, and vaccinated women should be advised to avoid pregnancy for 1 month after each dose because of concern about possible fetal effects. Surveillance data to date on fetal outcomes after inadvertent vaccine exposures, however, have not found any cases of fetal varicella syndrome. Women who do not have varicella immunity should receive the first dose of VZV vaccine in the postpartum period before discharge from the birthing facility. A pregnant household member is not a contraindication to vaccination of a child. (For the most current immunization schedules and recommendations, please visit the CDC's "Vaccines & Immunizations" web page at http://www.cdc.gov/vaccines.)

West Nile Virus

West Nile virus is associated with fever, rash, arthritis, myalgias, weakness, lymphadenopathy, and meningoencephalitis. This virus is carried by mosquitoes and birds and can be transmitted through blood transfusion or organ transplant. To date, outcomes of 72 pregnancies have been published, and there has been only one fetus with proven intrauterine infection and subsequent bilateral chorioretinitis. It is unclear whether pregnant women are more susceptible to West Nile virus and whether the disease is more severe. Transmission through breast milk also is possible, but most infants infected by this route are asymptomatic or have mild symptoms. Women with symptoms should not be discouraged from breastfeeding. Pregnant and breastfeeding mothers should be encouraged to wear protective clothing, minimize their outdoor exposure at dawn and dusk when mosquitoes are most active, and use insect repellant containing N,N-diethyl-3-methylbenzamide (known as DEET) as a preventive measure.

Bacterial Infections

Anthrax Exposure

Anthrax infections are diagnosed by isolating *Bacillus anthracis* from body fluids or by measuring specific antibodies in the blood of persons suspected to have the disease. It is recommended that asymptomatic pregnant and lactating women who have been exposed to a confirmed environmental contamination or a high-risk source as determined by the local Department of Health (not the women's health care provider) receive prophylactic treatment. A variety of antimicrobial regimens are available. Although some of these drugs may present risks to the developing fetus, these risks are clearly outweighed by the potential morbidity and mortality from anthrax. Guidelines for prophylactic treatment of anthrax and treatment of suspected active cases of anthrax are changing continually, and the CDC's web site (http://emergency.cdc.gov/agent/anthrax/) should be consulted for the latest recommendations.

Chlamydial Infection

Chlamydia trachomatis is the most common reportable STI in the United States, with high rates among sexually active adolescents and young adults. Important risk factors for chlamydial infection include unmarried status, recent change in sexual partner, multiple concurrent partners, age 25 years or younger, inner-city residence, history or presence of other STIs, and little or no prenatal care. Most infected women have few symptoms, but *C trachomatis* may cause urethritis and mucopurulent (nongonococcal) cervicitis. Chlamydial infection also is associated with postpartum endometritis and infertility. Infection may be transmitted from the genital tract of infected women to their neonates during birth.

Antepartum Management

All pregnant women should be screened for chlamydial infection during the first prenatal care visit, and women at increased risk should be tested again in the third trimester (see also "Routine Laboratory Testing in Pregnancy" in Chapter 5). The diagnosis of *C trachomatis* infection is based on a cell culture, direct fluorescent antibody staining, enzyme immunoassay, DNA probe, or NAATs (eg, PCR). Nucleic acid amplification tests are the most sensitive diagnostic measure.

Treatment should be administered to women who have known *C trachomatis* infection (ie, with mucopurulent cervicitis) or whose neonates are infected. Women whose sexual partners have nongonococcal urethritis or epididymitis are presumed to be infected and also should be treated. Simultaneous treatment of partners is an important component of the therapeutic regimen. Doxycycline and ofloxacin are contraindicated in pregnancy. Recommended regimens for treating *C trachomatis* infection in pregnant women include 1 g azithromycin orally in a single dose or amoxicillin 500 mg orally three times daily for 7 days. Alternative regimens in pregnant women include erythromycin base (500 mg orally four times a day for 7 days or 250 mg orally four times daily for 14 days) or erythromycin ethylsuccinate (800 mg orally four times daily for 7 days or 400 mg orally four times daily for 14 days). Erythromycin estolate is contraindicated during pregnancy because of drug-related hepatotoxicity. A test of cure is recommended in pregnancy 3–4 weeks after completion of treatment regimens to confirm successful treatment.

Neonatal Management

Approximately 50% of infants born to women who have untreated chlamydial infection become colonized with *C trachomatis*. Of these, 25–50% will manifest a purulent conjunctivitis a few days to several weeks after delivery, and 5–20% will develop pneumonia 2–19 weeks after delivery. Infections generally are mild and responsive to antimicrobial therapy. Infants with chlamydial conjunctivitis or pneumonia should be treated with oral azithromycin for 5 days or erythromycin base or ethylsuccinate for 14 days. Topical treatment of conjunctivitis is ineffective. If hospitalized, infants should be managed with standard precautions.

Gonorrhea

Gonorrhea, caused by the gram-negative bacterium *Neisseria gonorrhoeae* is one of the most commonly reported bacterial STIs. Women younger than 25 years are at highest risk of gonorrhea infection, as are those of black, Hispanic, American Indian, or Alaska Native ethnicity. Other risk factors for gonorrhea include a previous gonococcal infection, other STIs, new or multiple sexual partners, inconsistent condom use, commercial sex work, and illicit drug use. Gonococcal infection of the genital tract in females often is asymptomatic, and common clinical syndromes are vaginitis, urethritis, endocervicitis, and salpingitis. Asymptomatic infection in females can progress to pelvic inflammatory disease, with tubal scarring that can result in ectopic pregnancy or infertility. Perinatal transmission also can occur, which results in neonatal gonococcal infection.

Antepartum Management

All pregnant women with risk factors for gonorrhea or living in an area in which the prevalence of *N gonorrhoeae* is high should be screened for *N gonorrhoeae* at the first prenatal visit (see also "Routine Laboratory Testing in Pregnancy" in Chapter 5). A repeat test should be obtained in the third trimester for women at increased risk of gonorrhea and other STIs. Nucleic acid amplification tests (eg, PCR) are highly sensitive and specific for detecting *N gonorrhoeae* when used on endocervical or vaginal swab and urine specimens. Cultures are the most widely used tests for identifying *N gonorrhoeae* from nongenital sites.

Because of the prevalence of pencicillin-resistant, tetracycline-resistant and fluoroquinolone-resistant *N gonorrhoeae*, the recommended treatment is combination therapy with a single intramuscular dose of ceftriaxone plus oral azithromycin. A test-of-cure is not recommended routinely in individuals with uncomplicated gonorrhea who are treated with this first-line therapy. If ceftriaxone is unavailable, second-line therapy would be a single oral dose of cefixime plus oral azithromycin; however, a test-of-cure 1 week after treatment is required. If penicillin allergy prohibits the use of a cephalosporin, a single oral dose of azithromycin may be used but a test of cure is required 1 week after treatment. Because concurrent infection with *C trachomatis* is common, patients with gonococcal infections should be treated for chlamydial infection (unless it has been excluded) and should be evaluated for co-infection with syphilis, HIV, and other STIs. All cases of gonorrhea must be reported to public health officials.

Neonatal Management

Gonococcal infection in the newborn usually involves the eyes. Antimicrobial prophylaxis soon after delivery is recommended for all neonates (see also "Conjunctival (Eye) Care" in Chapter 8). Infants born to women with active gonorrhea should receive a single dose of cefotaxime (100 mg/kg given intravenously or intramuscularly). Single-dose systemic antibiotic therapy is effective treatment for gonococcal ophthalmia and prophylaxis for disseminated disease.

In addition to ophthalmia, neonatal disease may include scalp abscess, vaginitis, and systemic disease with bacteremia, arthritis, meningitis, or endocarditis. Infants with clinical gonococcal disease should be hospitalized, and cultures of blood, cerebrospinal fluid, eye discharge, or other sites of infection should be obtained. For infants with positive cultures (ie, disseminated infection), the recommended antimicrobial therapy is cefotaxime (50–100 mg/kg per day, divided into two doses given every 12 hours). The duration of antibiotic treatment depends on the site of infection; 7 days is recommended for disseminated infection; 10–14 days is recommended for meningitis and 14 days is recommended for arthritis. Infected infants should be managed with standard precautions. Tests for concomitant infection with *C trachomatis*, congenital syphilis, and HIV infection should be performed.

Group B Streptococci

Group B streptococci (GBS), also known as *Streptococcus agalactiae*, emerged as an important cause of perinatal morbidity and mortality in the 1970s. Between 10% and 40% of pregnant women are colonized with GBS in the vagina or rectum. Group B streptococci can cause maternal urinary tract infection, amnionitis, endometritis, sepsis, or, rarely, meningitis. Vertical transmission of GBS during labor or delivery can result in invasive infection in the newborn during the first 6 days after birth (early-onset group B streptococcal infection) characterized primarily by sepsis or pneumonia, or, less frequently, meningitis. Implementation of national guidelines for intrapartum antibiotic prophylaxis since the 1990s has resulted in an approximate 80% reduction in the incidence of early-onset neonatal sepsis due to GBS. Yet, GBS remains the leading cause of infectious mortality and morbidity in neonates.

The primary risk factor for early-onset group B streptococcal neonatal infection is maternal intrapartum colonization with GBS. Other clinical risk factors include gestational age of less than 37 weeks, rupture of membranes for 18 or more hours, intra-amniotic infection, young maternal age, and black race. Infants born to women who have previously given birth to a GBS-infected neonate or who have heavy GBS colonization, such as that seen with group B streptococcal bacteriuria, are at substantial risk of early-onset infection.

In 2010, the CDC revised its guidelines for the prevention of early-onset group B streptococcal disease in newborns. The updated recommendations continue to focus on universal antenatal GBS screening at 35–37 weeks of gestation and intrapartum antibiotic prophylaxis for GBS-positive women and for women with threatened preterm labor but include important changes for clinical practice, which are summarized here. For more information on screening, see "Routine Laboratory Testing in Pregnancy" in Chapter 5. The complete CDC guidelines are available at http://www.cdc.gov/groupbstrep/guidelines/guidelines.html.

Intrapartum Management

Indications for intrapartum antibiotic prophylaxis are summarized in Table 10-4. Intrapartum prophylaxis for GBS is not recommended for women undergoing a planned cesarean delivery in the absence of labor and rupture of membranes, regardless of the gestational age, even in GBS-positive women. All patients undergoing cesarean delivery should have prophylactic antibiotics administered before the incision to reduce the risk of postoperative infections (see also "Cesarean Delivery" in Chapter 6). When culture results are not available, intrapartum antibiotic prophylaxis should be offered only on the basis of the presence of intrapartum risk factors for early-onset GBS disease (see Table 10-4). The administration of intrapartum antibiotic prophylaxis to a woman with rupture of membranes for 18 hours or more with a culture negative for GBS at 35–37 weeks of gestation is strongly discouraged; in these clinical scenarios, antibiotics should be administered only if there is chorioamnionitis or other indications, such as pyelonephritis.

Intrapartum antibiotic prophylaxis is most effective if administered at least 4 hours before delivery at recommended doses. However, no medically necessary obstetric procedure should be delayed in order to achieve 4 or more

Table 10–4. Indications and Nonindications for Intrapartum Antibiotic Prophylaxis to Prevent Early-Onset Group B Streptococcal Disease

Intrapartum GBS Prophylaxis Indicated	Intrapartum GBS Prophylaxis Not Indicated
Previous infant with invasive GBS disease	Colonization with GBS during a previous pregnancy (unless an indication for GBS prophylaxis is present for current pregnancy)
GBS bacteriuria during any trimester of the current pregnancy	
Positive GBS screening culture during current pregnancy* (unless a cesarean delivery, is performed before onset of labor on a woman with intact amniotic membranes)	GBS bacteriuria during previous pregnancy (unless another indication for GBS prophylaxis is present for current pregnancy)
Unknown GBS status at the onset of labor (culture not done, incomplete, or results unknown) and any of the following:	Cesarean delivery performed before onset of labor on a woman with intact amniotic membranes, regardless of GBS colonization status or gestational age
• Delivery at less than 37 weeks of gestation[†]	Negative vaginal and rectal GBS screening culture result in late gestation* during the current pregnancy, regardless of intrapartum risk factors
• Amniotic membrane rupture greater than or equal to 18 hours	
• Intrapartum temperature greater than or equal to 100.4°F (greater than or equal to 38.0°C)[‡]	
• Intrapartum NAAT[§] positive for GBS	

Abbreviations: GBS, group B streptococci; NAAT, nucleic acid amplification test.
*Optimal timing for prenatal GBS screening is at 35–37 weeks of gestation.
[†]Recommendations for the use of intrapartum antibiotics for prevention of early-onset GBS disease in the setting of preterm delivery are included in the complete guidelines, which are available at http://www.cdc.gov/groupbstrep/guidelines/guidelines.html .
[‡]If amnionitis is suspected, broad-spectrum antibiotic therapy that includes an agent known to be active against GBS should replace GBS prophylaxis.
[§]NAAT testing for GBS is optional and may not be available in all settings. If intrapartum NAAT result is negative for GBS but any other intrapartum risk factor (delivery at less than 37 weeks of gestation, amniotic membrane rupture at 18 hours or more, or temperature greater than or equal to 100.4°F [greater than or equal to 38.0°C]) is present, then intrapartum antibiotic prophylaxis is indicated.
Verani JR, McGee L, Schrag SJ. Prevention of perinatal group B streptococcal disease—revised guidelines from CDC, 2010. Division of Bacterial Diseases, National Center for Immunization and Respiratory Diseases, Centers for Disease Control and Prevention (CDC). MMWR Recomm Rep 2010;59(RR-10): 1–36.

hours of GBS prophylaxis before delivery. Penicillin is the agent of choice, with ampicillin as an acceptable alternative. Cefazolin is the drug of choice for penicillin allergy without anaphylaxis, angioedema, respiratory distress, or urticaria. Erythromycin is no longer recommended under any circumstances because nearly 50% of GBS strains are resistant to this drug. Group B streptococcal isolates from women at high risk of anaphylaxis should be tested for susceptibility to clindamycin and erythromycin, and clindamycin can be used for prophylaxis if susceptibility to both drugs is documented. Vancomycin use is recommended only if the isolate is resistant to clindamycin and erythromycin. However, neither clindamycin nor vancomycin has been evaluated in the prevention of early-onset GBS disease.

Neonatal Management

The 2010 CDC guidelines for the prevention of early-onset GBS disease among newborns are summarized in Figure 10-1. Recommended management continues to be based on clinical signs, the presence of maternal risk factors, and the likely efficacy of intrapartum antibiotic prophylaxis (or maternal antimicrobial treatment in the case of clinical chorioamnionitis) in preventing early-onset

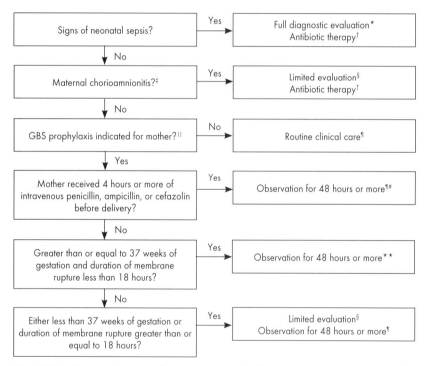

Fig. 10-1. Algorithm for secondary prevention of early-onset group B streptococcal disease among newborns. Abbreviation: GBS, group B streptococci.

*Full diagnostic evaluation includes a blood culture, a complete blood count, including white blood cell differential, platelet counts, chest radiograph (if respiratory abnormalities are present), and lumbar puncture (if patient is stable enough to tolerate procedure and sepsis is suspected).

†Antibiotic therapy should be directed toward the most common causes of neonatal sepsis, including intravenous ampicillin for GBS and coverage for other organisms (including *Escherichia coli* and other gram-negative pathogens) and should take into account local antibiotic resistance patterns.

‡Consultation with obstetric providers is important to determine the level of clinical suspicion for chorioamnionitis. Chorioamnionitis is diagnosed clinically and some of the signs are nonspecific.

§Limited evaluation includes blood culture (at birth), and complete blood count with differential and platelets (at birth, 6–12 hours of life, or both).

‖GBS prophylaxis is indicated if one or more of the following is present: 1) mother is GBS positive within preceding 5 weeks; 2) GBS status unknown, with one or more intrapartum risk factors, including less than 37 weeks of gestation, duration of rupture of membranes for 18 hours or more, or temperature greater than or equal to 100.4°F (greater than or equal to 38.0°C); 3) group B streptococcal bacteriuria during current pregnancy; 4) history of a previous infant with group B streptococcal disease.

¶If signs of sepsis develop, a full diagnostic evaluation should be conducted and antibiotic therapy initiated.

#If greater than or equal to 37 weeks of gestation, observation may occur at home after 24 hours if other discharge criteria have been met, access to medical care is readily available, and a person who is able to comply fully with instructions for home observation will be present. If any of these conditions is not met, the infant should be observed in the hospital for at least 48 hours and until discharge criteria are achieved.

**Some experts recommend a complete blood count with differential and platelets at 6–12 hours of age.

Verani JR, McGee L, Schrag SJ. Prevention of perinatal group B streptococcal disease—revised guidelines from CDC, 2010. Division of Bacterial Diseases, National Center for Immunization and Respiratory Diseases, Centers for Disease Control and Prevention (CDC). MMWR Recomm Rep 2010;59(RR-10):1–36.

disease. (Please refer to the CDC web site, http://www.cdc.gov/groupbstrep/index.html, for the latest recommendations to help prevent early onset GBS infection in neonates.) There is no known method for the prevention of late-onset neonatal GBS infection.

Listeriosis

The major cause of epidemic and sporadic listeriosis infection is food-borne transmission of the bacterium *Listeria monocytogenes*. Incriminated foods include unpasteurized milk, cheese, and other dairy products; undercooked poultry; and prepared meats, such as hot dogs, deli meats, and pâté, and some contaminated fresh fruits and vegetables. Asymptomatic fecal and vaginal carriage can result in sporadic neonatal disease, which can cause early-onset neonatal infections from transplacental or ascending intrauterine infection or from exposure during delivery. Maternal infection has been associated with preterm delivery and other obstetric complications. Late-onset neonatal infection results from acquisition of the organism during passage through the birth canal or possibly from environmental sources. To prevent pregnancy-related listeria infections, pregnant women are advised not to eat unpasteurized dairy products, undercooked foods, or unwashed fresh fruits and vegetables.

Listeria monocytogenes can be recovered on blood agar media from cultures of usually sterile body sites (eg, blood or cerebrospinal fluid). Special techniques may be needed to recover *L monocytogenes* from sites with mixed flora (eg, vagina, rectum). Because of morphologic similarity to diphtheroids and streptococci, a culture isolate of *L monocytogenes* mistakenly can be considered a contaminant or saprophyte.

Prompt diagnosis and antibiotic treatment of maternal listeriosis may prevent fetal or perinatal infection. *Listeria monocytogenes* is uniformly sensitive to ampicillin, but there may be a synergistic benefit from adding gentamicin. Signs of listeriosis in the newborn vary widely and often are nonspecific. The clinical picture is similar to that of GBS infection with early-onset and late-onset syndromes. Therapy with intravenous ampicillin and an aminoglycoside is recommended for neonatal infections. (For additional information and resources, please visit the CDC online at http://www.cdc.gov/ncbddd/pregnancy_gateway/infections-listeria.html.)

Pertussis

Pertussis, commonly known as whooping cough, is a respiratory infection that initially is manifested as coryza before the onset of paroxysms of cough that last for weeks. Complications in adults include pneumonia, sleep disturbance, rib fracture, and incontinence. In the first 6 months of life, illness is more severe, and infant complications include pneumonia, seizures, encephalopathy, and death. Newborns are thought to be protected from infection if high concentrations of passively transferred pertussis-specific antibodies are present.

Immunization During Pregnancy

Universal immunization is recommended to prevent transmission of pertussis. Women should ideally receive the tetanus toxoid, reduced diphtheria toxoid, and acellular pertussis vaccine (Tdap) before conception. However, there is no evidence that antenatal vaccination with Tdap causes any adverse effects specific to pregnancy. Moreover, immunization with Tdap during pregnancy has been associated with an increase in diphtheria and pertussis antibody levels in newborns of vaccinated mothers. Women's health care providers should implement a Tdap vaccination program for pregnant women who previously have not received Tdap. Health care providers should administer Tdap during pregnancy, preferably during the third trimester or late second trimester (ie, after 20 weeks of gestation). Alternatively, if not administered during pregnancy, Tdap should be administered immediately postpartum to ensure pertussis immunity and reduce the risk of transmission to the newborn. Regardless of the trimester, health care providers are encouraged to report Tdap administration to the appropriate manufacturer's pregnancy registry.

Additional guidelines for the administration of Tdap during pregnancy are outlined in the following paragraphs. Extensive information for health care providers and consumers about Tdap and other vaccines can be obtained at www.cdc.gov/vaccines and on the American College of Obstetricians and Gynecologists' immunization web site at www.immunizationforwomen.org/.

Tetanus Booster. If a tetanus and diphtheria (TD) booster vaccination is indicated during pregnancy (ie, more than 10 years since the previous TD vaccination) for a woman who has previously not received Tdap, then health care providers should administer the Tdap vaccine during pregnancy, preferably during the third or late second trimester (ie, after 20 weeks of gestation).

Wound Management. As part of standard wound management care to prevent tetanus, a tetanus toxoid-containing vaccine might be recommended for a pregnant woman if 5 years or more have elapsed since the previous TD booster vaccination. If a TD booster is indicated for a pregnant woman who previously has not received Tdap, health care providers should administer Tdap.

Unknown or Incomplete Tetanus Vaccination. To ensure protection against maternal and neonatal tetanus, pregnant women who never have been vaccinated against tetanus should receive three vaccinations containing tetanus and reduced diphtheria toxoids during pregnancy. The recommended schedule is 0, 4 weeks, and 6–12 months. One dose of the TD booster vaccine should be replaced by Tdap, preferably during the third trimester or late second trimester (ie, after 20 weeks of gestation).

Vaccination of Adolescents and Adults in Contact With Infants

The CDC Advisory Committee on Immunization Practices recommends that adolescents and adults (eg, siblings, parents, grandparents, child care providers, including individuals aged 65 years and older) who have or who anticipate having contact with an infant younger than 12 months and who have not received Tdap previously should receive a single dose of Tdap to protect against pertussis and reduce the likelihood of transmission. Ideally, these adolescents and adults should receive Tdap at least 2 weeks before they have contact with the infant.

Neonatal and Infant Management

Infected infants younger than 6 months of age frequently require hospitalization for supportive care and to manage complications, but those less than 3 months of age account for most of the pertussis-related mortality. Antimicrobial agents given during the catarrhal stage may lessen the severity of the disease. Azithromycin is the drug of choice in all age groups.

Tuberculosis

Tuberculosis is caused by infection with organisms of the *Mycobacterium tuberculosis* complex, which primarily affects the lungs. Clinical manifestations include feelings of sickness or weakness, weight loss, fever, and night sweats. The symptoms of tuberculosis also include coughing, chest pain, and the coughing up of blood. The risk of developing tuberculosis is highest during the 6 months after infection and remains high for 2 years; however, many years can elapse between initial tuberculosis infection and the onset of tuberculosis. Once considered rare in the United States, the incidence of tuberculosis has increased considerably in women of childbearing age. In endemic areas, the incidence of tuberculosis may approach 0.1% of pregnant women.

Tuberculosis is diagnosed in an individual with infection who also has signs, symptoms, positive cultures, or radiographic manifestations of *M tuberculosis*. Isolation of *M tuberculosis* by culture from early morning gastric aspirate, sputum, pleural fluid, or other body fluids establishes the diagnosis of active disease. *Mycobacterium tuberculosis* is slow growing, usually requiring 2–10 weeks for isolation from cultured materials. Smears to demonstrate acid-fast bacilli should be performed on sputum and body fluids.

Latent tuberculosis infection is defined by a positive Mantoux tuberculin skin test or interferon-gamma release assay in an individual with no physical findings of disease and either a normal chest X-ray or only granuloma or calcification in the lung parenchyma, or regional lymph nodes, or both. The purpose of treating latent tuberculosis infection is to prevent progression to disease.

Antepartum Management

All pregnant women who are at high risk of tuberculosis should be screened with a Mantoux tuberculin skin test with purified protein derivative (PPD) or an interferon-gamma release assay when they begin receiving prenatal care (see also "Routine Laboratory Testing in Pregnancy" in Chapter 5). When the result of a tuberculin skin test or interferon-gamma release assay is positive, the time of conversion usually is not known. If a chest X-ray is normal, some experts prefer to delay treatment of latent tuberculosis infection until after delivery because pregnancy itself does not increase the risk of progression to disease and because of an increased risk of drug-induced hepatotoxicity during pregnancy and immediately postpartum. Other experts recommend treatment with monthly monitoring for hepatotoxicity. Although isoniazid is not known to be teratogenic, most experts recommend waiting to start therapy until the second trimester of pregnancy.

Treatment regimens for tuberculosis are based on the presence or absence of tuberculosis disease, primarily determined by chest X-ray findings and sputum culture and, in the absence of disease, the likelihood of progressing to disease. The risk of progression to disease is highest in the 2 years after conversion to positive PPD. For this reason, the recommended medication in women known to have converted within the previous 2 years (such as known contacts of other tuberculosis cases) but with no evidence of disease is isoniazid (300 mg per day) starting after the first trimester and continuing for 9 months. For women who are infected with HIV, some experts would recommend 12 months of isoniazid therapy. All pregnant women receiving isoniazid also should take pyridoxine (50 mg daily) to mitigate the risk of peripheral neuritis.

If tuberculosis is diagnosed in a pregnant woman (by positive cultures, compatible clinical findings, or X-ray findings), prompt, multidrug therapy is recommended to protect both the woman and the fetus. Isoniazid and rifampin, supplemented initially by ethambutol are recommended drugs. Pyrazinamide frequently is used for the first 2 months in a three-drug or four-drug regimen. Although safety data in pregnancy have not been published, many experts have used the drug in pregnant women with no apparent problems for the woman or the fetus. Therapy with isoniazid and rifampin is continued for at least 6 months for drug-susceptible disease.

Neonatal Management

In utero infection can occur as a result of hematogenous dissemination, which seeds the placenta; or as a result of aspiration of infected amniotic fluid in utero. Neonatal infection may occur at the time of delivery as a result of aspiration of tubercle bacilli in women with tuberculosis endometritis. On the rare occasions in which congenital tuberculosis is suspected, diagnostic evaluations and treatment of the infant and the mother should be initiated promptly.

Management of a newborn whose mother (or other household contact) is suspected of having tuberculosis is based on individual considerations. Whenever possible, separation of the mother and the infant should be minimized. Differing circumstances and resulting recommendations are listed as follows:

- The mother has a positive tuberculin skin test or interferon-gamma release assay result but a negative X-ray result. If the mother is asymptomatic, the infant needs no special evaluation or therapy and no separation of the mother and the infant is required. Because the tuberculin skin test or interferon-gamma release assay result could be a marker of an unrecognized case of contagious tuberculosis within the household, other household members should be tested and have further evaluation, as needed.

- The mother has an abnormal chest X-ray but no evidence of current tuberculosis. If the mother's chest X-ray is abnormal but the history, physical examination, sputum smear, and X-ray indicate no evidence of current tuberculosis, the infant can be assumed to be at low risk of *M tuberculosis* infection. The radiographic abnormality in this circumstance probably is because of another cause or because of a quiescent focus of tuberculosis. In the latter case, the mother may develop contagious, pulmonary tuberculosis, if untreated, and should receive appropriate therapy if not treated previously. She and her infant should receive follow-up care. Other household members should be tested and appropriately evaluated.

- The mother has clinical or radiographic evidence of contagious tuberculosis. The mother should be reported immediately to the public health department so that investigation of all household members can be performed within several days. All contacts should have a tuberculin skin test or interferon-gamma release assay, chest X-ray, and physical examination. The infant should be evaluated for congenital tuberculosis and should be tested for HIV infection. The mother and the infant should be separated until both are receiving appropriate therapy and the mother is deemed to be not contagious. Women with tuberculosis disease who have been treated appropriately for 2 or more weeks and who are not considered contagious can breastfeed. Other household members should be tested and appropriately evaluated.

If congenital tuberculosis is excluded, isoniazid is given until the infant is 3–4 months of age, at which time a tuberculin skin test should be performed. If the tuberculin skin test result is positive, the infant should be reassessed for tuberculosis disease. If disease is not present, isoniazid should be continued for a total of 9 months; children infected with HIV should be treated for 12 months. If the skin test result is negative and the mother and other family members with tuberculosis have good adherence and response to treatment, and are no longer infectious, isoniazid may be discontinued.

- The mother has disease caused by multidrug-resistant (MDR) *M tuberculosis* or has poor adherence to treatment and directly observed therapy is not possible. The infant should be separated from the ill family member. Bacille Calmette–Guérin vaccination may be considered for the infant, especially if the family member has MDR tuberculosis (see the following paragraph on "Bacille Calmette–Guérin Vaccine"). Because the response to the vaccine in infants may be delayed, the infant should be separated from the ill family member for at least several weeks after vaccination. In general, in the United States directly observed therapy of the infant is preferred. The efficacy of any therapy for contacts of MDR tuberculosis is unknown. An expert in childhood tuberculosis should be consulted when this is a consideration.

Isoniazid Therapy. Breastfeeding is considered safe during maternal antituberculosis therapy. Breastfed infants of women taking isoniazid therapy should receive a multivitamin supplement, including pyridoxine.

Bacille Calmette-Guérin Vaccine. Bacille Calmette–Guérin vaccine is a live vaccine prepared from attenuated strains of *Mycobacterium bovis*. Bacille Calmette–Guérin immunization in the United States should be considered only for individuals with a negative tuberculin skin test result who are not infected with HIV and who are at high risk of intimate and prolonged exposure to patients with persistently infectious pulmonary tuberculosis or MDR tuberculosis, cannot be removed from the source of exposure, and cannot be placed on long-term preventive therapy.

Spirochetal Infections

Syphilis

Syphilis is a systemic disease caused by infection with the spirochete *Treponema pallidum*. Rates of infection are highest in urban areas and the rural South. In adults, syphilis is more common in individuals with HIV infection. Acquired syphilis almost always is contracted through direct sexual contact with ulcer-ative lesions of the skin or mucous membranes of infected people. Congenital syphilis most often is acquired through hematogenous transplacental infection of the fetus, although direct contact of the infant with infectious lesions during or after delivery also can result in infection. Transplacental infection can occur throughout pregnancy and at any stage of maternal infection.

Antepartum Management

All pregnant women should be serologically screened for syphilis as early as possible in pregnancy. False-negative serologic test results may occur in early primary infection, and infection after the first prenatal visit is possible. For communities and populations with a high prevalence, serologic testing also is recommended at 28–32 weeks of gestation and at delivery (as well as after exposure to an infected partner). Some states require all women to be screened for syphilis at delivery.

The specificity of serologic testing is high if both a nontreponemal screening test (Venereal Disease Research Laboratories [VDRL] or rapid plasma reagin [RPR] test result) and a subsequent treponemal serologic test result are reactive. Microscopic dark-field and histologic examinations for spirochetes are most reliable when lesions are present.

Pregnant women with syphilis should be treated with a penicillin regimen appropriate to the stage of infection. Women who are allergic to penicillin should be desensitized and then treated with the drug. Tetracycline and doxycy-cline are contraindicated during pregnancy. Erythromycin and azithromycin are suboptimal treatment options because neither reliably cures maternal infection nor treats an infected fetus. Women should be observed for signs of a Jarisch–Herxheimer reaction (an immune response to toxins released when spirochetes die), which may cause fever, nonreassuring fetal status, and preterm labor.

Women with syphilis should be queried about illicit substance use, espe-cially cocaine. Results of the maternal serologic tests and treatment, if given, should be recorded in the neonate's medical record or be made available to the neonate's pediatrician.

Neonatal Management

An infant should be evaluated for congenital syphilis if he or she is born to a mother with a positive treponemal test result who has one or more of the fol-lowing conditions:

- Syphilis and HIV infection

- Untreated or inadequately treated syphilis
- Syphilis during pregnancy treated with a nonpenicillin regimen and inadequate regimen, such as erythromycin
- Syphilis during pregnancy treated with an appropriate penicillin regimen that failed to produce the expected fourfold decrease in nontreponemal antibody titer after therapy
- Syphilis treated less than 1 month before delivery (because treatment failures occur, and the efficacy of treatment cannot be assumed without sufficient time for an expected decrease in nontreponemal antibody titer)
- Syphilis treatment not documented
- Syphilis treated before pregnancy but with insufficient serologic follow-up during pregnancy to assess the response to treatment and current infection status

The diagnostic and therapeutic approach to infants delivered to mothers with syphilis is outlined in Figure 10-2. Management decisions are based on the three possible maternal situations: 1) maternal treatment before pregnancy, 2) adequate maternal treatment and response during pregnancy, or 3) inadequate maternal treatment or inadequate maternal response to treatment (or reinfection) during pregnancy.

For proven or probable congenital syphilis (based on the infant's physical examination and radiographic and laboratory testing), the preferred treatment is aqueous crystalline penicillin G, administered intravenously. The dosage should be based on chronologic age rather than gestational age and is 50,000 units/kg, intravenously, every 12 hours (for infants 1 week of age or younger) or every 8 hours (for infants older than 1 week). Alternatively, procaine penicillin G, 50,000 units/kg, intramuscularly, can be administered as a single daily dose for 10 days; no treatment failures have occurred with this formulation despite its low cerebrospinal fluid concentrations. When the infant is at risk of congenital syphilis because of inadequate maternal treatment or response to treatment (or reinfection) during pregnancy but the infant's physical examination, radiographic imaging, and laboratory analyses are normal (including infant RPR/VDRL either the same as or less than fourfold the maternal RPR/VDRL), some experts would treat the infant with a single dose of penicillin G benzathine (50,000 units/kg intramuscularly), but most still would prefer 10 days of treatment. If more than 1 day of therapy is missed, the entire course should be restarted. Data supporting use of other antimicrobial agents (eg, ampicillin) for

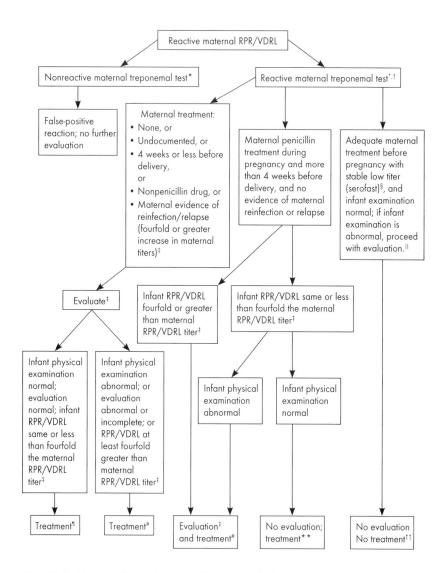

Fig. 10-2. Algorithm for evaluation and treatment of infants born to mothers with reactive serologic test results for syphilis. Abbreviations: FTA-ABS, fluorescent treponemal antibody absorption; MHA-TP, microhemagglutination test for antibodies to *Treponema pallidum*; RPR, rapid plasma regain; TP-EIA, *T pallidum* enzyme immunoassay; TP-PA, *T pallidum* particle agglutination; VDRL, Venereal Disease Research Laboratory.

*FTA-ABS, MHA-TP, TP-EIA, or TP-PA.

†Test for human immunodeficiency virus (HIV) antibody. Infants of HIV-infected mothers do not require different evaluation or treatment.

‡A fourfold change in titer is the same as a change of 2 dilutions. For example, a titer of 1:64 is fourfold greater than a titer of 1:16, and a titer of 1:4 is fourfold lower than a titer of 1:16.

§Women who maintain a VDRL titer 1:2 or less or an RPR 1:4 or less beyond 1 year after successful treatment are considered serofast.

‖Complete blood cell and platelet count; cerebrospinal fluid examination for cell count, protein, and qualitative VDRL; other tests as clinically indicated (eg, chest radiographs, long-bone radiographs, eye examination, liver function tests, neuroimaging, and auditory brainstem response).

¶Treatment (option 1 or option 2, below), with many experts recommending treatment option 1. If a single dose of benzathine penicillin G is used, then the infant must be fully evaluated, full evaluation must be normal, and follow-up must be certain. If any part of the infant's evaluation is abnormal or not performed, or if the cerebrospinal fluid analysis is rendered uninterpretable, then a 10-day course of penicillin is required.

#Treatment option 1: Aqueous penicillin G, 50,000 units/kg, intravenously, every 12 hours (1 week of age or younger) or every 8 hours (older than 1 week); or procaine penicillin G, 50,000 units/kg, intramuscularly, as a single daily dose for 10 days. If 24 or more hours of therapy are missed, the entire course must be restarted.

**Treatment option 2: Benzathine penicillin G, 50,000 units/kg, intramuscularly, single dose.

††Some experts would consider a single intramuscular injection of benzathine penicillin (treatment option 2), particularly if follow-up is not certain.

American Academy of Pediatrics. Red book: report of the Committee on Infectious Diseases, 29th. Elk Grove Village (IL): American Academy of Pediatrics; 2012.

treatment of congenital syphilis are not available. When possible, a full 10-day course of penicillin is preferred, even if ampicillin initially was provided for possible sepsis. Use of agents other than penicillin requires close serologic follow-up to assess adequacy of therapy.

Infants who have a normal physical examination and a serum quantitative nontreponemal serologic titer either the same as or less than fourfold (eg, 1:4 is fourfold lower than 1:16) the maternal titer are at minimal risk of syphilis if they are born to mothers who completed appropriate penicillin treatment for syphilis during pregnancy and more than 4 weeks before delivery, and if the mother had no evidence of reinfection or relapse. Although a full evaluation may be unnecessary, these infants should be treated with a single intramuscular injection of penicillin G benzathine because fetal treatment failure can occur despite adequate maternal treatment during pregnancy. Alternatively, these infants may be examined carefully, preferably monthly, until their nontreponemal serologic test results are negative.

Infants who have a normal physical examination and a serum quantitative nontreponemal serologic titer either the same as or less than fourfold the maternal titer, whose mothers' treatment was adequate before pregnancy, and whose mothers' nontreponemal serologic titer remained low and stable before and during pregnancy and at delivery (VDRL less than 1:2; RPR less than 1:4) require no evaluation. Some experts, however, would treat with penicillin G benzathine as a single intramuscular injection if follow-up is uncertain.

Lyme Disease

Lyme disease is caused by a spirochete (*Borrelia burgdorferi*) transmitted by the bite of a deer tick. The early localized stage of the disease is characterized by a distinctive "bull's-eye" skin lesion (erythema migrans) that occurs in 60–80% of patients and nonspecific, flu-like symptoms. Early disseminated disease can result in multiple erythema migrans several weeks after a tick bite, cranial nerve palsies (especially cranial nerve VII) or carditis within 4–6 weeks after the onset of early signs and symptoms. A late manifestation of Lyme disease is relapsing arthritis, usually pauciarticular and affecting large joints. Patients in the later stages of Lyme disease usually will be seropositive, but false-positive and false-negative test results are common.

Suspicion of early maternal infection is based on a history of exposure to tick bites, the presence of the distinctive erythema migrans rash, and nonspecific, flu-like symptoms. Adequately treated patients may never develop antibodies to spirochetes. Because congenital infection occurs with other spirochetal infections, there has been concern that an infected pregnant woman could transmit *B burgdorferi* to her fetus. No causal relationship between maternal Lyme disease and congenital abnormalities caused by *B burgdorferi* has been documented. No evidence shows that Lyme disease can be transmitted via breast milk. The neonate's health care provider should be informed when maternal disease is suspected.

Recommended treatment of suspected early disease in pregnant women is amoxicillin, 500 mg three times per day, for 2–3 weeks. For women who are allergic to penicillin, erythromycin is recommended for 2–3 weeks. For patients who are unable to tolerate erythromycin, cefuroxime axetil is an alternative for patients with immediate and anaphylactic hypersensitivity to penicillin who have undergone penicillin desensitization.

The best preventive measure is to avoid heavily wooded areas. If entrance into such areas is necessary, long-sleeved shirts and long pants tucked in at the ankle are helpful. Prophylactic antibiotic therapy for deer tick bites is not recommended routinely.

Parasitic Infections

Malaria

Although malaria mainly is confined to tropical areas of Africa, Asia, and Latin America, international travel and migration have made malaria a disease to consider in developed countries. The classic symptoms are high fever with chills, rigors, sweats, and headache.

Malaria infection may be more severe in pregnant women and also may increase the risk of adverse outcomes of pregnancy, including spontaneous abortion, stillbirth, preterm birth, and low birth weight. Because of the risk to both the woman and the fetus, and because no chemoprophylactic regimen is completely effective, pregnant women (or women likely to become pregnant) should avoid travel to malaria-endemic areas. If travel to a malaria-endemic area is necessary, appropriate consultation should be sought for chemoprophylaxis recommendations based on the malaria species and drug-resistance patterns prevalent in that area. (For current information and recommendations from the CDC, visit www.cdc.gov/travel.)

Congenital malaria is rare. Signs and symptoms resemble those of neonatal sepsis. Definitive diagnosis (of the mother and the infant) relies on identification of the parasite on stained blood films. Both thick and thin films should be examined. Treatment of infection is based on the infecting species, possible drug resistance, and severity of disease. If malaria is a diagnostic consideration in a pregnant woman or newborn, consultation with appropriate specialists is recommended for optimal patient management.

Toxoplasmosis

Toxoplasmosis is a protozoan infection caused by *Toxoplasma gondii*. Infection is acquired by foodborne transmission (consuming cysts in undercooked meat of infected animals or insect contamination of food), zoonotic transmission (by contact with oocysts from the feces of infected cats or by contact with contaminated soil or water), or through mother-to-child transmission during pregnancy. Infected women generally are asymptomatic. In the immunocompetent adult, the clinical course is benign and self-limited.

Congenital infection is more common after maternal infection in the third trimester; however, the sequelae from first-trimester fetal infection are more severe. Congenitally infected infants are healthy appearing at birth in 70–90%

of cases. Signs of congenital infection at birth may include maculopapular rash, generalized lymphadenopathy, hepatosplenomegaly, chorioretinitis, hydrocephaly, microcephaly, and intracranial calcifications. Neonates of women who are infected with both HIV and *T gondii* should be evaluated for congenital toxoplasmosis.

Antepartum Management

Routine serologic screening of pregnant women is not indicated, except in the presence of HIV infection. Because the presence of antibodies before pregnancy indicates immunity, the appropriate time to test for immunity to toxoplasmosis in women at risk is before conception.

The diagnosis of maternal infection is based on serologic test results for the detection of *Toxoplasma*-specific antibodies. Both immunoglobulin G (IgG) and IgM testing should be used for the initial evaluation of patients suspected to have toxoplasmosis. A positive IgG titer indicates infection with the organism at some time in the past. A negative IgM test essentially excludes recent infection, but a positive IgM test is difficult to interpret because *Toxoplasma*-specific IgM antibodies may be detected for as long as 18 months after acute acquired infection. In addition, false-positive test results are common with commercially available kits. Before making treatment recommendations, confirmation of diagnosis should be made based on results obtained in a reference laboratory. (Additional information on laboratory diagnosis of toxoplasmosis is available from the CDC web site at http://www.dpd.cdc.gov/dpdx/HTML/Toxoplasmosis.htm.)

Treatment of the pregnant woman with acute toxoplasmosis reduces but does not eliminate the risk of congenital infection. Identification of acute maternal infection necessitates immediate institution of treatment until results of fetal testing are known. Spiramycin, which concentrates in the placenta, may reduce the risk of fetal transmission by 60%, but as a single agent, it does not treat established fetal infection. Spiramycin is available only through the U.S. Food and Drug Administration after serologic confirmation at a reference laboratory; it is recommended for pregnant women at risk unless fetal infection is documented. If fetal infection is established, pyrimethamine, sulfonamides, and folinic acid are added to the regimen because they more effectively eradicate parasites in the placenta and in the fetus than spiramycin alone. With treatment, even early fetal infection with toxoplasmosis can result in successful pregnancy outcomes.

Neonatal Management

A definitive diagnosis of congenital toxoplasmosis can be made prenatally by either detecting parasite DNA in amniotic fluid by PCR, or documenting anti-toxoplasma IgM and immunoglobulin A antibodies in fetal blood. Congenital toxoplasmosis can be diagnosed serologically by the detection of anti–toxoplasma-specific IgM or immunoglobulin A antibodies soon after birth or by the persistence of anti-toxoplasma IgG beyond 12 months of age. If the diagnosis is suspected (but unconfirmed) at the time of birth, ophthalmologic, auditory, and neurologic examinations should be performed.

For healthy appearing infants and those with clinical signs of congenital toxoplasmosis, pyrimethamine and sulfadiazine (supplemented with folinic acid) are recommended for approximately 1 year. Infants with congenital toxoplasmosis should be managed in consultation with infectious disease specialists. (Additional professional and patient information is available on the CDC web site at http://www.cdc.gov/parasites/toxoplasmosis/.)

Bibliography

American Academy of Pediatrics. Red book: report of the Committee on Infectious Diseases. 29th. Elk Grove Village (IL): American Academy of Pediatrics; 2012.

American College of Obstetricians and Gynecologists. Perinatal viral and parasitic infections. ACOG Practice Bulletin 20. Washington, DC: ACOG; 2000.

American College of Obstetricians and Gynecologists. Scheduled cesarean delivery and the prevention of vertical transmission of HIV infection. ACOG Committee Opinion 234. Washington, DC: ACOG; 2000.

Antiviral therapy and prophylaxis for influenza in children. American Academy of Pediatrics Committee on Infectious Diseases. Pediatrics 2007;119:852–60.

Havens PL, Mofenson LM. Evaluation and management of the infant exposed to HIV-1 in the United States. American Academy of Pediatrics Committee on Pediatric AIDS. Pediatrics 2009;123:175–87.

HIV testing and prophylaxis to prevent mother-to-child transmission in the United States. American Academy of Pediatrics Committee on Pediatric AIDS. Pediatrics 2008;122: 1127–34.

Human immunodeficiency virus. ACOG Committee Opinion No. 389. American College of Obstetricians and Gynecologists. Obstet Gynecol 2007;110:1473–8.

Human milk, breastfeeding, and transmission of human immunodeficiency virus in the United States. American Academy of Pediatrics Committee on Pediatric AIDS. Pediatrics 1995;96:977–9.

Human papillomavirus vaccination. Committee Opinion No. 467. American College of Obstetricians and Gynecologists. Obstet Gynecol 2010;116:800–3.

Management of herpes in pregnancy. ACOG Practice Bulletin No. 82. American College of Obstetricians and Gynecologists. Obstet Gynecol 2007;109:1489–98.

Meningococcal vaccination for adolescents. ACOG Committee Opinion No. 314. American College of Obstetricians and Gynecologists. Obstet Gynecol 2005;106:667–9.

Nigro G, Adler SP, La Torre R, Best AM. Passive immunization during pregnancy for congenital cytomegalovirus infection. Congenital Cytomegalovirus Collaborating Group. N Engl J Med 2005;353:1350–62.

Policy statements—Modified recommendations for use of palivizumab for prevention of respiratory syncytial virus infections. American Academy of Pediatrics Committee on Infectious Diseases. Pediatrics 2009;124:1694–701.

Premastication of food by caregivers of HIV-exposed children—nine U.S. sites, 2009–2010. MMWR Morb Mortal Wkly Rep 2011;60:273–75.

Prenatal and perinatal human immunodeficiency virus testing: expanded recommendations. ACOG Committee Opinion No. 418. American College of Obstetricians and Gynecologists. Obstet Gynecol 2008;112:739–42.

Prevention of early-onset group B streptococcal disease in newborns. ACOG Committee Opinion No. 485. American College of Obstetricians and Gynecologists. Obstet Gynecol 2011;117:1019–27.

Prevention of varicella: recommendations for use of varicella vaccines in children, including a recommendation for a routine 2-dose varicella immunization schedule. American Academy of Pediatrics Committee on Infectious Diseases. Pediatrics 2007;120:221–31.

Read JS. Diagnosis of HIV-1 infection in children younger than 18 months in the United States. American Academy of Pediatrics Committee on Pediatric AIDS. Pediatrics 2007;120:e1547–62.

Recommendations for use of antiretroviral drugs in pregnant HIV-1-infected women for maternal health and interventions to reduce perinatal HIV transmission in the United States. Panel on Treatment of HIV-Infected Pregnant women and Prevention of Perinatal Transmission. Rockville (MD): National Institutes of Health; 2011. Available at: http://aidsinfo.nih.gov/contentfiles/PerinatalGL.pdf. Retrieved January 3, 2012.

Sheffield JS, Hollier LM, Hill JB, Stuart GS, Wendel GD. Acyclovir prophylaxis to prevent herpes simplex virus recurrence at delivery: a systematic review. Obstet Gynecol 2003;102:1396–403.

Sweet RL, Gibbs RS. Infectious diseases of the female genital tract. 5th. Philadelphia (PA): Wolters Kluwer/Lippincott Williams & Wilkins; 2009.

Update on immunization and pregnancy: tetanus, diphtheria, and pertussis vaccination. Committee Opinion No. 521. American College of Obstetricians and Gynecologists. Obstet Gynecol 2012;119:690–1.

Update to CDC's Sexually Transmitted Diseases Treatment Guidelines, 2010: Oral cephalosporins no longer a recommended treatment for gonococcal infections. MMWR Morb Mortal Wkly Rep 2012;61:590–4.

Updated recommendations for use of tetanus toxoid, reduced diphtheria toxoid and acellular pertussis (Tdap) vaccine from the Advisory Committee on Immunization Practices, 2010. Centers for Disease Control and Prevention. MMWR Morb Mortal Wkly Rep 2011;60:13–5.

Verani JR, McGee L, Schrag SJ. Prevention of perinatal group B streptococcal disease—revised guidelines from CDC, 2010, Centers for Disease Control and Prevention. MMWR Recomm Rep 2010;59(RR-10):1-36. Available at: http://www.cdc.gov/groupbstrep/guidelines/guidelines.html. Retrieved January 3, 2012.

Viral hepatitis in pregnancy. ACOG Practice Bulletin No. 86. American College of Obstetricians and Gynecologists. Obstet Gynecol 2007;110:941–56.

Zaman K, Roy E, Arifeen SE, Rahman M, Raqib R, Wilson E, et al. Effectiveness of maternal influenza immunization in mothers and infants. N Engl J Med 2008;359:1555–64.

Resources

AIDSinfo: offering information on HIV/AIDS treatment, prevention, and research. Rockville (MD): National Institutes of Health; 2011. Available at: http://www.aidsinfo.nih.gov/. Retrieved January 3, 2012.

Cytomegalovirus (CMV) and Congenital CMV Infection. Atlanta (GA): CDC; 2010. Available at: http://www.cdc.gov/cmv/index.html. Retrieved January 3, 2012.

Food and Drug Administration. Silver Spring (MD): FDA; 2011. Available at: http://www.fda.gov. Retrieved December 22, 2011.

Immunization for women. Washington, DC: American College of Obstetricians and Gynecologists; 2011. Available at: http://immunizationforwomen.org/. Retrieved December 20, 2011.

Listeriosis (Listeria) and pregnancy. Atlanta, GA: CDC; 2011. Available at: http://www.cdc.gov/ncbddd/pregnancy_gateway/infections-listeria.html. Retrieved December 20, 2011.

Non-polio Enterovirus infections. Atlanta (GA): CDC; 2011. Available at: http://www.cdc.gov/ncidod/dvrd/revb/enterovirus/non-polio_entero.htm. Retrieved January 3, 2012.

Parasites - Toxoplasmosis (Toxoplasma infection). Atlanta (GA): CDC; 2010. Available at: http://www.cdc.gov/parasites/toxoplasmosis/. Retrieved January 3, 2012.

Protect your baby and yourself from listeriosis: fact sheet. Washington, DC: USDA; 2011. Available at: http://www.fsis.usda.gov/Fact_Sheets/Protect_Your_Baby/index.asp. Retrieved January 3, 2012.

Seasonal Influenza (Flu): information for health professionals. Atlanta (GA): CDC; 2011. Available at: http://www.cdc.gov/flu/professionals/. Retrieved January 3, 2012.

Toxoplasmosis. Atlanta (GA): CDC; 2009. Available at: http://www.dpd.cdc.gov/dpdx/ HTML/Toxoplasmosis.htm. Retrieved January 3, 2012.

Travelers' health. Atlanta (GA): CDC; 2011. Available at: http://wwwnc.cdc.gov/travel/. Retrieved January 3, 2012.

Vaccines & immunizations. Atlanta (GA): CDC; 2011. Available at: http://www.cdc.gov/ vaccines/. Retrieved January 3, 2012.

Workowski KA, Berman S. Sexually transmitted diseases treatment guidelines, 2010. Centers for Disease Control and Prevention [published erratum appears in MMWR Morb Mortal Wkly Rep 2011;60:18]. MMWR Recomm Rep 2010;59(RR-12):1–110.

Chapter 11
Infection Control

Serious infection of the mother–newborn dyad is rare. However, when colonization with certain organisms occurs, the outcome may be devastating for the neonate, the mother, or both. Many of the nosocomial infections that occur in intensive care units are caused by pathogens acquired from the hospital environment (ie, health care-associated infections). Health care-associated infections result in increased morbidity and mortality, prolonged lengths of hospital stay, and increased medical costs.

Definition of Health Care-Associated Infection

Health care-associated infection is defined as an infection that is acquired in the hospital while receiving treatment for other conditions. This definition should be applied consistently to allow uniform reporting and analysis of health care-associated infections. The infection-control committee of each hospital should work with perinatal care personnel to ensure that appropriate surveillance of health care-associated infection is being performed. For obstetric patients, a health care-associated infection can be defined broadly as one that is not present or incubating when the patient is admitted to the hospital and occurs more than 48 hours after hospitalization. Many cases of urinary tract infection that occur postpartum are health care-associated. Risk factors associated with health care-associated infection in the infant include preterm birth, the presence of invasive devices (intravascular catheters, endotracheal tubes, orogastric tubes, urinary catheters, drains), exposure to broad-spectrum antibiotic agents, parenteral nutrition, overcrowding and poor staffing ratios, administration of steroids and histamine-2 receptor blockers, and acuity of underlying illness.

Prevention and Control of Infections

Prevention of infections requires a multifaceted approach. This includes cleaning and decontamination of the environment, using meticulous patient care techniques, practicing hand hygiene, promoting breastfeeding (unless contraindicated because of maternal infection; see also "Contraindications to Breastfeeding" in Chapter 8), limiting the number of invasive procedures (eg, central lines), limiting the number of visitors, grouping together (cohorting) infants colonized with the same pathogen, the judicious use of antimicrobial therapy.

Labor and Delivery Admission Policy

The pediatric health care provider should be notified of all mothers admitted to the antepartum obstetrics unit who are colonized with or are chronic carriers of a potentially infectious organism that may be transmitted vertically to the neonate (eg, human immunodeficiency virus, hepatitis B or hepatitis C virus, herpes simplex virus, influenza, methicillin-resistant staphylococcus, vancomycin-resistant enterococcus) or may be associated with a congenital infection. Both group A streptococci and group B streptococci are pathogens that may be indigenous to the female genital tract, and both may cause serious, life-threatening infection in the mother and newborn. There are national guidelines for the management of group B streptococci colonization in the mother (see also "Group B Streptococci" in Chapter 10).

Nursery Admission Policies

Infants transferred from another hospital and those who require rehospitalization a few days after being discharged home ideally should be admitted to the newborn unit. Infants with suspected infectious diseases should be admitted to specialized areas where additional transmission precautions (airborne, contact, droplet) can be provided to minimize the risks of spreading the infection to others.

Routine culturing of infants' respiratory or gastrointestinal tract or skin for surveillance purposes is not recommended, but cultures from lesions or sites of infection should be taken to identify the etiology. When clusters of infections caused by a single strain of bacteria are noted, appropriate personnel, such as hospital infection-control professionals, should be notified. Routine surveillance cultures of infants and nursery staff can be useful to characterize and to control an outbreak of infection with a common organism. During an outbreak of infection, it is important to document organisms colonizing all infants residing in the area where the outbreak occurred so that appropriate isolation and cohorting procedures can be undertaken.

Standard Precautions

The Centers for Disease Control and Prevention (CDC) recommend that standard precautions be used for all patients. Standard precautions are intended to prevent transmission of bloodborne pathogens, recognizing the importance of all body fluids, secretions, excretions, and contaminated items in the transmission of health care-associated pathogens. These precautions apply to the following: blood, semen, vaginal secretions, cerebrospinal fluid, synovial fluid, pleural fluid, pericardial fluid, peritoneal fluid, amniotic fluid, saliva in dental procedures, any body fluid that is visibly contaminated with blood, and all body fluids in situations in which it is difficult or impossible to differentiate between body fluids, except sweat; nonintact skin; and mucous membranes. Standard precautions include practicing hand hygiene before and after examining patients; wearing gloves (in addition to practicing hand hygiene); using masks, eye protection, and face shields; and wearing nonsterile gowns.

Disposal of equipment or materials contaminated with blood or other potentially infectious material always should be accomplished using standard precautions and careful hand hygiene practices. Instruments should not be shared, and each patient's bedside should be considered a separate, clean environment.

The federal Occupational Safety and Health Administration (OSHA) has issued regulations designed to minimize the transmission of human immunodeficiency virus (HIV), hepatitis B virus (HBV), and other potentially infectious organisms in the workplace. The OSHA guidelines are discussed extensively in Appendix H. The regulations apply to all employees in physicians' offices, hospitals, medical laboratories, and other health care facilities where workers reasonably could be anticipated to come into contact with blood and other potentially infectious material. The OSHA regulations require employers to implement an exposure-control plan to minimize employees' exposure to bloodborne and infectious pathogens. The plan must contain the following components:

- Personal protective equipment for employees exposed to blood and other body fluids
- Housekeeping requirements
- Provision of HBV vaccination to employees
- Postexposure evaluation and follow-up procedures

- Employee training
- Use of warning labels
- Record-keeping requirements
- Adoption of certain work practice controls (eg, hand hygiene facilities, safer medical devices, such as needleless systems and sharps with engineered sharps protection)

These requirements are enforced by OSHA or, in the case of states with OSHA-approved comparable job safety and health plans, by state agencies. Violations are punishable by fines.

Health Standards for Personnel

Obstetric, nursery, and neonatal intensive care unit (NICU) personnel, as well as others who have significant contact with newborns, should be as free of transmissible infectious diseases as possible. Each hospital should establish written policies and procedures for assessing the health of personnel assigned to perinatal care services, restricting their contact with patients when necessary, maintaining their health records, and requiring staff to report any potentially infectious illness they may have. These policies and procedures should address screening for immunity to measles, rubella, mumps, varicella zoster virus, HBV, pertussis, tetanus, diphtheria, and exposure to tuberculosis. The frequency of and need for screening employees should be determined by local epidemiologic data. Personnel with active tuberculosis should be restricted from patient contact until adequate treatment has occurred and noninfective status has been verified.

Vaccinations protect both staff and patients and may reduce health care costs. All susceptible, nonpregnant hospital personnel should be offered immunization against measles, mumps, rubella, varicella, tetanus, diphtheria, pertussis, and HBV. Susceptible pregnant hospital personnel should be offered tetanus, diphtheria, pertussis, HBV, and inactivated influenza vaccines. Offering annual influenza immunization to all health care providers is strongly encouraged. Given the communicability of influenza, obstetric and pediatric care practices should consider alternative prevention strategies (eg, wearing a mask) during peak influenza season for staff who are unable or unwilling to receive influenza vaccination.

Bloodborne pathogens, such as HBV, hepatitis C virus, and HIV may be transmitted from infected patients to health care workers as well as from infected health care workers to patients. To reduce the risk of transmission, all practicing obstetric and neonatal care providers should receive the HBV vaccine. Health care providers infected with HBV, hepatitis C virus, or HIV are advised to follow the updated recommendations from the Society for Healthcare Epidemiology of America regarding infection-control measures, supervision, and periodic testing (see "Bibliography" in this chapter). The recommendations provide a framework within which to consider such cases; however, each case should be independently considered by an expert review panel. Such an expert panel may include the following: the health care provider's personal physician, an infectious disease specialist with expertise in disease transmission, a health care professional with expertise in the procedures performed by the health care provider, state or local public health official(s), and a hospital epidemiologist or other member of the infection-control committee of the hospital.

Individuals with a respiratory, cutaneous, mucocutaneous, or gastrointestinal infection should not have direct contact with newborns. Personnel with exudative skin lesions or weeping dermatitis should refrain from all direct patient care and should not handle patient care equipment until the condition resolves. Personnel in contact with newborns should report personal infections, inability to perform adequate hand hygiene (eg, because of casts or braces), and other conditions to their immediate supervisors and should be medically examined by employee health to determine suitability for patient contact. Decisions regarding the exclusion of staff members from obstetric and nursery areas should be made on an individual basis. Employee health policies should be worded and applied in a way to ensure that personnel feel free to report infectious problems without fear of repercussions.

Transmission of herpes simplex virus from infected personnel to infants in newborn nurseries is rare. Personnel with cold sores who have direct contact with newborns should cover their lesions and carefully observe hand hygiene policies. Transmission of herpes simplex virus infection from personnel with genital lesions is not likely. Personnel with herpetic hand infections (herpetic whitlow) should not participate in patient care until the lesions have healed.

Nursery personnel can be exposed to infants excreting cytomegalovirus. Acquisition of cytomegalovirus infection from infants is minimized by compliance with standard precautions. Women of childbearing age who work in neonatal units should be counseled about the relatively low risk of exposure should they become pregnant. A routine program of serologic testing of obstetric and nursery hospital employees for immunity to cytomegalovirus is not recommended.

Employee education regarding standard precautions and other proper infection control techniques should occur regularly. All personnel should be required to follow strictly established infection-control procedures.

Personnel who care for women during pregnancy and the postpartum period and their infants should collaborate with hospital infection-control personnel in conducting and reviewing the results of surveillance programs for health care-associated infections. This type of monitoring provides information about any unusual problems or clusters of infection, the risks associated with certain procedures or techniques, and the success of specific preventive measures. It also can reveal temporal trends, allow comparison with other obstetric and neonatal units by using standard definitions, and provide feedback to responsible personnel working in these units.

Hand Hygiene

Proper hand hygiene before and after each patient contact is the single most effective method for reducing health care-associated infections. In 2009, the World Health Organization (WHO) published new consensus recommendations for hand hygiene. The WHO guidelines provide a comprehensive overview of hand hygiene in health care and evidence-based and consensus-based recommendations for successful implementation and are available at http://whqlibdoc. who.int/publications/2009/9789241597906_eng.pdf. The American Academy of Pediatrics has also published guidance on infection control and hand hygiene based on the WHO recommendations (see "Bibliography" in this chapter).

Dress Codes

Each hospital should establish dress codes for personnel who enter the labor, delivery, and nursery areas. Sterile, long-sleeved gowns should be worn by all personnel who have direct contact with the sterile field during vaginal deliveries, obstetric surgical procedures, and surgical procedures in the nursery or NICU (eg, central line insertion). Hospital policies regarding sterile areas should be established and maintained. It has become commonplace for medical care providers to wear surgical scrubs to and from work. This has engendered controversy regarding the efficacy and safety of laundering surgical scrubs at home versus the hospital. According to the CDC, "the risk of actual disease transmission from soiled linen is negligible." It is further stated by the CDC that, "in the home, normal washing and drying cycles including 'hot' and 'cold' cycles are adequate to ensure patient safety." To date, there are no data indicating that there is any significant difference between home and hospital laundering of scrubs.

Some hospitals have approved more flexible dress codes for personnel who work in birthing rooms; however, based on the CDC's standard precautions for the prevention of infection with bloodborne pathogens, it is recommended that all health care workers who perform or assist in deliveries wear sterile gloves, gowns, surgical masks, caps, and eye protection during the procedure. Wearing aprons or gowns made of impervious material during cesarean delivery may provide additional protection. Gloves should be worn when handling the placenta or the neonate until blood and amniotic fluid have been removed from the neonate's skin. Hands should be washed immediately before putting gloves on and after gloves are removed or when skin surfaces are contaminated with blood.

Studies have demonstrated that the routine use of cover gowns is not necessary in the nursery or NICU. However, regular personnel in the nursery or NICU should wear a cover gown with long sleeves whenever they hold an infant. The gown can be discarded after use or maintained exclusively for reuse when holding the same infant and changed on a regular basis.

Gowns and gloves should be worn when an infant is colonized with a resistant or invasive pathogen, consistent with appropriate isolation requirements. Additional personal protective equipment may be required on the basis of isolation requirements of the specific pathogen or clinical condition and the activity or procedure to be performed.

Caps, beard bags, and masks should be worn during certain surgical procedures, including umbilical vessel catheterization and insertion of central lines. Long hair should be restrained so that it does not touch the neonate or equipment during patient examinations or treatments. Masks should be worn so that they cover both the nose and the mouth, and they should be discarded as soon as they are removed from the nose and mouth. High-efficiency, disposable masks should be used, but even these masks remain effective only for a few hours.

Sterile gloves should be used during deliveries and all invasive procedures performed in either the obstetric or the nursery area. Disposable, nonsterile gloves may be useful in the care of patients in isolation or in the performance of procedures that may result in contamination of the hands.

Obstetric Considerations

The areas where cesarean deliveries and tubal ligations are performed are operating rooms and are subject to all policies pertaining to such facilities. Therefore, all individuals present should wear appropriate operating room attire. For those close to the sterile surgical field, this attire includes clean scrub clothing, sterile operating room gowns, caps, masks, eye protection, gloves, and shoe covers. For those not involved with the surgical field, a sterile operating room gown is not required, but caps, masks, and shoe covers should be worn. The surgical field should be prepared and draped according to standard recommendations. Preoperative clipping of hair very close to the skin is preferred to shaving.

Intrauterine pressure catheters (for monitoring contractions or for amnio-infusion) or internal fetal electrodes (for fetal heart rate monitoring) should be inserted and maintained in accordance with standard sterile techniques. Fluids used with pressure catheters should be sterile. To minimize the chance of contamination, the packages containing the devices should be opened only at the time of their use, and proper sterile techniques should be followed during their handling and insertion. Disposable items should be used whenever possible.

Neonatal Considerations

Prevention of Catheter-Related Bloodstream Infections

Catheter-related bloodstream infections are the most common hospital-acquired infections in the NICU. Maximum sterile barrier precautions (ie, cap, mask, sterile gown, sterile gloves, and sterile drapes) during the insertion of central venous catheters, including all umbilical catheters, substantially reduce the incidence of catheter-related bloodstream infections compared with standard precautions (ie, sterile gloves and small drapes).

Extraluminal contamination of the intracutaneous tract is believed to be responsible for catheter-related infections that occur in the week after placement. Catheters are more mobile during the first week after insertion and can slide in and out of the insertion site, drawing organisms down into the catheter tract. Techniques to reduce the likelihood of extraluminal contamination include proper hand hygiene, aseptic catheter insertion (including use of a maximal sterile barrier for catheter insertion and care), use of a topical antiseptic, and use of sterile dressing. Both chlorhexidine [2%] and povidone iodine are recommended for skin antisepsis in infants 2 months or older. However, chlorhexidine is not approved by the U.S. Food and Drug Administration for infants younger than 2 months. Although transparent dressings permit easier inspection of the catheter site, they have no proven benefit in reducing infection. Catheter sites must be monitored visually or by palpation on a daily basis and should be redressed and cleaned on a weekly basis. In infants, there are no data indicating that tunneled catheters have a lower risk of infection than nontunneled catheters.

After the first week of placement, intraluminal colonization after hub manipulation and contamination is responsible for most catheter-related bloodstream infections. Tubing used to administer blood products or lipid emulsions should be changed daily. Tubing used to infuse dextrose and amino acids should be replaced every 4–7 days. It is important to remove all central venous catheters when they are no longer essential. Many NICUs remove central catheters when the volume of enteral feedings reaches 80–100 mL/kg per day.

An intravascular catheter should be removed promptly if signs of device-associated infection occur. Each unit should have a written policy on the procedures governing the use of these catheters. Arterial cannulas and catheters present a risk of acquired infection, especially when used for obtaining blood samples. Samples should be obtained aseptically, with precautions to avoid contamination of the system and with the realization that the risk of infection is increased when using the cannula or catheter.

Meticulous attention should be given to aseptic techniques of fluid administration. Total parenteral nutrition generally is safe, but it has been associated with infection, including bacteremia and fungemia. A multidisciplinary team approach involving pharmacists, nurses, and physicians is strongly recommended to reduce the incidence of infections and other complications. The hospital pharmacy should establish a system to ensure a satisfactory and safe means of providing sterile, unpreserved fluids to the nursery areas. All solutions intended for parenteral infusion should be compounded in the hospital pharmacy, including those containing heparin. The CDC has no recommendations for the duration of infusion (hang time) of intravenous fluids, including lipid-free parenteral nutrition fluids. Infusion of lipid-containing parenteral nutrition fluids should be completed within 24 hours of hanging the fluid. Infusion of lipid emulsions alone should be completed within 12 hours of hanging the fluid. Infusions of blood products should be completed within 4 hours of hanging the product. Flush solutions should be kept at room temperature no longer than 8 hours before being used or discarded. They should be labeled clearly with the time of opening or preparation. Single-use prefilled saline or heparin flushes also may be used. Solutions with benzyl alcohol are contraindicated in neonates because their use may lead to severe metabolic acidosis, encephalopathy, and death.

Care bundles have been shown to be an effective strategy for reducing the incidence of catheter-related bloodstream infections in NICU patients. Care bundles are groups of interventions (extrapolated from studies in adults or recommendations from professional organizations) that are likely to be effective.

This multifaceted approach has reduced the incidence of health care-associated sepsis in each center or groups of centers where it has been implemented.

Guidelines for the prevention of umbilical catheter-related infections have been published and are summarized as follows:

- Remove and do not replace umbilical artery catheters if any signs of central line-associated bloodstream infection, vascular insufficiency in the lower extremities, or thrombosis are present.

- Remove and do not replace umbilical venous catheters if any signs of central line-associated bloodstream infection or thrombosis are present.

- Cleanse the umbilical insertion site with an antiseptic before catheter insertion. Avoid tincture of iodine because of the potential effect on the neonatal thyroid. Other iodine-containing products (eg, povidone-iodine) can be used.

- Do not use topical antibiotic ointment or creams on catheter insertion sites because of the potential to promote fungal infections and antimicrobial resistance.

- Add low doses of heparin (0.25–1.0 unit/mL) to the fluid infused through an umbilical arterial catheter.

- Remove umbilical catheters as soon as possible when no longer needed. Optimally, umbilical artery catheters should not be left in place for more than 5 days.

- Umbilical venous catheters should be removed as soon as possible when no longer needed but can be used up to 14 days if managed aseptically.

A malfunctioning umbilical catheter may be replaced if there is no other indication for catheter removal and the total duration of catheterization has not exceeded 5 days for an umbilical artery catheter or 14 days for an umbilical vein catheter.

Prevention of Health Care-Associated Pneumonia

The CDC published guidelines for preventing health care-associated pneumonia in all patient populations in 2003. Although these guidelines were not specifically designed to address the unique issues facing mechanically ventilated neonates and the definition of health-care associated pneumonia in neonates is controversial, many of the recommendations are relevant to all patient populations. General concepts in the CDC document are as follows:

- Staff education and involvement in infection prevention—All health care providers should receive appropriate information relating to the epidemiology of and infection-control procedures for preventing health care-associated pneumonia. There should be procedures in place, including performance of appropriate infection-control activities, to ensure worker competency. Staff should be involved with implementation of interventions to prevent health care-associated pneumonia using performance-improvement tools and techniques.

- Infection and microbiologic surveillance—Surveillance for health care-associated pneumonia should be performed to determine trends and help identify outbreaks or other problems. Routine surveillance cultures of patients or equipment should not be performed.

- Prevention of transmission of microorganisms—Risks of acquisition of microorganisms that could result in health care-associated pneumonia can be reduced by proper sterilization or disinfection and maintenance of equipment and devices, and 2) prevention of person-to-person transmission of bacteria by use of standard precautions as well as other isolation practices, when appropriate.

- Modifying host risk of infection—Aspiration is a major risk for the development of health care-associated pneumonia. Devices, such as endotracheal tubes, tracheostomy tubes, or enteral tubes, should be removed from patients as soon as appropriate and clinically indicated. In the absence of medical contraindication(s), the head of the bed should be elevated at an angle of 30–45° for mechanically ventilated patients. A comprehensive oral-hygiene program should be followed for the patient.

Suctioning practices may influence tracheal colonization. The use of closed-suctioning systems allows endotracheal suctioning without disconnecting patients from the ventilator. Closed-suctioning methods reduce physiologic disruptions (hypoxia and decrease in heart rate), and NICU nurses judged them to be easier to use than an open system. Closed-suctioning systems provide an opportunity for bacterial contamination when pooled secretions in the lumen are reintroduced into the lower respiratory tract with repeat suctioning. On the other hand, closed-suctioning systems could potentially reduce environmental contamination of the endotracheal tube. In studies evaluating mechanically ventilated adults, airway colonization was more common when closed-suctioning systems were used, but ventilator-associated pneumonia rates were equal to or slightly less than the rates in patients cared for with open systems. The CDC recommendations do not endorse one system over the other, and there is no recommendation addressing the frequency at which closed-suctioning systems should be changed.

Using a nonsupine position may reduce the risk of ventilator-associated pneumonia. Tracheal colonization from oropharyngeal contamination is less common in infants on mechanical ventilation when the infants are placed in a lateral position on the bed as compared with the supine position. Keeping the endotracheal tube and the ventilator circuit in a horizontal position might reduce tracking of oropharyngeal sections down into the lower respiratory tract. The lateral position also is associated with reduced aspiration of gastric secretion into the trachea.

Prophylactic Antibiotic Therapy for Prevention of Health Care-Associated Infection

The efficacy of prophylactic antibiotic therapy for the prevention of infection in newborns has not been documented. Antibiotic prophylaxis in newborns is strongly discouraged except for specific indications (eg, ophthalmic antibiotics for prevention of ophthalmia neonatorum). The relative frequencies of documented infections in newborns, etiologic agents, and patterns of antimicrobial susceptibility should be monitored by the infection-control committee in collaboration with the unit's medical director. These data should guide the selection of antibiotics to be used for treating suspected infection while awaiting the results of cultures. The best tolerated, narrowest spectrum, and most effective antibiotic regimen should be selected for this purpose based on the accumulated data on the antibiotic sensitivity patterns of microbial isolates. Antibiotics should be discontinued (within 2–3 days) when culture results are negative and the probability of infection is thought to be low. The indiscriminate and injudicious use of either systemic or topical antibiotics promotes the emergence of resistant strains of bacteria, making subsequent therapy for clinical infections more difficult and dangerous.

Women With Postpartum Infections

The newborn need not be isolated from a mother with a postpartum infection in most circumstances. Women with abscesses or infected or draining wounds should have appropriate cover dressings. If it is not possible to cover the infected or draining wound completely, the infant should be placed in a separate room. Gloves and, if necessary, gowns should be worn by staff during all contact with infected patients.

Mothers with communicable diseases that are likely to be transmitted to their newborn should be separated from the newborn until the infection is no longer communicable, based on the natural history of the infection and the effectiveness of therapy in eliminating the contagion. A mother with postpartum fever that does not have a specific, communicable cause may feed and care for her newborn. With the exception of certain infections (see also "Contraindications to Breastfeeding" in Chapter 8), breastfeeding rarely is contraindicated because of maternal infection. A mother can care for her newborn if

• she feels well enough to handle the infant.

• she demonstrates effective hand hygiene techniques.

• she avoids contact of the infant with contaminated clothes, linen, dressings, or pads.

A woman with a respiratory tract infection should be made aware that the infection can be transmitted not only by droplets but also by contact with contaminated hands and fomites. Therefore, she should practice strict hand hygiene techniques and appropriately handle or dispose of contaminated tissues and any other items that may have come in contact with infectious secretions. If needed, she can wear a surgical mask to reduce the chance of droplet spread to her newborn.

Postpartum women who are infected with nonobstetric-related communicable diseases should be treated according to the precautions and isolation techniques required by the specific disease. If the required guidelines cannot be followed safely in the obstetric unit, the patient should be transferred to the appropriate unit where such care can be provided.

Cohorting During Epidemics

During hospital epidemics, a comprehensive program of infection control is required. Even if an intensive investigation is not indicated, the results of the control measures should be evaluated to ensure that they have been effective and that the problem has been resolved. Because many infections become apparent only after newborns leave the hospital, each hospital should establish procedures to be used during a suspected or confirmed epidemic for disease surveillance of recently discharged newborns. Hospital infection-control personnel and appropriate public health officials should be notified promptly about suspected or confirmed epidemics.

Newborns with overt infection and those who are colonized with that pathogen should be identified rapidly and placed in cohorts—separate areas where newborns with similar exposure or illness receive care. If rapid identification of these newborns is not possible, separate cohorts should be established for newborns with disease, those who have been exposed, those who have not been exposed, and those who are newly admitted. The success of cohort programs depends largely on the willingness and ability of nursery and ancillary personnel to adhere strictly to the cohort system and to follow established infection-control practices.

Newborns With Infections

The isolation requirements for a newborn who is infected or suspected of being infected depend on the type of infection, the condition of the newborn, the type of care required, the available space and facilities, the ratio of available nurses to patients, and the size and type of the clinical service. Other factors to be considered include the clinical manifestations of the infection, the source and possible modes of its transmission, and the number of colonized or infected newborns.

Isolation. In many instances (notable exceptions are neonatal varicella zoster virus infection or epidemics of bacterial infection), infected newborns do not need to be placed in a separate room, if certain criteria are met:

- Sufficient nursing and medical staff are on duty to provide comprehensive care.
- Adequate sinks for handwashing are available in each nursery room or area and alcohol-based hand hygiene solutions are available at all entry points and at each bed space.
- Continuing instruction is provided about the ways in which infections spread.
- If multiple infants are kept in a single room, a 4–6-foot aisle is open between infant stations.

Physical separation with assignment of separate health care personnel for each area is best. In 2007, the CDC recommended new isolation guidelines for hospitalized patients (see "Bibliography" in this chapter). These guidelines outline transmission-based precautions for patients who are infected or colonized with pathogens that are spread by airborne, droplet, or contact routes. Isolation categories, with examples, are listed in Table 11-1.

Forced-air incubators filter incoming air, but they do not filter the air that is discharged from the incubator into the nursery. Therefore, they are satisfactory for limited protective isolation of infants, but they should not be relied on to prevent transmission of microorganisms from infected infants to others.

Table 11-1. Transmission-Based Precautions for Hospitalized Patients*

Category of Precautions	Single-Patient Room	Respiratory Tract and Mucous Membrane Protection	Gowns	Gloves
Airborne	Yes, with negative air-pressure ventilation, 6–12 air exchanges per hour, ±HEPA filtration	Respirators: N95 or higher level	No[†]	No[†]
Droplet	Yes[‡]	Surgical masks[§]	No[†]	No[†]
Contact	Yes[‡]	No	Yes	Yes

Abbreviation: HEPA, high-efficiency particulate air

*These recommendations are in addition to those for standard precautions for all patients.

[†]Gowns and gloves may be required as a component of standard precautions (eg, for blood collection or during procedures likely to cause blood splashes or if there are skin lesions containing transmissible infectious agents).

[‡]Preferred. Cohorting of children infected with the same pathogen is acceptable if a single-patient room is not available, a distance of more than 3 feet between patients can be maintained, and precautions are observed between all contacts with different patients in the room.

[§]Masks should be donned on entry into the room.

American Academy of Pediatrics. Red book: report of the Committee on Infectious Diseases. 29th ed. Elk Grove Village (IL): AAP; 2012.

When an isolation room is deemed necessary (eg, for patients with highly contagious infections), blinds, windows, and other structural items must allow for ease of regular room cleaning. An intercom should be provided. Air from this room should be exhausted to the outside and not to the nursery or NICU.

Gastroenteritis, Abscess, Viral Respiratory Infection, or Cutaneous Infection. Contact precautions should be observed when treating patients with viral respiratory infection, gastroenteritis, cutaneous infections, or draining lesions or abscesses that cannot be contained adequately by a dressing. All personnel should use gowns and disposable gloves when providing direct patient care. If the patient has a viral respiratory infection, masks are also needed. Contaminated items should be properly discarded, and gowns and gloves should be discarded before leaving the room. The environment may be heavily contaminated with the infecting microorganism, and these organisms often are transmitted on the hands of personnel to other neonates. If more than one neonate is infected, a cohort approach should be taken (see also "Cohorting During Epidemics" earlier in this chapter).

Congenital Infections. Standard precautions provide adequate isolation for most congenital infections, with two exceptions: 1) congenital rubella, which requires droplet isolation, and 2) suspected herpetic infection, which requires contact isolation.

Viral Infections. Many viruses, such as respiratory syncytial virus, coxsackieviruses, or echoviruses, spread rapidly among infants and personnel in a nursery. Such viral infections can be serious in newborns, sometimes resulting in death. Because infants may shed selected viruses after their clinical illness has been resolved, they can be reservoirs of infection. It is believed that the enteroviruses and respiratory syncytial virus are transmitted predominantly by direct or indirect contact by the hands of personnel that become contaminated with virus-containing secretions or with contaminated environmental surfaces or fomites.

Newborns with confirmed or possible infections caused by a viral agent that could be transmitted by the airborne route should be separated from other infants by transfer from the nursery area, rooming-in with the mother, or enclosure of all other infants in the area in incubators.

Multidrug-Resistant (MDR) Organisms. Although the CDC reports a decrease in health care-associated infection with invasive methicillin-resistant *Staphylococcus aureus* (MRSA), infection with MRSA and other MDR organisms continues to be an important public health care problem. Infants infected with MDR organisms or MRSA should be isolated, and contact precautions should be observed.

Environmental Control

The responsible physicians and the nurse managers of the obstetric and nursery areas should work with infection-control personnel and other appropriate groups (eg, representatives of the respiratory therapy service, central supply, and housekeeping) to establish an environmental control program for the labor, delivery, and nursery areas. This program should include specific procedures in a written policy manual for cleaning and disinfection or sterilization of patient care areas, equipment, and supplies. Consultation for specific details and problems should be encouraged. Nursing supervisors should ensure that these procedures are carried out correctly.

Methods of Sterilization and Disinfection

All medical and hospital personnel should understand the difference between sterilization and disinfection. Sterilization is the destruction of all microorganisms, including spores. Disinfection is a reduction in the number of contaminating microorganisms. High-level disinfection is the elimination or destruction of all microorganisms except spores. Cleaning is the physical removal of organic material or soil, including microorganisms, from objects.

Devices that enter tissue or the vascular system should be sterile. For neonates, devices that come into contact with mucous membranes or that have prolonged or intimate contact with skin also should be sterile. Much of the equipment required in perinatal care areas, however, can be used safely if it is satisfactorily cleaned and disinfected; clean, dry surfaces do not support the growth of microorganisms.

Sometimes it is necessary to decontaminate equipment before it is cleaned and sterilized or disinfected to allow processing without exposing personnel to hazardous microbes. The equipment must be cleaned thoroughly to remove all blood, tissue, secretions, food, and other residue. Without thorough cleaning, no method of sterilization or disinfection can be effective. Furthermore, some chemical disinfectants are inactivated by organic materials.

Sterilization

Methods of sterilization include steam autoclaving, dry heat, and gaseous (ethylene oxide) or liquid chemical (eg, 2% glutaraldehyde) techniques. The preferred method of sterilization is steam autoclaving because it is the least expensive and provides the greatest margin of safety. Some equipment may be damaged by steam, however, and must be sterilized by another method. The best method for sterilization must be established for each piece of equipment.

Equipment made of material that absorbs ethylene oxide usually requires 8–12 hours of aeration after sterilization with ethylene oxide before it can be used again. Ethylene oxide sterilization of supplies or equipment should be preceded by a comprehensive review of data on the aeration time required for each material to be processed and the extent to which toxicity standards have been established. An ethylene oxide sterilization plan requires the presence of sufficient backup equipment to allow time for aeration.

Equipment that cannot be sterilized with steam or ethylene oxide may be satisfactorily sterilized after cleaning by immersion for 10 hours in acetic acid liquid sterilant or 2% glutaraldehyde or other acceptable liquid sporicide. This immersion should be followed by three rinses with sterile water (or tap water with at least 10 mg of hypochlorite per liter), thorough drying, and packaging in sterile wrappers.

High-Level Disinfection

Equipment that does not need to be sterilized may be subjected to high-level disinfection. Both hot-water disinfection and chemical disinfection are satisfactory. Hot water disinfection of equipment requires immersing it in water at 80–85°C (176–185°F) for 15 minutes or 75°C (167°F) for 30 minutes. After air drying (preferably in a cabinet with heated, filtered air), disinfected items should be wrapped aseptically and stored until needed. Although spores are not eradicated by this method, bacterial and viral decontamination is adequate. The recommendations of the equipment manufacturer should be consulted for a list of any parts or materials that may be warped or damaged at these temperatures.

The choice of liquid chemicals for high-level disinfection depends on the type of equipment to be disinfected. In many instances, immersion of the equipment for 20 minutes in 2% glutaraldehyde, followed by three rinses with sterile water (or tap water with at least 10 mg of hypochlorite per liter) and thorough drying is satisfactory.

Cleaning and Disinfecting Noncritical Surfaces

Selection of Disinfectants

Although numerous disinfectants are available, no single agent or preparation is ideal for all purposes. Consideration should be given to the agent and its special use, as well as to the types of organisms likely to be contaminating the object that is to be disinfected. Special attention should be given to the recommended concentration of each disinfectant and to its time of exposure. Unnecessary exposure of neonates to disinfectants should be avoided, and strict adherence to manufacturers' recommendations is essential.

Quaternary ammonias, chlorine compounds, and phenolic compounds are satisfactory disinfectants, although neonatal exposure to phenolic compounds has been associated with hyperbilirubinemia. Sodium hypochlorite has been suggested for disinfection of HIV-exposed surfaces. Use of any of these substances should be limited to disinfectant–detergent products registered with the U.S. Environmental Protection Agency and recommended by the manufacturer for nursery surfaces with which neonates have contact. Information about specific label claims of commercial germicides can be obtained from the U.S.

Environmental Protection Agency (www.epa.gov) or from the Association for Professionals in Infection Control and Epidemiology (http://www.apic.org//AM/Template.cfm?Section=Home1).

General Housekeeping

Cleaning should be conducted in the following time sequence:

1. Patient areas
2. Accessory areas
3. Adjacent halls

It is not known whether floor bacteria are a source of health care-associated infection, but regular cleaning prevents the accumulation of pathogenic bacteria. Disinfectant–detergents have been shown to be more effective than soap and water alone in cleaning floors, although hospital floors are recontaminated rapidly after disinfection. Available disinfectant–detergents may differ in effectiveness.

During the cleaning process, dust should not be dispersed into the air. Removal of dust by a dry vacuum machine followed by wet vacuuming is effective in cleaning and disinfecting hospital floors. Once dust has been removed, scrubbing with a mop and a disinfectant–detergent solution should be sufficient to clean and disinfect floors. Mop heads should be machine laundered and thoroughly dried daily.

Cabinet counters, work surfaces, and similar horizontal areas may be subject to heavy contamination during routine use. These areas should be cleaned once per day and between patient use with a disinfectant–detergent and clean cloths; application of friction during cleaning is important to ensure physical removal of dirt and contaminating microorganisms. Surfaces that are contaminated by patient specimens or accidental spills should be cleaned carefully and disinfected.

Walls, windows, and storage shelves may be reservoirs of pathogenic microorganisms if visibly soiled or if dust and dirt are allowed to accumulate. These areas and similar noncritical surfaces should be scrubbed periodically with a disinfectant–detergent solution as part of the general housekeeping program.

Faucet aerators may be useful to reduce water splashing in sinks, but they are extremely susceptible to contamination with a variety of hydrophilic bacteria. For this reason, removing aerators permanently may be preferred. Sinks should be sufficiently deep and have backsplashes to prevent splashing of hands with water pooled in the sink drain, a source of bacterial growth. Sinks should be scrubbed clean daily with a disinfectant–detergent; drain traps should not need routine cleaning or disinfection. The walls and floor surrounding the sinks should be covered with easily cleanable surfaces.

Written policies should be established for the removal and disposal of solid waste. Sturdy plastic liners should be used in trash receptacles; these liners should be sealed before they are removed from the trash receptacles. In patient care areas, trash receptacles should be cleaned and disinfected regularly. Potentially infectious material requires special handling and disposal.

Dedicated housekeeping personnel should be assigned to clean the nursery. If the nursery is small, they also may be assigned to work in the obstetric areas or other clean areas of the hospital. The nursery should be cleaned daily at an appropriate time. Intensive care units ideally should be cleaned when traffic is minimal.

Cleaning and Disinfecting Patient Care Equipment

Incubators, Open Care Units, and Bassinets

After an infant has been discharged, the care unit used by that infant should be thoroughly cleaned and disinfected. A disinfectant–detergent registered by the U.S. Environmental Protection Agency should be used for this purpose. Manufacturers' directions for use of a disinfectant–detergent should be followed carefully. A bassinet or incubator should never be cleaned when occupied. Infants who remain in the nursery for an extended period should be transferred periodically, as per hospital policy, to a different, disinfected unit.

When a care unit is being cleaned and disinfected, all detachable parts should be removed and scrubbed meticulously. If the incubator has a fan, it should be cleaned and disinfected; the manufacturer's instructions should be followed to avoid equipment damage. The air filter should be maintained as recommended by the manufacturer. Mattresses should be replaced when the surface covering is broken; such a break precludes effective disinfection or sterilization. Mattresses may be sterilized by heat or gas. Incubator portholes and porthole cuffs and sleeves are contaminated easily and often heavily; cuffs should be replaced on a regular schedule or cleaned and disinfected frequently with freshly prepared mild soap or quaternary ammonium disinfectant–detergent solution. Incubators not in use should be dried thoroughly by running the incubator hot without water in the reservoir for 24 hours after disinfection.

Evaporative humidifiers in incubators usually do not produce contaminated aerosols, but contaminated water reservoirs may be responsible for direct, rather than airborne, transmission of infection. Reservoirs should be filled with sterile water only, and they should be drained and refilled with sterile water every 24 hours. In many areas of the United States and in hospitals with a central ventilation system, environmental humidity levels may be sufficiently high to eliminate the need for additional humidification in most cases, and water reservoirs may be left dry. If humidification is necessary, a source of humidity external to the incubator may be preferable to incubator humidifiers. An external humidifier can be changed daily and the equipment can then be sent for cleaning and sterilization or disinfection.

Nebulizers, Water Traps, and Respiratory Support Equipment

Nebulizers and attached tubing should be replaced by clean, sterile equipment (or equipment that has been subjected to high-level disinfection) in accordance with established hospital policy. Failure to replace tubing may result in contamination of freshly cleaned equipment. Water traps also should be replaced regularly by autoclaved or disinfected equipment. Only sterile water should be used for nebulizers or water traps; residual water should be discarded when these containers are refilled. Water condensed in tubing loops should be removed and discarded and should not be allowed to reflux into the container.

Other Equipment

Cleaning and disinfection or sterilization of equipment should be performed between patients. Equipment that is used for only one patient should be replaced, cleaned, and disinfected or sterilized according to an established schedule. Disposable equipment should be replaced with approximately the same frequency as reusable equipment. Disposable equipment never should be reused.

Resuscitators, face masks, laryngoscopes, eye speculums, and other items used in direct contact with neonates should be dismantled, thoroughly cleaned, and sterilized, if possible. Alternately, the equipment may be subjected to high-level disinfection with liquid chemicals or by pasteurization. Equipment, such as tubing for respiratory or oxygen therapy, should be sterilized or discarded after use. In-line, closed suctioning systems are thought to reduce the risk of spreading potential pathogens from the airway of intubated patients. Stethoscopes and similar types of diagnostic instruments should be wiped with iodophor or alcohol before use. Standard precautions should be used when any type of suctioning is performed.

Nursery Linen

Procedures for laundering, making up linen packs, and delivering linen to the nursery should be established by the medical, nursing, laundry, and administrative staffs of the hospital. Each delivery of clean linen should contain sufficient linen for at least one nursing shift. Linen should be cleaned and transported in covered carts to the nursery areas. Autoclaving linen has not been shown to be effective in preventing infections in normal newborn nurseries or intensive care areas. New garments and linen for neonates should be laundered before use.

An established procedure for the disposal of soiled linen should be followed strictly. Chutes for the transfer of soiled linen from patient care areas to the laundry are not acceptable unless they are under negative air pressure. Soiled linen should be discarded into impervious plastic bags placed in hampers that are easy to clean and disinfect. Plastic bags of soiled linen should be sealed and removed from the nursery at least twice a day. Individuals who collect the bags of soiled linen need not enter the nursery if all bags are placed outside the nursery. Sealed bags of reusable, soiled nursery linens should be taken to the laundry at least twice each day.

Laundering

Nursery linens should be washed separately from other hospital linen and with products used to retain softness. Acidification neutralizes the alkalis used in the washing process and is responsible for the greatest bacterial destruction. Standard precautions should be taken in handling linen soiled with blood. Chlorine bleach should be used for any items that are contaminated with blood.

Trichlorocarbanilide and the sodium salt of pentachlorophenol should not be used in hospital laundering because they may be harmful. Therefore, caution should be exercised when new laundry or cleaning agents are introduced into the nursery or when procedures are changed.

Bibliography

American Academy of Pediatrics. Red book: report of the Committee on Infectious Diseases. 29th. Elk Grove Village (IL): American Academy of Pediatrics; 2012.

Antimicrobial pesticide products. EPA Fact Sheets. Washington, DC: EPA; 2004. Available at: http://www.epa.gov/pesticides/factsheets/antimic.htm. Retrieved January 3, 2012.

Belkin NL. Home laundering of soiled surgical scrubs: surgical site infections and the home environment. Am J Infect Control 2001;29:58–64.

Epidemiology and diagnosis of health care–associated infections in the NICU. American Academy of Pediatrics. Committee on Fetus and Newborn and Committee on Infectious Diseases. Pediatrics 2012;129:e1104–9.

Henderson DK, Dembry L, Fishman NO, Grady C, Lundstrom T, Palmore TN, et al. SHEA guideline for management of healthcare workers who are infected with hepatitis B virus, hepatitis C virus, and/or human immunodeficiency virus. Society for Healthcare Epidemiology of America. Infect Control Hosp Epidemiol 2010;31:203–32.

Hepatitis B, hepatitis C, and human immunodeficiency virus infections in obstetrician-gynecologists. Committee Opinion No. 489. American College of Obstetricians and Gynecologists. Obstet Gynecol 2011;117:1242–6.

Infection prevention and control in pediatric ambulatory settings. American Academy of Pediatrics. Committee on Infectious Diseases. Pediatrics 2007;120:650–665.

Jurkovich P. Home- versus hospital-laundered scrubs: a pilot study. MCN Am J Matern Child Nurs 2004;29:106–10.

Laundry: washing infected material. Preventing healthcare-associated infections. Atlanta (GA): CDC; 2011. Available at: http://www.cdc.gov/HAI/prevent/laundry.html. Retrieved January 3, 2012.

Methicillin-resistant Staphylococcus Aureus (MRSA) Infections. MRSA Statistics. Atlanta (GA): Centers for Disease Control and Prevention; 2012. Available at: http://www.cdc.gov/mrsa/statistics/index.html. Retrieved January 23, 2012.

O'Grady NP, Alexander M, Burns LA, Dellinger EP, Garland J, Heard SO, et al. Guidelines for the prevention of intravascular catheter-related infections. Healthcare Infection Control Practices Advisory Committee. Clin Infect Dis 2011;52:e162–93.

Pittet D, Allegranzi B, Boyce J. The World Health Organization Guidelines on Hand Hygiene in Health Care and their consensus recommendations. World Health Organization World Alliance for Patient Safety First Global Patient Safety Challenge Core Group of Experts. Infect Control Hosp Epidemiol 2009;30:611–22.

Polin RA. Management of neonates with suspected or proven early-onset bacterial sepsis. American Academy of Pediatrics. Committee on Fetus and Newborn. Pediatrics 2012;129:1006–15.

Polin RA, Denson S, Brady MT. Strategies for prevention of health Care–associated infections in the NICU. American Academy of Pediatrics. Committee on Fetus and Newborn and Committee on Infectious Diseases. Pediatrics 2012; 129:e1085–93.

Polizzi J, Byers JF, Kiehl E. Co-bedding versus traditional bedding of multiple-gestation infants in the NICU. J Healthc Qual 2003;25:5,10; quiz 10-1.

Sehulster L, Chinn RY. Guidelines for environmental infection control in health-care facilities. Recommendations of CDC and the Healthcare Infection Control Practices Advisory Committee (HICPAC). MMWR Recomm Rep 2003;52(RR-10):1–42.

Siegel JD, Rhinehart E, Jackson M, Chiarello L. 2007 guideline for isolation precautions: preventing transmission of infectious agents in healthcare settings. Healthcare Infection Control Practices Advisory Committee (HICPAC). Atlanta (GA): Centers for Disease Control and Prevention; 2007. Available at: http://www.cdc.gov/hicpac/pdf/isolation/Isolation2007.pdf. Retrieved January 3, 2012.

Resources

Association for Professionals in Infection Control and Epidemiology. Washington, DC: APIC; 2011. Available at: http://www.apic.org//AM/Template.cfm?Section=Home1. Retrieved January 3, 2012.

United States Environmental Protection Agency (EPA). Washington, DC: EPA; 2011. Available at: http://www.epa.gov. Retrieved January 3, 2012.

World Health Organization. WHO guidelines on hand hygiene in health care: first global patient safety challenge clean care is safer care. Geneva: WHO; 2009. Available at: http://whqlibdoc.who.int/publications/2009/9789241597906_eng.pdf. Retrieved January 3, 2012.

Appendix A

American College of Obstetricians and Gynecologists' Antepartum Record and Postpartum Form

Patient Addressograph

DATE: _____

NAME: _____
     LAST   FIRST   MIDDLE

ID #: _____ HOSPITAL OF DELIVERY: _____

NEWBORN CARE PROVIDER: _____ REFERRED BY: _____

PRIMARY PROVIDER/GROUP: _____

FINAL EDD: _____	ADDRESS: _____	

BIRTH DATE:	AGE:	RACE:	MARITAL STATUS: S M W D SEP	ADDRESS:	
MONTH DAY YEAR				ZIP: _____ PHONE: _____ (1)_____ (2)_____	
OCCUPATION:		EDUCATION: (LAST GRADE COMPLETED)		E-MAIL:	
LANGUAGE:		ETHNICITY:		INSURANCE CARRIER/MEDICAID #:	
HUSBAND/DOMESTIC PARTNER:		PHONE:		POLICY #:	
FATHER OF BABY:		PHONE:		EMERGENCY CONTACT:	PHONE:

TOTAL PREG:	FULL TERM:	PREMATURE:	AB. INDUCED:	AB. SPONTANEOUS:	ECTOPICS:	MULTIPLE BIRTHS:	LIVING:

MENSTRUAL HISTORY

LMP ☐ DEFINITE   ☐ APPROXIMATE (MONTH KNOWN)   MENSES MONTHLY ☐ YES ☐ NO   FREQUENCY: Q _____ DAYS   MENARCHE: _____ (AGE ONSET)
   ☐ UNKNOWN   ☐ NORMAL AMOUNT/DURATION   PRIOR MENSES _____ DATE   ON BCP AT CONCEPT ☐ YES ☐ NO   hCG + ___/___/___
   ☐ FINAL: _____

PAST PREGNANCIES (LAST SIX)

DATE MONTH/ YEAR	GA WEEKS	LENGTH OF LABOR	BIRTH WEIGHT	SEX M/F	TYPE OF DELIVERY	ANES	PLACE OF DELIVERY	PRETERM LABOR YES/NO	COMMENTS/ COMPLICATIONS

MEDICAL HISTORY

	○ Neg. + Pos.	DETAIL POSITIVE REMARKS INCLUDE DATE & TREATMENT		○ Neg. + Pos.	DETAIL POSITIVE REMARKS INCLUDE DATE & TREATMENT
A. DRUG/LATEX ALLERGIES/ REACTIONS			18. OPERATIONS/HOSPITALIZATIONS (YEAR & REASON)		
B. ALLERGIES (FOOD, SEASONAL, ENVIRONMENTAL)			19. GYN SURGERY		
1. NEUROLOGIC/EPILEPSY			20. ANESTHETIC COMPLICATIONS		
2. THYROID DYSFUNCTION			21. HISTORY OF BLOOD TRANSFUSIONS		
3. BREAST DISEASE			22. INFERTILITY		
4. PULMONARY (TB, ASTHMA)			23. ASSISTED REPRODUCTIVE TECHNOLOGY		
5. HEART DISEASE			24. UTERINE ANOMALY/DES		
6. HYPERTENSION			25. HISTORY OF ABNORMAL PAP		
7. CANCER			26. HISTORY OF STI		
8. HEMATOLOGIC DISORDERS			27. PSYCHIATRIC ILLNESS		
9. ANEMIA			28. DEPRESSION/POSTPARTUM DEPRESSION		
10. GASTROINTESTINAL DISORDERS			29. TRAUMA/VIOLENCE		
11. HEPATITIS/LIVER DISEASE				PREPREG. PREG. # YEARS USE	
12. KIDNEY DISEASE/UTI			30. TOBACCO (AMT/DAY)		
13. VARICOSITIES/PHLEBITIS			31. ALCOHOL (AMT/WK)		
14. DIABETES (TYPE 1 OR TYPE 2)			32. ILLICIT/RECREATIONAL DRUGS (USES/WK)		
15. GESTATIONAL DIABETES			33. RELEVANT FAMILY HISTORY		
16. AUTOIMMUNE DISORDERS			34. OTHER		
17. DERMATOLOGIC DISORDERS					

COMMENTS: _____

PATIENT NAME:	BIRTH DATE: / /	ID NO.:	DATE: / /

GENETIC SCREENING/TERATOLOGY COUNSELING
INCLUDES PATIENT, BABY'S FATHER, OR ANYONE IN EITHER FAMILY WITH:

	YES	NO		YES	NO
1. THALASSEMIA (ITALIAN, GREEK, MEDITERRANEAN, OR ASIAN BACKGROUND): MCV LESS THAN 80			12. HUNTINGTON CHOREA		
			13. MENTAL RETARDATION/AUTISM		
2. NEURAL TUBE DEFECT (MENINGOMYELOCELE, SPINA BIFIDA, OR ANENCEPHALY)			IF YES, WAS PERSON TESTED FOR FRAGILE X?		
3. CONGENITAL HEART DEFECT			14. OTHER INHERITED GENETIC OR CHROMOSOMAL DISORDER		
4. DOWN SYNDROME			15. MATERNAL METABOLIC DISORDER (EG, TYPE 1 DIABETES, PKU)		
5. TAY-SACHS (ASHKENAZI JEWISH, CAJUN, FRENCH CANADIAN)			16. BIRTH DEFECTS NOT LISTED ABOVE		
6. CANAVAN DISEASE (ASHKENAZI JEWISH)			17. RECURRENT PREGNANCY LOSS OR A STILLBIRTH		
7. FAMILIAL DYSAUTONOMIA (ASHKENAZI JEWISH)			18. MEDICATIONS (INCLUDING SUPPLEMENTS, VITAMINS, HERBS, OR OTC DRUGS)/ILLICIT/RECREATIONAL DRUGS/ALCOHOL SINCE LAST MENSTRUAL PERIOD		
8. SICKLE CELL DISEASE OR TRAIT (AFRICAN)					
9. HEMOPHILIA OR OTHER BLOOD DISORDERS			IF YES, AGENT(S) AND STRENGTH/DOSAGE		
10. MUSCULAR DYSTROPHY			19. ANY OTHER		
11. CYSTIC FIBROSIS*					

*If a patient has been screened previously, cystic fibrosis screening results should be documented but the test should not be repeated.

COMMENTS/COUNSELING: _____

INFECTION HISTORY	YES	NO		
1. LIVE WITH SOMEONE WITH TB OR EXPOSED TO TB			5. HISTORY OF STIs: GONORRHEA, CHLAMYDIA, HPV, SYPHILIS, PID (CIRCLE ALL THAT APPLY)	
2. PATIENT OR PARTNER HAS HISTORY OF GENITAL HERPES			6. HISTORY OF HIV YES ☐ NO ☐	
3. RASH OR VIRAL ILLNESS SINCE LAST MENSTRUAL PERIOD			7. HISTORY OF HEPATITIS	
4. PRIOR GBS-INFECTED CHILD			8. OTHER (SEE COMMENTS)	

COMMENTS: _____

INTERVIEWER'S SIGNATURE: _____

IMMUNIZATIONS	YES (MONTH/YEAR) ___/___	NO	IF NO, POSTPARTUM VACCINE INDICATED?	IMMUNIZATIONS	YES (MONTH/YEAR) ___/___	NO	IF NO, POSTPARTUM VACCINE INDICATED?
TDAP or TD				HEPATITIS A (WHEN INDICATED)			
INFLUENZA*				HEPATITIS B (WHEN INDICATED)			
VARICELLA*				MENINGOCOCCAL (WHEN INDICATED)			
MMR*				PNEUMOCOCCAL (WHEN INDICATED)			

*All live vaccines are contraindicated in pregnancy, including the live intranasal influenza, MMR, and varicella vaccines. All women who will be pregnant during influenza season (October through May) should receive inactivated influenza vaccine at any point in gestation. Administer the MMR and varicella vaccines postpartum if needed.

INITIAL PHYSICAL EXAMINATION

DATE: ___/___/___   WEIGHT: _____   HEIGHT: _____   BMI: _____   BP: _____

1. HEENT	☐ NORMAL ☐ ABNORMAL	12. VULVA	☐ NORMAL	☐ CONDYLOMA	☐ LESIONS
2. TEETH	☐ NORMAL ☐ ABNORMAL	13. VAGINA	☐ NORMAL	☐ INFLAMMATION	☐ DISCHARGE
3. SYMPTOMS SINCE LMP	☐ NORMAL ☐ ABNORMAL	14. CERVIX	☐ NORMAL	☐ INFLAMMATION	☐ LESIONS
4. THYROID	☐ NORMAL ☐ ABNORMAL	15. UTERUS SIZE	_____ WEEKS		☐ FIBROIDS
5. BREASTS	☐ NORMAL ☐ ABNORMAL	16. ADNEXA	☐ NORMAL	☐ MASS	
6. LUNGS	☐ NORMAL ☐ ABNORMAL	17. RECTUM	☐ NORMAL	☐ ABNORMAL	
7. HEART	☐ NORMAL ☐ ABNORMAL	18. DIAGONAL CONJUGATE	☐ REACHED	☐ NO	_____ CM
8. ABDOMEN	☐ NORMAL ☐ ABNORMAL	19. SPINES	☐ AVERAGE	☐ PROMINENT	☐ BLUNT
9. EXTREMITIES	☐ NORMAL ☐ ABNORMAL	20. SACRUM	☐ CONCAVE	☐ STRAIGHT	☐ ANTERIOR
10. SKIN	☐ NORMAL ☐ ABNORMAL	21. SUBPUBIC ARCH	☐ NORMAL	☐ WIDE	☐ NARROW
11. LYMPH NODES	☐ NORMAL ☐ ABNORMAL	22. GYNECOID PELVIC TYPE	☐ YES	☐ NO	

COMMENTS (Number and explain abnormals): _____

EXAM BY: _____

Version 7. Copyright 2011 The American College of Obstetricians and Gynecologists   (AA128)   12345/54321

ANTEPARTUM RECORD (FORM B, page 2 of 12)

Patient Addressograph

PATIENT NAME:		BIRTH DATE: / /	ID NO:	DATE: / /

DRUG ALLERGY:_____	LATEX ALLERGY ☐ YES ☐ NO	POSTPARTUM CONTRACEPTION METHOD:_____
IS BLOOD TRANSFUSION ACCEPTABLE? ☐ YES ☐ NO	ANTEPARTUM ANESTHESIA CONSULT PLANNED ☐ YES ☐ NO	

PROBLEMS   **PLANS**

1.
2.
3.
4.
5.

MEDICATION LIST   Start date   Stop date

1. _____ / _____ / _____   _____ / _____ / _____
2. _____ / _____ / _____   _____ / _____ / _____
3. _____ / _____ / _____   _____ / _____ / _____
4. _____ / _____ / _____   _____ / _____ / _____
5. _____ / _____ / _____   _____ / _____ / _____

EDD CONFIRMATION

INITIAL EDD
LMP: _____ / _____ / _____   =   EDD _____ / _____ / _____
INITIAL EXAM: _____ / _____ / _____ = _____ WKS = EDD _____ / _____ / _____
ULTRASONOGRAPHY: _____ / _____ / _____ = _____ WKS = EDD _____ / _____ / _____
INITIAL EDD: _____ / _____ / _____   INITIALED BY: _____

18–20-WEEK EDD UPDATE

QUICKENING   _____ / _____ / _____   +22 WKS = _____ / _____ / _____
FUNDAL HT.
AT UMBIL: _____ / _____ / _____   +20 WKS = _____ / _____ / _____
ULTRASONOGRAPHY: _____ / _____ / _____ = _____ WKS = _____ / _____ / _____
FINAL EDD: _____ / _____ / _____   INITIALED BY: _____

PREPREGNANCY WEIGHT

BMI

WEEKS GEST. (BEST EST.)	FUNDAL HEIGHT (CM)	PRESENTATION	FHR	FETAL MOVEMENT	PRETERM LABOR SIGNS/SYMPTOMS +PRESENT -ABSENT	CERVIX EXAM (DIL/EFF STA) LENGTH ON ULTRASONOGRAPHY	BLOOD PRESSURE	WEIGHT	URINE (ALBUMIN/GLUCOSE)	EDEMA	PAIN SCALE * (0-10)	NEXT APPOINTMENT	PROVIDER (INITIALS)	COMMENTS

ANTEPARTUM RECORD (FORM C, page 3 of 12)

*Describe the intensity of discomfort ranging from 0 (no pain) to 10 (worst possible pain).

Version 7. Copyright 2011 The American College of Obstetricians and Gynecologists   (AA128)   12345/54321

Patient Addressograph

PATIENT NAME		BIRTH DATE / /	ID NO:	DATE / /

LABORATORY AND SCREENING TESTS

INITIAL LABS	DATE	RESULT	REVIEWED
BLOOD TYPE	/ /	A B AB O	
D (Rh) TYPE	/ /		
ANTIBODY SCREEN	/ /		
COMPLETE BLOOD COUNT	/ /	HCT/HGB: _____ % _____ g/dL	
		MCV:_____	
		PLT:_____	
VDRL/RPR	/ /		
URINE CULTURE/SCREEN	/ /		
HBsAg	/ /		
HIV TESTING*	/ /	POS. NEG. DECLINED	
CHLAMYDIA	/ /		
GONORRHEA (WHEN INDICATED)	/ /		
OTHER:			

SUPPLEMENTAL LABS	DATE	RESULT
HEMOGLOBIN	/ /	AA AS SS AC SC AF ↑A₂ POS. NEG. DECLINED
PPD/QUANTA	/ /	
PAP TEST	/ /	
CYSTIC FIBROSIS	/ /	
HPV	/ /	POS. NEG. DECLINED
TAY–SACHS/CANAVAN DISEASE	/ /	POS. NEG. DECLINED
EARLY DIABETES SCREEN	/ /	POS. NEG. DECLINED
FAMILIAL DYSAUTONOMIA	/ /	POS. NEG. DECLINED
GENETIC SCREENING TESTS (SEE FORM B)	/ /	
OTHER:		

8–20-WEEK SCREENING (WHEN INDICATED/ELECTED)	DATE	RESULT
1ST TRIMESTER ANEUPLOIDY AND NEURAL TUBE DEFECT SCREENING	/ /	
2ND TRIMESTER SERUM SCREENING	/ /	
AMNIO/CVS	/ /	
KARYOTYPE	/ /	46,XX OR 46,XY/OTHER_____
AMNIOTIC FLUID (AFP)	/ /	NORMAL_____ ABNORMAL_____
OTHER:	/ /	

COMMENTS/ADDITIONAL LABS

*Check state requirements before recording results.   (continued)

PROVIDER SIGNATURE (AS REQUIRED): _____

Version 7. Copyright 2011 The American College of Obstetricians and Gynecologists   (AA128)   12345/54321

ANTEPARTUM RECORD (FORM D, page 4 of 12)

Patient Addressograph

PATIENT NAME		BIRTH DATE / /	ID NO	DATE / /

LABORATORY AND SCREENING TESTS *(continued)*

24–28-WEEK LABS	DATE	RESULT	REVIEWED	COMMENTS/ADDITIONAL LABS
COMPLETE BLOOD COUNT	/ /	HCT/HGB _____ % _____ g/dL MCV: _____ PLT: _____		
DIABETES SCREEN	/ /			
GTT (IF SCREEN ABNORMAL)	/ /	_____FBS _____1 HOUR _____2 HOUR _____3 HOUR		
D (Rh) ANTIBODY SCREEN (WHEN INDICATED)	/ /			
ANTI-D IMMUNE GLOBULIN (RhIG) GIVEN (28 WKS OR GREATER) (WHEN INDICATED)	/ /	SIGNATURE _____		
OTHER:	/ /			
32–36-WEEK LABS AND SCREENING TESTS (WHEN INDICATED)	**DATE**	**RESULT**		
COMPLETE BLOOD COUNT	/ /	HCT/HGB _____ % _____ g/dL MCV: _____ PLT: _____		
ULTRASONOGRAPHY (WHEN INDICATED)	/ /			
HIV (WHEN INDICATED)*				
VDRL/RPR (WHEN INDICATED)	/ /			
GONORRHEA (WHEN INDICATED)	/ /			
CHLAMYDIA (WHEN INDICATED)	/ /			
DEPRESSION SCREENING (WHEN INDICATED)	/ /			
OTHER:	/ /			
35–37-WEEK LABS	**DATE**	**RESULT**		
GROUP B STREP	/ /			
RESISTANCE TESTING IF PENICILLIN ALLERGIC	/ /			

*Check state requirements before recording results.

COMMENTS

PROVIDER SIGNATURE (AS REQUIRED) _____

ANTEPARTUM RECORD (FORM D, page 5 of 12)

Patient Addressograph

PATIENT NAME:	BIRTH DATE: / /	ID NO:	DATE: / /

PLANS/EDUCATION
(COUNSELED ☐)—BY TRIMESTER INITIAL AND DATE WHEN DISCUSSED

FIRST TRIMESTER	COMPLETED	NEED FOR FURTHER DISCUSSION
☐ HIV AND OTHER ROUTINE PRENATAL TESTS		☐ FOLLOW-UP IF NEEDED ☐ REFERRAL NEEDED
☐ RISK FACTORS IDENTIFIED BY PRENATAL HISTORY		
☐ ANTICIPATED COURSE OF PRENATAL CARE		
☐ NUTRITION COUNSELING, SPECIAL DIET, DIETARY PRECAUTIONS (MERCURY, LISTERIOSIS)		
☐ WEIGHT GAIN COUNSELING		
☐ TOXOPLASMOSIS PRECAUTIONS (CATS/RAW MEAT)		
☐ SEXUAL ACTIVITY		
☐ EXERCISE		
☐ DENTAL CARE		
☐ ENVIRONMENTAL/WORK HAZARDS		
☐ AVOIDANCE OF SAUNAS OR HOT TUBS		
☐ TERATOGENS		
☐ TRAVEL		
☐ TOBACCO/SMOKING CESSATION COUNSELING (ASK, ADVISE, ASSESS, ASSIST, AND ARRANGE)		
☐ ALCOHOL		
☐ ILLICIT/RECREATIONAL DRUGS		
☐ BREASTFEEDING		
☐ SCREENING FOR ANEUPLOIDY		
☐ USE OF ANY MEDICATIONS (INCLUDING SUPPLEMENTS, VITAMINS, HERBS, OR OTC DRUGS)		
☐ INDICATIONS FOR ULTRASONOGRAPHY		
☐ INTIMATE PARTNER VIOLENCE		
☐ SEAT BELT USE		
☐ CHILDBIRTH CLASSES/HOSPITAL FACILITIES		
SECOND TRIMESTER		
☐ SIGNS AND SYMPTOMS OF PRETERM LABOR		
☐ ABNORMAL LAB VALUES		
☐ SELECTING A NEWBORN CARE PROVIDER		
☐ TOBACCO/SMOKING CESSATION COUNSELING (ASK, ADVISE, ASSESS, ASSIST, AND ARRANGE)		
☐ DEPRESSION SCREENING (WHEN INDICATED)		
☐ INTIMATE PARTNER VIOLENCE		
☐ POSTPARTUM FAMILY PLANNING/TUBAL STERILIZATION		

(continued)

COMMENTS

Version 7. Copyright 2011 The American College of Obstetricians and Gynecologists

(AA128)   12345/54321

Patient Addressograph

PATIENT NAME	BIRTH DATE / /	ID NO	DATE / /

PLANS/EDUCATION (continued)
(COUNSELED ☐)—BY TRIMESTER. INITIAL AND DATE WHEN DISCUSSED.

THIRD TRIMESTER	COMPLETED	NEED FOR FURTHER DISCUSSION
☐ ANESTHESIA PLANS		
☐ FETAL MOVEMENT MONITORING		
☐ LABOR SIGNS		
☐ TRIAL OF LABOR AFTER CESAREAN (TOLAC) COUNSELING		
☐ SIGNS AND SYMPTOMS OF PREECLAMPSIA		
☐ POSTTERM COUNSELING		
☐ CIRCUMCISION		
☐ BREASTFEEDING		
☐ POSTPARTUM DEPRESSION		
☐ TOBACCO/SMOKING CESSATION COUNSELING (ASK, ADVISE, ASSESS, ASSIST, AND ARRANGE)		
☐ INTIMATE PARTNER VIOLENCE		
☐ NEWBORN EDUCATION (NEWBORN SCREENING, JAUNDICE, SIDS/SAFE SLEEPING POSITION, CAR SEAT)		
☐ FAMILY MEDICAL LEAVE OR DISABILITY FORMS		

REQUESTS
_____
_____
_____

TUBAL STERILIZATION CONSENT SIGNED (IF DESIRED).   DATE   INITIALS
                                                          __/__/__   _____

HISTORY AND PHYSICAL HAVE BEEN SENT TO HOSPITAL, IF APPLICABLE.   DATE   INITIALS
                                                          __/__/__   _____

UPDATE WITH GROUP B STREPTOCOCCUS RESULTS SENT.   DATE   INITIALS
                                                          __/__/__   _____

COMMENTS
_____
_____
_____
_____
_____
_____
_____
_____
_____
_____
_____
_____
_____
_____

ANTEPARTUM RECORD (FORM E, page 7 of 12)

(AA128)   12345/54321

PATIENT NAME	BIRTH DATE / /	ID NO.	DATE / /

Plans/Education Notes

_____

_____

_____

_____

_____

_____

_____

_____

_____

_____

_____

_____

_____

_____

_____

_____

_____

_____

_____

_____

_____

_____

_____

_____

_____

_____

_____

_____

_____

_____

_____

_____

_____

_____

_____

_____

_____

Version 7. Copyright 2011 The American College of Obstetricians and Gynecologists   (AA128)   12345/54321

Patient Addressograph

NAME: _____
LAST   FIRST   MIDDLE

ID #: _____

EDD: _____

Prenatal Visits

PREPREGNANCY
WEIGHT
_____

BMI
_____

WEEKS GEST. (BEST EST.)	FUNDAL HEIGHT (CM)	PRESENTATION	FHR	FETAL MOVEMENT	PRETERM LABOR SIGNS/SYMPTOMS + = PRESENT O = ABSENT	CERVIX EXAM (IF INDICATED)	BLOOD PRESSURE	WEIGHT	URINE (ALBUMIN/GLUCOSE)	EDEMA	PAIN SCALE* (0–10)	NEXT APPOINTMENT	PROVIDER (INITIALS)

ALLERGIES   YES ☐   NO ☐
IF YES, PLEASE LIST
_____
_____
_____
_____
_____

COMMENTS
_____
_____
_____
_____
_____
_____
_____
_____
_____
_____

*Describe the intensity of discomfort ranging from 0 (no pain) to 10 (worst possible pain)

Progress Notes

_____
_____
_____
_____
_____
_____
_____
_____
_____

PROVIDER SIGNATURE (AS REQUIRED) _____

Version 7. Copyright 2011 The American College of Obstetricians and Gynecologists   (AA128)   12345/54321

ANTEPARTUM RECORD (FORM F, page 9 of 12)

NAME: _____
        LAST   FIRST   MIDDLE

ID #: _____

EDD: _____

Prenatal Visits

PREPREGNANCY
WEIGHT
_____

BMI
_____

WEEKS GEST. (BEST EST.)	FUNDAL HEIGHT (CM)	PRESENTATION	FHR	FETAL MOVEMENT	PRETERM LABOR SIGNS/SYMPTOMS + PRESENT – ABSENT	CERVIX EXAM (IF INDICATED)	BLOOD PRESSURE	WEIGHT	URINE (ALBUMIN/GLUCOSE)	EDEMA	PAIN SCALE* (0–10)	NEXT APPOINTMENT	PROVIDER (INITIALS)

ALLERGIES   YES ☐   NO ☐
IF YES, PLEASE LIST:
_____
_____
_____
_____
_____

COMMENTS
_____
_____
_____
_____
_____
_____
_____

*Describe the intensity of discomfort ranging from 0 (no pain) to 10 (worst possible pain).

Progress Notes

_____
_____
_____
_____
_____
_____
_____
_____

PROVIDER SIGNATURE (AS REQUIRED): _____

(AA128)   12345/54321

NAME: _____
LAST   FIRST   MIDDLE

ID #: _____

EDD: _____

Progress Notes

_____
_____
_____
_____
_____
_____
_____
_____
_____
_____
_____
_____
_____
_____
_____
_____
_____
_____
_____
_____
_____
_____
_____
_____
_____
_____
_____
_____
_____
_____
_____
_____
_____
_____
_____
_____
_____
_____

PROVIDER SIGNATURE (AS REQUIRED) _____

Version 7. Copyright 2011 The American College of Obstetricians and Gynecologists

(AA128)   12345/54321

ANTEPARTUM RECORD (FORM G, page 11 of 12)

NAME: _____
        LAST   FIRST   MIDDLE

ID #: _____

EDD: _____

Progress Notes

_____
_____
_____
_____
_____
_____
_____
_____
_____
_____
_____
_____
_____
_____
_____
_____
_____
_____
_____
_____
_____
_____
_____
_____
_____
_____
_____
_____
_____
_____
_____
_____
_____
_____

PROVIDER SIGNATURE (AS REQUIRED) _____

Version 7. Copyright 2011 The American College of Obstetricians and Gynecologists   (AA128)   12345/54321

ANTEPARTUM RECORD (FORM G, page 12 of 12)

POSTPARTUM FORM

NAME: _____
LAST   FIRST   MIDDLE

DELIVERY DATE: _____   HOSPITAL: _____

DISCHARGE DATE: _____

DELIVERY INFORMATION

DELIVERY AT_____WEEKS

☐ VAGINAL   ☐ CESAREAN
  ☐ SVD   ☐ PRIMARY (For _____)
  ☐ VACUUM   ☐ REPEAT - ELECTIVE
  ☐ FORCEPS   ☐ REPEAT - UNSUCCESSFUL TOLAC
  ☐ EPISIOTOMY   ☐ INCISION
  ☐ LACERATIONS ☐ LOW TRANSVERSE
  ☐ TOLAC   ☐ LOW VERTICAL
           ☐ CLASSICAL

LABOR
☐ NONE
☐ SPONTANEOUS
☐ INDUCED
☐ AUGMENTED

ANESTHESIA
☐ NONE
☐ LOCAL/PUDENDAL
☐ EPIDURAL
☐ SPINAL
☐ GENERAL
☐ OTHER: _____

POSTPARTUM CONTRACEPTION

	YES	NO
TUBAL STERILIZATION	☐	☐
INTRAUTERINE DEVICE (IUD)	☐	☐
DEPOT MEDROXYPROGESTERONE ACETATE (DMPA)	☐	☐
IMPLANT	☐	☐
ORAL CONTRACEPTIVES	☐	☐

OTHER : _____
NOTES : _____
_____
_____

DELIVERED BY : _____

POSTPARTUM INFORMATION

COMPLICATIONS
☐ NONE   ☐ HEMORRHAGE   ☐ INFECTION   ☐ HYPERTENSION   ☐ DIABETES   ☐ OTHER: _____

DISCHARGE INFORMATION

NEONATAL INFORMATION

NAME OF BABY: _____

SEX
☐ FEMALE   ☐ MALE
    CIRCUMCISION ☐ YES ☐ NO

BIRTH WEIGHT: _____

DISPOSITION
☐ HOME WITH MOTHER   ☐ IN HOSPITAL
☐ TRANSFER   ☐ NEONATAL DEATH
☐ STILLBIRTH   ☐ OTHER_____

COMPLICATIONS/ANOMALIES: _____
_____
_____
_____

NEWBORN CARE PROVIDER: _____
_____

SEEN BY NEWBORN CARE PROVIDER BEFORE
DISCHARGE ☐ YES ☐ NO

MATERNAL INFORMATION

MATERNAL AGE:_____   GRAVITY AND PARITY:_____
☐ NONSMOKER   ☐ QUIT SMOKING DURING PREGNANCY
☐ CURRENT SMOKER
HGB/HCT LEVEL: _____

MEDICATIONS: _____
_____

HIV STATUS* KNOWN ☐ YES   ☐ NO

FEEDING METHOD   ☐ BREAST   ☐ BOTTLE
DIAGNOSTIC STUDIES PENDING: _____
_____
_____
_____

SECONDARY DIAGNOSIS/PRE-EXISTING CONDITIONS
☐ ASTHMA   ☐ HYPERTENSION
☐ DIABETES   ☐ OTHER: _____

IMMUNIZATIONS GIVEN
☐ ANTI-D IMMUNE GLOBULIN
☐ TDAP or TD   ☐ HPV (WHEN INDICATED)
  ☐ NO, RECEIVED DURING PREGNANCY
☐ INFLUENZA   ☐ VARICELLA
  ☐ NO, RECEIVED   ☐ OTHER: _____
                   DURING PREGNANCY
☐ MMR (WHEN INDICATED)

INFANT STATUS: _____
_____
_____

☐ IF NEONATAL DEATH, BEREAVEMENT COUNSELING
FOLLOW-UP APPT: _____
  DATE: _____
  LOCATION: _____
  OTHER: _____
_____

*Check state requirements before recording results.

INTERIM CONTACTS OR HOSPITALIZATIONS

DATE	COMMENT
_____	_____
_____	_____
_____	_____
_____	_____
_____	_____

PROVIDER SIGNATURE (AS REQUIRED): _____

Version 5. Copyright 2011 The American College of Obstetricians and Gynecologists

(AA197)   12345/54321

POSTPARTUM VISIT

DATE: _____

FEEDING METHOD: _____

CONTRACEPTION METHOD

TUBAL STERILIZATION	☐ YES	☐ NO
INTRAUTERINE DEVICE (IUD)	☐ YES	☐ NO
DEPOT MEDROXYPROGESTERONE ACETATE (DMPA)	☐ YES	☐ NO
IMPLANT	☐ YES	☐ NO
ORAL CONTRACEPTIVES	☐ YES	☐ NO

OTHER: _____

POSTPARTUM DEPRESSION SCREENING: _____

INTIMATE PARTNER VIOLENCE SCREENING: _____

DISCUSS SMOKING RELAPSE
PREVENTION TECHNIQUES: _____

INFANT HEALTH: _____

INTERIM HISTORY: _____
_____
_____

FOLLOW-UP LAB STUDIES ORDERED

☐ YES ☐ NO   POSTPARTUM HGB/HCT: _____

☐ YES ☐ NO   POSTPARTUM GLUCOSE SCREENING IF PATIENT HAD
                GESTATIONAL DIABETES: _____

☐ YES ☐ NO   OTHER STUDIES REQUESTED: _____

PHYSICAL EXAM

BP:_____   WT:_____   BMI:_____

BREASTS	☐ NORMAL	☐ ABNORMAL: _____
ABDOMEN	☐ NORMAL	☐ ABNORMAL: _____
EXTERNAL GENITALIA	☐ NORMAL	☐ ABNORMAL: _____
VAGINA	☐ NORMAL	☐ ABNORMAL: _____
CERVIX	☐ NORMAL	☐ ABNORMAL: _____
UTERUS	☐ NORMAL	☐ ABNORMAL: _____
ADNEXA	☐ NORMAL	☐ ABNORMAL: _____
RECTAL-VAGINAL	☐ NORMAL	☐ ABNORMAL: _____

PAP TEST   ☐ YES ☐ NO   IF NO, DUE: _____

COMMENT
_____
_____
_____
_____
_____
_____
_____
_____
_____
_____
_____
_____
_____
_____
_____
_____
_____
_____

ALLERGIES: _____
_____

IMMUNIZATION UPDATE: _____
_____
_____
_____

MEDICATIONS/CONTRACEPTION: _____
_____
_____
_____

☐ DISPENSED

INTERVAL CARE RECOMMENDATIONS

FOR GENERAL HEALTH PROMOTION: _____
_____
_____
_____
_____

PLANS FOR FUTURE PREGNANCIES: _____

FOR REPRODUCTIVE HEALTH PROMOTION: _____
_____
_____
_____

REPEAT GLUCOSE SCREENING NEEDED? ☐ YES ☐ NO
IF YES, HAS PATIENT BEEN COUNSELED? ☐ YES ☐ NO
DATE OF REPEAT TESTING: _____

RETURN VISIT: _____

REFERRALS: _____
_____
_____

EXAMINED BY: _____

PROVIDER SIGNATURE (AS REQUIRED): _____

Appendix B
Early Pregnancy Risk Identification for Consultation

Risk Factor	Recommended Consultation*
Medical history and conditions	
Asthma	
Symptomatic on medication	Obstetrician-gynecologist
Severe (multiple hospitalizations)	MFM subspecialist
Cardiac disease	
Cyanotic, prior MI, aortic stenosis, pulmonary hypertension, Marfan syndrome, prosthetic valve,	MFM subspecialist
AHA Class II or greater	
Other	Obstetrician-gynecologist
Pregestational diabetes	MFM subspecialist
Drug and alcohol use	Obstetrician-gynecologist
Epilepsy (on medication)	Obstetrician-gynecologist
Family history of genetic problems (Down syndrome, Tay-Sachs disease, PKU)	MFM subspecialist
Hemoglobinopathy (SS, SC, S-thal)	MFM subspecialist
Hypertension	
Chronic, with renal or heart disease	MFM subspecialist
Chronic, without renal or heart disease	Obstetrician-gynecologist
Prior pulmonary embolus or deep vein thrombosis	MFM subspecialist
Psychiatric illness	Obstetrician-gynecologist
Pulmonary disease	
Severe obstructive or restrictive	MFM subspecialist
Moderate	Obstetrician-gynecologist
Renal disease	
Chronic, creatinine 3 or greater with or without hypertension	MFM subspecialist

(continued)

Early Pregnancy Risk Identification for Consultation (*continued*)

Risk Factor	Recommended Consultation*
Renal disease (*continued*)	
Chronic, other	MFM subspecialist
Requirement for prolonged anticoagulation	MFM subspecialist
Severe systemic disease	MFM subspecialist
Obstetric history and conditions	
Age 35 years or older at delivery	Obstetrician-gynecologist
Cesarean delivery, prior classical or vertical incision	Obstetrician-gynecologist
Cervical insufficiency	Obstetrician-gynecologist
Prior fetal structural or chromosomal abnormality	MFM subspecialist
Prior neonatal death	Obstetrician-gynecologist
Prior fetal death	Obstetrician-gynecologist
Prior preterm delivery or preterm PROM	Obstetrician-gynecologist
Prior low birth weight (less than 2,500 g)	Obstetrician-gynecologist
Second-trimester pregnancy loss	Obstetrician-gynecologist
Uterine leiomyomata or malformation	Obstetrician-gynecologist
Initial laboratory tests	
HIV	
Symptomatic or low CD4 count	MFM subspecialist
CDE (Rh) or other blood group isoimmunization (excluding ABO, Lewis)	MFM subspecialist
Initial examination—condylomata (extensive, covering vulva or vaginal opening)	Obstetrician-gynecologist

Abbreviations: AHA, American Heart Association; HIV, human immunodeficiency virus; MFM, maternal-fetal medicine; MFM, maternal-fetal medicine; MI, myocardial infarction; PKU, phenylketonuria; PROM, premature rupture of membranes; SC, sickle cell C disease; SS, sickle cell disease; S-thal, sickle cell-thalassemia disease.

*At the time of consultation, continued patient care should be established either by collaboration with the referring health care provider or by transfer of care.

Modified with permission from March of Dimes Birth Defects Foundation, Committee on Perinatal Health. Toward improving the outcome of pregnancy: the 90s and beyond. White Plains, New York: March of Dimes Birth Defects Foundation, 1993.

Appendix C

Ongoing Pregnancy Risk Identification for Consultation

Risk Factor	Recommended Consultation*
Medical history and conditions	
Drug and alcohol use	Obstetrician-gynecologist
Proteinuria (2+ or greater by catheter sample, unexplained by urinary tract infection)	Obstetrician-gynecologist
Pyelonephritis	Obstetrician-gynecologist
Severe systemic disease that adversely affects pregnancy	MFM subspecialist
Obstetric history and conditions	
Blood pressure elevation (diastolic 90 mm Hg or greater), no proteinuria	Obstetrician-gynecologist
Fetal growth restriction suspected	Obstetrician-gynecologist
Fetal abnormality suspected by ultrasonography	MFM subspecialist
Fetal demise	Obstetrician-gynecologist
Gestational age 41 weeks (to be seen by 42 weeks)	Obstetrician-gynecologist
Gestational diabetes mellitus	Obstetrician-gynecologist
Herpes, active lesions 36 weeks	Obstetrician-gynecologist
Hydramnios by ultrasonography	Obstetrician-gynecologist; if severe, MFM subspecialist
Hyperemesis, persisting beyond first trimester	Obstetrician-gynecologist
Multiple gestation	Obstetrician-gynecologist
Oligohydramnios by ultrasonography	Obstetrician-gynecologist
Preterm labor, threatened, less than 37 weeks	Obstetrician-gynecologist
Premature rupture of membranes	Obstetrician-gynecologist
Vaginal bleeding 14 weeks or greater	Obstetrician-gynecologist
Examination and laboratory findings	
Abnormal MSAFP (low or high)	Obstetrician-gynecologist
Abnormal Pap test result	Obstetrician-gynecologist

(continued)

Ongoing Pregnancy Risk Identification for Consultation *(continued)*

Risk Factor	Recommended Consultation
Examination and laboratory findings (continued)	
Anemia (Hct less than 28%, unresponsive to iron therapy)	Obstetrician–gynecologist
Condylomata (extensive, covering labia and vaginal opening)	Obstetrician–gynecologist
HIV	
Symptomatic or low CD4 count	MFM subspecialist
CDE (Rh) or other blood group isoimmunization (excluding ABO, Lewis)	MFM subspecialist

Abbreviations: Hct, hematocrit; HIV, human immunodeficiency virus; MFM, maternal–fetal medicine; MSAFP, maternal serum alpha-fetoprotein.

*At the time of consultation, continued patient care should be determined to be by collaboration with the referring care provider or by transfer of care.

Modified with permission from March of Dimes Birth Defects Foundation, Committee on Perinatal Health. Toward improving the outcome of pregnancy: the 90s and beyond. White Plains, New York: March of Dimes Birth Defects Foundation, 1993.

Appendix D
Granting Obstetric Privileges*

Privileging defines what procedures a credentialed practitioner is permitted to perform at the facility. The granting of privileges is based on training, experience, and demonstrated current clinical competence. The educational requirements assume that applicants have achieved a doctor of medicine or doctor of osteopathy degree. Each staff member must be assessed at the time of initial application and on an ongoing basis. In addition to routine requests for privileges, a physician also may request privileges to perform a new technology.

The granting of privileges at any level in obstetrics and gynecology is based on satisfaction of criteria for the specified procedures. Criteria for granting privileges must be applied consistently regardless of the applicant's specialty. As new technologies evolve, processes for granting privileges for them will need to be formulated.

Granting Privileges

The following list has been developed to aid in granting privileges to those health care providers within the facility to perform obstetric and gynecologic procedures. Hospitals using this material may adapt it to conform to the specific situations at these facilities. This information is not intended to be all inclusive or exclusive. It is intended primarily for educational purposes. Except as otherwise noted, prerequisites for each category of privileges are listed as follows:

Training
- Successful completion of an Accreditation Council for Graduate Medical Education-accredited residency program in obstetrics–gynecology

Certification
- Board certification (or active candidate) by the American Board of Obstetrics and Gynecology or the American Osteopathic Board of Obstetrics and Gynecology
- Maintenance of certification, if applicable

---

*Data from Quality and Safety in Women's Health Care. 2nd ed. Washington, DC: American College of Obstetricians and Gynecologists; 2010.

Reappraisal (recredentialing and reprivileging) (2-year cycle) should require the following:

- Review of quality improvement file including the following:
  — Trending
  — Sentinel events
  — Other problems with specific procedures
- Review of level of activity including the following:
  — Total number of cases
  — Total number of complications
  — Outcomes
- If the credentials committee determines that the number of cases performed within the cycle is insufficient for adequately assessing competency, it may recommend that the individual be proctored and evaluated for a designated period until competency is demonstrated. However, if the physician has privileges at another institution for the particular procedure, then the individual must provide credentialing data from that hospital for review by the credentials committee and may not require proctoring.

I. Obstetric Privileges

A. Basic Level Obstetric Privileges
1. Privileges may include the following:
   a. Management of labor
   b. Pudendal and local anesthesia
   c. Fetal assessment, antepartum and intrapartum, including limited obstetric ultrasound examination
   d. Induction of labor
   e. Internal fetal monitoring
   f. Normal cephalic delivery, including use of vacuum extraction and outlet forceps
   g. Episiotomy and repair, including third-degree lacerations
   h. Management of common intrapartum problems
   i. Exploration of vagina, cervix, and uterus
   j. Emergency breech delivery
   k. Management of common postpartum problems
   l. First-assist at cesarean delivery
   m. Circumcision

B. Specialty Level Obstetric Privileges
  1. Privileges may include the following:
     a. All basic level obstetric privileges
     b. Management of normal and abnormal labor and delivery (including premature labor, breech presentation, cesarean delivery, vaginal delivery after previous cesarean delivery, cephalopelvic disproportion, nonreassuring fetal status, use of amniotomy and oxytocin, and midforceps delivery)
     c. Management of medical or surgical complications of pregnancy
     d. Diagnostic amniocentesis
     e. Cesarean hysterectomy
     f. Hypogastric artery ligation
     g. Vaginal cerclage or treatment of incompetent cervix
     h. External version of breech presentation
     i. Obstetric ultrasonography—complete
     j. Midforceps rotation
     k. Regional anesthesia as determined by training and local practice
  2. Board certification (or active candidate) by the American Board of Obstetrics and Gynecology in maternal–fetal medicine may be considered
C. Subspecialty Level Obstetric Privileges
  1. Privileges may include the following:
     a. All basic and specialty obstetric privileges
     b. Intrauterine fetal transfusion
     c. Intrauterine fetal surgery
     d. Chorionic villous sampling
     e. Percutaneous umbilical sampling
  2. Training should include documentation of specialized postresidency training
  3. Subspecialty certification (or active candidate) by the American Board of Obstetrics and Gynecology in maternal–fetal medicine may be considered

II. Credentialing for Family Physicians

A. Obstetric Privileges for Family Physicians
   1. Privileges may include the following:
      a. Labor induction or augmentation
      b. Management of labor
      c. Pudendal and local block anesthesia
      d. Fetal assessment, antepartum and intrapartum, including limited obstetric ultrasound examination
      e. Internal fetal monitoring
      f. Normal cephalic delivery
      g. Management of common intrapartum problems
      h. Exploration of vagina, cervix, and uterus
      i. Emergency breech delivery
      j. Episiotomy/laceration repair
      k. Management of common postpartum problems
      l. First-assist at cesarean delivery
      m. Circumcision
   2. Family physicians requesting these privileges must demonstrate the following:
      a. Successful completion of obstetric training as delineated in the special requirements for residency training in Family Medicine by the Accreditation Council for Graduate Medical Education
      b. If transferring from another institution, documentation of current competence as supported by ongoing clinical practice and quality review data
      c. Maintenance of board certification (or active candidate) by the American Board of Family Physicians
B. Advanced Obstetric Privileges for Family Physicians
   1. Privileges may include the following:
      a. Management of high-risk pregnancy
      b. Operative vaginal delivery, including low forceps or vacuum extraction
      c. Cesarean delivery
      d. Third-degree and fourth-degree laceration repair
   2. Family physicians requesting these privileges must demonstrate the following:
      a. Additional intensive experience taught by or in collaboration with obstetrician–gynecologists (1). In programs where

obstetrician–gynecologists are not available, these skills should be taught by appropriately skilled and credentialed family physicians.

b. The assignment of hospital privileges is a local responsibility, and privileges should be granted on the basis of training, experience, and demonstrated current clinical competence. All physicians should be held to the same standards for granting privileges, regardless of specialty, in order to ensure the provision of high-quality patient care. Prearranged, collaborative relationships should be established to ensure ongoing consultations, as well as consultations needed for emergencies.

The standard of training should allow any physician who receives training in a cognitive or surgical skill to meet the criteria for privileges in that area of practice. Provisional privileges in primary care, obstetric care, and cesarean delivery should be granted regardless of specialty as long as training criteria and experience are documented. All physicians should be subject to a proctorship period to allow demonstration of ability and current competence. These principles should apply to all health care systems.

c. Privileges recommended by the department of family practice shall be the responsibility of the department of family practice. Similarly, privileges recommended by the department of obstetrics and gynecology shall be the responsibility of the department of obstetrics and gynecology. When privileges are recommended jointly by the departments of family practice and obstetrics and gynecology, they shall be the joint responsibility of the two departments.

Requests for New Privileges

New Equipment and Technology

New equipment or technology usually improves health care, provided that practitioners and other hospital staff understand the proper indications for usage. Problems can arise when staff perform duties or use equipment for which they are not trained. It is imperative that all staff be properly trained in the use of the advanced technology or new equipment.

Privileges for new skills should only be granted when the appropriate training has been completed and documented and the competency level has been achieved with adequate supervision. That is, each physician requesting additional privileges for new equipment or technology should be evaluated by answering the following three questions:

1. Does the hospital have a mechanism in place to ensure that necessary support for the new equipment or technology is available?

2. Has the physician been adequately trained, including hands-on experience, to use the new equipment or to perform the new technology?

3. Has the physician adequately demonstrated an ability to use the new equipment or perform the new technology? This may require that the physician undergo a period of proctoring or supervision, or both. If no one on staff can serve as a proctor, the hospital may either require reciprocal proctoring at another hospital or grant temporary privileges to someone from another hospital to supervise the applicant.

Specifically, if the new privileges were not included in residency training, the applicant must do the following:

• Complete a preceptorship with a physician already credentialed to perform the procedures of that skill level; the preceptorship should require the applicant to perform the designated surgery with the preceptor acting as first assistant.

• Provide a list of cases satisfactorily completed under supervision at each skill level, as defined by the local institution.

• Submit a letter from the preceptor documenting that the procedures were completed in a satisfactory manner and that the applicant is competent to perform the procedures independently at the designated skill level.

If there is no experienced surgeon on the hospital staff who is able to serve as a preceptor for advanced or new surgical procedures, a supervised preceptorship must be arranged. This may be done by scheduling a number of cases from physicians requiring credentialing and inviting a credentialed surgeon from another institution to serve as a surgical consultant.

After a Period of Inactivity

The American Medical Association defines *physician reentry* as "a return to clinical practice in the discipline in which one has been trained and certified following an extended period of inactivity" (2). This section will not address inactivity that results from discipline or impairment.

There are several reasons why a physician might take a leave of absence from clinical practice, such as family leave (maternity and paternity leave and child care); personal health reasons; career dissatisfaction; alternate careers, such as administration; military service; or humanitarian leave. Traditionally, women were more likely to experience career interruptions; however, recent research shows that younger cohorts of male physicians also take on multiple roles and express intentions to adjust their careers accordingly (2).

When physicians request reentry after a period of inactivity, a general guideline for evaluation would be to consider the physician as any other new applicant for privileges. This would include evaluation of the following three aspects:

1. Demonstration that a minimum number of hours of continuing medical education has been earned during the period of inactivity. It is also important to meet any board certification requirements during the absence.

2. In accordance with the medical staff bylaws, supervision by a proctor appointed by the department chair for a minimum number and defined breadth of cases during the provisional period, evaluating and documenting proficiency.

3. A time-sensitive, focused review of cases as required by the departmental quality improvement committee may be completed as appropriate.

The area of skills assessment may prove challenging if the previous guidelines, number 2 and number 3, are not felt to be adequate. But, there are three options to consider:

1. Residency Training Programs

    Benefits: More locations are available, providing structured didactic programs, and implementing competency assessment. Participating in these programs can provide a source of manpower to help compensate for restricted residency work hours.

    Drawbacks: Many hospitals with residency programs have only a limited number of cases available for training. Reentry programs must not negatively affect the residency training program (ie, if someone is being brought into a reentry program in an institution that has a residency program, the Residency Review Committee must be notified with an explanation as to how it will not negatively affect the residents).

2. Simulation Centers

   Benefits: These centers can help supplement hands-on clinical experience and may be more geographically accessible. The use of simulation centers for reentry into practice is a new concept. This training may precede and supplement proctored clinical experience.

   Drawbacks: Currently there is a limited number of functioning simulation centers, though this number should continue to expand. Cost is another drawback.

3. Physician Reentry Program

   Benefits: Well-designed physician reentry program systems should be consistent with the current continuum of medical education and meet the needs of the reentering physician.

   Drawbacks: Only a few physician reentry program systems are offered nationally; thus, cost and location are considerable obstacles in utilizing these programs.

An underlying assumption is that physicians do not necessarily lose competence in all areas of practice with time. Competencies, such as patient communication and professionalism, may not decline. Therefore, a reentry program should target those areas where physicians are more likely to have lost relevant skills or knowledge, or where skills and knowledge need to be updated (3).

Finally, it is extremely important for physicians considering a leave of absence or major change in practice activities to think in advance about options should they wish to return. When possible, physicians should strongly consider the option of limited clinical activity rather than none at all. Because there is no national standard for practice departure and reentry and because all credentialing and privileging is local, each physician and hospital will ultimately have to determine the process by which the hospital and professional liability carriers will credential and privilege physicians reentering practice (4).

References

1. American Academy of Family Physicians, American College of Obstetricians and Gynecologists. AAFP-ACOG joint statement on cooperative practice and hospital privileges. Leawood (KS): AAFP; Washington, DC: ACOG; 1998.

2. Mark S, Gupta J. Reentry into clinical practice: challenges and strategies. JAMA 2002; 288:1091–6.

3. American Medical Association. Report 6 of the Council on Medical Education (A-08): physician reentry. Chicago (IL): AMA; 2008. Available at: http://www.ama-assn.org/ama1/pub/upload/mm/377/cmerpt_6a-08.pdf. Retrieved June 24, 2009.

4. Re-entering the practice of obstetrics and gynecology. Committee Opinion No. 523. American College of Obstetricians and Gynecologists. Obstet Gynecol 2012;119: 1066–9.

Appendix E
Glossary of Midwifery Organizations and Terms*

There is wide variability in the legal status and level of practice authority of midwives across the United States. The different titles for midwives—certified nurse–midwives (CNMs), certified midwives, direct-entry midwives, licensed midwives, licensed direct-entry midwives, and certified professional midwives—can be confusing, as can the different credentialing standards for midwives and different professional associations and grassroots organizations. This glossary is provided for information and reference purposes to clarify these various requirements, qualifications and standards. It is inclusive of the range of midwifery terms, including nurse–midwifery, and is representative of current activity across the country. Listings are alphabetical and include a web site address where applicable. The year an organization was formed and when a term first came into use is also noted.

American Association of Birth Centers: A nonprofit, multidisciplinary membership organization founded by Childbirth Connection (formerly Maternity Center Association) over 25 years ago. It was formerly known as the National Association of Childbearing Centers. The American Association of Birth Centers establishes national standards and accreditation for birth centers and advocates federally and in the states for birth center reimbursement and other concerns. www.birthcenters.org

American College of Nurse-Midwives (ACNM): Professional organization for CNMs and certified midwives established in 1955. The American College of Nurse–Midwives sets standards for academic preparation and clinical practice. www.midwife.org

---

*Data from the American College of Obstetricians and Gynecologists' Midwifery Work Group. www.acog.org/About_ACOG/ACOG_Departments/State_Legislative_Activities/Midwifery_Legislation.

ACNM Division of Accreditation: The group that accredits CNM and certified midwife education programs. From 1982 to 1997, ACNM Division of Accreditation only accredited educational programs for nurse–midwives.

American Midwifery Certification Board, Inc.: The certification organization affiliated with ACNM. This board was formerly called the ACNM Certification Council, Inc. Certification by the American Midwifery Certification Board, Inc is equivalent to certification by the ACNM Certification Council, Inc. In 1997, the American Midwifery Certification Board, Inc. opened its national certification examination to nonnurse graduates of midwifery education programs and issued the first certified midwife credential. Beginning in 2010, a graduate degree will be required for entry into clinical practice for both CNMs and certified midwives. www.amcbmidwife.org

Certified Midwife: A midwife who undergoes the same certification process as a CNM, but whose training does not include education in nursing. In 1996, the ACNM adopted standards for the certification of direct-entry midwives to be known as certified midwives. Certified midwives must pass the same certification exam as CNMs and must have a master's degree. They are licensed in only three states: 1) New Jersey, 2) New York, and 3) Rhode Island. New York had the first certified midwife training program and was the first state to recognize the certified midwife credential. It is the only state that has one unified framework for licensing all midwives, both CNMs and certified midwives.

Certified Nurse-Midwife: A midwife who is educated at the baccalaureate level or higher in the two disciplines of nursing and midwifery. A master's degree is required for certification. These midwives typically have prescriptive authority for most drugs, third-party reimbursement, including Medicaid, and practice independently or in collaborative practice with physicians. The professional organization for CNMs is the ACNM.

Certified Professional Midwife (also licensed midwives, licensed direct-entry midwives, and registered midwives): In the mid-1990s, the certified professional midwife credential was developed jointly by the Midwives Alliance of North America, the North American Registry of Midwives and the Midwifery Education Accreditation Council. There is no single standard for education, and both apprentice-only trained midwives and midwives who undergo a university-affiliated training use the title certified professional midwife. A certified professional midwife can learn through a structured program, through apprenticeship, or through self study. Another route to the credential is current legal recognition to practice in Britain. These midwives must pass a written and practical examination for certification. According to the Midwives Alliance of North America, in 2009, 24 states recognized the certified professional midwife credential as the basis for licensure or used the North American Registry of Midwives written examination. Some of these states use a different nomenclature. For example, licensed midwife is used in California, Idaho, Oregon, and Washington; licensed direct-entry midwife is used in Utah, and registered midwife is used in Colorado.

Childbirth Connection: Established in 1918, Childbirth Connection (formerly Maternity Center Association) is a national nonprofit organization whose mission is to improve the quality of maternity care through research, education, advocacy, and policy. www.childbirthconnection.org

Citizens for Midwifery, Inc.: A nonprofit, volunteer, grassroots organization founded by several mothers in 1996 to promote certified professional midwives and the Midwives Model of Care™ (see also Midwives Model of Care™). The organization is active federally and in the states. www.cfmidwifery.org

Collaborative Practice: A comprehensive, dynamic system of patient-centered health care delivered by a multidisciplinary team. [NOTE: This definition is from the glossary section of the 1995 document, the American College of Obstetricians and Gynecologists' *Guidelines for Implementing Collaborative Practice*. The following definition, approved by the American College of Obstetricians and Gynecologists' Executive Board, appears on page one of that document: Collaborative practice in the health care of women is a comprehensive, dynamic system of patient-centered health care delivered by a multidisciplinary team. The team consists of obstetrician–gynecologists and other health care professionals who function within their educational preparation and scope of practice. These team members work together, utilizing mutually agreed upon guidelines and policies that define the individual and shared responsibilities of each member. Although the responsibilities of obstetrician–gynecologists place them in the role of ultimate authority because of their education and training, the contributions of each team member are valued and important to the quality of patient outcomes. The concept of a team guided by one of its own members and the acceptance of shared responsibility for outcomes promote shared accountability.]

Direct-Entry Midwives (licensed direct-entry midwives, licensed midwives, registered midwives): A midwife who enters the profession of midwifery directly without earning a nursing degree. Both certified professional midwives and certified midwives are considered direct-entry midwives, although their level of education and training varies markedly. According to the Midwives Alliance of North America, direct-entry midwives can practice legally in 26 states. Some states prohibit, by statute or judicial interpretation, direct-entry midwifery practice. Other states allow midwifery practice without licensure or have statutes that require licensure but do not have a mechanism in place to issue the license (see also "Lay Midwife").

International Confederation of Midwives: The International Confederation of Midwives, in collaboration with the International Federation of Gynecology and Obstetrics (FIGO), first published a definition of midwife in 1972; it was later endorsed by the World Health Organization (WHO). In 2005, the definition was updated and revised. It defines a *midwife* as an individual who, "having been regularly admitted to a midwifery education program duly recognized in the country in which it is located, has successfully completed the prescribed course of studies in midwifery and acquired the requisite qualifications to be registered and/or legally licensed to practice midwifery." The International Confederation of Midwives, WHO, and FIGO stress the importance of a formal education and accreditation process as a means to ensure skilled practitioners. www.internationalmidwives.org

Lay Midwife: Often used incorrectly, this term refers to an unlicensed midwife. In some states still today, any lay person may attend or assist a woman giving birth, but in a gratuitous, nonprofessional, nonbusiness capacity. These lay midwives act outside of state recognition and oversight and, in fact, are not licensed by the state.

MAMA Campaign (Midwives & Mothers in Action): This is a grassroots advocacy effort to gain federal government recognition of certified professional midwives. www.mamacampaign.org

Midwives Alliance of North America: A broad-based alliance founded in 1982 representing midwives of diverse educational backgrounds. In the 1980s, the Midwives Alliance of North America developed the first national certifying examination for direct-entry midwives and in 1986 launched a national registry of midwives. Its members include certified professional midwives, CNMs, licensed midwives, and lay midwives; over one third are certified professional midwives. Midwives Alliance of North America's *Core Competencies* delineate the clinical skills for direct-entry midwife practice. In the 1990s, Midwives Alliance of North America initiated data collection on out-of-hospital births and in 2000, required all certified professional midwives to participate in a year-long prospective study that was published in the *BMJ* in 2005. Midwives Alliance of North America conducts consumer education and grassroots lobbying campaigns nationally and in individual states. www.mana.org

Midwifery Education Accreditation Council: Agency that accredits programs leading to a certified professional midwife credential. Standards for accreditation were developed in the 1990s. The Midwifery Education Accreditation Council requires that midwifery schools incorporate the *Core Competencies* adopted by Midwives Alliance of North America and the clinical experience requirements and essential knowledge and skills identified by the North American Registry of Midwives, an international certifying agency. The Midwifery Education Accreditation Council is recognized by the U.S. Secretary of Education as a national accrediting agency for direct-entry midwifery educational programs and institutions. www.meacschools.org

Midwives Model of Care™: The standard of care for certified professional midwives established by the Midwives Alliance of North America, the North American Registry of Midwives, and the Midwifery Education Accreditation Council.

National Association of Certified Professional Midwives: A professional organization for certified professional midwives created in 2001 that advocates for the removal of legal barriers to certified professional midwife practice at the federal and state levels. www.nacpm.org

North American Registry of Midwives: The credentialing agency for certified professional midwives established in 1987 by the Midwives Alliance of North America. The North American Registry of Midwives is accredited by the National Commission for Certifying Agencies, the accrediting body of the National Organization for Competency Assurance. The National Commission for Certifying Agencies accredits many health care credentials including the CNM. The North American Registry of Midwives administers certification for certified professional midwives who are qualified to provide the Midwives Model of Care™. In many states, midwifery licensure laws and regulations refer to and adopt the North American Registry of Midwives and Midwives Alliance of North America standards of practice. www.narm.org

North American Registry of Midwives Portfolio Evaluation Process: This is the North American Registry of Midwives alternative certification route for certified professional midwives who have not participated in a formal education program. Certification is based on clinical experience and understanding of core competencies. The Portfolio Evaluation Process meets National Commission for Certifying Agencies recommendations stating that programs have an education evaluation process so that candidates who have been educated outside of established pathways can have their qualifications evaluated for credentialing.

Skilled Birth Attendant: The WHO, International Confederation of Midwives, and FIGO define the *skilled birth attendant* as "an accredited health professional who has been educated and trained to proficiency in the skills needed to manage normal (uncomplicated) pregnancies, childbirth and the immediate postnatal period, and in the identification, management and referral of complications in women and newborns." (See their 2004 joint statement, *The Critical Role of the Skilled Attendant.*) www.internationalmidwives.org

Traditional Birth Attendant: These practitioners lack formal education and credentials. The WHO, International Confederation of Midwives, and FIGO define the *traditional birth attendant* as the "traditional, independent (of the health care system), non-formally trained and community-based provider of care during pregnancy, childbirth and the postnatal period." www.international midwives.org

Appendix F

Standard Terminology for Reporting of Reproductive Health Statistics in the United States*

The adoption of standard definitions and reporting requirements for reproductive health statistics will provide an improved basis for standardization and uniformity in the design, implementation, and evaluation of intervention strategies. The reduction of maternal and infant mortality and the improvement of the health of our nation's women and infants are the ultimate goals. The collection and analysis of reliable statistical data are an essential part of in-depth investigations and incorporate case finding, individual review, and analysis of risk factors. These studies could then yield valuable clinical information for practitioners, aiding them in improved case management for patients at high risk, which would result in decreased morbidity and mortality.

Both the collection and the use of statistics have been hampered by lack of understanding of differences in definitions, statistical tabulations, and reporting requirements among state, national, and international bodies. Misapplication and misinterpretation of data may lead to erroneous comparisons and conclusions. For example, specific requirements for reporting of fetal deaths often have been misinterpreted as implying a weight or gestational age for viability. Distinctions can and should be made among the definition of an event, the reporting requirements for the event, and the statistical tabulation and interpretation of the data. The definition indicates the meaning of a term (eg, live birth, fetal death, or maternal death). A reporting requirement is that part of the defined event for which reporting is mandatory or desired. Statistical tabulations connote the presentation of data for the purpose of analysis and

---

*Different states use different birth weight and gestational age criteria to define fetal death. The Committee on Obstetric Practice of the American College of Obstetricians and Gynecologists recommends that perinatal mortality statistics be based on a gestational weight of 500 g.

497

interpretation of existing and future conditions. The data should be collected in a manner that will allow them to be presented in different ways for different users. Adjustments should be made for variations in reporting before comparisons among data are attempted.

If information is collected and presented in a standardized manner, comparisons between the new data and the data obtained by previous reporting requirements can be delineated clearly and can contribute to improved public understanding of reproductive health statistics. For ease in assimilating this information, this appendix is divided into three sections: 1) definitions, 2) statistical tabulations, and 3) reporting requirements and recommendations. Some of the definitions and recommendations are a departure from those currently or historically accepted; however, these recommendations were agreed on by an interorganizational group that was brought together in the mid 1980s to review terminology related to reproductive health issues.

Definitions*

Birth Weight: The weight of a neonate determined immediately after delivery or as soon thereafter as feasible. It should be expressed to the nearest gram.

Fetal Death: Death before the complete expulsion or extraction from the mother of a product of human conception, irrespective of the duration of pregnancy that is not an induced termination of pregnancy. The death is indicated by the fact that, after such expulsion or extraction, the fetus does not breathe or show any other evidence of life, such as beating of the heart, pulsation of the umbilical cord, or definite movement of voluntary muscles. Heartbeats are to be distinguished from transient cardiac contractions; respirations are to be distinguished from fleeting respiratory efforts or gasps.

For statistical purposes, fetal deaths are further subdivided as early (20–27 weeks of gestation) or late (28 weeks of gestation). The term stillbirth also is used to describe fetal deaths at 20 weeks of gestation or more. Fetuses that die in utero before 20 weeks of gestation are categorized specifically as miscarriages.

---

*These definitions are for statistical purposes and are not intended to affect clinical management. Appropriate assessment of fetal maturity for purposes of clinical management is delineated in Chapter 7.

Gestational Age: The number of weeks that have elapsed between the first day of the last normal menstrual period (not the presumed time of conception) and the date of delivery, irrespective of whether the gestation results in a live birth or a fetal death.

Infant Death: A live birth that results in death within the first year (less than 365 days) is defined as an infant death. Infant deaths are further subdivided as early neonatal (less than 7 days), late neonatal (7–27 days), neonatal (less than 28 days), or postneonatal (28–364 days).

Live Birth: The complete expulsion or extraction from the mother of a product of human conception, irrespective of the duration of pregnancy, which, after such expulsion or extraction, breathes or shows any other evidence of life, such as beating of the heart, pulsation of the umbilical cord, or definite movement of voluntary muscles, regardless of whether the umbilical cord has been cut or the placenta is attached. Heartbeats are to be distinguished from transient cardiac contractions; respirations are to be distinguished from fleeting respiratory efforts or gasps.

Neonatal Death: Death of a liveborn neonate before the neonate becomes age 28 days (up to and including 27 days, 23 hours, and 59 minutes from the moment of birth).

Neonate:

Low birth weight—Any neonate, regardless of gestational age, whose weight at birth is less than 2,500 g.

Postterm—Any neonate whose birth occurs from the beginning of the first day (295th day) of the 43rd week after the onset of the last menstrual period.

Preterm*—Any neonate whose birth occurs through the end of the last day of the 37th week (259th day) following the onset of the last menstrual period.

---

*To ensure comparable calculations with the medical community, statisticians making a determination of the status of a neonate, namely preterm or term, should define preterm as a neonate who is born after less than 259 days of gestation and term as a neonate who is born after 259 days to less than 294 days of gestation. Statisticians, by formula, subtract the date of the first day of the last menstrual period from the date of birth, whereas physicians include the first day, thus accounting for the difference.

Term—Any neonate whose birth occurs from the beginning of the first day (260th day) of the 38th week through the end of the last day of the 42nd week (294th day) after the onset of the last menstrual period.

Maternal Death*: The death of a woman from any cause related to or aggravated by pregnancy or its management (regardless of the duration or site of pregnancy), but not from accidental or incidental causes.

Direct obstetric death—The death of a woman resulting from obstetric complications of pregnancy, labor, or the puerperium; from interventions, omissions, or treatment; or from a chain of events resulting from any of these.

Indirect obstetric death—The death of a woman resulting from a previously existing disease or a disease that developed during pregnancy, labor, or the puerperium that did not have direct obstetric causes, although the physiologic effects of pregnancy were partially responsible for the death.

In 1987, the Centers for Disease Control and Prevention (CDC) collaborated with the Maternal Mortality Special Interest Group of the American College of Obstetricians and Gynecologists (the College), the Association of Vital Records and Health Statistics, and state and local health departments to initiate the National Pregnancy Mortality Surveillance System. The CDC–College Maternal Mortality Study Group introduced two terms, which are being used by the CDC and increasingly by some states and researchers. The study group differentiates between pregnancy-associated and pregnancy-related deaths.

Pregnancy-Associated Death: The death of any woman, from any cause, while pregnant or within 1 calendar year of termination of pregnancy, regardless of the duration and the site of pregnancy.

Pregnancy-Related Death: A pregnancy-associated death resulting from complications of the pregnancy itself, the chain of events initiated by the pregnancy that led to death, or aggravation of an unrelated condition by the physiologic or pharmacologic effects of the pregnancy that subsequently caused death.

Induced Termination of Pregnancy: The purposeful interruption of an intrauterine pregnancy with the intention other than to produce a liveborn infant, and

---

*Death occurring to a woman during pregnancy or after its termination from causes not related to the pregnancy or to its complications or management is not considered a maternal death. Nonmaternal deaths may result from accidental causes (eg, auto accident or gunshot wound) or incidental causes (eg, concurrent malignancy).

which does not result in a live birth. This definition excludes management of prolonged retention of products of conception after fetal death.

Statistical Tabulations

Statistical tabulations for vital events related to pregnancy provide the medical and statistical community with valuable information on reproductive health and generate data on trends apparent in this country and worldwide. This information often is disaggregated and used to examine specific events over time or within selected geographic locations. In informing the public about health issues, media sources often report various statistical measures. Heightened public interest in health-related issues makes it essential that the medical community understand and have the capacity to interpret these statistics.

The following explanations of statistical tabulations are intended to provide the reader with a better understanding of the measures used for events related to reproduction:

Rate: A measure of the frequency of some event in relation to a unit of population during a specified time period, such as a year; events in the numerator of the rate occur to individuals in the denominator. Rates express the risk of the event in the specified population during a particular time. Rates generally are expressed as units of population in the denominator (eg, per 1,000, per 100,000). For example, the 2008 teenage birth rate was 41.5 live births per 1,000 women aged 15–19 years.

Ratios: A term that expresses a relationship of one element to a different element (where the numerator is not necessarily a subset of the denominator). A ratio generally is expressed per 1,000 of the denominator element. For example, the sex ratio of live births for 2008 was 1,048 males per 1,000 females.

In the formulae that follow, the term *period* refers to a calendar year.

Live Birth Measures

These measures are designed to show the rate at which childbearing is occurring in the population. The crude birth rate, which relates the total number of births to the total population, indicates the effect of fertility on population growth. The general fertility rate is a more specific measure of fertility because it relates the number of births to the population at risk, namely, women of childbearing age (assumed to be aged 15–44 years). An even more specific set of rates, the age-specific birth rate, relates the number of births to women of specific ages directly to the total number of women in that age group. Formulae for these measures are as follows:

$$\text{Crude birth rate} = \frac{\substack{\text{Number of live births to women} \\ \text{of all ages during a calendar year} \times 1,000}}{\text{Total estimated mid-year population}}$$

$$\text{General fertility rate} = \frac{\substack{\text{Number of live births to women} \\ \text{of all ages during a calendar year} \times 1,000}}{\substack{\text{Estimated mid-year population} \\ \text{of women aged } 15\text{-}44 \text{ years}}}$$

$$\text{General pregnancy rate} = \frac{\substack{\text{Number of live births} + \text{number of fetal} \\ \text{deaths} + \text{number of induced terminations of} \\ \text{pregnancy during a calendar year} \times 1,000}}{\substack{\text{Estimated mid-year population} \\ \text{of women aged } 15\text{-}44 \text{ years}}}$$

$$\text{Age-specific birth rate} = \frac{\substack{\text{Number of live births to women in a specific} \\ \text{age group during a calendar year} \times 1,000}}{\substack{\text{Estimated mid-year population} \\ \text{of women in same age group}}}$$

$$\text{Total fertility rate} = \substack{\text{The sum of age-specific birth rates of women} \\ \text{at each age group } 10\text{-}14 \text{ through } 45\text{-}49.}$$

Five-year age groups are used; therefore, the sum is multiplied by 5. This rate also can be computed by using single years of age.

Because the birth weight of the infant is included on the birth certificate, it is possible to tabulate and focus an analysis on selected groups of live births, for example, those weighing 500 g or more. Births can be tabulated by where they occur. Therefore, they can be shown by place of occurrence, by place of residence, and by kind of setting of delivery, such as at a hospital or home. Most tabulations of vital statistics are routinely calculated by place of residence of the mother, but they could be tabulated on another basis as well. What is essential, however, is that the classification be the same for all events under consideration for a specific measure.

Fetal Mortality Measures

The population at risk of fetal mortality is the number of live births plus the number of fetal deaths in a year. Fetal death indices, defined by a minimum weight and gestational age, indicate the magnitude of late pregnancy losses.

It is recognized that most states report fetal deaths on the basis of gestational age. However, birth weight can be more accurately measured than can gestational age. Therefore, it is recommended that states adopt minimum reporting requirements of fetal deaths based on and labeled as specific birth weight rather than gestational age (see also "Fetal Death" later in this appendix). In addition, statistical tabulations of fetal deaths should include, at a minimum, fetal deaths of those weighing 500 g or more.

It is recognized that states will not be able to immediately translate data from gestational age to weight, and, for comparative purposes, it may be desirable to know fetal death rates for various gestational periods. Therefore, the collection of both weight and gestational age is recommended to allow for these comparisons. When calculating fetal death rates based on gestational age, the number of weeks or more of stated or presumed gestation can be substituted for weight in the previous formulae.

$$\text{Fetal death rate} = \frac{\text{Number of fetal deaths (x weight or more) during a period} \times 1{,}000}{\text{Number of fetal deaths (x weight or more)} + \text{number of live births during the same period}}$$

$$\text{Fetal death ratio} = \frac{\text{Number of fetal deaths (x weight or more) during a period} \times 1{,}000}{\text{Number of live births during the same period}}$$

Perinatal Mortality Measures

Perinatal death is not a reportable vital event, per se, but is used for statistical purposes. Indices of perinatal mortality combine fetal deaths and live births with only brief survival (up to a few days or weeks) on the assumption that similar factors are associated with these losses. The population at risk is the total number of live births plus fetal deaths, or alternatively, the number of live births. Perinatal mortality indices can vary as to age of the fetus and the infant who is included in the particular tabulation. However, the concept itself cuts across all the calculations.

It is recommended that perinatal mortality measures be based on and labeled with specific weight rather than gestational age (see also "Reporting Requirements and Recommendations," later in this appendix):

$$\text{Perinatal mortality rate} = \frac{\begin{array}{c}\text{Number of infant deaths of less than x days}\\ \text{+ number of fetal deaths (with stated or}\\ \text{presumed weight of y or more)}\\ \text{during the same period} \times 1{,}000\end{array}}{\text{Number of live births during the same period}}$$

It is recognized that states will not be able to immediately translate data from gestational age to weight, and for purposes of comparability, knowledge of gestational age (based on last menstrual period) may be required and should be collected. When perinatal death rates based on gestational age are calculated, the number of weeks of a stated or presumed gestational age can be substituted for weight in the formulae. When comparisons based on gestational age are desired, the generally accepted breakdown is as follows:

• Perinatal period I includes infant deaths occurring at less than 7 days and fetal deaths with a stated or presumed period of gestation of 28 weeks or more.

• Perinatal period II includes infant deaths occurring at less than 28 days and fetal deaths with a stated or presumed period of gestation of 20 weeks or more.

• Perinatal period III includes infant deaths occurring at less than 7 days and fetal deaths with a stated or presumed gestation of 20 weeks or more.

Perinatal measures can be specific for race and other characteristics. Perinatal events can be tabulated by where they occur. Therefore, they can be shown by place of occurrence, by place of residence, and by place of delivery, such as at a hospital or home. Most tabulations of vital statistics are routinely calculated by place of residence of the woman, but they could be tabulated by place of occurrence. What is essential, however, is that the classification be the same for all events under consideration for a specific measure.

Indices of infant mortality are designed to show the likelihood that live births with certain characteristics will survive the first year of life or, conversely, will die during the first year of life. For infant mortality, the population at risk is approximated by live births that occur in a calendar year. The infant mortality rate of different population groups can be compared, such as that between white and black infants. Interest sometimes focuses on two different periods in the first year of an infant's life, such as the very early period when the infant is younger than 28 days (up through 27 days, 23 hours, and 59 minutes from the moment of birth), called the neonatal period; and the later period starting at the end of the 28th day up to, but not including, age 1 year (364 days, 23 hours, and 59 minutes), called the postneonatal period. Accordingly, two indices reflect these differences, namely, the neonatal mortality rate and the postneonatal mortality rate. The neonatal period can be divided further for statistical tabulations:

- Neonatal period I is from the moment of birth through 23 hours and 59 minutes.

- Neonatal period II starts at the end of the 24th hour of life through 6 days, 23 hours, and 59 minutes.

- Neonatal period III starts at the end of the 7th day of life through 27 days, 23 hours, and 59 minutes.

The denominator for the postneonatal mortality rate also can be calculated by subtracting the number of neonatal deaths from the number of live births. This denominator more accurately defines the population at risk of death in the postneonatal period. In addition, it should be noted that infant deaths can be broken down into birth weight categories, if desired, for comparative purposes when birth and death records are linked (see also "Reporting Requirements and Recommendations," later in this appendix):

$$\text{Infant mortality rate} = \frac{\text{Number of infant deaths (neonatal and postneonatal) during a period} \times 1{,}000}{\text{Number of live births during the same period}}$$

$$\text{Neonatal mortality rate} = \frac{\text{Number of neonatal deaths during a period} \times 1{,}000}{\text{Number of live births during the same period}}$$

$$\text{Postneonatal mortality rate} = \frac{\text{Number of postneonatal deaths during a period} \times 1{,}000}{\text{Number of live births during the same period}}$$

Maternal Mortality Measures

Measures of maternal mortality are designed to indicate the likelihood that a pregnant woman will die from complications of pregnancy, childbirth, or the puerperium. Accordingly, the population at risk is an approximation of the population of pregnant women in a year; the approximation usually is taken to be the number of live births. Maternal mortality can be examined in terms of characteristics of the woman, such as age, race, and cause of death. The maternal mortality rate measures the risk of death from deliveries and complications of pregnancy, childbirth, and the puerperium.

The group exposed to risk consists of all women who have been pregnant at some time during the period. Therefore, the population at risk should theoretically include all fetal deaths (reported and unreported), all induced terminations of pregnancy, and all live births. Because most states do not require the reporting of all fetal deaths and a large number of states still do not require reporting of induced terminations of pregnancy, the entire population at risk cannot be included in the denominator. Therefore, the total number of live births has become the generally accepted denominator. It is recommended that when complete ascertainment of the denominator (ie, the number of pregnant women) is achieved, a modified maternal mortality rate should be defined, in addition to the traditional rate. The rate is most frequently expressed per 100,000 live births:

$$\text{Maternal mortality rate} = \frac{\text{Number of deaths attributed to maternal conditions during a period} \times 100,000}{\text{Number of live births during the same period}}$$

Death rates for specified maternal causes are computed by restricting the numerator to the specified cause. The maternal mortality rates specific for race and age groups are computed by appropriately restricting both the numerator and the denominator to the specified group. Caution should be used in interpreting rates in small geographic areas; it may not be possible to generate race-specific and age-specific rates.

For statistical comparisons with the World Health Organization (WHO), it is recommended that two tabulations of statistics be prepared: 1) maternal deaths within 42 days of the end of pregnancy (WHO); and 2) maternal deaths with no time limitation for comparison within the United States.

The CDC uses the following statistical measures of pregnancy-related mortality:

$$\text{Pregnancy mortality ratio} = \frac{\text{Number of pregnancy-related deaths during a period} \times 100,000}{\text{Number of live births during the same period}}$$

$$\text{Pregnancy mortality rate} = \frac{\text{Number of pregnancy-related deaths during a period} \times 100{,}000}{\substack{\text{Number of pregnancies (live births, fetal deaths,} \\ \text{induced and spontaneous abortions, ectopic} \\ \text{pregnancies, and molar pregnancies)}}}$$

Measures of Induced Termination of Pregnancy

Measures of induced pregnancy termination parallel those of fetal deaths but refer to induced events. The population at risk of induced termination of pregnancy is taken to be live births in a year, which is used as a surrogate measure of pregnancies. Because this is not actually the total population at risk, this measure generally is considered to be a ratio.

$$\substack{\text{Induced termination} \\ \text{of pregnancy ratio I}} = \frac{\substack{\text{Number of induced terminations} \\ \text{occurring during a period} \times 1{,}000}}{\substack{\text{Number of live births occurring} \\ \text{during the same period}}}$$

Another measure is one that, by also including an estimate of pregnancies that do not result in live births, more closely approximates the population at risk:

$$\substack{\text{Induced termination} \\ \text{of pregnancy ratio II}} = \frac{\substack{\text{Number of induced terminations} \\ \text{occurring during a period} \times 1{,}000}}{\substack{\text{Number of induced terminations of} \\ \text{pregnancies + live births + reported} \\ \text{fetal deaths during the same period}}}$$

Still a third measure is a rate that provides information on the probability that a woman of a certain age or race will have an induced termination of pregnancy:

$$\substack{\text{Induced termination} \\ \text{of pregnancy rate}} = \frac{\substack{\text{Number of induced terminations} \\ \text{occurring during a period} \times 1{,}000}}{\text{Female population aged 15–44 years}}$$

Sometimes indices for induced termination are specific for certain characteristics of the woman; that is, they can refer to women of particular age or race groups.

Reporting Requirements and Recommendations

Reporting requirements for vital events related to reproductive health enable the collection of data that are essential to the calculation of statistical tabulations to examine trends and changes at the local, state, and national levels. The data used in statistical tabulations may be only a portion of those collected, because of the need for consistency in a tabulation and because of the variations in reporting requirements from state to state. For instance, although a few states require that all fetal deaths, regardless of length of gestation, be reported, statistical tabulations of fetal death rates by the National Center for Health Statistics use only those fetal deaths occurring at 20 weeks or more of gestation.

Live Birth

It generally is recognized that all states report all live births, as defined in the definitions section of this document. It is recommended that all live births be reported, regardless of birth weight, length of gestation, or survival time.

Fetal Death

Reporting requirements for fetal deaths now vary from state to state. At present, most states require reporting of fetal deaths by gestational age. It generally is recognized that birth weight can be measured more accurately than can gestational age. The 1992 revision of the Model State Vital Statistics Act and Regulations* recommends reporting of all spontaneous losses occurring at 20 weeks or more of gestation or weighing 350 g or more. It must be emphasized that a specific birth weight criterion for reporting of fetal deaths does not imply a point of viability and should be chosen instead for its feasibility in collecting useful data.

Current statistical tabulations of fetal deaths include, at a minimum, fetal deaths at 500 g or more. Furthermore, 25 states have adopted the requirement of reporting deaths of 20 weeks or more of gestation. Therefore, it is recommended that all state fetal death report forms include birth weight and gestational age.

Perinatal Mortality

Perinatal mortality indices generally combine fetal deaths and live births that survive only briefly (up to a few days or weeks). Because reporting requirements of fetal deaths vary from state to state, perinatal mortality reporting also will vary (see definitions of perinatal periods in "Perinatal Mortality Measures" earlier in this appendix).

As with fetal deaths, it is recommended that perinatal mortality be weight specific. However, for purposes of comparability, knowledge of gestational age (based on last menstrual period) should be collected.

---

*In 2011, the Model Law Revision workgroup completed its work on evaluating and revising the 1992 Model State Vital Statistics Act and Regulations. The proposed revision of the Model Law was still under review by the U.S. Department of Health and Human Services at the time of printing of Guidelines for Perinatal Care, Seventh Edition.

Infant Mortality

All states require that all infant deaths (neonatal plus postneonatal), as defined in the section "Definitions" in this appendix, be reported. Infant deaths by birth weight are not routinely available for the United States as a whole because birth weight information is not collected on the death certificate. However, because birth weight is reported on the birth certificate, it is possible to obtain information on infant deaths by birth weight by linking together the birth certificate and the death certificate for the same infant. At present, most states link birth and death certificates. A national linked birth certificate and infant death certificate file is now available. In addition, it is recommended that infant death reports include the exact interval from birth rather than categories, such as "neonatal" or "postneonatal." This, too, will allow for more specific age-related death analyses.

Maternal Mortality

Every state is required to report all maternal deaths. Case finding, together with individual review and analysis of risk factors contributing to maternal deaths, is of the highest importance. Collection of data regarding these rare events is critical, when combined, as it should be, with educational review by those closest to the case, usually the obstetrician–gynecologists in the hospital and the surrounding region. Such analysis can yield clinical information about risk factors associated with, for example, detection and treatment of ectopic pregnancies or with anesthesia. This clinical information can then be gathered and exchanged to help practitioners identify risk factors that contribute to maternal death and associated conditions.

The CDC–College Maternal Mortality Study Group also has designed a new system of classifying pregnancy-related deaths after review of the case. This system differentiates between the immediate and underlying causes of death as stated on the death certificate, associated obstetric and medical conditions or complications, and the outcome of pregnancy. For example, if a woman died of a hemorrhage that resulted from a ruptured ectopic pregnancy, the immediate cause of death would be classified as "hemorrhage," the associated obstetric condition would be classified as "ruptured fallopian tube," and the outcome of pregnancy would be "ectopic pregnancy." This classification scheme allows analysis of the chain of events that led to the death.

Induced Termination of Pregnancy

The United States has no national system for reporting induced termination of pregnancy. State health departments vary greatly in their approaches to the compilation of these data, from compiling no data to periodically requesting hospitals, clinics, and physicians performing the procedures to voluntarily report total number of procedures performed; requiring (by legislative or regulatory authority) hospitals, clinics, and physicians to periodically report aggregate level data on number or number and characteristics of procedures; or requiring (by legal or regulatory authority) hospitals, clinics, and physicians to periodically report individual data on each procedure performed.

Since 1969, the CDC Division of Reproductive Health has published an annual Abortion Surveillance Report based on data provided from state health departments, when available, and from data voluntarily provided to the CDC from hospitals and clinics in states with no data available from health departments. In addition to information on the number and characteristics of induced terminations of pregnancy, the Abortion Surveillance Report contains information from the CDC abortion mortality surveillance, which was begun with the cooperation of state health departments in 1972. Investigation and review of each related death by epidemiologists in the Division of Reproductive Health result in improved detailed nosological identification of abortion mortality by type of risk.*

Since 1977, the National Center for Health Statistics has analyzed the induced terminations of pregnancy occurring in states in which individual reports of induced termination are submitted to state vital registration offices. In addition, the Alan Guttmacher Institute, a private organization, publishes information on induced termination that it obtains from a nationwide survey of health care providers of induced termination.

Collecting information on the number of induced terminations of pregnancy, the characteristics of women having such procedures, and the number and characteristics of all deaths related to induced termination of pregnancy would be extremely valuable in identifying and evaluating risk factors for specific population groups and for the public in general. By gathering these data, studies could be instituted that would examine clinical issues and then results could be shared with practitioners. Knowing the outcomes could further the body of knowledge and ultimately reduce the risks.

---

*The CDC Abortion Surveillance Report includes information on events categorized by the CDC as abortions (legal, illegal, and spontaneous). Although this terminology predates the recommendations in this document and is at variance with the definition herein, it has been commonly used and understood to include induced termination of pregnancy.

Rates of Vaginal Births After Cesarean Delivery

Two methods for defining vaginal birth after cesarean delivery (VBAC) rates are proposed:

$$1.\ \text{VBAC rate} = \frac{\text{Total number of VBACs}}{\begin{array}{c}\text{Total number of women with prior cesarean}\\\text{deliveries, including women who were}\\\text{candidates for a trial of labor but declined}\\\text{and women who were not candidates}\end{array}} \times 100$$

$$2.\ \begin{array}{c}\text{Trial of labor}\\\text{success rate} =\end{array}\frac{\text{VBAC}}{\begin{array}{c}\text{Number of women who had a trial}\\\text{of labor after cesarean delivery}\end{array}} \times 100$$

Clearly, these rates are interrelated. However, calculations based on the rates as defined allow a more accurate comparison of practice between health care providers and institutions.

Current Reporting Requirements

The general fetal death reporting requirements, as of 2005 (Table F-1), should be brought into conformity with the recommendations in this report.

Table F-1. Reporting Requirements for Fetal Death According to State or Reporting Area, 2005

Criteria	State and Reporting Area
Gestational age criteria only	
All periods	Arkansas, Colorado, Georgia, Hawaii, New York,* Rhode Island, Virginia, Virgin Islands
16 weeks or greater	Pennsylvania
20 weeks or greater	Alabama, Alaska, California, Connecticut, Florida, Illinois, Indiana, Iowa, Maine, Maryland,[†] Minnesota, Nebraska, Nevada, New Jersey, North Carolina, North Dakota, Ohio, Oklahoma, Oregon, Texas, Utah, Vermont,[‡] Washington, West Virginia, Wyoming
5 months or greater	Puerto Rico

(continued)

Table F-1. Reporting Requirements for Fetal Death According to State or Reporting Area, 2005 *(continued)*

Criteria	State and Reporting Area
Both gestational age and birth weight criteria	
20 weeks or greater or 350 g or more	Arizona, Idaho, Kentucky, Louisiana, Massachusetts, Mississippi, Missouri, New Hampshire, South Carolina, Wisconsin, Guam
20 weeks or greater or 400 g or more	Michigan
20 weeks or greater or 500 g or more	District of Columbia
Birth weight criteria only	
350 g or more	Delaware,[§] Kansas, Montana[§]
500 g or more	New Mexico, South Dakota, Tennessee[ll]

*Includes New York City, which has separate reporting.

[†]If gestational age is unknown, weight of 500 g or more.

[‡]If gestational age is unknown, weight of 400 g or more, 15 oz or more.

[§]If weight is unknown, 20 weeks of completed gestation or more.

[ll]If weight is unknown, 22 completed weeks of gestation or more.

Data from Barfield WD. Standard terminology for fetal, infant, and perinatal deaths. American Academy of Pediatrics Committee on Fetus and Newborn. Pediatrics 2011; 128:177–81.

Bibliography

Barfield WD. Standard terminology for fetal, infant, and perinatal deaths. American Academy of Pediatrics Committee on Fetus and Newborn. Pediatrics 2011;128:177–181.

Centers for Disease Control and Prevention. National Center for Health Statistics. State definitions and reporting requirements for live births, fetal deaths, and induced terminations of pregnancy. Hyattsville, MD: National Center for Health Statistics; 1997. Available at: www.cdc.gov/nchs/data/misc/itop97.pdf. Retrieved January 27, 2012.

International statistical classification of diseases and related health problems, Tenth Revision (ICD-10). Vol 2. Geneva, Switzerland: World Health Organization; 2006.

Appendix G

Federal Requirements for Patient Screening and Transfer*

In 1986, the United States Congress first enacted legal requirements specifying how Medicare-participating hospitals with emergency services must handle individuals with emergency medical conditions or women who are in labor. Since then, the patient screening and transfer law has undergone numerous refinements and revisions. Physicians should expect that this law will continue to evolve and that there will be additional modifications to it in the future.

Requirements for an Appropriate Medical Screening Examination

Federal law requires that all Medicare-participating hospitals with a dedicated emergency department must provide an "appropriate medical screening examination" for any individual who comes to the emergency department for medical treatment or examination to determine whether the patient has an emergency medical condition. This examination must be made within the capability of the hospital's emergency department, including ancillary services routinely available to the emergency department. For example, "[i]f a hospital has a department of obstetrics and gynecology, the hospital is responsible for adopting procedures under which the staff and resources of that department are available to treat a woman in labor who comes to its emergency department."

Medical screening examinations also must "...be conducted by individuals determined qualified by hospital by-laws or rules and regulations." Therefore, it is up to a hospital to designate who is a qualified medical person to provide an appropriate medical screening examination. The law does not require that physicians perform all screening examinations. Therefore, a hospital can determine

---

*Data from Emergency Medical Treatment and Labor Act. P.L. 99-272, 100 Stat.164 (1986) codified at 42 U.S.C. SS 1395dd et seq. (2010). Available at: http://www.gpo.gov/fdsys/pkg/USCODE-2010-title42/pdf/USCODE-2010-title42-chap7-subchapXVIII.pdf. Retrieved March 21, 2012.

under what circumstances a physician is required to provide medical screening and when screening can be done by a nonphysician.

Determining Whether a Patient Has an Emergency Medical Condition

The legal definition of *emergency medical condition* is not the same as the medical one. Under the law, it is defined as:

"A medical condition manifesting itself by acute symptoms of sufficient severity (including severe pain, psychiatric disturbances and/or symptoms of substance abuse) such that the absence of immediate attention could reasonably be expected to result in—

(A) Placing the health of the individual (or, with respect to a pregnant woman, the health of the woman or her unborn child) in serious jeopardy;

(B) Serious impairment to bodily functions; or

(C) Serious dysfunction of any bodily organ or part."

It is important to note that, in the case of a pregnant woman, the health of the fetus also must be considered in determining whether an "emergency medical condition" exists.

Special Determination of Emergency Medical Conditions for Pregnant Women

The definition of an emergency medical condition also makes specific reference to a pregnant woman who is having contractions. It provides that an emergency medical condition exists if a pregnant woman is having contractions and "… there is inadequate time to effect a safe transfer to another hospital before delivery; or that transfer may pose a threat to the health or safety of the woman or the unborn child." An emergency medical condition does not exist, even when a woman is having contractions, as long as there is adequate time to effect a safe transfer before delivery and the transfer will not pose a threat to the health or safety of the mother or the fetus. *Labor* is defined as the process of childbirth beginning with the latent phase of labor or early phase of labor and continuing through delivery of the placenta. A woman experiencing contractions is in true labor unless a physician, certified nurse-midwife, or other qualified medical person acting within his or her scope of practice as defined in hospital medical staff bylaws and State law, certifies that, after a reasonable time of observation, the woman is in false labor. Under this definition, a qualified medical person must certify that a woman is in false labor before she can be released.

Patients With Emergency Medical Conditions

Once a patient comes to an emergency department, is appropriately screened, and is determined to have an emergency medical condition, the physician may do one of two things:

1. Treat the patient and stabilize her condition.
2. Transfer the patient to another medical facility in accordance with specific procedures outlined later.

In situations in which a pregnant woman is in true labor, her condition will be considered stabilized once the newborn and the placenta have been delivered.

Patients Can Refuse to Consent to Treatment

If a patient refuses to consent to treatment, the hospital has fulfilled its obligations under the law. If a patient refuses to consent to treatment, however, the following three steps must be taken:

1. The patient must be informed of the risks and benefits of the examination or treatment or both.
2. The medical record must contain a description of the examination and treatment that was refused by the patient.
3. The hospital must take all reasonable steps to secure the patient's written informed refusal. The written document must indicate that the individual has been informed of the risks and benefits of the examination or treatment or both.

Procedures for Transferring a Patient to Another Medical Facility

In general, a patient who meets the criteria of an emergency medical condition may not be transferred until he or she is stabilized. There are, however some exceptions to this prohibition.

The patient may request a transfer, in writing, after being informed of the hospital's obligations under the law and the risks of transfer. The unstabilized patient's written request for transfer must indicate the reasons for the request and that the patient is aware of the risks and benefits of transfer.

An unstabilized patient also may be transferred if a physician signs a written certification that based upon the information available at the time of transfer, the medical benefits reasonably expected from the provision of appropriate medical treatment at another medical facility outweigh the increased risks to the individual or, in the case of a woman in labor, to the woman or the unborn child, from being transferred. The certification must contain a summary of the risks and benefits of transfer.

If a physician is not physically present in the emergency department at the time of the transfer of a patient, a qualified medical person can sign the certification described previously after consulting with a physician who authorizes the transfer. The physician must countersign the certification as contemporaneously as possible.

Patients Can Refuse to Consent to Transfer

If the hospital offers to transfer a patient, in accordance with the appropriate procedures, and the patient refuses to consent to transfer, the hospital also has fulfilled its obligations under the law. When a patient refuses to consent to the transfer, the hospital must take the following three steps:

1. The patient must be informed of the risks and benefits of the transfer.

2. The medical record must contain a description of the proposed transfer that was refused by the patient.

3. The hospital must take all reasonable steps to secure the patient's written informed refusal. The written document must indicate that the individual has been informed of the risks and benefits of the transfer and the reasons for the patient's refusal.

Additional Requirements of the Transferring and Receiving Hospitals

The transferring hospital must comply with the following three requirements to ensure that the transfer was appropriate:

1. The receiving hospital must have space and qualified personnel to treat the patient and must have agreed to accept the transfer. A hospital with specialized capabilities, such as a neonatal intensive care unit, may not refuse to accept patients if space is available.

2. The transferring hospital must minimize the risks to the patient's health, and the transfer must be executed through the use of qualified personnel and transportation equipment.

3. The transferring hospital must send to the receiving hospital all medical records related to the emergency condition that are available at the time of transfer. These records include available history, records related to the emergency medical condition, observations of signs or symptoms, preliminary diagnosis, results of diagnostic studies or telephone reports of the studies, treatment provided, results of any tests and informed written consent or certification, and the name of any on-call physician who has refused or failed to appear within a reasonable time to provide necessary stabilizing treatment. Other records not yet available must be sent as soon as possible.

General Requirements

The following seven general requirements should be met:

1. Medical records related to transfers must be retained by both the transferring and receiving hospitals for 5 years from the date of the transfer.

2. Hospitals are required to report to the Centers for Medicare and Medicaid Services or the state survey agency within 72 hours from the time of the transfer any time they have reason to believe they may have received a patient who was transferred in an unstable medical condition.

3. Hospitals are required to post signs in areas, such as entrances, admitting areas, waiting rooms, and emergency departments, with respect to their obligations under the patient screening and transfer law.

4. Hospitals also are required to post signs stating whether the hospital participates in the Medicaid program under a state-approved plan. This requirement applies to all hospitals, not only those that participate in Medicare.

5. Hospitals must keep a list of physicians who are on call after the initial examination to provide treatment to stabilize a patient with an emergency medical condition.

6. Hospitals must keep a central log of all individuals who come to the emergency department seeking assistance and the result of each individual's visit.

7. A hospital may not delay providing appropriate medical screening to inquire about payment method or insurance status.

Enforcement and Penalties

Physicians and hospitals violating these federal requirements for patient screening and transfer are subject to civil monetary penalties of up to $50,000 for each violation and to termination from the Medicare program. Hospitals are prohibited from penalizing physicians who report violations of the law or who refuse to transfer an individual with an unstabilized emergency medical condition.

Appendix H

Occupational Safety and Health Administration Regulations on Occupational Exposure to Bloodborne Pathogens*

In 1970, the U.S. Congress enacted the Occupational Safety and Health Act to protect workers from unsafe and unhealthy conditions in the workplace. To oversee this effort, the law also created the Occupational Safety and Health Administration (OSHA) within the U.S. Department of Labor. The Occupational Safety and Health Administration has the responsibility for developing and implementing job safety and health standards and regulations. Its standards and regulations apply to all employers and employees. To promote and ensure compliance with its standards, OSHA has the authority to conduct unannounced workplace inspections. It also maintains a reporting and record-keeping system to monitor job-related injuries and illnesses. Failure to comply with OSHA standards may result in the assessment of civil or criminal penalties.

In December 1991, OSHA issued new regulations on occupational exposure to bloodborne pathogens that are designed to minimize the transmission of human immunodeficiency virus (HIV), hepatitis B virus (HBV), and other potentially infectious materials in the workplace. The regulations cover all employees in physician offices, hospitals, medical laboratories, and other health care facilities where workers could be "reasonably anticipated" as a result of performing their job duties to come into contact with blood and other potentially infectious materials. The regulations were revised, effective April 2001, to comply with the Needlestick Safety and Prevention Act of 2000.

---

*Data from Occupational Safety and Health Administration. Washington, DC: OSHA; 2012. Available at: http://www.osha.gov/. Retrieved January 20, 2012.

Approved State Plans

Under the federal law that created OSHA, states are encouraged to develop and operate—under OSHA guidance—state job safety and health plans. Currently, 25 states and two other jurisdictions have OSHA-approved plans, which require them to provide standards and enforcement programs that are at least as effective as the federal standards. These states and jurisdictions are as follows:

Alaska	Maryland	Puerto Rico
Arizona	Michigan	South Carolina
California	Minnesota	Tennessee
Connecticut	Nevada	Utah
Hawaii	New Jersey	Vermont
Illinois	New Mexico	Virgin Islands
Indiana	New York	Virginia
Iowa	North Carolina	Washington
Kentucky	Oregon	Wyoming

A list of these state OSHA offices is available on the OSHA web site at http://www.osha.gov/; call the number listed to receive a copy of the state's standards on occupational exposure to blood-borne pathogens. In Connecticut, Illinois, New Jersey, New York, and the Virgin Islands the state plans cover state and local government employees only; the private sector is covered by the federal OSHA standard. In addition, states with an OSHA-approved state plan must comply with the federal OSHA standard.

Complying With the Regulations

Exposure Control Plan

In order to comply with the regulations, health care employers are required to prepare a written Exposure Control Plan designed to eliminate or minimize employee exposure to bloodborne pathogens. This plan must list all job classifications in which employees are likely to be exposed to infectious materials and the relevant tasks and procedures performed by these employees. Infectious materials include blood, semen, vaginal secretions, peritoneal fluid, amniotic fluid, any body fluid visibly contaminated with blood, all body fluids in which it is impossible to differentiate between the body fluids, any unfixed human tissue or organ (living or dead), as well as HIV-containing cell or tissue cultures, organ cultures, and HIV-containing or HBV-containing culture medium or other solutions.

Under the plan, employers are required to adopt universal precautions, engineering and work practice controls, and personal protective equipment requirements. Employers also must establish a schedule for implementing the following controls:

- Housekeeping requirements
- Employee training and record-keeping requirements
- Hepatitis B virus vaccination for employees and postexposure evaluation and follow-up procedures
- Communication of hazards

A detailed discussion of each of these requirements follows. The plan must be accessible to employees and made available to OSHA upon request. The Exposure Control Plan must be reviewed annually and updated to reflect changes in technology that eliminate or reduce exposure to bloodborne pathogens. The employer must document this annual consideration and use of appropriate effective safer medical procedures and devices that are commercially available. In designing and reviewing the Exposure Compliance Plan, the employer must solicit input from nonmanagerial employees who are potentially exposed to injuries from contaminated sharps. Employers must document, in the Exposure Control Plan, how they received input from employees.

Mandatory Universal Precautions

The regulations require that universal precautions must be used to prevent contact with blood or other potentially infectious materials. It is OSHA's intention to follow the Centers for Disease Control and Prevention's guidelines on universal precautions. As defined by the Centers for Disease Control and Prevention, the concept of universal precautions requires the employer and employee to assume that blood and other body fluids are infectious and must be handled accordingly.

Engineering and Work Practice Controls

Specific engineering and work practice controls for the workplace must be implemented and examined for effectiveness on a regular schedule. These include the following seven controls:

1. Employers are required to provide hand-washing facilities that are readily accessible to employees; when this is not feasible, employees must be provided with an antiseptic hand cleanser with clean cloth/paper towels

or antiseptic towelettes. It is the employer's responsibility to ensure that employees wash their hands immediately after gloves and other protective garments are removed.

2. Contaminated needles and other contaminated sharp objects shall not be bent, recapped, or removed unless the employer can demonstrate that no alternative is feasible or that a specific medical procedure requires such action. Shearing or breaking of contaminated needles is prohibited. Recapping or needle removal must be accomplished by a mechanical device or a one-handed technique. Contaminated reusable sharp objects shall be placed in appropriate containers until properly reprocessed; these containers must be puncture resistant, leakproof, and labeled or color-coded in accordance with the regulations for easy identification.

3. Eating, drinking, smoking, applying cosmetics or lip balm, and handling contact lenses are prohibited in work areas where there is a reasonable likelihood of exposure to potentially infectious materials.

4. Food and drink must not be kept in refrigerators, freezers, shelves, cabinets, or on countertops where blood or other potentially infectious materials are present.

5. All procedures involving blood or other infectious materials shall be performed in a manner to minimize splashing, spraying, spattering, and creating droplets; mouth pipetting and suctioning of blood or other potentially infectious materials is prohibited.

6. Specimens of blood or other potentially infectious materials must be placed in closed containers that prevent leakage during collection, handling, processing, storage, transport, or shipping; containers must be labeled or color-coded in accordance with the regulations for easy identification. However, when a facility uses universal precautions in the handling of all specimens, the required labeling or color coding of specimens is not necessary as long as containers are recognizable as containing specimens; this exemption applies only while the specimens and containers remain in the facility. If outside contamination of the primary container occurs, it must be placed within a second container that is leakproof, puncture resistant, and labeled or color-coded accordingly.

7. Equipment that could be contaminated with blood or other infectious materials must be examined before servicing or shipping and shall be decontaminated as necessary, unless the employer can demonstrate that decontamination of the equipment or parts of the equipment is not

feasible. A visible label must be attached to the equipment stating which parts remain contaminated. The employer must ensure that this information is conveyed to all affected employees, the servicing representative or the manufacturer or both before handling, servicing, or shipping so that the necessary precautions will be taken.

Personal Protective Equipment

The regulations also stress the importance of appropriate personal protective equipment that employers are required to provide at no cost to employees whose job duties expose them to blood and other infectious materials. Appropriate personal protective equipment includes but is not limited to gloves, gowns, laboratory coats, face shields or masks, eye protection, mouthpieces, resuscitation bags, pocket masks, or other ventilation devices. As defined by OSHA, *personal protective equipment* is considered appropriate if it prevents blood or other potentially infectious materials from reaching an employee's work clothes and skin, eyes, mouth, or other mucous membranes under normal conditions of use.

Employers must ensure that the employee uses appropriate personal protective equipment unless the employer can demonstrate that the employee temporarily declined to use the equipment, when under rare and extraordinary circumstances, it was the employee's professional judgment that use of personal protective equipment would have prevented the delivery of health care services or would have posed an increased hazard to the safety of the worker or co-worker. When an employee makes this judgment, the circumstances shall be investigated and documented in order to determine whether changes can be made to prevent such situations in the future.

Personal protective equipment in the appropriate sizes must be accessible at the worksite or issued to employees. Hypoallergenic gloves, glove liners, powderless gloves, or other similar alternatives, shall be accessible to those employees who are allergic to the gloves normally provided. The employer shall provide for laundering and disposal of personal protective equipment, as well as repair and replace this equipment when necessary to maintain its effectiveness, at no cost to the employee. If a garment(s) is penetrated by blood or other infectious materials, it must be removed immediately or as soon as feasible. All personal protective equipment must be removed before leaving the work area, whereupon it shall be placed in a designated area or storage container for washing or disposal.

Gloves must be worn when it reasonably can be anticipated that the employee may have hand contact with blood, other potentially infectious materials, mucous membranes, and nonintact skin; when performing vascular access procedures; and when handling or touching contaminated surfaces. Disposable gloves shall be replaced as soon as practical when contaminated or when torn or punctured; they shall not be washed or decontaminated for reuse. Utility gloves may be decontaminated for reuse but must be discarded if a glove is cracked, peeling, torn, punctured, or shows other signs of deterioration.

Masks in combination with goggles or protective eye shields must be worn whenever splashes, spray, spatter, or droplets of blood may be created and eye, nose, or mouth contamination can reasonably be anticipated. Gowns and other protective body clothing, such as, but not limited to, gowns, aprons, lab coats, clinic jackets, or similar outer garments, shall be worn in occupational exposure situations. The type and characteristics will depend upon the task and degree of exposure anticipated. Surgical caps or hoods, or shoe covers, or both must be worn in situations in which gross contamination can reasonably be anticipated (eg, autopsies, orthopedic surgery).

Housekeeping

Employers must ensure that the worksite is maintained in a clean and sanitary condition and shall develop and implement a written schedule for cleaning and method of decontamination based upon the location within the facility, type of surface to be cleaned, type of soil present, and tasks or procedures being performed in the area. All equipment and working surfaces shall be cleaned and decontaminated after contact with blood or other potentially infectious materials.

Contaminated work surfaces shall be decontaminated with an appropriate disinfectant after tasks and procedures are completed; immediately or as soon as feasible when surfaces are contaminated or after any spill of blood or other potentially infectious materials; and at the end of the work shift if the surface may have become contaminated since the last cleaning. Protective covering (eg, plastic wrap, aluminum foil, or imperviously backed absorbent paper used to cover equipment and environmental surfaces) must be removed and replaced as soon as feasible upon contamination or at the end of the work shift if they may have become contaminated during the shift. All bins, pails, cans, and similar containers intended for reuse shall be inspected and decontaminated on a regularly scheduled basis and cleaned immediately or as soon as feasible upon visible contamination.

Broken glassware that may be contaminated must not be picked up directly with the hands; it must be cleaned up using a brush and dustpan, tongs, or forceps. Contaminated reusable sharp objects must not be stored or processed in a manner that requires employees to reach by hand into the containers in which these sharp objects have been placed. Containers for contaminated sharp objects must be closable, puncture resistant, leakproof on the sides and bottom, and labeled or color-coded in accordance with the regulations. During use, containers for contaminated sharp objects shall be easily accessible to personnel and located as close as possible to the immediate area where sharp objects are used. Additionally, these containers must be maintained upright throughout use, replaced routinely, and not be allowed to be overfilled. Reusable containers shall not be opened, emptied, or cleaned manually or in any other manner that would expose employees to the risk of percutaneous injury. Containers of contaminated disposable sharp objects and personal protective equipment are defined as regulated waste; such containers must prevent the spillage or protrusion of contents during handling, storage, transport, or shipping.

Contaminated laundry shall be handled as little as possible and must be placed in bags or containers at the location where it was used; it must not be sorted or rinsed in the location of use. Contaminated laundry shall be transported in clearly labeled or color-coded bags or containers in accordance with the regulations. Employers shall ensure that employees who have contact with contaminated laundry wear protective gloves and other appropriate personal protective equipment. When a facility ships contaminated laundry offsite to a second facility that does not use universal precautions in handling all laundry, the facility generating the contaminated laundry must clearly mark or color-code the bags or containers with appropriate biohazard labels.

Hepatitis B Vaccination

Employers are required to provide the vaccination for HBV free of charge to all employees who are at risk of occupational exposure. The vaccine must be provided within 10 days of an employee's initial assignment, except in the following cases:

- The employee has previously received the complete HBV vaccination series.
- Antibody testing has revealed that the employee is immune.
- The vaccine is contraindicated for medical reasons.

The regulations prohibit employers from making employees participate in a prescreening program as a prerequisite for receiving the vaccination. Employees who refuse the vaccination must sign a Hepatitis B Vaccine Declination form stating that they have declined the vaccine. If the U.S. Public Health Service ever recommends booster doses of HBV vaccine they also must be provided to employees free of charge. The employee, however, is allowed to change his or her mind and elect to receive the vaccine at any time at the employer's expense.

Postexposure Evaluation and Follow-up

Following a report of an employee exposure incident, the employer must make immediately available to the exposed employee a confidential medical evaluation at no cost to the employee and at a reasonable time and place, and follow-up, including at least the following information and follow-up care:

- Documentation of the route(s) of exposure and the circumstances under which the exposure occurred.

- Identification and documentation of the individual who is the source of the blood or potentially infectious material, unless the employer can establish that such identification is not feasible or is prohibited by state or local law. The source individual's blood shall be tested as soon as possible and after consent is obtained, in order to determine HBV or HIV infectivity. If consent is not obtained, the employer must document that legally required consent cannot be obtained. If the source individual's consent is not required by law, the source individual's blood if available must be tested and the results documented. However, when the source individual is already known to be infected with HBV or HIV, blood testing for HBV or HIV is not required. Results of the source individual's blood test must be made available to the exposed employee, and the employee shall be informed of all applicable laws concerning the disclosure of the source individual's identity and infectious status.

- Collection and testing of the exposed employee's blood for HBV and HIV serologic status as soon as feasible after the employee gives consent. If the employee consents to baseline blood collection but does not give consent at that time for HIV serologic testing, the sample shall be preserved for 90 days. Testing of the blood shall take place within the 90 days if the employee decides to do so.

- Postexposure prophylaxis when medically indicated, as recommended by the U.S. Public Health Service

- Counseling

- Evaluation of reported illnesses

The employer must ensure that the health professional responsible for the employee's HBV vaccination is provided a copy of the OSHA regulation on bloodborne pathogens. In the case of a health professional evaluating an exposed employee, the employer shall ensure that the health professional is provided the following information:

- A copy of the OSHA bloodborne pathogens regulations
- A description of the exposed employee's duties as they relate to the exposure incident
- Documentation of the routes of exposure and circumstances under which exposure occurred
- Results of the source individual's blood testing, if available
- All medical records relevant to the appropriate treatment of the exposed employee, including vaccination status, which is the employer's responsibility to maintain

The employer must obtain and provide the employee with a copy of the evaluating health professional's written opinion within 15 days of completion. The health professional's written opinion for HBV vaccination shall be limited to whether HBV vaccination is indicated for the employee and if the employee has received such vaccination. The health professional's written opinion for postexposure evaluation and follow-up shall be limited to the following information:

- The employee has been informed of the results of the evaluation.
- The employee has been told about any medical conditions resulting from exposure to blood or other potentially infectious materials that require further evaluation or treatment.

All other findings or diagnoses must remain confidential and shall not be included in the written report.

Communication of Hazards to Employees

Warning Labels and Signs

The regulations require warning labels on containers of regulated waste and refrigerators and freezers containing blood or other potentially infectious materials. Warning labels also must be affixed to containers used to store, transport, or ship blood or other potentially infectious materials. The warnings must be fluorescent orange or orange red; however, red bags or red containers may be substituted for labels.

Employee Training

Employers must ensure that all employees at risk of occupational exposure participate in a training program at no cost to employees and during working hours. Training shall take place at the time of an employee's initial assignment to tasks that risk exposure and at least annually thereafter. Annual training for employees shall be provided within 1 year of their previous training. Additional training must be provided when changes, such as modifications of tasks or procedures or introduction of new tasks and procedures, affect the worker's exposure risk. The training must be conducted by an individual knowledgeable about the subject matter, and the material shall be presented at an educational level appropriate to the employees. The training program at a minimum must include the following information:

- A copy of the bloodborne pathogens regulations and an explanation of their contents
- A general explanation of the epidemiology and symptoms of bloodborne diseases
- An explanation of the modes of transmission of bloodborne diseases
- An explanation of the employer's Exposure Control Plan and information on how the employee can obtain a copy of the plan
- An explanation of the appropriate methods for identifying tasks and other activities that may involve exposure
- An explanation of the methods that will prevent or reduce exposure (including appropriate engineering controls, work practices, and personal protective equipment)
- Information on the types, proper use, location, removal, handling, decontamination, and disposal of personal protective equipment
- An explanation of the basis for selection of personal protective equipment
- Information on the HBV vaccine (efficacy, safety, method of administration, benefits of being vaccinated, and that the vaccine will be offered free of charge)
- Information on the appropriate actions to take and individuals to contact in an emergency involving blood or other infectious materials

- An explanation of the procedure for follow-up if an exposure incident occurs (including the method for reporting incident and the medical follow-up that may be available)
- Information on the postexposure evaluation and follow-up that the employer is required to provide for the employee
- An explanation of the signs and label requirements, or color-coding requirements, or both
- An opportunity for interactive questions and answers with the individual conducting the training session

Record-Keeping Requirements

The employer shall maintain an accurate record for each employee at risk of occupational exposure that includes the following information:

- The name and social security number of the employee
- The employee's HBV vaccination status (dates and any medical information relative to the employee's ability to receive the vaccination)
- The results of examinations, medical testing, and follow-up procedures
- The employer's copy of the health professional's written evaluation as required after an exposure incident
- A copy of the information provided to the health professional as required after an exposure incident

The employer shall ensure the confidentiality of employee records; information shall not be disclosed without the employee's written consent. The employer is required to maintain records for the duration of employment plus 30 years. The employer also must maintain records of the training sessions that include the dates, the names and qualifications of individuals who conducted training sessions, and the names and job titles of employees who attended sessions. These records shall be maintained for 3 years from the date the training session occurred.

All records shall be made available to the assistant secretary of OSHA for examination and copying, including employee medical records, for which the employee's consent is not needed. In the event of an employer going out of business, these records must be transferred to the new owner or must be offered to the National Institute for Occupational Safety and Health.

Sharps Injury Log

An employer with more than 10 employees shall maintain a "sharps injury log" to record percutaneous injuries from contaminated sharps. The information in the log shall be kept in a way to protect the confidentiality of the injured employee. The log must contain the following:

- The type and brand of device involved in the incident
- The department or work area where the exposure incident occurred
- An explanation of how the incident occurred

The bloodborne pathogens regulations are just one of the OSHA standards that physician offices must follow to be in compliance. Other OSHA regulations include standards on the hazards of chemicals in the workplace, compressed gases, office equipment, and an action plan in case of fire. An emergency hotline number has been established by OSHA to report emergencies: 1-800-321-OSHA (6742).

Appendix I

American Academy of Pediatrics Policy Statements and American College of Obstetricians and Gynecologists' Committee Opinions and Practice Bulletins

American Academy of Pediatrics Policy Statements

Committee on Adolescence

Counseling the adolescent about pregnancy options. American Academy of Pediatrics. Committee on Adolescence. Pediatrics 1998;101:938–40.

Klein JD. Adolescent pregnancy: current trends and issues. American Academy of Pediatrics Committee on Adolescence. Pediatrics 2005;116:281–6.

Committee on Bioethics

American Academy of Pediatrics Committee on Bioethics: Guidelines on foregoing life-sustaining medical treatment. Pediatrics 1994;93:532–6.

Committee on Children With Disabilities

Guidelines for home care of infants, children, and adolescents with chronic disease. American Academy of Pediatrics Committee on Children with Disabilities. Pediatrics 1995;96(1 Pt 1):161–4.

Committee on Drugs

Neonatal drug withdrawal. American Academy of Pediatrics Committee on Drugs, Committee on Fetus and Newborn. Pediatrics 2012;129:e540–60.

Cote CJ, Wilson S. Guidelines for monitoring and management of pediatric patients during and after sedation for diagnostic and therapeutic procedures: an update. Work Group on Sedation American Academy of Pediatrics and American Academy of Pediatric Dentistry. Pediatrics 2006;118:2587–602.

Committee on Early Childhood, Adoption, and Dependent Care

Families and adoption: the pediatrician's role in supporting communication. American Academy of Pediatrics Committee on Early Childhood, Adoption, and Dependent Care. Pediatrics 2003;112:1437–41.

Committee on Fetus and Newborn

Hospital stay for healthy term newborns. American Academy of Pediatrics. Committee on Fetus and Newborn. Pediatrics 2010;125:405–9.

The Apgar score. American Academy of Pediatrics, Committee on Fetus and Newborn. Pediatrics 2006;117:1444–7.

Controversies concerning vitamin K and the newborn. American Academy of Pediatrics Committee on Fetus and Newborn. Pediatrics 2003;112(1 Pt 1):191–2.

Apnea, sudden infant death syndrome, and home monitoring. American Academy of Pediatrics Committee on Fetus and Newborn. Pediatrics 2003;111(4 Pt 1):914–7.

Adamkin DH. Postnatal glucose homeostasis in late-preterm and term infants. American Academy of Pediatrics Committee on Fetus and Newborn. Pediatrics 2011;127:575–9.

Barfield WD. Standard Terminology for Fetal, Infant, and Perinatal Deaths. American Academy of Pediatrics Committee on Fetus and Newborn. Pediatrics 2011;128:177–181.

Batton DG. Clinical report--Antenatal counseling regarding resuscitation at an extremely low gestational age. American Academy of Pediatrics Committee on Fetus and Newborn. Pediatrics 2009;124:422–7.

Batton DG, Barrington KJ, Wallman C. Prevention and management of pain in the neonate: an update. American Academy of Pediatrics Committee on Fetus and Newborn; American Academy of Pediatrics Section on Surgery; Canadian Paediatric Society Fetus and Newborn Committee. Pediatrics 2006;118:2231–41.

Bell EF. Noninitiation or withdrawal of intensive care for high-risk newborns. American Academy of Pediatrics Committee on Fetus and Newborn. Pediatrics 2007;119:401–3.

Engle WA. Surfactant-replacement therapy for respiratory distress in the preterm and term neonate. American Academy of Pediatrics Committee on Fetus and Newborn. Pediatrics 2008;121:419–32.

Levels of neonatal care. Policy statement. American Academy of Pediatrics. Committee on Fetus and Newborn. Pediatrics 2012;130:587–97.

Wallman C. Advanced practice in neonatal nursing. American Academy of Pediatrics Committee on Fetus and Newborn. Pediatrics 2009;123:1606–7.

Epidemiology and diagnosis of health care–associated infections in the NICU. American Academy of Pediatrics. Committee on Fetus and Newborn and Committee on Infectious Diseases. Pediatrics 2012; 129:e1104–9.

Polin RA. Management of neonates with suspected or proven early-onset bacterial sepsis. American Academy of Pediatrics. Committee on Fetus and Newborn. Pediatrics 2012;129:1006–15.

Polin RA, Denson S, Brady MT. Strategies for prevention of health care–associated infections in the NICU. American Academy of Pediatrics. Committee on Fetus and Newborn and Committee on Infectious Diseases. Pediatrics 2012;129:e1085–93.

Committee on Genetics

Maternal Phenylketonuria. American Academy of Pediatrics Committee on Genetics. Pediatrics 2008;122:445–9.

Folic acid for the prevention of neural tube defects. American Academy of Pediatrics. Committee on Genetics. Pediatrics 1999;104(2 Pt 1):325–7.

Kaye CI, Accurso F, La Franchi S, Lane PA, Northrup H, Pang S, et al. Newborn screening fact sheets. American Academy of Pediatrics Committee on Genetics. Pediatrics 2006;118:e934–63.

Committee on Infectious Diseases

Policy statement: recommendations for the prevention of perinatal group b streptococcal (GBS) disease. American Academy of Pediatrics Committee on Infectious Diseases and Committee on Fetus and Newborn. Pediatrics 2011;128:611–6.

American Academy of Pediatrics. Red book: report of the Committee on Infectious Diseases. 29th. Elk Grove Village (IL): AAP; 2012.

Infection prevention and control in pediatric ambulatory settings. American Academy of Pediatrics. Committee on Infectious Diseases. Pediatrics 2007;120:650–65.

Committee on Injury and Poison Prevention

Bull M, Agran P, Laraque D, Pollack SH, Smith GA, Spivak HR, et al. Safe transportation of newborns at hospital discharge. American Academy of Pediatrics. Committee on Injury and Poison Prevention. Pediatrics 1999;104(4 Pt 1):986–7.

Bull MJ, Engle WA. Safe transportation of preterm and low birth weight infants at hospital discharge. American Academy of Pediatrics Committee on Injury, Violence, and Poison Prevention and Committee on Fetus and Newborn. Pediatrics 2009;123:1424–9.

Committee on Nutrition

American Academy of Pediatrics. Pediatric nutrition handbook. 6th. Elk Grove Village (IL): American Academy of Pediatrics; 2009.

Baker RD, Greer FR. Diagnosis and prevention of iron deficiency and iron-deficiency anemia in infants and young children (0-3 years of age). Committee on Nutrition American Academy of Pediatrics. Pediatrics 2010;126:1040–50.

Bhatia J, Greer F. Use of soy protein-based formulas in infant feeding. American Academy of Pediatrics Committee on Nutrition. Pediatrics 2008;121:1062–8.

Greer FR, Sicherer SH, Burks AW. Effects of early nutritional interventions on the development of atopic disease in infants and children: the role of maternal dietary restriction, breastfeeding, timing of introduction of complementary foods, and hydrolyzed formulas. American Academy of Pediatrics Committee on Nutrition; American Academy of Pediatrics Section on Allergy and Immunology; Pediatrics 2008;121: 183–91.

Committee on Pediatric AIDS

HIV testing and prophylaxis to prevent mother-to-child transmission in the United States. American Academy of Pediatrics Committee on Pediatric AIDS. Pediatrics 2008;122: 1127–34.

Human milk, breastfeeding, and transmission of human immunodeficiency virus in the United States. American Academy of Pediatrics Committee on Pediatric AIDS. Pediatrics 1995;96(5 Pt 1):977–9.

Havens PL, Mofenson LM. Evaluation and management of the infant exposed to HIV-1 in the United States. American Academy of Pediatrics Committee on Pediatric AIDS. Pediatrics 2009;123:175–87.

Committee on Practice and Ambulatory Medicine

Eye examination in infants, children, and young adults by pediatricians. Committee on Practice and Ambulatory Medicine, Section on Ophthalmology, American Association of Certified Orthoptists, American Association for Pediatric Ophthalmology and Strabismus, American Academy of Ophthalmology. Pediatrics 2003;111(4 Pt 1):902–7.

Recommendations for preventive pediatric health care (periodicity schedule). Elk Grove Village (IL): AAP; 2008. Available at: http://practice.aap.org/content.aspx?aid=1599. Retrieved December 22, 2011.

Committee on Psychosocial Aspects of Child and Family Health

American Academy of Pediatrics. Guidelines for health supervision III. 3rd, updated 2002. Elk Grove Village (IL): AAP; 2002.

Cohen GJ. The prenatal visit. Committee on Psychosocial Aspects of Child and Family Health. Pediatrics 2009;124:1227–32.

Joint Committee on Infant Hearing

Principles and guidelines for early hearing detection and intervention programs. American Academy of Pediatrics, Joint Committee on Infant Hearing. Pediatrics 2007;120: 898–921.

Medical Home Initiatives for Children With Special Needs Project Advisory Committee

The medical home. Medical Home Initiatives for Children With Special Needs Project Advisory Committee. American Academy of Pediatrics. Pediatrics 2002;110(1 Pt 1): 184–6.

Neonatal Resuscitation Steering Committee

American Academy of Pediatrics, American Heart Association. Textbook of neonatal resuscitation. 6th ed. Elk Grove Village (IL): AAP; Dallas (TX): AHA; 2011.

Section on Breastfeeding

Breastfeeding and the use of human milk. American Academy of Pediatrics. Section on Breastfeeding. Pediatrics 2012;129:e827–41.

Section on Cardiology and Cardiac Surgery

Endorsement of health and human services recommendation for pulse oximetry screening for critical congenital heart disease. American Academy of Pediatrics. Section on Cardiology and Cardiac Surgery Executive Committee. Pediatrics 2012;129:190–192.

Section on Endocrinology

Rose SR, Brown RS, Foley T, Kaplowitz PB, Kaye CI, Sundararajan S, et al. Update of newborn screening and therapy for congenital hypothyroidism. American Academy of Pediatrics Section on Endocrinology and Committee on Genetics; American Thyroid Association; Public Health Committee, Lawson Wilkins Pediatric Endocrine Society. Pediatrics 2006;117:2290–303.

Section on Home Care

American Academy of Pediatrics. Guidelines for pediatric home health care. 2nd. Elk Grove Village (IL): AAP; 2009.

Section on Ophthalmology

Screening examination of premature infants for retinopathy of prematurity. Section on Ophthalmology American Academy of Pediatrics; American Academy of Ophthalmology; American Association for Pediatric Ophthalmology and Strabismus [published erratum appears in Pediatrics 2006;118:1324]. Pediatrics 2006;117:572–6.

Section on Transport Medicine

Woodward GA, Insoft RM, Kleinman ME, editors. Guidelines for air and ground transport of neonatal and pediatrics. American Academy of Pediatrics. Section on Transport;Medicine. 3rd ed. Elk Grove Village (IL): American Academy of Pediatrics; 2007. p. 515.

Subcommittee on Hyperbilirubinemia

Bhutani VK, Committee on Fetus and Newborn, American Academy of Pediatrics. Phototherapy to prevent severe neonatal hyperbilirubinemia in the newborn infant 35 or more weeks of gestation. Pediatrics 2011;128:e1046–52.

Management of hyperbilirubinemia in the newborn infant 35 or more weeks of gestation. American Academy of Pediatrics Subcommittee on Hyperbilirubinemia. Pediatrics 2004;114:297–316.

Task Force on Circumcision

Circumcision policy statement. American Academy of Pediatrics. Task Force on Circumcision. Pediatrics 2012;130:585–6.

Task Force on Infant Positioning and SIDS

Moon RY. SIDS and other sleep-related infant deaths: expansion of recommendations for a safe infant sleeping environment. American Academy of Pediatrics. Task Force on Sudden Infant Death Syndrome. Pediatrics 2011;128:1030–9.

American College of Obstetricians and Gynecologists' Committee Opinions

Committee on Adolescent Health Care

Human papillomavirus vaccination. Committee Opinion No. 467. American College of Obstetricians and Gynecologists. Obstet Gynecol 2010;116:800–3.

Committee on Ethics

Multifetal pregnancy reduction. ACOG Committee Opinion No. 369. American College of Obstetricians and Gynecologists. Obstet Gynecol 2007;109:1511–5.

Human immunodeficiency virus. ACOG Committee Opinion No. 389. American College of Obstetricians and Gynecologists. Obstet Gynecol 2007;110:1473–8.

At-risk drinking and illicit drug use: ethical issues in obstetric and gynecologic practice. ACOG Committee Opinion No. 422. American College of Obstetricians and Gynecologists. Obstet Gynecol 2008;112:1449–60.

Informed consent. ACOG Committee Opinion No. 439. American College of Obstetricians and Gynecologists. Obstet Gynecol 2009;114:401–8.

Adoption. Committee Opinion No. 528. American College of Obstetricians and Gynecologists. Obstet Gynecol 2012;119:1320–4.

Committee on Genetics

Umbilical cord blood banking. ACOG Committee Opinion No. 399. American College of Obstetricians and Gynecologists. Obstet Gynecol 2008;111:475–7.

Preconception and prenatal carrier screening for genetic diseases in individuals of Eastern European Jewish descent. ACOG Committee Opinion No. 442. American College of Obstetricians and Gynecologists. Obstet Gynecol 2009;114:950–3.

Family history as a risk assessment tool. Committee Opinion No. 478. American College of Obstetricians and Gynecologists. Obstet Gynecol 2011;117:747–50.

Newborn screening. Committee Opinion No. 481. American College of Obstetricians and Gynecologists. Obstet Gynecol 2011;117:762–5.

Update on carrier screening for cystic fibrosis. Committee Opinion No. 486. American College of Obstetricians and Gynecologists. Obstet Gynecol 2011;117:1028–31.

Committee on Gynecologic Practice

The importance of preconception care in the continuum of women's health care. ACOG Committee Opinion No. 313. American College of Obstetricians and Gynecologists. Obstet Gynecol 2005;106:665–6.

Hepatitis B, hepatitis C, and human immunodeficiency virus infections in obstetrician-gynecologists. Committee Opinion No. 489. American College of Obstetricians and Gynecologists. Obstet Gynecol 2011;117:1242–6.

Understanding and using the U.S. Medical Eligibility Criteria For Contraceptive Use, 2010. Committee Opinion No. 505. American College of Obstetricians and Gynecologists. Obstet Gynecol 2011;118:754–60.

Committee on Health Care for Underserved Women

Smoking cessation during pregnancy. Committee Opinion No. 471. American College of Obstetricians and Gynecologists. Obstet Gynecol 2010;116:1241–4.

Substance abuse reporting and pregnancy: the role of the obstetrician-gynecologist. Committee Opinion No. 473. American College of Obstetricians and Gynecologists. Obstet Gynecol 2011;117:200–1.

Methamphetamine abuse in women of reproductive age. Committee Opinion No. 479. American College of Obstetricians and Gynecologists. Obstet Gynecol 2011;117:751–5.

Health literacy. Committee Opinion No. 491. American College of Obstetricians and Gynecologists. Obstet Gynecol 2011;117:1250–3.

Cultural sensitivity and awareness in the delivery of health care. Committee Opinion No. 493. American College of Obstetricians and Gynecologists. Obstet Gynecol 2011;117:1258–61.

At-risk drinking and alcohol dependence: obstetric and gynecologic implications. Committee Opinion No. 496. American College of Obstetricians and Gynecologists. Obstet Gynecol 2011;118:383–8.

Tobacco use and women's health. Committee Opinion No. 503. American College of Obstetricians and Gynecologists. Obstet Gynecol 2011;118:746–50.

Health care for pregnant and postpartum incarcerated women and adolescent females. Committee Opinion No. 511. American College Obstetricians and Gynecologists. Obstet Gynecol 2011;118:1198–202.

Intimate partner violence. Committee Opinion No. 518. American College of Obstetricians and Gynecologists. Obstet Gynecol 2012;119:412–7.

Opioid abuse, dependence, and addiction in pregnancy. Committee Opinion No. 524. American College of Obstetricians and Gynecologists. Obstet Gynecol 2012:119: 1070–6.

Access to postpartum sterilization. Committee Opinion No. 530. American College of Obstetricians and Gynecologists. Obstet Gynecol 2012;120:212–15.

Committee on Obstetric Practice

American College of Obstetricians and Gynecologists. Scheduled cesarean delivery and the prevention of vertical transmission of HIV infection. ACOG Committee Opinion 234. Washington, DC: ACOG; 2000.

American College of Obstetricians and Gynecologists. Statement on surgical assistants. ACOG Committee Opinion 240. Washington, DC: ACOG; 2000.

Circumcision. ACOG Committee Opinion No. 260. American College of Obstetricians and Gynecologists. Obstet Gynecol 2001;98:707–8.

Exercise during pregnancy and the postpartum period. ACOG Committee Opinion No. 267. American College of Obstetricians and Gynecologists. Obstet Gynecol 2002;99:171–3.

Obstetric management of patients with spinal cord injuries. ACOG Committee Opinion: No. 275. American College of Obstetricians and Gynecologists. Obstet Gynecol 2002;100:625–7.

Pain relief during labor. ACOG Committee Opinion No. 295. American College of Obstetricians and Gynecologists. Obstet Gynecol 2004;104:213.

Obesity in pregnancy. ACOG Committee Opinion No. 315. American College of Obstetricians and Gynecologists. Obstet Gynecol 2005;106:671–5.

Inappropriate use of the terms fetal distress and birth asphyxia. ACOG Committee Opinion No. 326. American College of Obstetricians and Gynecologists. Obstet Gynecol 2005;106:1469–70.

The Apgar score. ACOG Committee Opinion No. 333. American College of Obstetricians and Gynecologists. Obstet Gynecol 2006;107:1209–12.

Analgesia and cesarean delivery rates. ACOG Committee Opinion No. 339. American College of Obstetricians and Gynecologists. Obstet Gynecol 2006;107:1487–8.

Mode of term singleton breech delivery. ACOG Committee Opinion No. 340. American College of Obstetricians and Gynecologists. Obstet Gynecol 2006;108:235–7.

Nalbuphine hydrochloride use for intrapartum analgesia. ACOG Committee Opinion No. 376. American College of Obstetricians and Gynecologists. Obstet Gynecol 2007;110:449.

Subclinical hypothyroidism in pregnancy. ACOG Committee Opinion No. 381. American College of Obstetricians and Gynecologists. Obstet Gynecol 2007;110:959–60.

Fetal monitoring prior to scheduled cesarean delivery. ACOG Committee Opinion No. 382. American College of Obstetricians and Gynecologists. Obstet Gynecol 2007; 110:961–2.

Late-preterm infants. ACOG Committee Opinion No. 404. American College of Obstetricians and Gynecologists. Obstet Gynecol 2008;111:1029–32.

Prenatal and perinatal human immunodeficiency virus testing: expanded recommendations. ACOG Committee Opinion No. 418. American College of Obstetricians and Gynecologists. Obstet Gynecol 2008;112:739–42.

Use of progesterone to reduce preterm birth. ACOG Committee Opinion No. 419. American College of Obstetricians and Gynecologists. Obstet Gynecol 2008;112: 963–5.

Optimal goals for anesthesia care in obstetrics. ACOG Committee Opinion No. 433. American College of Obstetricians and Gynecologists and American Society of Anesthesiologists. Obstet Gynecol 2009;113:1197–9.

Postpartum screening for abnormal glucose tolerance in women who had gestational diabetes mellitus. ACOG Committee Opinion No. 435. American College of Obstetricians and Gynecologists. Obstet Gynecol 2009;113:1419–21.

Oral intake during labor. ACOG Committee Opinion No. 441. American College of Obstetricians and Gynecologists. Obstet Gynecol 2009;114:714.

Air travel during pregnancy. ACOG Committee Opinion No. 443. American College of Obstetricians and Gynecologists. Obstet Gynecol 2009;114:954–5.

Influenza vaccination during pregnancy. Committee Opinion No. 468. American College of Obstetricians and Gynecologists. Obstet Gynecol 2010;116:1006–7.

Antenatal corticosteroid therapy for fetal maturation. Committee Opinion No. 475. American College of Obstetricians and Gynecologists. Obstet Gynecol 2011;117: 422–4.

Planned home birth. Committee Opinion No. 476. American College of Obstetricians and Gynecologists. Obstet Gynecol 2011;117:425–8.

Prevention of early-onset group B streptococcal disease in newborns. Committee Opinion No. 485. American College of Obstetricians and Gynecologists. Obstet Gynecol 2011;117:1019–27.

Vitamin D: screening and supplementation during pregnancy. Committee Opinion No. 495. American College of Obstetricians and Gynecologists. Obstet Gynecol 2011; 118:197–8.

Screening and diagnosis of gestational diabetes mellitus. Committee Opinion No. 504. American College of Obstetricians and Gynecologists. Obstet Gynecol 2011;118:751–3.

Update on immunization and pregnancy: tetanus, diphtheria, and pertussis vaccination. Committee Opinion No. 521. American College of Obstetricians and Gynecologists. Obstet Gynecol 2012;119:690–1.

Placenta accreta. Committee Opinion No. 529. American College of Obstetricians and Gynecologists. Obstet Gynecol 2012;120:207–11.

Lead screening during pregnancy and lactation. Committee Opinion No. 533. American College of Obstetricians and Gynecologists. Obstet Gynecol 2012;120:416–20.

Committee on Patient Safety and Quality Improvement

Patient safety in obstetrics and gynecology. ACOG Committee Opinion No. 447. American College of Obstetricians and Gynecologists. Obstet Gynecol 2009;114:1424–7.

Patient safety in the surgical environment. Committee Opinion No. 464. American College of Obstetricians and Gynecologists. Obstet Gynecol 2010;116:786–90.

Preparing for clinical emergencies in obstetrics and gynecology. Committee Opinion No. 487. American College of Obstetricians and Gynecologists. Obstet Gynecol 2011; 117:1032–4.

Partnering with patients to improve safety. Committee Opinion No. 490. American College of Obstetricians and Gynecologists. Obstet Gynecol 2011;117:1247–9.

Effective patient-physician communication. Committee Opinion No. 492. American College of Obstetricians and Gynecologists. Obstet Gynecol 2011;117:1254–7.

Communication strategies for patient handoffs. Committee Opinion No. 517. American College of Obstetricians and Gynecologists. Obstet Gynecol 2012;119:408–11.

Fatigue and patient safety. Committee Opinion No. 519. American College of Obstetricians and Gynecologists. Obstet Gynecol 2012;119:683–5.

Disclosure and discussion of adverse events. Committee Opinion No. 520. American College of Obstetricians and Gynecologists. Obstet Gynecol 2012;119:686–9.

Re-entering the practice of obstetrics and gynecology. Committee Opinion No. 523. American College of Obstetricians and Gynecologists. Obstet Gynecol 2012;119: 1066–9.

American College of Obstetricians and Gynecologists' Practice Bulletins

American College of Obstetricians and Gynecologists. Prevention of Rh D alloimmunization. ACOG Practice Bulletin 4. Washington, DC: ACOG; 1999.

American College of Obstetricians and Gynecologists. Antepartum fetal surveillance. ACOG Practice Bulletin 9. Washington, DC: ACOG; 1999.

American College of Obstetricians and Gynecologists. Intrauterine growth restriction. ACOG Practice Bulletin 12. Washington, DC: ACOG; 2000.

American College of Obstetricians and Gynecologists. External cephalic version. ACOG Practice Bulletin 13. Washington, DC: ACOG; 2000.

American College of Obstetricians and Gynecologists. Operative vaginal delivery. ACOG Practice Bulletin 17. Washington, DC: ACOG; 2000.

American College of Obstetricians and Gynecologists. Perinatal viral and parasitic infections. ACOG Practice Bulletin 20. Washington, DC: ACOG; 2000.

Gestational diabetes. ACOG Practice Bulletin No. 30. American College of Obstetricians and Gynecologists. Obstet Gynecol 2001;98:525–38.

Assessment of risk factors for preterm birth. ACOG Practice Bulletin No. 31. American College of Obstetricians and Gynecologists. Obstet Gynecol 2001;98:709–16.

Diagnosis and management of preeclampsia and eclampsia. ACOG Practice Bulletin No. 33. American College of Obstetricians and Gynecologists. Obstet Gynecol 2002; 99:159–67.

Obstetric analgesia and anesthesia. ACOG Practice Bulletin No. 36. American College of Obstetricians and Gynecologists. Obstet Gynecol 2002;100:177–91.

Thyroid disease in pregnancy. ACOG Practice Bulletin No. 37. American College of Obstetricians and Gynecologists. Obstet Gynecol 2002;100:387–96.

Perinatal care at the threshold of viability. ACOG Practice Bulletin No. 38. American College of Obstetricians and Gynecologists. Obstet Gynecol 2002;100:617–24.

Dystocia and augmentation of labor. ACOG Practice Bulletin No. 49. American College of Obstetricians and Gynecologists. Obstet Gynecol 2003;102:1445–54.

Nausea and vomiting of pregnancy. ACOG Practice Bulletin No. 52. American College of Obstetricians and Gynecologists. Obstet Gynecol 2004;103:803–14.

Multiple gestation: complicated twin, triplet, and high-order multifetal pregnancy. ACOG Practice Bulletin No. 56. American College of Obstetricians and Gynecologists. Obstet Gynecol 2004;104:869–83.

Pregestational diabetes mellitus. ACOG Practice Bulletin No. 60. American College of Obstetricians and Gynecologists. Obstet Gynecol 2005;105:675–85.

Episiotomy. ACOG Practice Bulletin No. 71. American College of Obstetricians and Gynecologists. Obstet Gynecol 2006;107:957–62.

Management of alloimmunization during pregnancy. ACOG Practice Bulletin No. 75. American College of Obstetricians and Gynecologists. Obstet Gynecol 2006;108: 457–64.

Postpartum hemorrhage. ACOG Practice Bulletin No. 76. American College of Obstetricians and Gynecologists. Obstet Gynecol 2006;108:1039–47.

Screening for fetal chromosomal abnormalities. ACOG Practice Bulletin No. 77. American College of Obstetricians and Gynecologists. Obstet Gynecol 2007;109:217–27.

Hemoglobinopathies in pregnancy. ACOG Practice Bulletin No. 78. American College of Obstetricians and Gynecologists. Obstet Gynecol 2007;109:229–37.

Premature rupture of membranes. ACOG Practice Bulletin No. 80. American College of Obstetricians and Gynecologists. Obstet Gynecol 2007;109:1007–19.

Management of herpes in pregnancy. ACOG Practice Bulletin No. 82. American College of Obstetricians and Gynecologists. Obstet Gynecol 2007;109:1489–98.

Viral hepatitis in pregnancy. ACOG Practice Bulletin No. 86. American College of Obstetricians and Gynecologists. Obstet Gynecol 2007;110:941–56.

Invasive prenatal testing for aneuploidy. ACOG Practice Bulletin No. 88. American College of Obstetricians and Gynecologists. Obstet Gynecol 2007;110:1459–67.

Asthma in pregnancy. ACOG Practice Bulletin No. 90. American College of Obstetricians and Gynecologists. Obstet Gynecol 2008;111:457–64.

Use of Psychiatric Medications During Pregnancy and Lactation. ACOG Practice Bulletin No. 92. American College of Obstetricians and Gynecologists. Obstet Gynecol 2008; 111:1001–20.

Anemia in pregnancy. ACOG Practice Bulletin No. 95. American College of Obstetricians and Gynecologists. Obstet Gynecol 2008;112:201–7.

Critical care in pregnancy. ACOG Practice Bulletin No. 100. American College of Obstetricians and Gynecologists. Obstet Gynecol 2009;113:443–50.

Ultrasonography in pregnancy. ACOG Practice Bulletin No. 101. American College of Obstetricians and Gynecologists. Obstet Gynecol 2009;113:451–61.

Management of stillbirth. ACOG Practice Bulletin No. 102. American College of Obstetricians and Gynecologists. Obstet Gynecol 2009;113:748–61.

Bariatric surgery and pregnancy. ACOG Practice Bulletin No. 105. American College of Obstetricians and Gynecologists. Obstet Gynecol 2009;113:1405–13.

Intrapartum fetal heart rate monitoring: nomenclature, interpretation, and general management principles. ACOG Practice Bulletin No. 106. American College of Obstetricians and Gynecologists. Obstet Gynecol 2009;114192–202.

Induction of labor. ACOG Practice Bulletin No. 107. American College of Obstetricians and Gynecologists. Obstet Gynecol 2009;114:386–97.

Vaginal birth after previous cesarean delivery. Practice Bulletin No. 115. American College of Obstetricians and Gynecologists. Obstet Gynecol 2010;116:450–63.

Management of intrapartum fetal heart rate tracings. Practice bulletin No. 116. American College of Obstetricians and Gynecologists. Obstet Gynecol 2010;116:1232–40.

Antiphospholipid syndrome. Practice Bulletin No. 118. American College of Obstetricians and Gynecologists. Obstet Gynecol 2011;117:192–9.

Use of prophylactic antibiotics in labor and delivery. Practice Bulletin No. 120. American College of Obstetricians and Gynecologists. Obstet Gynecol 2011;117:1472–83.

Long-acting reversible contraception: implants and intrauterine devices. Practice bulletin no. 121. American College of Obstetricians and Gynecologists. Obstet Gynecol 2011;118:184–96.

Thromboembolism in pregnancy. Practice Bulletin No. 123. American College of Obstetricians and Gynecologists. Obstet Gynecol 2011;118:718–29.

Inherited thrombophilias in pregnancy. Practice bulletin No. 124. American College of Obstetricians and Gynecologists. Obstet Gynecol 2011;118:730–40.

Chronic hypertension in pregnancy. Practice Bulletin No. 125. American College of Obstetricians and Gynecologists. Obstet Gynecol 2012;119:396–407.

Management of preterm labor. Practice Bulletin No. 127. American College of Obstetricians and Gynecologists. Obstet Gynecol 2012;119:1308–17.

Other Publications

American College of Obstetricians and Gynecologists. Quality and safety in women's health care. 2nd. Washington, DC: American College of Obstetricians and Gynecologists; 2010.

Appendix J
Web Site Resources

Agency for Healthcare Research and Quality	www.ahrq.gov
American Academy of Pediatrics	www.aap.org
American College of Obstetricians and Gynecologists	www.acog.org
American College of Medical Genetics and Genomics	www.acmg.net
College of American Pathologists	www.cap.org
American Dental Association	www.ada.org
American Medical Association	www.ama-assn.org
American Psychiatric Association	www.psych.org
Association for Professionals in Infection Control and Epidemiology, Inc	www.apic.org
Association of Air Medical Services	www.aams.org
Association of Women's Health, Obstetric and Neonatal Nurses	www.awhonn.org
Centers for Disease Control and Prevention	www.cdc.gov
ECRI Institute	www.ecri.org
Guttmacher Institute	www.guttmacher.org
HRSA's Heritable Disorders in Newborns and Children	www.hrsa.gov/advisorycommittees/mchbadvisory/heritabledisorders
Immunization for Women	www.immunizationforwomen.org
Institute for Healthcare Improvement	www.ihi.org
Institute for Patient-and Family-Centered Care	www.ipfcc.org

The Joint Commission	www.jointcommission.org
Managing Obstetrical Risk Efficiently	www.moreob.com
March of Dimes	www.marchofdimes.com
National Association of Neonatal Nurses	www.nann.org/
National Center for Health Statistics	www.cdc.gov/nchs/
National Heart Lung and Blood Institute	www.nhlbi.nih.gov/
National Institutes of Health	www.nih.gov

Index

Page numbers followed by italicized letters
b, *f*, and *t* indicate boxes, figures, and tables,
respectively.

A

AAP. *See* American Academy of Pediatrics
Abdominal distention, neonatal, 284*b*
Abdominal pain
 acute, admission policies on, 171
 bariatric surgery and, 219
Abdominal trauma during pregnancy, 246
ABO blood group screening, 237–238
Abortion
 antibody testing and, 116
 Centers for Disease Control and Prevention
  Surveillance Report on, 510
 early pregnancy blood sugar control and, 100
 incarcerated women and, 151
 multifetal reduction, 242
 radiation exposure anxiety and, 142
 spontaneous
  drug use in pregnancy and, 338
  malaria and, 433
  parvovirus B19 and, 407
  sickle cell disease and, 215
 unintended pregnancy and, 4
 unwanted pregnancy and, 127
Abruptio placentae
 breech presentation and, 158
 cesarean delivery and, 192
 chronic hypertension and, 232
 inherited thrombophilias and, 215–216
 intrauterine drug exposure and, 338
 preeclampsia and HELLP syndrome and, 231
 premature rupture of membranes and, 176, 260
 tobacco use and smoke exposure and, 128
 trauma during pregnancy and, 247–248
Abscess, precautions for, 453
Academy of Breastfeeding Medicine, 292
Accountability, 5
Accreditation Association for Ambulatory Health
  Care, 169
Accreditation Commission for Midwifery
  Education, 23
Accreditation Manual for Hospitals, 185
Acetaminophen, 363
Acetic acid liquid sterilant, 455
Acetylcholinesterase, neural tube defects and, 126
Acidosis, as reversible, 347–348

Acidosis, retinopathy of prematurity and, 353
Acoustic stimulation, fetal, 145, 147
Acoustics, in neonatal functional units, 57
ACT sheets, 298
Acute bilirubin encephalopathy, 325
Acyclovir, 394, 396, 397, 413
Adjustable gastric banding, 218
Admission and observation area, in neonatal
  functional units, 47–48
Admission policies
 for intrapartum care, 170–175
 labor and delivery, 171, 440
 nursery, 440–441
Adolescents
 in contact with infants, Tdap for, 423–424
 as mothers
  discharge readiness and, 153
  medical record of, 279
  newborn care and, 314
  preconception counseling after bariatric surgery
   in, 218
 pregnant
  antepartum care for, 151
  nutrition, 134–136*t*
Adoption, 314–315
Adults in contact with infants, Tdap immunization for, 423–424
Advance directives, informed consent and, 156
Advanced maternal age. *See* Maternal age
Advanced practice registered nurses, 27–29
Advisory Committee on Immunization Practices.
  See Centers for Disease Control and
  Prevention
African American ethnicity
 hemoglobin and hematocrit levels and, 224
 preeclampsia and eclampsia and, 231
 preterm births and, 257
African descent
 anemia and, 113*t*
 genetic screening for, 121*t*
 hemoglobinopathies and, 214
Agency for Healthcare Research and Quality, 64
Age-specific birth rate, 502
Air quality, in neonatal functional units, 54–55
Air transport medical equipment, 85
Air travel, during pregnancy, 143–144
Airway management equipment, emergency, 187,
  267, 269*f*
Alcohol, in umbilical cord care, 285–286

Alcohol use. *See also* Substance use and abuse
early postpartum discharge and, 173
incarcerated women and, 152
maternal, neonatal withdrawal and, 335,
336–337*t*
postpartum counseling on, 208
postpartum follow-up on, 207
in pregnancy, 100
psychosocial risk screening and counseling on,
129
recommended consultation for, 477, 479
stillbirth and, 261
Allergies, history of, 172
Alloimmunization, 237
Alpha-thalassemia screening, 121*t*
Ambulation
during labor, 174
postpartum, 196–197
Ambulatory prenatal care, 6–8, 7*t*
American Academy of Pediatrics (AAP)
on Apgar scores, 274
Committee on Drugs, 291
on critical congenital heart disease screening,
304
on hand hygiene, 444
on hepatitis B virus vaccine in low-risk preterm
infants, 390
on immunizations, 366, 423
on neonatal hearing screening, 298
Neonatal Resuscitation Program, 24, 266–268,
269*f*, 271, 273
parent-education site, 309–310
on patient safety, 67
on phototherapy and exchange transfusion,
326
on phototherapy for hyperbilirubinemia, 332
policy statements, 531–536
on preventive health care, 314
on respiratory syncytial virus prophylaxis,
408–409, 410*t*
American Association of Birth Centers, 169, 491
American College of Cardiology, 251
American College of Medical Genetics and
Genomics ACT sheets and confirmatory algorithms, 298
American College of Nurse–Midwives, 491
Division of Accreditation, 492
American College of Obstetricians and
Gynecologists
Antepartum Record and Postpartum Form,
463–476
on collaborative practice, 493
committee opinions, 536–540
on contraceptive use, 203
Immunization for Women web site, 406
National Pregnancy Mortality Surveillance
System and, 500
other publications, 543
practice bulletins, 540–543
American College of Radiology, 142
American Dental Association, 139

American Diabetes Association, 207, 229, 230
American Heart Association
on infective endocarditis prophylaxis, 251
Neonatal Resuscitation Program, 24, 266–268,
269*f*
American Midwifery Certification Board, Inc.,
23, 492
American Society of Regional Anesthesia and Pain
Medicine, 223
Aminoglycosides, 253–254, 422
Ammonias, quaternary, 456
Amniocentesis
for aneuploidy, 124, 125–126
birth defects caused by teratogens and, 142
fetal-to-maternal bleeding and, 116
for hemoglobinopathies, 214
multiple gestations and, 239–240
for neural tube defects, 125
for premature rupture of membranes diagnosis,
176
serial, twin–twin transfusion syndrome and,
242
Amnioinfusion, 181–182
Amnionitis, 417
Amniotic fluid
meconium aspiration, 255
meconium staining, 271, 279
pooling in vagina, 176
Amniotic fluid index, 145, 149–150
Amniotic fluid volume, 149, 256
Amniotomy, 177, 181
Amoxicillin, 415, 417, 432
Ampicillin, 251, 419, 422
Analgesia and anesthesia
administration of, 185–186
cesarean deliveries and, 192
cesarean delivery on maternal request and,
193
for circumcision, 286
critical care in pregnancy and, 245
general, 184–185
labor and delivery and, 173, 174
local, 185
for newborns, 362–365
for operative vaginal delivery, 192
parenteral agents for, 182–183
personnel, 24, 25, 26, 30
postpartum, 195, 197, 198
regional, 183–184
risk factors and complications, 186–187
Analyte, serum levels, 121
Anemia
antepartum management, 224–225
common causes in pregnancy and puerperium,
223–224
fetal, non–Rh-D alloimmunization, 237
fetal and neonatal, trauma and, 248
iron-deficiency, in pregnancy, 133, 215, 224
microcytic, 113*t*, 121*t*
pregnant adolescents and, 151
of prematurity, 321–322

Anemia *(continued)*
  recommended consultation for, 480
  retinopathy of prematurity and, 353
  screening and diagnosis, 224, 224*t*
  zidovudine and, 403
Aneuploidy
  diagnostic tests for, 125–126
  intrauterine growth restriction and, 235
  screening, 120–121, 122*t*, 123–124
Angiotensin-converting enzyme inhibitors, 234
Angiotensin receptor blockers, 234
Ankyloglossia, 290
Anogenital carcinomas, HPV and, 404
Antepartum care. *See also* Pregnancy
  ACOG's Antepartum Record and Postpartum
      Form, 463–476
  anemia, 224–225
  antenatal testing strategy, 145–146
  bariatric surgery and, 218–219
  chlamydial infections, 415
  chronic hypertension, 233–234
  fetal well-being tests, 144–145
    biophysical profile, 149
    fetal movement assessment, 146–147
    modified biophysical profile, 149–150
    nonstress test, 147–148
  first-trimester patient education
    air travel, 143–144
    dental care, 138–139
    exercise, 137–138
    nausea and vomiting, 139
    nutrition, 132–133, 134–136*t*, 136
    teratogens, 141–143
    vitamin and mineral toxicity, 139–141
    weight gain, 136–137, 137*t*
  genetic screening and diagnosis, 119–126
  gestational diabetes mellitus, 228–229
  gonorrhea, 416–417
  herpes simplex virus, 393–394
  illicit drug use and lack of, 337, 338
  immunizations, 117–119
  informed consent and, 155–156
  intrauterine growth restriction, 235–237
  isoimmunization, 238
  laboratory testing, 112, 113–114*t*, 114–117
  multiple gestations, 239–242
  preeclampsia and eclampsia, 231–232
  pregestational diabetes mellitus, 220–221
  prenatal visits
    first, 107–108
    frequency, 106–107
    group, 108–109
  psychosocial risk screening and counseling,
      126–132
  routine laboratory testing, 112–117
  routine visits, 108
    estimated date of delivery, 109–110
    fetal magnetic resonance imaging, 111–112
    fetal ultrasound imaging, 110–111, 111*b*
  rubella screening, 410–411
  scope of, 95, 105–106

Antepartum care *(continued)*
  second-trimester and third-trimester patient
      education
    anticipating labor, 157–158
    breastfeeding, 161
    breech presentation at term, 158–159
    cesarean delivery on maternal request, 160
    childbirth education classes, 157
    choosing newborn care providers, 157
    discharge preparation, 161
    elective delivery, 160
    neonatal interventions, 161
    preterm labor, 158
    trial of labor after cesarean delivery,
        159–160
    umbilical cord blood banking, 160–161
    working, 156–157
  special populations and considerations, 150–155
    adolescents, 151
    homeless women, 153
    incarcerated women, 151–153
    women with disabilities, 154–155
  syphilis, 428
  toxoplasmosis, 434
  tuberculosis, 425
  varicella zoster virus, 412–413
Antepartum hospitalization, 243–244
Antepartum Record and Postpartum Form,
      ACOG's, 463–476
Anthrax infections, 414
Anti-β_2-glycoprotein I, 211
Antibiotics
  breastfeeding and, 290
  catheters and, 448
  for chorioamnionitis, 260
  deer tick bites and, 432
  for dental care, 139
  for endocarditis, 251
  for gonorrhea, 284, 417
  for group B streptococci, 117, 251, 418–420,
      419*t*
  health care-associated infection and, 439, 450
  for hypoxic cardiorespiratory failure, 348
  in infection control, 450
  for late preterm infants, 281
  for listeriosis, 422
  neonatal care and, 279
  for postpartum endometritis, 253–254
  preterm labor and, 258
  prophylaxis for cesarean delivery, 69, 194
Antibody screen, 113*t*, 116, 174
Anticardiolipin, 211
Anticoagulation, therapeutic, 226, 227
Antidepressant drugs, 206
Anti-D immune globulin, 116, 126, 198, 237.
      See also D immune globulin
Antihypertensive therapy, 233
Antimetabolites, breastfeeding and, 290
Antimicrobial agents
  prophylaxis for cesarean deliveries, 194
  for syphilis, 429, 431

Antioxidants, bronchopulmonary dysplasia and, 352
Antiphospholipids, thrombosis and, 225
Antiphospholipid syndrome, 144, 211–212, 231, 236b
Antiretroviral drugs, 398, 402
Antiseptics, during intrapartum period, 177
Antithrombin deficiency, 227
Anxiety, in newborns, 362
Apgar scores, 256, 274, 275f, 281
Apnea
  late preterm infants and, 280, 309, 312
  of prematurity, 322–323
  retinopathy of prematurity and, 353
Arthritis
  gonococcal, 417
  relapsing, 432
Artificial insemination, 105
Aseptic techniques, 447
Ashkenazi Jews, genetic screening of, 101, 121t
Asian ethnicity. See also East Asian ethnicity
  anemia and, 113t
  late preterm infants and, 281
  postpartum hemorrhage and, 254
  rehospitalization or neonatal mortality and, 281
Aspiration
  in anesthetic-related maternal morbidity and, 187
  of meconium, 255, 347
Aspiration pneumonitis, 158
Assisted reproductive technology, 105
Association for Professionals in Infection Control and Epidemiology, 457
Asthma, 212–213, 214b
  children of mothers smoking during pregnancy and, 128
  preconception control of, 101
  recommended consultation for, 477
Audiovisual materials, for new parent education, 309–310
Autoclaving, for sterilization, 455
Autoimmune thrombocytopenia, 212
Autopsy
  fetal, 261
  neonatal, 369
Azithromycin, 415, 416, 417, 424, 428

B
Baby blues, 206
Bacille Calmette–Guérin vaccine, 427
Back to Sleep national campaign positioning recommendation, 312
Bacterial infections, 414–427, 452. See also specific infections
Bacteroides bivius, 252
Ballard Score, 282–283f
Barbiturates, neonatal withdrawal and, 335, 336–337t
Bariatric surgery, 101, 218–219
Barlow test, 302–303
Barrier contraception methods, 205

Basic care facilities, prenatal, 6, 7t, 10t. See also Level I care facilities
Basic Level Obstetric Privileges, 482
Bassinet cleaning, 458–459
β-blockers, 213
Beard bags, infection control and, 445
Bed need analysis, 43–45
Bed rest
  in multiple gestations, 241
  postpartum, 196–197
  preterm labor and, 258
Bed sharing instructions, 307, 311–312
Bedside reagent test-strip glucose analyzers, 300
Behavioral health risks, 4–5
β-endorphin, 362
Benzodiazepines
  acquired dependency on, 342–343
  neonatal withdrawal and, 335, 336–337t
Benzyl alcohol contraindications, 447
Bereavement counseling, 367–369, 370
Beta-mimetics, preterm labor and, 258
Beta-thalassemia screening for, 121t
Bevacizumab, 356
Bilirubin encephalopathy, 325, 326
Bilirubin toxicity. See Hyperbilirubinemia
Biophysical profile, 145, 146, 149
  intrauterine growth restriction and, 236
  modified, 145, 149–150
  multiple gestations and, 240
Birth defects, teratogens and, 141–143
Birthing centers, 169
Birth plan, 174
Births at threshold of viability, 249–250
Birth weight. See also Low birth weight infants
  definition of, 498
  fetal death reporting and, 497
  live birth statistics and, 502
  measurement of, 280
Bivalent human papillomavirus vaccine, 118
Bladder, postpartum care of, 197, 201
Bloodborne pathogens, transmission of, in health care setting, 442–443. See also Occupational exposure to bloodborne pathogens
Blood clotting, 215–216
Blood loss, acute, and anemia in pregnancy and, 224
Blood pressure. See also Hypertension, in pregnancy
  postpartum monitoring, 195
  preeclampsia and eclampsia and, 232
  in pregnancy, recommended consultation for, 479
Blood products
  for blood transfusion, 174, 254
  obese mother and need for, 217
  Occupational Safety and Health Administration guidelines on, 522
Blood transfusion
  anemia of prematurity and, 321–322
  blood products for, 174, 254
  for postpartum hemorrhage, 255

Blood type. *See also* Rh D blood type
  mother's, medical record of, 279
  of neonate, discharge and, 307
  recommended consultation for, 478, 480
  screening, 113*t*, 174, 237–238
Bloom syndrome screening, 121*t*
Body cooling, total, 324–325
Body length, at birth, 280
Body mass index
  postpartum, 200
  preconception, 102
  underweight prepregnancy, preterm birth and,
    257
  weight gain during pregnancy and, 136–137,
    137*t*
Body temperature. *See also* Core body temperature
  admission policies on, 171
  instability, and late preterm infants and, 280,
    284*b*
  neonatal
    maintenance of, 270
    mother's understanding of, 307
    parent education on, 310
    skin care and, 285
    techniques for, 202
  postpartum monitoring, 195
  during pregnancy, 143
Bottle-feeding, 288, 307, 309
Bouncers, occiput pressure and, 312
BPD. *See* Bronchopulmonary dysplasia
Bradycardia
  apnea of prematurity and, 322
  late preterm infants and, 309, 312
Brain injury, 323–325
Breastfeeding
  advantages of, 287
  antepartum counseling on, 161
  banked donor milk, 293
  contraindications, 290
  cytomegalovirus and, 383
  in delivery room, 265, 276
  discharge readiness and, 307
  formula marketing packages and, 293
  groups supporting, 311
  hepatitis B surface antigen-positive mother and,
    390
  human immunodeficiency virus transmission
    and, 402
  human papillomavirus vaccine and, 404
  hyperbilirubinemia and, 303*b*, 329–330, 331
  by incarcerated women, 152
  initiation of, 287–288
  isoniazid therapy and, 427
  jaundice and, 329–330
  lactational amenorrhea and, 202
  late preterm infants and, 281, 309
  Lyme disease and, 432
  maternal conditions compatible with,
    290–291
  maternal infections and, 450–451
  milk collection and storage, 291–293, 292*t*

Breastfeeding *(continued)*
  monitoring, 288–290
  parent education on, 310
  postpartum follow-up on, 207
  postpartum immunizations and, 198
  pregestational diabetes mellitus and, 221–222
  progestin-only contraceptives and, 205
  situations compromising, 279
  substance abuse and, 337–338
  West Nile virus and, 414
Breast pump, 292
Breasts, postpartum care of, 197, 201
Breathing assessment, neonatal, 268, 269*f*, 270,
    280, 284*b*
Breech presentation at term
  counseling on, 158–159
  developmental dysplasia of the hip and, 303
Britain, recognition of midwifery practice in, 493
Bronchopulmonary dysplasia (BPD)
  apnea and, 322
  characteristics of, 349–350, 351*t*
  infants on extracorporeal membrane oxygen-
    ation and, 349
  surfactant therapy and, 345–346
  therapeutic approaches, 350–353
  treatment, 353
Bronchospasm, asthma medications and, 213
Bruising, significant, hyperbilirubinemia and,
    303*b*, 331
"Bull's-eye" skin lesion, 432

C
Caffeine
  neonatal withdrawal and, 336–337*t*
  supplementation, bronchopulmonary dysplasia
    and, 351
Cajun ethnicity, genetic screening for, 121*t*
Calcium
  antepartum, after bariatric surgery, 218–219
  postpartum, 200
  preconception supplementation, 104*t*, 105
  for pregnant and lactating adolescents and
    women, 135–136*t*
Calcium channel blockers, 234, 258
Caloric intake. *See also* Diet; Weight gain
  follow-up assessment, 378
  hyperbilirubinemia and, 329
  neonatal drug withdrawal and, 342
  postpartum, 200
  pregestational diabetes mellitus and, 221–222
Canavan disease screening, 101, 121*t*
Caps
  infection control and, 445, 446
  as personal protective equipment, 524
Carbon dioxide, exhaled, 273
Cardiac disease. *See* Heart disease
Cardiac lesions, ductal-dependent, 306
Cardiopulmonary resuscitation, 196, 310
Care bundles, 447–448
Carpenter and Coustan, on glucose level, 228,
    228*t*

Car safety seats, 307, 309, 312. *See also* Car-seat
    carriers
Car-seat carriers, 312. *See also* Car safety seats
Category I FHR tracing results, 178, 179*b*
Category II FHR tracing results, 178, 179*b*
Category III FHR tracing results, 178, 180*b*
Catheter-related bloodstream infections, 446–448
Caucasian ethnicity, genetic screening for, 101
CDC. *See* Centers for Disease Control and
    Prevention
CDE blood group. *See* Isoimmunization
Cefazolin, 253, 419
Cefixime, 416
Cefotaxime, 417
Ceftriaxone, 416
Cefuroxime axetil, 432
Centers for Disease Control and Prevention
    (CDC)
    Abortion Surveillance Report, 510
    on anthrax exposure, 414
    on contraceptive use, 203
    on dress codes, 444–445
    on folic acid supplementation, 102–103
    on group B streptococcal disease, 418, 420–421,
        420–421*f*
    of health care-associated pneumonia prevention,
        448–449
    on human immunodeficiency virus treatment,
        400
    on immunizations, 98, 118, 366–367, 406
    on influenza vaccine for pregnant women, 405
    isolation guidelines, 452
    on maternal retroviral therapy, 400
    on medications during pregnancy, 141–142
    National Pregnancy Mortality Surveillance
        System and, 500
    Pregnancy Risk Assessment Monitoring System,
        64–65
    on prenatal lead exposure, 141
    on routine laboratory testing in pregnancy,
        112–117
    on standard precautions, 441
    on Tdap for infant caregivers, 423–424
    on universal precautions, 521
Centers for Medicare and Medicaid Services, 517
Central nervous system dysfunction, fetal alcohol
    syndrome and, 129
Cephalohematoma, 190, 303*b*, 331
Cephalohematomata, 190
Cephalosporins, 253, 416
Cerclage, in multiple gestation, 241. *See also*
    Cervical insufficiency
Cerebral atrophy, diffuse, 323
Cerebral energy deficiency, neonatal hypoglycemia
    and, 300
Cerebral palsy, 326, 343
Cerebrovascular accidents, drug use in pregnancy
    and, 338
Certified midwives, 491, 492
Certified nurse–midwives, 491, 492–493
Certified professional midwives, 491, 492–493

Cervical carcinomas, human papillomavirus and,
    404
Cervical dilation, 172, 257
Cervical insufficiency, exercise during pregnancy
    and, 138. *See also* Cerclage
Cervical ripening, 180–181
Cervicitis, 415
Cervix
    favorable, postterm pregnancy and, 256
    short length, preterm birth and, 257
Cesarean deliveries
    anesthesia choices for, 185
    asthma and need for, 212
    bariatric surgery and, 218
    breech presentation and, 159
    chronic hypertension and, 232
    considerations, 192–194
    convalescence after, 201
    of extremely preterm neonates, 250
    genital human papillomavirus infections and,
        404
    gestational diabetes mellitus and, 227
    group B streptococcal testing, 117
    herpes simplex virus and, 395
    human immunodeficiency virus viral load and,
        401
    infection control and, 445–446
    in intensive care unit, 245
    on maternal request, 160, 193
    of multiple gestations, 194
    nutrition during, 158
    obese mother and, 216
    postanesthesia care and, 196
    postpartum care, 201
    postpartum endometritis and, 253
    postterm pregnancy and, 256
    pregestational diabetes mellitus and, 221
    prior, recommended consultation for, 478
    sickle cell disease and, 215
    vaginal birth after, 159, 188–190, 189*b*, 208,
        511
    venous thromboembolism and, 226–227
Checklists, genetic testing and, 119, 120
Cheeses, unpasteurized soft, listeria infections and,
    140–141
Chemical disinfection, 456
Chemotherapy, breastfeeding and, 290
Chest compressions, neonatal, 268, 269*f*, 273
Chest drain placement and removal, 364
Chest syndrome, sickle cell disease and, 215
Chest X-ray, for tuberculosis, 424, 425, 426
Chickenpox, 305, 412
Child abuse
    factors associated with, 314
    high-risk infants at risk for, 375, 377
    intimate partner violence and, 131, 132
    or neglect
        discharge readiness and, 307
        medical record of, 279
        neonatal withdrawal and, 337
Childbirth Connection, 493

Childbirth education classes, 157
Childhood obesity, gestational diabetes mellitus and, 227
Chlamydia (*Chlamydia trachomatis*)
    early pregnancy screening for, 112, 114*b*, 115
    gonorrhea and, 416–417
    incidence and management, 415–416
    preconception testing for, 99
    premature rupture of membranes and, 176, 260
    topical agents and, 284
Chlordiazepoxide, neonatal withdrawal and, 336–337*t*
Chlorhexidine, 285–286, 446
Chlorine bleach, 460
Chlorine compounds, 456
Chorioamnionitis
    breastfeeding and, 291
    genetic amniocentesis and, 126
    group B streptococci and, 418–419
    neonatal medical record of, 279
    peripartum, 204
    postpartum hemorrhage and, 254
    premature rupture of membranes and, 259–260
    signs, symptoms and treatment, 250–251
Chorionic villus sampling (CVS)
    for aneuploidy, 124, 125
    anti-D immune globulin and, 116
    birth defects caused by teratogens and, 142
    multiple gestations and, 239–240
    prenatal diagnosis of hemoglobinopathies with, 214
Chorioretinitis, toxoplasmosis and, 434
Chromosomal abnormalities, 124
Circumcision, 286–287, 307
Cirrhosis, hepatitis C virus and, 392
Citizens for Midwifery, Inc., 493
Cleaning and disinfecting, 455–458
Clerical areas, 54
Clindamycin, 253–254, 420
Clinical and Laboratory Standards Institute, 297
Clinical nurse specialists, 28
Clinical protocols, quality improvement and, 63–64
Clomipramine, neonatal withdrawal and, 336–337*t*
Clothing, for newborn, 287
Cocaine, 337, 428
Cohort programs during epidemics, 451–452
Coitus
    genital herpes simplex virus infection and, 394
    postpartum, 201
    preterm labor and, 258
Cold sores, 398
Colic, infantile, 128
Collaborative practice, 493
Collagen-vascular disease, 236*b*
Combined units, 39–43
Comfort measures, for stress and pain management, 362–363
Committee on Perinatal Health, 1

Communication
    barriers, adequate follow-up and, 153
    of fetal autopsy results, 261
    informed consent and, 156
    of neonatal information, 278–279
    of occupational exposure hazards, 521, 527–529
    patient safety and, 70
    women with disabilities and, 154
Complete blood count, 113*t*, 214
Complications. *See also* Obstetric and medical complications
    neonatal, instructions to follow for, 307
    postnatal, birth weight correlation to gestational age and, 280
    postpartum, information for mother on, 201, 202
Comprehensive perinatal health care services, 2
Compressed-air outlets, 56–57
Computed tomography, 365–366
    angiography, 225–226
    spiral, 142
Condoms, male and female, 205
Condylomata acuminata, 404, 478, 480
Congenital cretinism, 223
Congenital diaphragmatic hernia, 347
Congenital heart defect screening, 124
Congenital heart disease
    cyanotic, 304
    respiratory syncytial virus and, 408, 409
Congenital malaria, 433
Congenital rubella syndrome, 409, 410, 411, 454
Congenital syphilis, 428–429
Congenital toxoplasmosis, 433–434, 435
Congenital tuberculosis, 426–427
Congenital varicella syndrome, 412
Conjunctival care, for neonate, 284
Conjunctivitis
    chlamydial, 416
    phototherapy and, 333
Connective tissue disease, preeclampsia and eclampsia and, 231
Consent. *See* Informed consent
Continuous positive airway pressure, bronchopulmonary dysplasia and, 352
Contraception
    oral
        after bariatric surgery, 218
        breastfeeding and, 291
    postpartum
        for adolescents, 151
        antepartum counseling on, 161
        barrier methods, 205
        benefits and choices for, 202–203
        hormonal, 205
        for incarcerated women, 152
        long-acting reversible, 203–204
        parent education on, 310
        sterilization, 203–204
Contraceptive implants, 204
Contractions. *See* Uterine contractions
Contraction stress test, 146, 148–149, 236

Contrast agents, iodinated, 142
Convalescence length, 201
Coombs test result, 307
Copper intrauterine device, 204
Cord blood. *See also* Umbilical cord
  banking, 160–161, 174
  human immunodeficiency virus testing, 402
  newborn blood spot screening and, 297
  specimens, identification of, 278
  type, 307
Core body temperature. *See also* Body temperature
  hypoxic–ischemic encephalopathy care at,
    324–325
  during pregnancy, 143
Cor pulmonale, bronchopulmonary dysplasia
    and, 350
Corticosteroids
  antenatal therapy with
    bronchopulmonary dysplasia risk and, 350
    preterm labor and, 258
    respiratory distress syndrome and, 248–249,
      346
  delivery of extremely preterm neonates and,
    250
  inhaled, bronchopulmonary dysplasia and, 352
  postnatal, bronchopulmonary dysplasia and,
    351–352
  pregestational diabetes mellitus and, 221
  prenatal, for brain injury prevention, 324
Cortisol, pain response and, 362
Co-sleeping, 311–312
Counseling, bereavement, 367–369, 370. *See also*
    Education; Preconception care, coun-
    seling and interventions; Psychosocial
    risk screening and counseling
Cow's milk, 293
Coxsackie viruses, 385–386, 454
Cranial asymmetry, 312
Cranial ultrasonography, portable bedside,
    323
Credentialing. *See also* Privileges
  family physicians, 484–485
  of medical providers, 21–22
  obstetricians, 482–483
  physician assistants, 33
Critical care. *See also* Intensive care unit
  interhospital transfer for, 89
  in pregnancy, 244–245
Crude birth rate, 501–502
Cuddle time, upright, 312
Culturally appropriate care, 3–4
Culture of safety, 67–68, 73
Cutaneous infections, precautions for, 453
CVS. *See* Chorionic villus sampling
Cyanosis, 276, 345
Cyanotic congenital heart disease, 304
Cystic fibrosis carrier testing, 101, 120,
    121*t*
Cytomegalovirus, 383–385
  breastfeeding and, 291
  health care-associated, 444

D
D (Rh) type. *See* Rh D blood type
Death
  fetal. *See* Fetal death
  maternal. *See* Maternal death
  neonatal. *See* Neonatal death
Deep vein thrombosis
  antepartum management, 226
  evaluation and diagnosis, 225–226
  intrapartum management, 226–227
  postpartum management, 227
  pulmonary embolism and, 225
  recommended consultation for, 477
Deferoxamine, 215
Dehydration, 281, 307, 330. *See also* Hydration
Dehydrogenase, 300
Delivery
  before 39 weeks, fetal pulmonary maturation
    and, 248
  after fetal death, 261
  cesarean
    anesthesia choices for, 185
    asthma and need for, 212
    bariatric surgery and, 218
    breech presentation and, 159
    breech presentation at term and, 159
    chronic hypertension and, 232
    considerations, 192–194
    convalescence after, 201
    of extremely preterm neonates, 250
    genital human papillomavirus infections
      and, 404
    gestational diabetes mellitus and, 227
    group B streptococcal testing, 117
    herpes simplex virus and, 395
    human immunodeficiency virus viral load
      and, 401
    infection control and, 445–446
    in intensive care unit, 245
    on maternal request, 160, 193–194
    multiple gestations, 194
    nutrition during, 158
    obese mother and, 216
    postanesthesia care and, 196
    postpartum care, 201
    postpartum endometritis and, 253
    postterm pregnancy and, 256
    pregestational diabetes mellitus and, 221
    prior, recommended consultation for,
      478
    sickle cell disease and, 215
    vaginal birth after, 159, 188–190, 189*b*,
      208, 511
    venous thromboembolism and, 226–227
  cytomegalovirus and, 383–384
  elective, 160
  facilities for, 41–43
  gestational diabetes mellitus and, 229–230
  human immunodeficiency virus and route of,
    401
  intrauterine growth restriction and, 236–237

Delivery *(continued)*
    medical record of, 279
    preregistration for, 173
    public insurance at, late preterm infants and, 281
    safety considerations, 169
    support persons, 195
    at threshold of viability, 249–250
    transfer of responsibility for neonatal care after, 268
    vaginal
        after cesarean delivery, 159, 188–190, 189*b*, 208, 511
        chronic hypertension and, 234
        of extremely preterm neonates, 250
        herpes simplex virus and, 396
        human immunodeficiency virus and, 401
        multiple gestations, 194
        obese mother and, 217
        operative, 190–192
        risk assessment, 187–188
Dental care
    endocarditis prophylaxis and, 251, 252*b*
    during pregnancy, 138–139
Dentoalveolar dysplasia, hyperbilirubinemia and, 326
Depression
    follow-up on, 207–208
    postpartum, 130–131, 201, 206
Dermopathy, 223
Developmental delay
    cytomegalovirus and, 383
    early intervention programs and, 378–379
    infants on extracorporeal membrane oxygenation and, 349
Developmental disabilities, pregnant women with, 155
Developmental dysplasia of the hip, 302–303
Dexamethasone, postnatal, bronchopulmonary dysplasia and, 351–352
Diabetes mellitus. *See also* Gestational diabetes mellitus
    insulin-treated, fetal well-being tests and, 144
    intrauterine growth restriction and, 236*b*
    neonatal hypoglycemia and, 299–300, 333, 334*f*
    neonatal respiratory distress syndrome and, 345
    postpartum follow-up on, 208
    preconception control of, 100–101
    pregestational
        antepartum assessment, 220–221
        fetal and neonatal complications, 220
        intrapartum management, 221–222
        maternal complications, 219–220
        preeclampsia and eclampsia and, 231
        recommended consultation for, 477
    screening during pregnancy, 116–117
    stillbirth and, 261
Diaphragm, for contraception, 205
Diazepam, neonatal withdrawal and, 336–337*t*

Diet. *See also* Caloric intake; Nutrition
    gestational diabetes mellitus and, 229
    postpartum, 196–197
Dietary Folate Equivalents, 133
Dietary supplements, preconception, 102–103, 103–104*t*, 105
Digital photographic retinal image capture, 355
Dilation and evacuation, of stillbirth, 261
D immune globulin, 248. *See also* Anti-D immune globulin
Diphtheria, 442
Direct-entry midwives, 491, 494
Director of interhospital transfer program, 81–82
Disabilities, pregnant women with, 154–155
Disaster preparedness plan, 54
Discharge
    adolescent mothers and, 153
    antepartum counseling on, 161
    of healthy newborns, 306–308
    of high-risk infants, 370–376
    of late preterm infants, 309
    maternal illicit drug or alcohol use and, 173
    neonatal drug withdrawal and, 342
Disclosure of medical errors, 70
Discordant growth, multiple gestations and, 241
Disinfection
    disinfectant selection, 456–457
    general housekeeping, 457–458
    high-level, 455, 456, 459
    noncritical surfaces, 456–458
Dispatching units, interhospital transfer responsibilities of, 84
Disposable equipment, 459
Diuretics, bronchopulmonary dysplasia and, 353
Documentation, neonatal resuscitation, 267
Domestic violence, 131–132, 247, 279, 307
Donor milk, banked, 293
Doppler ultrasonography
    of intrauterine growth restriction, 236
    severe fetal anemia predictions using, 238
    of umbilical artery blood flow velocity, 146, 150
Down syndrome, 120–121, 122*t*, 123–124
Doxycycline, 415, 428
Dress codes, infection control and, 444–445
Drugs. *See also* Illicit drugs; Medications; Neonatal drug withdrawal
    misuse and abuse during pregnancy, 100
    mood-altering, 129–130
Dry heat, for sterilization, 455
Durable power of attorney for health care, 156
Dust removal methods, 457
Dysautonomia, familial, 101, 121*t*

E
Early Hearing Detection and Intervention programs, 299
Early-onset group B streptococcal disease in newborns, 418, 420–421*f*
East Asian ethnicity, hyperbilirubinemia and, 303*b*, 331. *See also* Asian ethnicity
Echoviruses, 385–386, 454

Eclampsia. *See also* Preeclampsia
  antepartum management, 231–232
  cesarean delivery and, 192
  definition of, 230
  diagnosis, 231
  intrapartum care, 232
  risk factors for, 231
ECMO. *See* Extracorporeal membrane oxygenation
Ectopic pregnancy risks, 128, 416
EDD. *See* Estimated date of delivery
Education
  on antepartum issues, 108
  on family assistance, 310–311
  first-trimester patient
    air travel, 143–144
    dental care, 138–139
    exercise, 137–138
    nausea and vomiting, 139
    nutrition, 132–133, 134–136t, 136
    teratogens, 141–143
    vitamin and mineral toxicity, 139–141
    weight gain, 136–137, 137t
  for inpatient perinatal care providers, 35–36
  on interhospital transfer program, 91
  for new parents, 309–310, 313
  perinatal outreach, 36–37
  quality improvement and, 62
  on reproductive health, 4–5
  on safe sleep position and sudden infant death syndrome, 311–312
  on safe transportation of preterm and low birthweight infants, 312
  second-trimester and third-trimester patient
    anticipating labor, 157–158
    breastfeeding, 161
    breech presentation at term, 158–159
    cesarean delivery on maternal request, 160
    childbirth education classes, 157
    choosing newborn care providers, 157
    discharge preparation, 161
    elective delivery, 160
    neonatal interventions, 161
    preterm labor, 158
    trial of labor after cesarean delivery, 159–160
    umbilical cord blood banking, 160–161
    working, 156–157
  on standard precautions, 444
Education areas, 54
Elective delivery, 160, 193
Electrical equipment
  electrical outlets and, 57
  interhospital transfer, 86
Electrolyte disturbances, uncontrolled pregestational diabetes mellitus and, 220
Electronic fetal heart rate monitoring. *See* Fetal heart rate, monitoring
Electronic medical records, 38, 173
Emergency department
  log of patients seeking assistance at, 517
  management of pregnant patients in, 244

Emergency drills, patient safety and, 71–72
Emergency medical conditions, 307, 313, 514–515
Emergency Medical Treatment and Labor Act, 77, 87, 89, 513–518
Emotional responses, postpartum, 201
Encephalitis, 412
Encephalopathy
  bilirubin, 325, 326
  hypoxic–ischemic, 324–325
  pertussis and, 422
Endocarditis, 251, 252b
Endocervicitis, 416
Endometritis
  breastfeeding and, 290
  discharge of healthy newborns and, 306
  group B streptococci and, 417
  peripartum, 204
  postpartum, 252–254, 415
  tuberculosis, 426
Endotracheal intubation, 272–273, 364
Enteral nutrition, 359, 360–361t, 361
Enteroviruses, 385–386
Environmental control and monitoring, 54–55, 454–460
Environmental exposures, 141–143
Epidemics, cohort programs during, 451–452
Epidural anesthesia, 173, 184
Epilepsy, 477
Epinephrine, 268, 269f, 273, 362
Episiotomy, 188, 197, 198, 201, 254
Equipment
  cleaning and disinfecting, 455–456, 458–459
  decontamination, Occupational Safety and Health Administration guidelines on, 522–523
  electrical, electrical outlets and, 57
  interhospital transfer, 84–86
  new, obstetric privileges and, 485–486
Equivocal contraction stress test, 148
Erythema migrans, 432
Erythroblastosis fetalis, 238, 326
Erythrocyte antibodies, 237
Erythromycin
  for bronchopulmonary dysplasia, 352
  for chlamydia, 415
  for group B streptococci, 419, 420
  for Lyme disease, 432
  as ophthalmic prophylaxis, 284
  for syphilis, 428, 429
Erythropoietin, recombinant human, 322
Escherichia coli, 251, 252
Estimated date of delivery (EDD), evaluation of, 109–110
Estriol, aneuploidy and, 123
Estrogen–progestin combination contraceptives, 205, 212
Ethambutol, 425
Ethchlorvynol, neonatal withdrawal and, 336–337t

Ethnic groups
  genetic screening and, 101, 121*t*
  nonwhite, trial of labor after cesarean delivery
    and, 189*b*
  single-gene disorders and, 120
Ethylene oxide sterilization, 455–456
Etonogestrel single-rod contraceptive implant, 204
Eunice Kennedy Shriver National Institute
  of Child Health and Human
  Development, 178, 249, 325
Evacuation plan, 54
Exanthem erythema infectiosum, 406, 407
Exchange transfusion guidelines, 327–328, 328*f*,
  333
Exercise
  postpartum, 200, 201
  preconception, 102
  during pregnancy, 137–138, 229
External cephalic version
  breech presentation at term and, 159
Extracorporeal membrane oxygenation (ECMO)
  infants and health risks, 349
  therapy, 343, 348–349
Eyes. *See also* Retinopathy of prematurity
  chlamydial infection in newborns and, 416
  congenital rubella syndrome and, 410
  covered, phototherapy and, 332–333
  gonococcal infection in newborns and, 417
  initial examination of, 354, 355*t*
  neonatal care for, 284
  protection for, infection control and, 445

F

Facial abnormalities, anesthesia risks and, 186–187
Facial clefting, obese mother and, 217
Falls, trauma during pregnancy and, 246
False labor, 175, 515
Family. *See also* Family-centered health care;
    Father; Partner; Support persons
  conflict, admission evaluation of, 173
  definition of, 95
  in delivery room, 174, 195
  history
    developmental dysplasia of the hip and,
      303
    genetic screening and, 101, 119, 120
  and infant death, 367–370
  newborn care and, 307, 310, 313–314
  plans for newborn and, 276
  postpartum adjustments for, 206–207
Family and Medical Leave Act, 157
Family-centered health care, 2–3, 95
Family physician credentialing, 484–485
Family physicians. *See* Physicians, family
Family planning. *See* Contraception
Fanconi anemia group C screening, 121*t*
Fasting plasma glucose test, 230
Father. *See also* Family; Parents; Partner; Support
    persons
  labor and delivery and, 169, 195
  postpartum period and, 304

Faucet aerators, cleaning, 457–458
FDA. *See* U.S. Food and Drug Administration
Feeding. *See also* Bottle-feeding; Breastfeeding
  difficulties
    infants on extracorporeal membrane oxygen-
      ation and, 349
    late preterm infants and, 280–281
  follow-up review on, 313
  gavage, 334, 374–375
  neonatal, discharge and, 307
  neonatal refusal of, 284*b*
  supplemental, breastfeeding and, 288
Female condoms, 205
Female gender, developmental dysplasia of the hip
  and, 303
Fern testing, premature rupture of membranes
  diagnosis and, 176
Ferritin, iron-deficient anemia and, 224
Fetal alcohol syndrome, 129
Fetal anemia
  non–Rh-D alloimmunization and, 237
  screening for, 238
Fetal anomalies
  medical record of, 279
  postpartum follow-up on, 208
  recommended consultation for, 479
Fetal breathing movements
  biophysical profile and, 149
Fetal compromise
  postterm pregnancy and, 256
  premature rupture of membranes and, 260
Fetal death (demise, loss)
  antiphospholipid syndrome and, 211
  chronic hypertension and, 232
  current reporting requirements, 511–512
  definition, 498
  delivery methods, 261
  evaluation of, 261
  fetal–maternal hemorrhage and, 248
  incidence of, 260–261
  inherited thrombophilias and, 215–216
  intrauterine drug exposure and, 338
  intrauterine growth restriction and, 236
  malaria and, 433
  maternal rubella during pregnancy and, 410
  measures of, 503
  multiple gestations and risk of, 240
  obese mother and, 217
  of one fetus in multiple gestations, 241–242
  parvovirus B19 and, 406–407
  preeclampsia and HELLP syndrome and,
    231
  prior
    fetal well-being tests and, 145
    recommended consultation for, 478
  recommended consultation for, 479
  recurrence counseling, 262
  reporting requirements and recommendations,
    508
  risk factors and comorbidities, 261
  sickle cell disease and, 215

Fetal death (demise, loss) *(continued)*
spontaneous, increased nuchal transparency
measurement and, 124
state differences in definition of, 497
twin–twin transfusion syndrome and, 242
uncontrolled pregestational diabetes mellitus
and, 220
Fetal growth restriction. *See also* Growth restriction; Intrauterine growth restriction
chronic hypertension and, 232, 233
inherited thrombophilias and, 215
medical record of, 279
recommended consultation for, 479
Fetal heart rate. *See* Heart rate, fetal
Fetal heart tones
elective cesarean delivery and, 193–194
elective delivery and, 160
Fetal hemolysis, isoimmunization and, 238
Fetal imaging. *See also* Ultrasonography
magnetic resonance, 111–112
ultrasonography, 110–111, 111*b*
Fetal loss. *See* Fetal death
Fetal movement
admission evaluation of, 172
assessment of, 144, 145, 146–147
biophysical profile and, 149
Fetal nonstress test. *See* Nonstress test
Fetal presentation and station, labor and, 172
Fetal pulmonary maturation, assessment and management of, 248
Fetal scalp monitoring, 179, 180, 395
Fetal surveillance
antepartum management in multiple gestations
and, 240
critical care in pregnancy and, 245
trauma during pregnancy and, 247–248
Fetal-to-maternal bleeding, amniocentesis or chorionic villus sampling and, 116, 126
Fetal tone, biophysical profile and, 149
Fetal well-being
discordant growth in multiple gestations and,
241
postterm pregnancy and, 255–256
premature rupture of membranes and, 175–176
tests, 144–150
abnormal results, 279
biophysical profile, 149
fetal movement assessment, 146–147
gestational diabetes mellitus and,
228–229
labor and, 172
modified biophysical profile, 149–150
nonstress test, 147–148
Fibronectin, fetal, preterm birth and, 257
Fifth disease, 406–407
Fingerprints, patient identification and, 278
Finnegan's Neonatal Abstinence Scoring Tool,
340–341*f*
Fish, mercury levels in, 140
Fluoride supplementation, 294
Flush solutions, 447

Flu vaccine, 98, 118, 198, 295, 442. *See also*
Influenza viruses
Folic acid (folate), 102–103
antepartum, after bariatric surgery, 218–219
Dietary Folate Equivalents, 133
preconception supplementation, 103*t*
during pregnancy, 133
for pregnant and lactating adolescents and
women, 134*t*
sickle cell disease and, 215
Folinic acid, for toxoplasmosis, 434, 435
Follow-up care
appointment for healthy newborns, 308
appointment for late preterm infants, 309
functions of, 313–314
for high-risk infants
components, 376–377
early intervention programs, 378–379
surveillance and assessment, 377–378
Food and drink safety, Occupational Safety and
Health Administration guidelines on,
522
Food-borne infections, 421–422, 433–435
Footprints, patient identification and, 278
Forceps extraction, 190–192
Formula milk preparations, 293–294
area for, 51
preterm, 359, 361–362
Fraction of inspired oxygen, 343
French Canadian ethnicity, genetic screening for,
121*t*
Frenotomy, 290
Frozen milk, thawing, 292–293, 292t
Fulminant hepatitis, 387
Fundal height, intrauterine growth restriction
and, 235

G
G6PD. *See* Glucose-6-phosphate dehydrogenase
Galactosemia, 290
Ganciclovir, 385
Gastroenteritis, precautions for, 453
Gastroesophageal reflux, infants on extracorporeal
membrane oxygenation and, 349
Gastroesophageal reflux disease, 312
Gastrointestinal obstruction, 306
Gastrostomy feedings, 374–375
Gaucher disease screening, 121*t*
Gavage feeding, 334, 374–375
General anesthesia. *See also* Analgesia and anesthesia
labor and delivery and, 173, 184–185
postpartum monitoring of, 196
General fertility rate, 501–502
Genetic screening
antepartum, 119–125
Down syndrome, 122*t*
ethnic groups and, 121*t*
multiple gestations and, 239
for hemoglobinopathies, 213–214
preconception, 101
Genital warts, 404

Gentamicin, 251, 253–254, 422
Gestational age
    advanced, 256
    antenatal corticosteroid therapy and, 249
    body weight at birth and, 280
    definition, 499
    determination of, discharge and, 309
    elective cesarean delivery and, 193
    elective delivery and, 160
    fetal death reporting and, 497
    of 41 weeks, recommended consultation for, 479
    group B streptococci and, 418
    hyperbilirubinemia and, 303b, 325, 331
    initial eye examination based on, 354, 355t
    intrauterine growth restriction and, 237
    labor induction and, 181
    low, resuscitation and, 277–278
    multiple gestation testing and, 240
    optimal neonatal intensive care unit care and,
        11–12t, 78
    pharmacokinetics and, 363
    premature rupture of membranes and, 175–176
    trial of labor after cesarean delivery and, 189b
Gestational diabetes mellitus
    antepartum management, 228–229
    bariatric surgery and, 218
    definition of, 227
    diagnosis, 228
    exercise during pregnancy, 229
    intrapartum management, 229–230
    malabsorption-type bariatric surgery and, 219
    obese mother and, 216
    postpartum follow-up on, 202, 207
    postpartum screening and, 230
    recommended consultation for, 479
    screening during pregnancy, 116–117
Gestational hypertension, 230
Gloves
    infection control and, 445, 453t
    as personal protective equipment, 523–524
Glucose
    control of, pregestational diabetes mellitus and,
        219–221
    pain response and, 362
    screening
        for gestational diabetes mellitus, 116–117,
            229
        in newborns, 299–300, 333, 334f
Glucose-6-phosphate dehydrogenase (G6PD)
    deficiency, 303b, 331
Glucose tolerance test, 228, 228t, 230
Glutaraldehyde, 455–456, 456
Glutethimide, neonatal withdrawal and, 336–337t
Glycoprotein G, herpes simplex virus-specific, 394
Goiter, anesthesia risks and, 186–187
Golden minute, 268, 269f
Gonorrhea
    antepartum management, 416–417
    antibiotics for, 284
    early pregnancy screening for, 112, 114b, 115
    incidence and characteristics, 416

Gonorrhea (continued)
    neonatal management, 417
    preconception testing for, 99
    premature rupture of membranes and, 176, 260
Gowns
    infection control and, 445, 453t
    as personal protective equipment, 524
Gram-negative bacteria
    chorioamnionitis and, 251
    endometritis, 252
Graves disease, 100–101, 143, 222–223
Group A streptococci, 440
Group B β-hemolytic streptococci, 252
Group B streptococci (GBS)
    cesarean deliveries and, 117
    chorioamnionitis and, 251
    incidence and characteristics, 417–418
    intrapartum care, 418–420, 419t
    mothers admitted with, 440
    neonatal management, 420, 420–421f
    premature rupture of membranes and, 176,
        260
Group prenatal care visits, 108–109
Growth abnormalities, obese mother and, 217
Growth assessment, in high-risk infants, 378
Growth restriction. See also Fetal growth restric-
        tion; Intrauterine growth restriction
    asthma and, 212
    fetal alcohol syndrome and, 129
    multiple gestations and, 241

H
Hand hygiene
    gloves and, 445
    herpes simplex virus and, 395, 398
    human immunodeficiency virus transmission
        and, 402
    maternal, 307
    Occupational Safety and Health Administration
        guidelines on, 521–522
    postpartum visits and, 304, 305
    respiratory syncytial virus and, 409
    World Health Organization guidelines on,
        444
HBsAg. See Hepatitis B surface antigen
Head circumference, neonatal, 280
Head cooling, hypoxic–ischemic encephalopathy
        and, 324
Health care-associated infection
    catheter-related bloodstream, 446–448
    definition of, 439
    labor and delivery admissions policy on, 440
    pneumonia, 448–450
    transmission of, 443–444
Health care delivery system, 1–5
Health care workers. See Personnel
Health literacy, 69–70
Health Professional Shortage Areas, 17
Hearing loss
    cytomegalovirus and, 383
    hyperbilirubinemia and, 326

Hearing loss *(continued)*
  infants on extracorporeal membrane oxygen-
    ation and, 349
Hearing screening, 298–299, 307
Heart disease
  cyanotic
    congenital, screening for, 304
    fetal conditions and, 144
    intrauterine growth restriction and, 236*b*
  exercise during pregnancy and, 138
  maternal, anesthesia risks and, 186–187
  recommended consultation for, 477
  respiratory syncytial virus and, 408
Heart rate
  fetal
    admission policies on, 171
    intrapartum monitoring, 177–180, 179–180*b*
    nonstress test of, 147–148
    parenteral pain medications and, 183
    trauma during pregnancy and, 247–248
  neonatal
    abnormal, 284*b*
    in resuscitation assessment, 269*f*, 270
Heel pricks or sticks, 297, 365
HELLP. *See* Hemolysis, elevated liver enzymes,
    low platelets
Hematocrit, 197. *See also* Complete blood count
  anemia screening and, 224
  third trimester measurement of, 116
Hemodynamic status, postpartum, 196–197
Hemoglobin. *See also* Complete blood count
  anemia screening and, 224
  third trimester measurement of, 116
Hemoglobin electrophoresis, 214
Hemoglobin H disease, 215
Hemoglobinopathies, 213–215. *See also* Sickle
    cell disease
  intrauterine growth restriction and, 236*b*
  parvovirus B19 and, 407
  preconception control of, 101
  recommended consultation for, 477
  venous thromboembolism in pregnancy and,
    225
Hemolysis, elevated liver enzymes, low platelets
    (HELLP) syndrome, 231, 232
Hemolytic disease in the newborn, 237
Hemorrhage
  fetal–maternal, trauma and, 248
  intensive care admission and, 244–245
  intrapartum, sickle cell disease and, 215
  intraventricular, surfactant therapy and, 346
  maternal, 254–255
Hemorrhagic and periventricular white matter
    brain injury, 323–324
Hemorrhagic disease of the newborn, 285
Hemorrhagic infarction, 323
Heparin, 212, 217–218, 226, 448
Hepatitis, illicit drug use and risk of, 337
Hepatitis A virus, 99, 118, 386
Hepatitis B core antigen, 386
Hepatitis B e antigen, 386

Hepatitis B immune globulin, 290, 295, 387,
    390
Hepatitis B surface antigen (HBsAg)
  breastfeeding and, 290
  in early pregnancy, 113*t*
  hepatitis B virus and, 386
  milk collection and storage and, 292
  milk donor testing for, 293
  neonatal immunizations for, 295
  testing for, 172–173, 174, 307, 387
Hepatitis B virus
  early pregnancy screening for, 112, 113*b*, 114,
    387
  health care worker vaccination, 442–443, 521,
    525–526
  internal fetal monitoring and, 179
  maternal immunization, 99, 113*t*, 118, 387
  mother's test result, 279
  newborn immunization, 202, 290, 295, 307
    by birth weight, 388, 388–389*t*
    HBsAg-negative mother, 388–390
    HBsAg-positive mother, 390
    HBsAg-status unknown mother, 390, 392
    recommended dosages, 391*t*
  Occupational Safety and Health Administration
    guidelines on, 441–442, 519
  perinatal transmission of, 386–387
  postexposure evaluation and follow-up,
    526–527
  screening, intrauterine drug exposure and, 338
Hepatitis C virus, 392–393
  breastfeeding and, 290–291
  health care worker vaccination, 442–443
  internal fetal monitoring and, 179
  milk donor testing for, 293
  screening, intrauterine drug exposure and, 338
Hepatosplenomegaly, 383, 434
Hernia, congenital diaphragmatic, 347
Heroin, nursing infants and, 337
Herpes, illicit drug use and risk of, 337
Herpes labialis, 398
Herpes simplex virus
  active at 36 weeks, recommended consultation
    for, 479
  antepartum management, 393–394
  breastfeeding and, 290
  circumcision and, 286
  congenital, precautions for, 454
  health care worker with, 443
  infant contact with infected mother, 397–398
  internal fetal monitoring and, 179
  intrapartum management, 395
  neonatal diagnosis, 395–397
  neonatal treatment, 397
  types and characteristics, 393
Hexokinase, 300
High-level disinfection, 455, 456, 459
High-risk infants
  compassionate and comfort care for, 277
  death of, 367–370
  follow-up care for, 376–379

High-risk infants *(continued)*
  hospital discharge
    anticipated early death, 375–376
    community and health care system readiness, 373
    family and home readiness, 372–373
    infant readiness, 371–372
    planning, 370–371
    preterm infants, 374
    risks due to family issues for, 375
    technology-dependent or special care needs, 374–375
  immunization of, 366–367
  pain prevention and management, 362–365
  parent counseling on resuscitation of, 277–278
  parents and decision-making for, 276–277
  preterm, nutritional needs of, 356–362
  radiation exposure, 365–366
  surgical procedures in neonatal intensive care unit, 366
Hip, developmental dysplasia of, 302–303
Hispanic ethnicity, postpartum hemorrhage and, 254
HIV. *See* human immunodeficiency virus
Home births, planned, 170
Home care services, 310–311
Homeless women
  antepartum care for, 153
  discharge readiness and, 307
Home oxygen therapy (ventilation), 375
Home phototherapy, 333
Home uterine monitoring, 241
Hormonal contraceptives, 205
Hospice care, 376
Hospital discharge. *See* Discharge
Hospitalists, 22
Hospitalization. *See also* Intensive care unit; Neonatal functional units; Obstetric functional units
  antepartum, 243–244
  intrapartum, 170–175
  postpartum, 198–200
  preterm labor and delivery with multiple gestations and, 241
Hot dogs, listeria infections and, 140–141
Hot tubs, during pregnancy, 143
Hot-water disinfection, 456
Housekeeping
  general, 457–458
  Occupational Safety and Health Administration guidelines on, 524–525
HPV. *See* Human papillomavirus
Human chorionic gonadotropin, 123, 160, 193
Human diploid vaccine RA 27/3, 411
Human immunodeficiency virus (HIV)
  antepartum management, 398–400
  breastfeeding and, 290
  circumcision and, 286
  gonorrhea and, 417
  health care worker vaccination, 442–443
  hepatitis C virus transmission and, 392

Human immunodeficiency virus (HIV) *(continued)*
  illicit drug use and risk of, 337
  incarcerated women and, 152
  internal fetal monitoring and, 179
  labor and delivery and, 400–401
  maternal retroviral therapy, 399–400
  mother's test result, 279
  Occupational Safety and Health Administration guidelines on, 441–442, 519
  postexposure evaluation and follow-up, 526–527
  postpartum management, 402
  recommended consultation for, 478, 480
  screening
    discharge readiness and, 307
    early pregnancy, 112, 113*t*, 114
    intrapartum, 174
    intrauterine drug exposure and, 338
    milk donor, 293
    neonatal, 402–403
    prenatal, 399
    rapid, 400–401
  syphilis and, 427
  toxoplasmosis and, 434
  transmission, 398
  tuberculosis treatment and, 425
Human papillomavirus (HPV), 99, 404
Human parvovirus B19, 406–407
Human T-cell lymphotrophic virus type I or II, 290
Hydramnios, 254, 479
Hydration. *See also* Dehydration
  preterm labor and, 258
Hydrocephalus (hydrocephaly)
  posthemorrhagic, 323
  toxoplasmosis and, 434
Hydrocortisone, postnatal, bronchopulmonary dysplasia and, 351–352
Hydrops, 238, 406
Hydroxyzine, neonatal withdrawal and, 336–337*t*
Hyperbilirubinemia. *See also* Jaundice
  assessment of, 330
  breastfeeding and jaundice, 329–330
  characteristics of, 325
  dehydration and, 330
  follow-up assessment, 331–332
  gestational diabetes mellitus and, 227
  hemolytic disease and, 326, 331
  laboratory evaluation, 330–331
  late preterm infants and, 280, 281
  newborn screening, 301, 302*f*, 303*b*
  phenolic compounds and, 456
  preterm infants and, 326–329
  risk assessment, 331
  treatment
    exchange transfusion, 333
    phototherapy, 332–333
  uncontrolled pregestational diabetes mellitus and, 220
Hypercapnia, permissive, bronchopulmonary dysplasia and, 352

Hypercarbia, as reversible, 347–348
Hyperemesis, recommended consultation for, 479
Hyperglycemia. *See* Diabetes mellitus
Hypertension
    admission policies on, 171
    adult-onset, small for gestational age infants and, 235
    bariatric surgery and, 218
    chronic, 230, 232
        antepartum management, 233–234
        diagnosis, 233
        intrapartum management, 234
    fetal well-being tests and, 144
    gestational, 230
    intensive care admission of obstetric patients and, 244–245
    intrauterine drug exposure and, 338
    postpartum follow-up on, 208
    preconception care for, 101
    preeclampsia and eclampsia and, 231
    in pregnancy
        chronic hypertension, 232–234
        exercise and, 138
        fetal well-being tests and, 144
        incidence and definitions, 230
        preeclampsia and eclampsia, 231–232
        routine testing and, 146
    recommended consultation for, 477
    stillbirth and, 261
    venous thromboembolism in pregnancy and, 225
Hyperthyroidism
    preconception control of, 100–101
    pregnancy and, 222–223
Hypervolemia, 269*f*
Hypocapnia, 324
Hypoglycemia
    gestational diabetes mellitus and, 227
    late preterm infants and, 280
    in newborns, 299–300, 333–335, 334*f*
    uncontrolled pregestational diabetes mellitus and, 220
Hypotension, multifetal pregnancy reduction and, 242
Hypothermia, 270
    mild, hypoxic–ischemic encephalopathy and, 324–325
Hypothyroidism
    neonatal, 142
    preconception control of, 100–101
    pregnancy and, 222, 223
Hypotonicity, neonatal, 284*b*
Hypoxemia, as reversible, 347–348
Hypoxic cardiorespiratory failure, 347–349
Hypoxic–ischemic encephalopathy, 324–325
Hysterectomy
    gravid, cesarean delivery on maternal request and, 193
    postpartum hemorrhage and, 254, 255
Hysteroscopic sterilization devices, 203–204

I
Identification of newborn, 265, 278
Illicit drugs. *See also* Neonatal drug withdrawal
    breastfeeding and, 290
    discharge readiness and, 153
    infants exposed to, 342
    medical risks with, 337
    milk donor testing for, 293
    recommended consultation for, 477, 479
    women with syphilis and, 428
Illumination, 55–56
Imiquimod, 404
Immunizations. *See also* Vaccines, live
    antepartum, 117–119, 413–414
    Bacille Calmette–Guérin, 427
    for health care workers, 442
    hepatitis A virus, 99, 118, 386
    human papillomavirus, 99, 404
    influenza viruses, 98, 118, 198, 295, 442
    measles, 99
    measles–mumps–rubella, 99, 118–119, 413–414
    meningococcus, 99, 118
    of neonate
        after discharge, 313
        counseling on, 202
        for hepatitis B. *See* Hepatitis B virus, newborn immunization
        for human immunodeficiency virus coinfections, 402–403
        hospitalized, 366–367
    pneumococcus, 99, 118
    postpartum maternal, 198
    postpartum monitoring, 208
    preconception, 98–99
    rotavirus, 366
    tetanus–diphtheria acellular pertussis, 98–99, 198, 422–423
    varicella zoster virus, 99, 413–414
    web sites on, 406
Immunoglobulin A, 435
Immunoglobulin G, 393, 434
Immunoglobulin M, 434, 435
Inactivity period, obstetric privileges after, 486–488
Incarcerated women, antepartum care for, 151–153
Incontinence, pertussis and, 422
Incubator cleaning, 458–459
Indomethacin, 324
Induced termination of pregnancy
    definition, 500–501
    measures of, 507
    reporting requirements and recommendations, 509–510
Induction of labor
    abnormal fetal well-being tests and, 146
    cervical ripening and, 180–181
    isoimmunization and, 238
    pregestational diabetes mellitus and, 221
    for premature rupture of membranes, 179, 260
    stillbirth and, 261

Infant abduction prevention, 305
Infant death. *See also* Neonatal death
    definition, 499
    reporting requirements and recommendations,
        509
Infection control. *See also* Occupational exposure
        to bloodborne pathogens
    antibiotics, 450
    cohort programs, 451–452
    dress codes, 444–445
    environmental, 454–460
        noncritical surfaces, 456–458
        nursery linen, 460
        patient care equipment, 458–459
        sterilization and disinfection, 455–456
    hand hygiene, 444
    health care-associated infections and, 439
    labor and delivery admissions policy, 440
    neonatal considerations, 446–454
    nursery admission policy, 440–441
    obstetric considerations, 445–446
    personnel health standards, 442–444
    postpartum infections and, 450–451
    prevention and, 440–454
    standard precautions, 441–442
    transmission-based precautions, 453*t*
Infections. *See also* Occupational exposure to
        bloodborne pathogens; *specific infections*
    admission policies and, 170–171
    anthrax, 414
    bacterial, 414–427
    catheter-related bloodstream, 446–448
    chlamydia, 415–416
    chorioamnionitis, 250–251
    cytomegalovirus, 383–385
    enteroviruses, 385–386
    gonorrhea, 416–417
    group B streptococci, 417–421
    health care-associated, 443–444, 448–450
    hepatitis A virus, 386
    hepatitis B virus, 386–392
    hepatitis C virus, 392–393
    herpes simplex virus, 393–398
    human immunodeficiency virus, 398–403
    human papillomavirus, 404
    human parvovirus B19, 406–407
    influenza A and B viruses, 404–406
    intrauterine, postterm pregnancy and, 255
    intrauterine, premature rupture of membranes
        and, 175–176
    intrauterine growth restriction and, 236*b*
    listeria, 140–141
    listeriosis, 421–422
    Lyme disease, 432
    malaria, 433
    neonates with, 452–454, 453*t*
    parasitic, 433–435
    pertussis, 422–424
    pneumocystis jiroveci pneumonia, 403
    postpartum, 450–451
    postpartum counseling on, 208

Infections *(continued)*
    postpartum hemorrhage and, 254
    postpartum visits and, 305
    rubella, 409–411
    sexually transmitted. *See* Sexually transmitted
        infections
    spirochetal, 427–433
    toxoplasmosis, 433–435
    transmissible, admissions policies on, 172
    tuberculosis, 424–427
    varicella zoster virus, 411–414
    viral, 383–414
    West Nile virus, 414
    workplace, Occupational Safety and Health
        Administration guidelines on, 441–442
Infertility
    abnormal body mass index and, 102
    sexually transmitted infections and, 99, 415, 416
    treatments
        assisted reproductive technology for, 105
        prenatal care visit frequency and, 107
Influenza viruses, 98, 118, 198, 295, 404–406,
        442
Informed consent
    for drug or metabolite testing, 129
    for interhospital transfer, 80–81
    power of attorney and, 155–156
    for return interhospital transfer, 90
    for vaginal breech deliveries, 159
    for women with intellectual and developmental
        disabilities, 155
Inhibin, aneuploidy and, 123
In-hospital perinatal care, 8–9, 10–13*t*
Inpatient perinatal care services
    education for medical providers, 35–36
    for incarcerated women, 152
    medical providers, 21–26
    neonatal functional units, 45–54
    nurse practitioners, 27–33
    obstetric functional units, 37–45
    physician assistants, 33–34
    quality improvement, 37
    support providers, 34–35
Institute for Clinical Systems Improvement, 63
Institute of Medicine
    on prepregnancy BMI and maternal weight
        gain, 136–137, 137*t*, 217
    on quality improvement, 61–62
    on unintended pregnancies, 4
    on vitamin D during pregnancy, 133
    on weight gain for twin pregnancy, 239
Instructional directives, 156
Insulin, 219, 220–221, 229
Intellectual disabilities, pregnant women with, 155
Intensive care unit, 50–51, 247. *See also* Critical
        care; Neonatal intensive care units
Intercostal drain placement and removal, 364
Intercourse
    genital herpes simplex virus infection and, 394
    postpartum, 201
    preterm labor and, 258

Interferon, pegylated, 393
Interferon-gamma release assay, 114*b*, 424, 425
Interhospital transfer
for critical care, 89
delivery of extremely preterm neonates and, 250
enforcement and penalties for violating federal patient screening and transfer requirements, 517
equipment, 84–86
federal general requirements, 517–518
federal requirements for patient screening and, 513
goals for high-risk patients, 77
of incarcerated women, 152–153
maternal, 78
medical–legal responsibilities, 80–81
neonatal, 78–79, 276
outreach education on, 91
patient care during, 88–89
personnel, 84
procedure, 87–88, 515–516
program components, 79–80
program evaluation, 91–92
refusal, 516
responsibilities, 80
dispatching unit, 84
program director, 81–82
receiving center, 83–84
referring hospital, 82–83
return transport, 79, 89–91
International Confederation of Midwives, 494
International Federation of Gynecology and Obstetrics, 494
Intimate partner violence, 131–132, 153
Intra-amniotic infection, 250–251
Intracerebral or intracranial calcifications
cytomegalovirus and, 383
toxoplasmosis and, 434
Intracytoplasmic sperm injection, 105
Intrapartum care
admission, 170–175
analgesia and anesthesia, 182–185
administration of, 185–186
for cesarean deliveries, 185
risk factors and complications, 186–187
chronic hypertension, 234
critical care and, 245
delivery
cesarean, 160, 192–194
elective, 160
multiple gestation, 194
support persons, 195
vaginal, 187–192, 189*b*
eclampsia, 232
gestational diabetes mellitus, 229–230
group B streptococci infections, 418–420
home births, 170
isoimmunization, 238
labor
amnioinfusion, 181–182
false, at term, 175

Intrapartum care, labor *(continued)*
fetal heart rate monitoring, 177–180, 179–180*b*
induction of, 180–181
management of, 176–177
onset of, 175
premature rupture of membranes, 175–176
multiple gestations, 243
planned home birth, 170
preeclampsia, 232
of pregestational diabetes mellitus, 221–222
safety considerations, 169
underwater births, 170
Intrauterine devices, 204
Intrauterine growth assessment, 280
Intrauterine growth restriction. *See also* Fetal growth restriction; Growth restriction
antepartum management, 235–237
antiphospholipid syndrome and, 211
asthma and, 213
cytomegalovirus and, 383
diagnosis, 235
Doppler ultrasonography of umbilical artery and, 150
fetal well-being tests and, 145
intrauterine drug exposure and, 338
multifetal pregnancy reduction and, 242
parvovirus B19 and, 406
postpartum follow-up on, 208
risk factors, 236*b*
screening for, 235
sickle cell disease and, 215
tobacco use and smoke exposure and, 128
use of term, 234–235
Intubation, endotracheal, 272–273, 364
In vitro fertilization, 105
Iodine
deficiency, hypothyroidism and, 223
for Graves disease, 143
povidone, 446, 448
preconception supplementation, 104*t*
for pregnant and lactating adolescents and women, 135–136*t*
Iron
anemia of prematurity and, 321–322
antepartum, after bariatric surgery, 218–219
deficiency, anemia in pregnancy and, 133, 224
multiple gestations and, 239
for neonates, 294
postpartum, 200
preconception supplementation, 104*t*, 105
for pregnant and lactating adolescents and women, 135–136*t*
supplementation during pregnancy, 133
thalassemias and, 215
Isoimmunization
fetal well-being tests and, 145
hyperbilirubinemia and, 331
in pregnancy, 237–238
recommended consultation for, 478, 480

Isolation room requirements, 452–453, 453*t*
Isoniazid, 425, 426–427

J

Jarisch–Herxheimer reaction, 428
Jaundice. *See also* Hyperbilirubinemia
    assessment of, 330–331
    breastfeeding and, 329–330
    cytomegalovirus and, 383
    follow-up assessment, 331–332
    follow-up plans for, 307
    hepatitis B and, 387
    in newborns, 301, 303*b*, 306
    parent education on, 310
    in preterm infants, 326
    vacuum extraction and, 190
Jehovah's Witnesses, 322
Jitteriness, neonatal, 284*b*
Joint Commission, 67, 70, 169, 186
Joint Committee on Infant Hearing, 298

K

Kell antibodies, alloimmunization and, 238
Kernicterus, 325, 326
Ketoacidosis, diabetes and, 219
Kick counts, 145, 146–147
Kleihauer–Betke test, 248

L

Labetalol, 233–234
Labor. *See also* Induction of labor
    amnioinfusion, 181–182
    anticipating, 157–158
    definition of, 514–515
    evaluation of, 171–172
    facilities for, 40–41
    fetal heart rate monitoring, 177–180, 179–180b
    management of, 176–177
    medical record of, 279
    onset of, 175
    options for early stages of, 174
    precipitous, intrauterine drug exposure and, 338
    premature, exercise during pregnancy and, 138
    premature rupture of membranes, 175–176
    preregistration for, 173
    preterm, 158
    preterm admission policies, 171
    safety considerations, 169
    trial of labor after cesarean delivery, 159–160
Labor and delivery health care providers
    birth plan and, 174
    labor management by, 176–177
    mother's arrival in labor area and, 173
Labor dystocia, 189*b*, 256
Laborists, 22
Lactation. *See* Breastfeeding
Lactational amenorrhea, 202
LactMed database of drugs, 291
Lactogenesis delays, 290

Large for gestational age, neonatal hypoglycemia and, 299–300
LATCH score, 288
Latent tuberculosis, 424, 425
Late preterm infants
    assessment of, 280–281
    definition of, 265
    follow-up after discharge, 374
    with hemolytic disease, hyperbilirubinemia and, 326
    hypoglycemia and, 299–300, 333–335, 334*f*
    safe transportation of, 312
Laundering, 54, 444–445, 457, 460, 523
Lay midwives, 494
Leadership, quality improvement and, 62–63
Lead exposure, prenatal, 141
Learning disability, infants on extracorporeal membrane oxygenation and, 349
Legal issues
    drug use testing during pregnancy, 338
    family and medical leave, 157
    interhospital transfer, 77, 80–81
    pregnant adolescents, 151
Lethargy, neonatal, 284*b*
Leukomalacia, periventricular, 323, 324
Level I care facilities. *See also* Basic care facilities
    advanced practice registered nurses for, 30–31
    medical providers for, 23–24
    personnel and equipment for, 13–14
Level II care facilities. *See also* Specialty care facilities
    advanced practice registered nurses for, 32–33
    medical providers for, 24–25
    personnel and equipment for, 14
Level III care facilities. *See also* Subspecialty care facilities
    advanced practice registered nurses for, 31–32
    hypoxic–ischemic encephalopathy care at, 324–325
    medical providers for, 25–26
    personnel and equipment for, 14–15
Level IV care facilities. *See also* Subspecialty care facilities
    advanced practice registered nurses for, 32–33
    hypoxic–ischemic encephalopathy care at, 324
    medical providers for, 25–26
    personnel and equipment for, 15–16
Level of consciousness, neonatal, 280
Levels of care, classification system, 30–33. *See also* Interhospital transfer
Levonorgestrel intrauterine device, 204, 205
Levothyroxine, 223
Licensed direct-entry midwives, 491, 492–493, 494
Licensed midwives, 491, 492–493, 494
Lidocaine, 286, 364–365
Lighting, 55–56, 366
Limited fetal ultrasonography, 110
Linen, cleaning and disinfecting, 460
Linguistically appropriate care, 3–4
Listeriosis, 140–141, 421–422

Live births
definition, 499
measures of, 501–502
reporting requirements and recommendations, 508
Liver disease, hepatitis C virus and, 392
Living wills, 156
Local anesthesia, 185
Lochia pattern, postpartum changes in, 200
Long-acting reversible contraception, 204
Lorazepam, 343
Low birth weight infants
definition, 499
hyperbilirubinemia and, 326–329, 327f, 328f
increased nuchal transparency measurement and, 124
malaria and, 433
perinatal morbidity and mortality and, 235
pregnant adolescents and, 151
prior, recommended consultation for, 478
retinopathy of prematurity and, 353
safe transportation of, 312
selective fetal termination and, 242
tobacco use and smoke exposure and, 128
very low birth weight
anemia of prematurity in, 321–322
formula milk preparations for, 359
immunizations in, 366
Low operative vaginal delivery, 191
Luncheon meats, listeria infections and, 140–141
Lung disease. See also Bronchopulmonary dysplasia
chronic, retinopathy of prematurity and, 353
restrictive
exercise during pregnancy and, 138
intrauterine growth restriction and, 236b
Lupus anticoagulant, antiphospholipid syndrome and, 211
Lupus erythematosus, systemic, 144
Lyme disease, 432
Lymphadenopathy, generalized, 434

M

Macrocytic anemia, 224
Macrosomia
bariatric surgery and, 218
gestational diabetes mellitus and, 227
postpartum hemorrhage and, 254
postterm pregnancy and, 256
pregestational diabetes mellitus and, 221
Maculopapular rash, toxoplasmosis and, 434
Magnesium sulfate
preeclampsia and eclampsia, 232
preterm labor and, 258–259
Magnetic resonance imaging, 111–112, 142, 323
Malaria, 433
Male condoms, 205
Malnutrition, severe, intrauterine growth restriction and, 236b
MAMA Campaign. See Midwives & Mothers in Action
Managed care, return transport and, 89–90

Mantoux tuberculin skin test, 114b, 116, 424, 425, 426, 427
March of Dimes Foundation, 1, 72, 73
Marijuana, nursing infants and, 337
Masks
infection control and, 445, 446
as personal protective equipment, 524
Mastitis, breastfeeding and, 290
Maternal age
aneuploidy and, 120–121, 122t
chromosomal abnormalities and, 123
multiple gestations and, 239
preeclampsia and eclampsia and, 231
preterm birth and, 257
stillbirth and, 261
35 years or older, recommended consultation for, 478
trial of labor after cesarean delivery and, 189b
Maternal care
postdischarge, 16
quality improvement indicators in, 65b
Maternal coagulopathy, postpartum hemorrhage and, 254
Maternal confidence, 205–206
Maternal death
definition, 500
measures of, 505–507
preeclampsia and HELLP syndrome and, 231
reporting requirements and recommendations, 509
Maternal–fetal medicine specialist
antepartum hospitalization and, 243
twin–twin transfusion syndrome and, 242
Maternal fever, uncomplicated, breastfeeding and, 291
Maternal hemorrhage, 254–255
Maternal morbidity and mortality. See also Maternal death
asthma and, 212
sickle cell disease and, 215
Maternal risks, postterm pregnancy and, 255–256
Maternal serum alpha-fetoprotein
aneuploidy and, 123, 124
neural tube defects and, 125, 126
recommended consultation for, 479
Maternal transport, 78. See also Interhospital transfer
Maternal vital signs, 171, 172, 196
Measles
screening health care workers for, 442
vaccine, 99
Measles–mumps–rubella vaccine, 118–119, 413–414
Meconium
analysis for intrauterine drug exposure, 338
staining of amniotic fluid
aspiration, hypoxic cardiorespiratory failure and, 347
aspiration, postterm pregnancy and, 255
management of, 279
nasopharyngeal suctioning, 271

Medicaid programs, 517
Medical complications before pregnancy, 211–223
  antiphospholipid syndrome, 211–212
  asthma, 212–213, 214b
  hemoglobinopathies, 213–215
  inherited thrombophilias, 215–216
  obesity and bariatric surgery, 216–218
  pregestational diabetes mellitus, 219–222
  thyroid disease, 222–223
Medical errors
  communication and, 69
  disclosure of, 70
  literacy and language barriers and, 5
  patient safety and, 67–68
Medical insurance
  hospital medical screening and, 517
  public, at late preterm infant delivery, 281
Medical record(s). See also Informed consent
  of abuse, 132
  of antepartum hospitalization, 244
  electronic, 38, 173
  of evaluation for labor, 172, 173
  interhospital transfer and, 517
  of intrauterine growth, 280
  of management of labor, 177, 178
  of neonatal information, 279
  on operative vaginal delivery, 191
  of physician to care for newborn, 175
  on postpartum orders, 196
  prenatal, 173–174
  of routine laboratory tests, 112
  of trial of labor after cesarean delivery and elec-
    tive repeat cesarean delivery, 190
  transfer to neonatal care of, 265
  of vaccines, 118
  vaginal birth after cesarean delivery and trial of
    labor after cesarean delivery consider-
    ations and, 159, 160
  of venous thromboembolic events, 225
Medical screening examination requirements, for
  transfer, 513–514
Medications. See also specific medications
  admission evaluation of, 172
  antenatal corticosteroid therapy and, 248–249
  assessment in high-risk infants, 378
  contraindications for breastfeeding and, 291
  critical care in pregnancy and, 245
  delivery of extremely preterm neonates and,
    250
  for genital human papillomavirus during preg-
    nancy, 404
  maternal, medical record of, 279
  milk donor testing for, 293
  misuse and abuse during pregnancy, 100, 152
  neonatal resuscitation, 273–274
  preconception history taking of, 101
  psychotropic, teratogenic effects of, 246
  safe practices for, 69
  teratogenic potential of, 141–142
  therapeutic drug level, bariatric surgery and,
    219

Mediterranean ethnicity
  anemia and, 113t
  genetic screening for, 121t
  hemoglobinopathies and, 214
Medroxyprogesterone acetate injections, 205
Membrane examination, fetal death and, 261
Membrane rupture. See Rupture of membranes
Membrane stripping, labor induction and, 181
Mendelian inheritance disorders, 120, 121t
Meningitis, 417
Meningococcus vaccine, 99, 118
Menstrual dates, for estimated date of delivery
  calculation, 109
Mental illness of parent, discharge readiness and,
  307
Meprobamate, neonatal withdrawal and,
  336–337t
Metabolite screening
  informed consent for, 129
  in newborns, 297
Methadone, 337, 343
Methamphetamine, nursing infants and, 337
Methemoglobinemia, 364
Methicillin-resistant Staphylococcus aureus, 454
Methyldopa, 234
Microcephaly, 383, 434
Microcytic anemia, 113t, 121t, 224
Midpelvis operative vaginal delivery, 191
Midwifery Education Accreditation Council,
  492–493, 495
Midwives, 23
Midwives, glossary of organizations and terms,
  491–496
Midwives & Mothers in Action, 494
Midwives Alliance of North America, 492–493,
  494–495
Midwives Model of Care, 493, 495
Mild chronic hypertension, 233
Milk
  banked human, 293
  collection and storage, 291–293, 292t
  human, for preterm infants, 359
  preparation area, 51
Minerals
  neonatal supplementation, 294
  preconception supplementation, 104t, 105
  for pregnant and lactating adolescents and
    women, 135–136t
  toxicity during pregnancy, 139–141
Miscarriage. See Fetal death
Misoprostol, 261
Model State Vital Statistics Act and Regulations
  (1992), 2011 revisions to, 508
Modified biophysical profile, 145, 149–150, 236
Monochorionic diamniotic multiple gestation,
  145
Monochorionic placentation, 241. See also
  Multiple gestations
Mood disorders, postpartum, 202–205. See also
  Emotional responses, postpartum;
  Psychosis, postpartum

Mood swings, severe, intrauterine drug exposure and, 338
Mother–infant relationship, 205–206, 313, 314
Motor vehicle crashes, trauma during pregnancy and, 246
Multidrug-resistant *M tuberculosis*, 427
Multidrug-resistant organisms, 454
Multifetal pregnancy reduction, 242
Multiple gestations
 antepartum management
  fetal surveillance, 240
  nutritional considerations, 239
  prenatal diagnosis, 239–240
 complications
  death of one fetus, 241–242
  discordant growth, 145, 241
  growth restriction, 241
  multifetal pregnancy reduction, 242
  preterm labor and delivery, 240–241
  twin–twin transfusion syndrome, 242
 delivery considerations, 194
 incidence of, 239
 infant identification in, 278
 intrapartum management, 243
 intrauterine growth restriction and, 236*b*
 neonatal resuscitation readiness and, 267
 preeclampsia and eclampsia and, 231
 prenatal care visit frequency and, 107
 recommended consultation for, 479
 retinopathy of prematurity and, 353
Multisystem organ dysfunction, surfactant therapy and, 347
Mumps, 99, 442. *See also* Measles–mumps–rubella vaccine
Muscle tone, neonatal, 268, 280
Mycobacterium bovis, 427
Mycobacterium tuberculosis, 424. *See also* Tuberculosis
Myocardial infarction, intrauterine drug exposure and, 338
Myxedema, 223

N
Naloxone, 274
Narcotics. *See* Opioids
Nasopharyngeal suctioning, 270–271
National Academy of Sciences, 133
National Association of Certified Professional Midwives, 495
National Center for Health Statistics, 64, 508, 510
National Commission for Certifying Agencies, 495
National Diabetes Data Group, 228, 228*t*
National Fetal and Infant Mortality Review, 66
National Heart, Lung, and Blood Institute, 350
National Institute of Child Health and Human Development, 178, 249, 325
National Institutes of Health, 216, 240–241
National Newborn Screening and Genetic Resource Center, 296

National Organization for Competency Assurance, 495
National Patient Safety Goals, 67
National Practitioner Data Bank, 21–22
National Pregnancy Mortality Surveillance System, 500
National Quality Measures Clearinghouse, 64
Nausea, in pregnancy, 139, 219
Nebulizer cleaning, 459
Necrotizing enterocolitis, 338, 346
Needle aspiration, of tension pneumothorax, 267
Needle safety, 442, 522
Needlestick Safety and Prevention Act (2000), 519
Neisseria gonorrhea. *See* Gonorrhea
Neonatal Abstinence Scoring System, 338, 340–341*f*
Neonatal care. *See also* Neonatal functional units
 for adopted infants, 314–315
 Ballard Score and, 282–283*f*
 breastfeeding, 287–293, 289*t*, 292*t*
 catheter-related bloodstream infections, 446–448
 for chlamydia, 415–416
 circumcision, 286–287
 classification system for, 13–16
 clothing, 287
 communication of information, 278–279
 congenital syphilis, 428–429, 430–431*f*, 431–432
 conjunctival care, 284
 in delivery room
  assessment, 268, 269*f*, 270, 274, 275*f*, 276
  body temperature maintenance, 270
  clearing the airway, 270–271
  positioning, 271
  resuscitation management plan, 266–268
  stimulation, 271
  supplemental oxygen administration, 271–272
  ventilation, 272–273
 facilities for, 43–45
 family-centered environment for, 265
 follow-up, 313–314
 for gonorrhea, 417
 health care-associated pneumonia, 448–450
 hospital discharge
  of healthy newborns, 306–308
  of late preterm infants, 309
 infant identification, 265, 278
 infant security, 305
 nurse–patient ratios, 30
 in nursery
  assessment, 280–283
  maturity assessments, 282–283*f*
  potential illness signs, 284*b*
 parent education and psychosocial factors, 309–312
 physician-directed follow-up, 308, 309
 postdischarge, 16
 postpartum counseling on, 201

Neonatal care *(continued)*
    preventive
        immunizations, 295
        scope of, 265–266
    quality improvement indicators in, 65*b*
    radiation exposure, 365–366
    screening
        blood spot, 296–298
        cyanotic congenital heart disease, 304
        developmental dysplasia of the hip,
            302–303
        glucose, 299–300
        hearing, 298–299
        hyperbilirubinemia, 301, 302*f*, 303*b*
        mandated, 295–296
    skin care, 285
    toxoplasmosis, 435
    transitional, 265, 284–287
    for tuberculosis, 425–427
    umbilical cord care, 285–286
    varicella zoster virus, 413
    visiting policies, 304–305
    vitamin K administration, 285
Neonatal clinical nurse specialists, 28
Neonatal complications
    anemia, 321–322
    apnea, 322–323
    assessment for, 281
    brain injury, 323–325
        hemorrhagic, 323
        periventricular white matter, 323
    hyperbilirubinemia, 325–333
    hypoglycemia, 333–335, 334*f*
    hypoxic–ischemic encephalopathy, 324–325
    neonatal drug withdrawal, 335–343
    radiation risk, 365–366
    respiratory
        bronchopulmonary dysplasia, 349–353,
            351*t*
        hypoxic cardiorespiratory failure, 347–349
        oxygen therapy, 343–345
        respiratory distress syndrome, 345–347
    retinopathy of prematurity, 353–356, 355*t*
Neonatal death
    anticipated, 375–376
    bereavement follow-up, 370
    definition, 499
    determining cause of, 369–370
    home births and, 170
    in-hospital support and counseling, 367–369
    pertussis and, 422, 424
    pregnant adolescents and, 151
    prior, recommended consultation for, 478
Neonatal drug withdrawal
    discharge and follow-up care, 342
    management of acquired opioid and benzodiaz-
        epine dependency, 342–343
    maternal nonnarcotic drugs causing, 336–337*t*
    screening, 338
    signs of, 335, 337–338, 339*b*
    treatment, 338–339, 340–341*f*, 342

Neonatal functional units
    acoustics, 57
    admission and observation, 47–48
    clerical areas, 54
    components, 45
    disaster preparedness and evacuation plan, 54
    education areas, 54
    electrical outlets and electrical equipment, 57
    illumination, 55–56
    neonatal intensive care unit, 50–51
    newborn nursery, 48–49
    nursing areas, 53–54
    oxygen and compressed-air outlets, 56–57
    resuscitation, 45–47
    safety and environmental control, 54–55
    scrub areas, 53
    special care nursery, 49–50
    supporting service areas, 51–52
    wall surfaces, 56
    windows, 56
Neonatal gonococcal infection, 416
Neonatal heart rate. *See* Heart rate, neonatal
Neonatal intensive care units (NICUs)
    acquired drug dependency and, 343
    components, 50–51
    gestational age and optimum care in, 11–12*t*,
        78
    immunizations in, 366–367
    known or anticipated needs for, 274, 276
    nosocomial hepatitis A virus infections in, 386
    quality improvement and patient safety in,
        72–73
    sleep position in, 312
    surgical procedures in, 366
Neonatal interventions, 161. *See also* Neonatal care
Neonatal narcotic abstinence syndrome, 335, 339*b*.
        See also Neonatal drug withdrawal
Neonatal Resuscitation Program (AAP), 24,
        266–268, 271, 273
Neonates. *See also* Neonatal care
    death. *See* Neonatal death
    definition, 499
    drug withdrawal in. *See* Neonatal drug with-
        drawal
    with infections, 452–454, 453*t*
    influenza viruses and, 405–406
    interhospital transfer of, 78–79
    pain prevention and management, 362–365
    parvovirus B19 and, 406–407
    pertussis in, 424
    rubella in, 409, 410, 411
    well-being assessment, information on, 202
Nephropathy, 219, 231
Neural tube defects, 124, 125, 217
Neurobehavioral abnormalities, intrauterine drug
        exposure and, 338
Neurologic diseases, maternal, anesthesia risks
        and, 186–187
Neuromuscular maturity, signs of, 282*f*
Newborn blood spot screening, 296–298
Newborn care. *See* Neonatal care

Newborn care providers
    choosing, 157
    identified, on maternal medical record, 175
Newborn nursery, 48–49. *See also* Nursery
Niacin, 134*t*
NICU. *See* Neonatal intensive care units
Niemann–Pick disease type A, 121*t*
Nifedipine, 234
Nitric oxide, inhaled, 348, 352
Non-English speaking parents, discharge readiness
    and, 153
Nonobstetric hospital services, pregnant patients
    in, 244
Nonobstetric surgery in pregnancy, 245–246
Nonreactive nonstress test, 147
Non–Rh-D alloimmunization, 237
Nonsteroidal antiinflammatory drugs, 258
Nonstress test, 145, 146, 147–148
    biophysical profile and, 149
    intrauterine growth restriction and, 236
    modified biophysical profile and, 149–150
    multiple gestations and, 240
    postterm pregnancy and, 256
Normocytic anemia, 224
North American Registry of Midwives, 492–493,
    495–496
    Portfolio Evaluation Process, 496
Nosocomial infections, surfactant therapy and,
    346
Nuchal translucency, aneuploidy and, 121, 123,
    124
Nuclear imaging, teratogenic potential of, 142
Nulliparity, stillbirth and, 261
Nurse–midwives, 23
Nurse–patient ratios, 30
Nurse practitioners, 27–33
Nursery
    admission policies, 440–441
    neonatal assessment, 280–283, 282–283*f*,
        284*b*
    newborn, 48–49, 458
    special care, 49–50, 276
Nursery linen cleaning and disinfecting, 460
Nursing areas, 53–54
Nutrition
    anemia of prematurity and, 321–322
    antepartum, after bariatric surgery, 218–219
    first-trimester patient education on, 132–133,
        134–136*t*, 136
    homelessness and, 153
    during labor, 158, 177
    multiple gestations and, 239
    neonatal, 265
    postpartum, 200, 201, 208
    preconception counseling, 102–103, 103–104*t*,
        105
    of preterm infants
        after discharge, 361–362
        enteral, 359, 360–361*t*, 361
        parenteral, 356, 357–358*t*, 358
    for technology-dependent infants, 374–375

O
Obesity and obese patients
    anesthesia risks and, 186–187
    childhood, gestational diabetes mellitus and, 227
    children of mothers smoking during pregnancy
        and, 128
    morbid, cesarean delivery and, 192
    obstetric functional units for, 39
    preconception care for, 101
    preconception weight loss and, 102
    preeclampsia and eclampsia and, 231
    pregestational diabetes mellitus and, 219
        before pregnancy, 216–218
    residual postpartum weight retention and, 200
    stillbirth and, 261
    trial of labor after cesarean delivery and, 189*b*
    venous thromboembolism in pregnancy and,
        225
    weight gain during pregnancy and, 136–137,
        137*t*, 239
Observation–admission–transition nursery, 276
Obstetric and medical complications
    anemia, 223–225
    antepartum hospitalization, 243–244
    critical care in pregnancy, 244–245
    labor and delivery
        antenatal corticosteroid therapy, 248–249
        births at threshold of viability, 249–250
        chorioamnionitis, 250–251
        endocarditis, 251, 252*b*
        endometritis, 252–254
        fetal pulmonary maturation, 248
        maternal hemorrhage, 254–255
        postterm pregnancy, 255–256
        premature rupture of membranes, 259–260
        preterm birth, 256–259
        stillbirth, 260–262
    late preterm infants and, 281
    medical complications before pregnancy,
        211–223
    neonatal resuscitation and, 267
    nonobstetric surgery, 245–246
    pregnancy-related complications, 223–243
    psychiatric disease, 246
    trauma during pregnancy, 246–248
Obstetric death, 500
Obstetric functional units
    bed need analysis, 43–45
    combined units, 39–43
    components, 37–39
    delivery, 41–43
    labor, 40–41
    postpartum and newborn care, 43
Obstetrician–gynecologists
    antepartum hospitalization and, 243
    granting privileges for, 481–482
    safety education by, 247
Obstetric nurse, vaginal delivery and, 187
Obstetric Privileges
    after inactivity period, 486–488
    Basic Level, 482

Obstetric Privileges *(continued)*
for family physicians, 484–485
new equipment or technology and, 485–486
Specialty Level, 483
Subspecialty Level, 483
Occupational exposure to bloodborne pathogens
approved state plans, 520
communication of hazards, 527–529
engineering and work practice controls, 521–523
exposure control plan, 520–521
hepatitis B vaccination, 525–526
housekeeping, 524–525
mandatory universal precautions, 521
Occupational Safety and Health Administration guidelines on, 519
personal protective equipment, 523–524
postexposure evaluation and follow-up, 526–527
record-keeping requirements, 529–530
Occupational Safety and Health Administration, 441–442
Ofloxacin, 415
Older women. *See also* Maternal age
aneuploidy and, 120–121, 122*t*
chromosomal abnormality screening and, 123
35 years or older, recommended consultation for, 478
Oligohydramnios, 145, 256, 479
Omphalitis, 285–286
Online education for new parents, 309–310
Open care units, cleaning, 458–459
Operative delivery
postpartum hemorrhage and, 254
venous thromboembolism in pregnancy and, 225
Operative vaginal delivery, 190–192
Ophthalmia, gonococcal, 284, 417
Ophthalmologic evaluation
chronic hypertension and, 233
retinopathy of prematurity and, 354–356, 355*t*
Ophthalmopathy, 223
Opioids
acquired dependency management, 342–343
neonatal drug withdrawal and, 335, 336–337*t*
for neonatal postoperative pain management, 363
pain of labor and, 182–183, 198
postpartum risks with, 202
Oral contraceptives, 218, 291
Oral nutrition, labor and, 158
Organization of Teratology Information Specialists, 141
Organomegaly, 220
Orgasm, preterm labor and, 258
Ortolani test, 302–303
Outcomes data, collection and analysis of, 64–66, 65*b*
Outlet operative vaginal delivery, 190–191
Outreach education, perinatal, 36–37
Oxygen and compressed-air outlets, 56–57

Oxygen desaturation, late preterm infants and, 309, 312
Oxygen saturation monitoring, neonatal
pain response and, 362
resuscitation and, 268, 269*f*, 270, 271–272
for special care infants, 375
Oxygen therapy
administration of, 268, 269*f*, 270, 271–272
bronchopulmonary dysplasia and, 350
equipment cleaning, 459
home, 375
retinopathy of prematurity and, 343–345, 353–354
Oxytocic agents
in labor induction, 180, 181
postpartum hemorrhage and, 254
Oxytocin challenge test, 146, 148–149

P
Pacific Island descent, late preterm infants and, 281
Pacifiers, safe sleeping and, 311
Pain management. *See also* Analgesia and anesthesia
nonpharmacologic, 354
Palivizumab, 295, 408
PaO_2, 344, 345, 353
Pap test, abnormal, 479
Paralysis of upward gaze, hyperbilirubinemia and, 326
Parasitic infections, 433–435
Parenteral nutrition
for preterm infants, 356, 357–358*t*, 358
for special care infants, 374–375
total, infection and, 447
Parenteral pain medications, 182–183
Parents
circumcision information for, 286
discharge education for, 310–311
of high-risk infants, decision-making for, 276–277
and infant death, 367–370
Partner, labor and delivery and, 169, 195. *See also* Family; Parents; Support persons
Parvovirus B19, 406–407
Patent ductus arteriosus, 346, 353, 410
Paternal age, 121
Patient-centered health care, 2–3
Patient handoffs, 70
Patient safety. *See also* Safety considerations
accountability and, 5
drills and simulator training, 71–72
Institute of Medicine on, 61–62
leadership on, 62–63
National Patient Safety Goals, 67
in neonatal intensive care units, 72–73
physician fatigue and, 70–71
physician–patient communication, 69–70
principles, 67–71
Patient self-care classes, postpartum, 310
Pedigree assessment, genetic testing and, 119–120
Peer review, quality improvement and, 63

Pelvic examination, labor and delivery and, 173
Pelvic inflammatory disease, 416
Penicillin, 419, 428
Penicillin G, 429, 431, 432
Penis, of newborn, 286–287
Peptococcus species, 252
Peptostreptococcus species, 252
Perinatal health care services
    clinical components, 6–9
    comprehensive, 2
Perinatal mortality
    measures, 503–505
    reporting requirements and recommendations,
        508
Perinatal outreach education, 36–37
Perineum, postpartum care of, 201
Peripheral artery catheters, 344, 446–448
Peripheral neuritis, tuberculosis treatment and,
        425
Periventricular–intraventricular hemorrhage,
        323–324
Personal protective equipment, 445, 521,
        523–524
Personnel
    distribution and supply of, 17
    education for, 35–36
    health standards for, 442–444
    inpatient perinatal care, 21–37
    interhospital transfer, 84
    medical providers, 21–26
    nurse practitioners, 27–33
    occupational exposure record-keeping by, 521,
        529–530
    occupational exposure training for, 521,
        528–529
    physician assistants, 33–34
    pregnant, parvovirus B19 and, 407
    quality improvement, 37
    standard precautions by, 441–442
    support providers, 34–35
Pertussis, 422–424, 442
pH
    oxygen therapy and, 345
    premature rupture of membranes diagnosis
        and, 176
    umbilical artery, postterm pregnancy and, 256
Pharmacologic interventions. *See* Medications
Phencyclidine, nursing infants and, 337
Phenolic compounds, 456
Phenylketonuria, 100–101
Phosphorus, 104t, 135–136t
Phototherapy
    guidelines, 326–328, 327f
    for hyperbilirubinemia, 332–333
    in previous sibling, hyperbilirubinemia and,
        303b
Physical disabilities, pregnant women with, ante-
        partum care for, 154–155
Physical facilities
    neonatal functional units, 45–54
    obstetric functional units, 37–45

Physical maturity, signs of, 282f
Physician assistants, 33–34
Physicians. *See also* Newborn care providers;
        Obstetrician–gynecologists
    credentialing, 21–22, 484–485
    distribution and supply of, 17
    list of, on call to stabilize emergency medical
        condition patients, 517
    patient safety and communication by, 69–70
    patient safety and fatigue of, 70–71
    primary care
        follow-up care for high-risk infants and,
            377
        newborn blood spot screening and,
            297–298
    reentry of, 486–488
Placenta
    fetal death and examination of, 261
    retained, postpartum hemorrhage and, 254
    retained fragments of, 290
Placenta accreta, 193, 254, 255
Placental abruption. *See* Abruptio placentae
Placenta previa
    assisted reproductive technology and, 105
    breech presentation and, 158
    cesarean delivery on maternal request and, 193
    contraction stress test and, 148
    exercise during pregnancy and, 138
    hemorrhage from, cesarean delivery and, 192
    tobacco use and smoke exposure and, 128
    vaginal birth after cesarean delivery and, 188
Pneumatic compression devices, 217–218, 227
Pneumococcus vaccine, 99, 118
Pneumonia
    chlamydial, 416
    group B streptococci and, 417
    health care-associated, 448–450
    hypoxic cardiorespiratory failure and, 347
    pertussis and, 422
    Pneumocystis jiroveci, prophylaxis, 403
    varicella zoster virus and, 412–413
Pneumothorax, 267, 269f
Podofilox, 404
Podophyllin, 404
Polioviruses, 385–386
Polycythemia, 220
Polyhydramnios, 145
Porencephaly, 323
Portfolio Evaluation Process, North American
        Registry of Midwives, 496
Positional plagiocephaly, 312
Positive pressure ventilation, neonatal, 268, 269f,
        270
Postdischarge care, 16. *See also* Follow-up care
Postpartum baby blues, 206
Postpartum care
    critical care in pregnancy and, 245
    facilities for, 43–45
    maternal, 102, 197
        analgesia, 198
        bed rest, ambulation, and diet, 196–197

Postpartum care, maternal *(continued)*
  of breasts, 197
  contraception, 202–205
  counseling issues, 200–202
  follow-up with physician, 207–208
  immediate, 195–196
  immunizations, 198
  length of hospital stay, 198–200
  mood disorders, 205–207
  nutritional guidelines, 200
  subsequent, 196
  urogenital, 197
Postpartum hemorrhage, 254–255
Postterm infant definition, 499
Postterm pregnancy (gestation), 255–256
Poverty, admission evaluation of, 173
Power of attorney, antepartum care and, 155–156
Preconception care, 95–105
  counseling and interventions, 96, 97*t*, 98
    assisted reproductive technology, 105
    chronic medical conditions, 100–101
    genetic screening, 101
    immunizations, 98–99
    medication use, 101
    nutrition, 102–103, 103–104*t*, 105
    postpartum care and, 208
    reproductive health plan, 98
    sexually transmitted infection testing, 99
    substance use and abuse, 99–100, 100*b*
  integrated perinatal services and, 6
  planning questions, 95–96
Preeclampsia
  anesthesia risks and, 186–187
  antepartum management, 231–232
  antiphospholipid syndrome and, 211
  asthma and, 212
  chronic hypertension vs., 233
  definition of, 230
  diagnosis, 231
  gestational diabetes mellitus and, 227
  inherited thrombophilias and, 215–216
  intrapartum management, 232
  obese mother and, 216
  postpartum hemorrhage and, 254
  pregnant adolescents and, 151
  premature, 138
  risk factors for, 231
  sickle cell disease and, 215
  trial of labor after cesarean delivery and, 189*b*
Pregestational diabetes mellitus. *See* Diabetes mellitus, pregestational
Pregnancy. *See also* Antepartum care
  body temperature during, 143
  breastfeeding discussions during, 287–288
  chlamydial infections in, 415
  complications related to
    anemia, 223–225, 224*t*
    deep vein thrombosis, 225–227
    gestational diabetes mellitus, 227–230
    hypertensive disorders, 230
    intrauterine growth restriction, 234–237

Pregnancy, complications related to *(continued)*
    isoimmunization, 237–238
    multiple gestations, 239–243
    pulmonary embolism, 225–227
  critical care in, 244–245
  desire for, 127
  emergency medical conditions in, 514–515
  genital human papillomavirus infections and, 404
  gonorrhea and, 417
  hepatitis A virus vaccine in, 386
  induced termination of, 500–501, 507
  influenza viruses and, 405–406
  informed consent and, 155–156
  listeriosis and, 422
  Lyme disease and, 432
  malaria and, 433
  maternal rubella during, 410
  medical complications before, 211–223
  nonobstetric surgery in, 245–246
  parvovirus B19 and, 406–407
  postterm
    fetal well-being tests and, 145
    routine testing and, 146
  psychiatric disease in, 246
  risk identification in
    early, 477–478
    on-going, 479–480
  syphilis medications during, 428
  Tdap immunization during, 422–423
  trauma during, 246–248
  tuberculosis treatment and, 425
  unintended, 4–5
  unwanted, intimate partner violence and, 131
  vaccine contraindications during, 118–119, 413–414
  varicella zoster virus and, 412
  West Nile virus and, 414
Pregnancy-associated death, 500
Pregnancy-associated plasma protein A, aneuploidy and, 123
Pregnancy-related death, 500
Pregnancy Risk Assessment Monitoring System, 64–65
Premature birth. *See* Preterm birth(s)
Premature labor, exercise and, 138
Premature rupture of membranes (PROM)
  antenatal corticosteroid therapy and, 249
  antibiotics and, 249
  contraction stress test and, 148
  definition of, 259
  diagnosis, 259
  herpes simplex virus and, 395
  interhospital transfer and, 87
  level II care facilities and, 14
  management of, 259–260
  preterm, admissions and, 171
  preterm birth and, 257
  prior, recommended consultation for, 478
  recommended consultation for, 479
  at term, 175–176

Premature rupture of membranes (continued)
tobacco use and smoke exposure and, 128
twin–twin transfusion syndrome and, 242
Prenatal care. See Antepartum care
Prenatal care visits
first, 107–108
frequency, 106–107
group, 108–109
routine, 108–112
Preterm birth(s)
adolescents and, 151
anemia and, 321–322
antiphospholipid syndrome and, 211
asthma and, 212
Ballard Score on, 282–283f
chronic hypertension and, 232, 234
family counseling for, 249–250
homeless women and, 153
increased nuchal transparency measurement
and, 124
intrauterine drug exposure and, 338
listeriosis and, 421–423
malaria and, 433
medical record of problems with, 279
multiple gestations and, 240–241
obese mother and, 216
oxygen therapy complications, 343–345
postpartum follow-up on, 208
preeclampsia and HELLP syndrome and, 231
prior, recommended consultation for, 478
respiratory syncytial virus and, 408
selective fetal termination and, 242
signs and symptoms of, 158
tobacco use and smoke exposure and, 128
very low birth weight, warming techniques
for, 270
Preterm infants. See also High-risk infants; Late
preterm infants
apnea of prematurity in, 322
blood spot screening in, 297
cytomegalovirus in, 384
definition, 499
discharge criteria for, 374
hemorrhagic and periventricular white matter
brain injury and, 323
high-risk, discharge considerations, 374
hyperbilirubinemia and, 326–329, 327f,
328f
immunizations for, 295
maternal cytomegalovirus and breastfeeding
for, 291
nutritional needs of, 356, 357–358t, 358–359,
360–361t, 361–362
Preterm labor
definition of, 158
diagnosis, 257
management of, 257–259
multiple gestations and, 240–241
recommended consultation for, 479
sickle cell disease and, 215
twin–twin transfusion syndrome and, 242

Preterm premature rupture of membranes, 260.
See also Premature rupture of mem-
branes
Preventive care, for newborns, 313
Prilocaine, 286, 364–365
Primary care providers. See also Physicians
follow-up care for high-risk infants and, 377
newborn blood spot screening and, 297–298
Primary cesarean delivery on maternal request, 193
Primary persistent pulmonary hypertension,
hypoxic cardiorespiratory failure and,
347
Primary placental disease, 236b
Primary support person. See Father; Partner;
Support persons
Printed materials, for new parent education,
309–310
Privileges. See also Credentialing
for anesthesia services personnel, 185–186
for forceps or vacuum extraction operations, 192
granting, prerequisites for, 481–482
granting obstetric, 481–489
Progesterone
preterm labor and delivery with multiple
gestations and, 241
prior preterm birth and, 257
Progestin-only contraceptives, 205
Program evaluation, interhospital transfer
program, 91–92
PROM. See Premature rupture of membranes
Proparacaine, 354
Propylthiouracil warnings, 223
Prostaglandins, in labor induction, 181
Proteinuria, gestational hypertension with, 479.
See Preeclampsia
Protocols, definition of, 63
Proxy directives, 156
Psychiatric disease in pregnancy, 246, 279, 477
Psychosis, postpartum, 206
Psychosocial risk screening and counseling,
126–132
clinical depression, 130–131
intimate partner violence, 131–132
pregnancy desire, 127
substance use and abuse, 127–130
alcohol, 129
mood-altering drugs, 129–130
tobacco, 128–129
Psychosocial support, postpartum, 202, 202–205
Psychotropic medication, 246
Public insurance at delivery, late preterm infants
and, 281
Puerperal sepsis, peripartum, 204
Pulmonary disease
maternal, anesthesia risks and, 186–187
recommended consultation for, 477
Pulmonary embolism (PE), 225–226, 477
Pulmonary hypertension, 343, 348, 350
Pulse oximeters, 344–345
Pulse rate, postpartum monitoring, 195
Purpura, cytomegalovirus and, 383

Pyelonephritis, 251, 418–419, 479
Pyrazinamide, 425
Pyridoxine, 425, 427
Pyrimethamine, 434, 435

Q
Quadrivalent human papillomavirus vaccine, 118
Quality improvement
  data collection and analysis, 64–66
  educational focus of, 62
  Institute of Medicine on, 61–62
  leadership, 62–63
  measures and indicators, 64, 65b
  neonatal intensive care unit budget for, 37
  in neonatal intensive care units, 72–73
  peer review, 63
  reducing variation, 63–64
Quaternary ammonias, 456
Questionnaires, genetic testing and, 119, 120

R
Radiation exposure
  breastfeeding and, 290
  critical care in pregnancy and, 245
  in neonatal function units, 55
  in neonates, 365–366
  teratogenic potential of, 142–143
Rate, in statistical tabulations, 501
Ratios
  nurse–patient, 30
  in statistical tabulations, 501
Reactive nonstress test, 147
Receiving center
  interhospital transfer responsibilities, 83–84
  requirements for, 516
Recommended Uniform Screening Panel, 296, 304
Record-keeping, on bloodborne pathogen exposure, 521, 529–530
Red blood cells, packed, 321
Red cell antibody sensitized women, chorionic villus sampling and, 126
Referring hospitals
  interhospital transfer responsibilities, 82–83
  requirements for, 517
Refusal of treatment, 515
Refusal to transfer, 516
Regional pain medications, 183–184, 186, 196, 245
Registered midwives, 492–493, 494
Relocation plan, disaster preparedness and, 54
Renal disease
  chronic, fetal well-being tests and, 144
  intrauterine growth restriction and, 236b
  recommended consultation for, 477–478
Renal function, chronic hypertension and, 233
Reproductive health
  definitions, 498–501
  education, 4–5
  plan for, 98
  reporting requirements and recommendations, 507–511

Reproductive health *(continued)*
  statistical tabulation measures, 501–507
  U.S. standard statistical reporting overview, 497–498
Residency training programs, physician reentry and, 487
Respiratory distress
  mild, 276
  neonatal herpes simplex virus infection and, 396
Respiratory distress syndrome, 345–347
  antenatal corticosteroid therapy and, 248–249
  gestational diabetes mellitus and, 227
  hypoxic cardiorespiratory failure and, 347
  uncontrolled pregestational diabetes mellitus and, 220
Respiratory failure therapy, acquired drug dependency and, 343
Respiratory papillomatosis, 404
Respiratory support equipment cleaning, 459
Respiratory syncytial virus, 407–409
  neonatal prophylaxis for, 295, 408–409, 410t
  precautions for, 454
Respiratory tract infections, maternal, 451
Resuscitation, neonatal
  delivery room management steps
    assessment, 268, 269f, 270
    stabilization, 270–274
  delivery room staff for, 265, 266–267
  facilities, 45–47
  of low gestational age infants, 277–278
  management plan, 266–268
  medical record of, 279
Retinal examinations, pain management for, 364
Retinal hemorrhages, 190
Retinitis, cytomegalovirus and, 383
Retinopathy, diabetic, 219
Retinopathy of prematurity, 343, 353–356, 355t
Retrolental fibroplasia, 343
Return transport, 79, 89–91
Rh (O) D-negative women, fetal–maternal hemorrhage and, 248
Rh alloimmunization, 237
Rh blood group, 480
Rh D blood type
  anti-D immune globulin therapy, 198
  early pregnancy screening for, 113t
  isoimmunization, 237
  negative, repeat antibody testing of, 116
  testing, admissions and, 174
Rib fracture, pertussis and, 422
Riboflavin, 103t, 134t
Rifampin, 425
Ring blocks, for circumcision, 286
Rockers, occiput pressure and, 312
Rotavirus vaccine, 366
Roux-en-Y gastric bypass, 218
Rubella, 409–411
  antepartum management, 410–411
  mother's test result, 279

Rubella *(continued)*
  screening health care workers for, 442
  vaccine, 99, 198, 411. *See also* Measles–
    mumps–rubella vaccine
Rupture of membranes. *See also* Premature
      rupture of membranes
  anticipating, 157–158
  cesarean deliveries and, 117
  duration of, 279
  group B streptococci and, 418
  labor and status of, 172
  signs and symptoms of, 107
  spontaneous, 177
  trauma during pregnancy and, 248

S
Safety considerations. *See also* Infection control;
      Occupational exposure to bloodborne
      pathogens
  birthing centers and, 169
  environmental control and, 54–55
Salpingitis, 416
Sarnat criteria, 324
Saunas, during pregnancy, 143
Scrub areas, 53
Sedatives, pain management and, 363, 364, 365
Seizures
  drug withdrawal-associated, 342
  infants on extracorporeal membrane oxygen-
    ation and, 349
  neonatal herpes simplex virus infection and,
    396
  pertussis and, 422
Selective fetal termination, multiple gestations
    and, 242
Selective serotonin reuptake inhibitors, neonatal
    withdrawal and, 336–337*t*
Selenium, 104*t*, 135–136*t*
Sepsis
  group B streptococci and, 417
  hypoxic cardiorespiratory failure and, 347
  neonatal herpes simplex virus infection and, 396
  retinopathy of prematurity and, 353
  suspected, late preterm infants and, 281
Septicemia, intrapartum, sickle cell disease and,
    215
Severe chronic hypertension, 233
Sexually transmitted infections (STIs)
  admission evaluation of, 173
  coinfections in mothers with human immuno-
    deficiency virus, 403
  gonorrhea and, 417
  hepatitis C virus and, 393
  postpartum counseling on, 208
  pregnant adolescents and, 151
  screening, intrauterine drug exposure and, 338
  testing, 99
Sexual relations
  genital herpes simplex virus infection and, 394
  postpartum, 201
  preterm labor and, 258

Shackling, of incarcerated women, 152–153
Shared decision making, 69
Sharps, disposal of, 522
Sharps injury log, 530
Shock, retinopathy of prematurity and, 353
Shoe covers, for infection control, 446, 524
Shoulder dystocia, gestational diabetes mellitus
    and, 227
Showers during labor, 174
Siblings
  previous jaundice in, hyperbilirubinemia and,
    331
  previous phototherapy in, 303*b*
  visits by, 304–305
Sickle cell disease, 213–215
Sickle hemoglobinopathies, 121*t*. *See also*
    Hemoglobinopathies
SIDS. *See* Sudden infant death syndrome
Signs, on infectious materials, 527–528
Simulation centers, physician reentry and, 487
Simulator training, patient safety and, 72, 73
Sinecatechins, 404
Single-gene disorders, 120, 121*t*
Single mothers, discharge readiness and social
    support for, 307
Single-patient room requirements, 452–453,
    453*t*
Skilled birth attendants, 496
Skin, neonatal
  appearance or color, 280, 284*b*
  care for, 285
  lesions, herpes simplex virus infection and,
    396
  parent education on, 310
Sleep
  deprivation, patient safety and, 70–71
  disturbance, pertussis and, 422
Sleep apnea, neonatal, sleep position and, 312.
    See also Apnea
Sleep position, neonatal, 161, 307, 311–312, 374
Small for gestational age, 235, 299–300,
    333–335, 334*f*
Smoking. *See also* Substance use and abuse
  discharge instructions on infant safety and, 307
  incarcerated women and, 152
  intrauterine growth restriction and, 235, 236*b*
  postpartum care and, 202
  postpartum counseling on, 208
  postpartum follow-up on, 207
  in pregnancy, 99–100, 100*b*
  preterm birth and, 257
  psychosocial risk screening and counseling on,
    128–129
  sudden infant death syndrome and, 311
  stillbirth and, 261
  venous thromboembolism in pregnancy and,
    225
Sniffing position, 271
Social services, in-hospital department for, 310
Society for Healthcare Epidemiology of America,
    443

Socioeconomic status, low, preterm birth and, 257
Sodium hypochlorite, 456
Soiled linen disposal, 460
Solid waste disposal, 458
Southeast Asian ethnicity
    genetic screening for, 121t
    hemoglobinopathies and, 214
Special care nursery, 49–50, 276
Specialized fetal ultrasonography, 111
Specialty care facilities, prenatal, 6, 7t, 10t. See
        also Level II care facilities
Specialty Level Obstetric Privileges, 483
Spinal anesthesia, 173, 184
Spiramycin, 434
Spirochetal infections, 427–433
Stabilization care area, 45–48
Standard fetal ultrasonography, 110
Standard precautions, 441–442. See also Universal
        precautions
    education on, 444
    human immunodeficiency virus transmission
        and, 402
Staphylococcus, chorioamnionitis and, 251
Staphylococcus aureus, methicillin-resistant, 454
Station, in operative vaginal delivery, 190–191
Statistical tabulations
    fetal mortality, 503
    of live births, 501–502
    measures for, 501
Statistics, U.S. standard reproductive health termi-
        nology reporting, 497–512
Steam autoclaving, for sterilization, 455
Sterile techniques, 446
Sterilization, for cleaning, 455–456, 459
Sterilization, reproductive, 203–204
Steroids, National Institutes of Health on preterm
        labor and, 240–241
Stillbirth. See Fetal death
STIs. See Sexually transmitted infections
Stools, neonatal, 284b, 307, 310
Storage areas, 52
Streptococcus agalactiae. See Group B streptococci
Stress reduction, for neonates, 362
Subcapsular hepatic hematoma, 231
Subspecialty care facilities, prenatal, 6, 7t, 10–11t.
        See also Level III care facilities; Level
        IV care facilities
Subspecialty Level Obstetric Privileges, 483
Substance use and abuse. See also Alcohol use;
        Illicit drugs
    admission evaluation of, 173
    anesthesia risks and, 186–187
    antepartum counseling on, 108
    high-risk infants at risk due to, 375
    history, medical record of, 279
    homelessness and, 153
    incarcerated women and, 152
    intimate partner violence and, 131
    intrauterine growth restriction and, 236b
    postpartum counseling on, 208
    postpartum follow-up on, 207

Substance use and abuse (continued)
    preconception counseling on, 99–100, 100b
    psychosocial risk screening and counseling on,
        127–130
    stillbirth and, 261
Sucrose, oral, for pain management, 286, 354, 363
Sudden infant death syndrome (SIDS), 128, 161,
        311–312, 322
Sulfonamides, 434, 435
Superimposed preeclampsia, 231, 233, 234
Superovulation drug therapy, 105
Superoxide dismutase, 352
Supplemental oxygen administration, neonatal,
        268, 269f, 270, 271–272
Support persons
    in delivery room, 174, 195
    newborn care and, 307
    postpartum period and, 304
    primary, labor and delivery and, 169
Support providers, medical care, 34–35
Surfactant replacement therapy, 345–347, 348,
        350
Surgery
    bariatric, 218–219
    neonatal, 363
    in neonatal intensive care units, 366
    nonobstetric, in pregnancy, 245–246
Surgical errors, patient safety and, 69–70
Surgical scrubs, infection control and, 444–445,
        446
Swaddling, for neonatal drug withdrawal, 342
Syphilis, 427–432
    antepartum management, 428
    early pregnancy screening for, 112, 113t,
        114–115
    gonorrhea and, 417
    illicit drug use and risk of, 337
    milk donor testing for, 293
    neonatal management, 428–429, 430–431f,
        431–432
    testing for, 174, 307
Systemic lupus erythematosus, 144
Systolic/diastolic ratio, 150

T
Tachysystole, contraction stress test and, 148
Task Force on Sudden Infant Death Syndrome,
        311–312
Tay–Sachs disease, testing for, 101, 121t
Tdap. See Tetanus–diphtheria acellular pertussis
Technetium Tc-99m scans, 142–143
Technology, new, obstetric privileges and,
        485–486
Technology-dependent infants, 374–375
Temperature, room, 46, 55. See also Body tem-
        perature
Tension pneumothorax decompression, 267.
        See also Pneumothorax
Teratogens
    alcohol as, 129
    first-trimester patient education on, 141–143

Teratogens *(continued)*
  intrauterine growth restriction and, 236*b*
  medications, 101
  mercury in fish, 140
  psychotropic medication, 246
Term, definition of, 265
Termination, selective fetal, multiple gestations
      and, 242
Term neonate, definition of, 500
Term premature rupture of membranes, 260
Tetanus, 442
Tetanus and diphtheria vaccination, 198, 423
Tetanus–diphtheria acellular pertussis (Tdap)
      vaccine, 98–99, 198, 422–423
Tetracycline, 284, 428
Thalassemias, 213–214, 215
Thiamin, 103*t*, 134*t*
Thiazide diuretic therapy, 234
Thimerosal preservative, 117, 405
Thioamide, 223
Thrombophilias
  inherited, 101, 215–216
  venous thromboembolism in pregnancy and,
      225
Thromboprophylaxis
  cesarean deliveries and, 194, 227
  obese women and, 217–218
Thrombosis, antiphospholipid syndrome and,
      212
Thrombotic events, multifetal pregnancy reduction
      and, 242
Thyroid disease, 100–101, 222–223
Thyroid-stimulating hormone, testing, 222, 223
Thyroid storm, 222
Tobacco. *See* Smoking
Tocolytics
  interhospital transfer and, 87
  preterm labor and, 258
  risks, multiple gestations and, 240
TOLAC. *See* Trial of labor after cesarean delivery
Tongue tie, 290
Topical anesthetics, 364–365
Toxoplasmosis, 433–435
Traditional birth attendants, 496
Transcutaneous oxygen analyzer, 344
Transferring hospitals, federal requirements for,
      516–517. *See also* Interhospital
      transfer; Referring hospitals
Transferritin, iron-deficient anemia and, 224
Transitional care area, 47–48
Transparent dressings, infection control and, 446
Transportation, lack of, discharge readiness and,
      153
Trauma
  fetal assessment, 247–248
  intimate partner violence and, 131
  during pregnancy, 246–248
Treatment rooms, 52
Triage principles, disaster preparedness and, 54
Trial of labor after cesarean delivery (TOLAC),
      159–160, 188–190, 189*b*

Triple dye, in umbilical cord care, 285–286
Triplet gestations, 242. *See also* Multiple gesta-
      tions
Trisomies, testing for, 120–121, 122*t*
Tubal ligation, 203–204, 445–446
Tuberculin skin test. *See* Mantoux tuberculin
      skin test
Tuberculosis
  antepartum management, 425
  early pregnancy screening for, 114*b*, 115–116
  incidence and characteristics, 424
  milk donor testing for, 293
  neonatal management, 425–427
  screening health care workers' exposure to,
      442
Tummy time, 312
Twins
  death of one fetus and, 242
  delivery of, 194
  discordant fetal growth in, 241
  postpartum hemorrhage and, 254
  recommended delivery for, 243
Twin–twin transfusion syndrome, 242

U
Ultrasonography
  for chromosomal abnormalities, 123
  compression, of proximal veins, for deep vein
      thrombosis, 225
  for developmental dysplasia of the hip, 302
  Doppler
    of intrauterine growth restriction, 236
    severe fetal anemia predictions using, 238
    of umbilical artery blood flow velocity, 146,
        150
  for estimated date of delivery evaluation,
      109–110
  elective cesarean delivery and, 193
  elective delivery and, 160
  fetal anomalies, 479
  as fetal imaging tool, 110–111
  first-trimester, indications for, 111*b*
  intrauterine growth restriction diagnosis using,
      235
  multiple gestations, 240
  multiple gestations and discordant growth,
      241
  obese mother and, 217
  portable bedside cranial, 323
  preterm labor diagnosis and, 257
  serial
    antiphospholipid syndrome and, 212
    chronic hypertension and, 233
    intrauterine growth restriction and,
        235–237
    multiple gestation and, 240
    pregestational diabetes mellitus and, 220
    sickle cell disease and, 215
    transvaginal, of cervical length, 172
Umbilical artery blood flow velocity, 146, 150
Umbilical artery catheters, 344, 446–448

Umbilical cord
    care for, 202, 285–286
    discharge readiness and, 307
    delayed clamping in preterm infants of, 321
    examination, fetal death and, 261
    prolapse, cesarean delivery and, 192
    pulse palpation at base of, 270
    sampling and transfusions, isoimmunization
        and, 238
Umbilical venous catheters, 267, 446–448
Underwater births, 170
Unintended pregnancies, 4–5
United States, standard reproductive health
        statistical reporting terminology in,
        497–512. *See also specific government
        departments and agencies*
Universal precautions, 521. *See also* Standard
        precautions
Universal Protocol to Prevent Wrong Site, Wrong
        Procedure, and Wrong Patient Surgery,
        70
Urethritis, 415, 416
Urinary tract infections, 257, 417
Urination, neonatal
    delayed, 284*b*
    discharge and, 307
    parent education on, 310
Urine culture (dipstick assessment), 108, 113*t*,
        257
Urogenital anomalies, intrauterine drug exposure
        and, 338
Urogenital care, postpartum, 197
U.S. Department of Health and Human Services
        AIDSinfo, 400
U.S. Environmental Protection Agency,
        456–457
U.S. Food and Drug Administration
    on chlorhexidine for infants, 446
    on in-flight medical devices, 85
    on herpes simplex virus antibody assays, 394
    on hysteroscopic sterilization devices,
        203–204
    on medications during pregnancy, 246
    propylthiouracil warnings by, 223
    spiramycin availability through, 434
U.S. Preventive Services Task Force, 133
U.S. Public Health Service, 526, 529
U.S. Secretary of Health and Human Services'
        Advisory Committee on Heritable
        Disorders in Newborns and Children,
        296, 304
Uterine atony, postpartum hemorrhage and,
        254
Uterine contractions
    admission policies on, 171
    during emergency care, 514–515
    false labor and, 175
    intrapartum monitoring of, 178–179
    labor and, 172, 177
    preterm labor and, 257
    trauma during pregnancy and, 247–248

Uterine inversion, 254
Uterine leiomyomata or malformation, 478
Uterine rupture, 159, 189, 192, 254, 255
Uteroplacental insufficiency, postterm pregnancy
        and, 255
Uterotonics, for postpartum hemorrhage, 254
Utility rooms, in neonatal functional units,
        51–52

V
Vaccinations. *See* Immunizations
Vaccines, live, 117–118
Vacuum extraction, 190–192
Vaginal birth after cesarean delivery (VBAC), 159,
        188–190, 189*b*, 208, 511
Vaginal bleeding
    admission policies on, 171
    at 14 weeks or later, recommended consultation
        for, 479
    prenatal care visit frequency and, 107
    preterm birth and, 257
    preterm labor and, 158
    transient, amniocentesis and, 126
    trauma during pregnancy and, 247–248
Vaginal breech deliveries, informed consent for,
        159. *See also* Breech presentation at
        term
Vaginal delivery
    after cesarean delivery, 159, 188–190, 189*b*,
        208, 511
    chronic hypertension and, 234
    of extremely preterm neonates, 250
    herpes simplex virus and, 396
    human immunodeficiency virus and, 401
    of multiple gestations, 194
    obese mother and, 217
    operative, 190–192
    risk assessment, 187–188
Vaginitis, gonorrhea and, 416
Valsalva maneuver, 177
Vancomycin, 420
Variation, quality improvement and reductions in,
        63–64. *See also* Clinical protocols
Varicella zoster virus, 411–414
    antepartum management, 412–413
    infection control, 413
    neonatal management, 413
    precautions for, 452
    screening health care workers for, 442
    vaccine, 99, 118, 413–414
Vascular disease
    preeclampsia and eclampsia and, 231
VBAC. *See* Vaginal birth after cesarean delivery
VDRL/RDR (nontreponemal tests), 113*t*. *See also*
        Syphilis
Vena cava filter, deep vein thrombosis before
        delivery and, 227
Venous thromboembolism
    cesarean deliveries and, 194
    combined hormonal contraceptives and, 205
    inherited thrombophilias and, 216

Ventilation. *See also* Oxygen therapy
    assisted, bronchopulmonary dysplasia and, 352
    equipment cleaning, 459
    home, 375
    of inpatient perinatal care building, 41, 55, 57
    mechanical, health care-associated pneumonia
        and, 448–450
    medication for, 365
    of neonate, 272–273
Ventilation–perfusion scanning, 142, 225–226
Ventriculomegaly, 323
Very low birth weight infants
    anemia of prematurity in, 321–322
    formula milk preparations for, 359
    immunizations in, 366
Viral infections, 383–414
    precautions for, 454
    respiratory, precautions for, 453
Visiting policies, 304–305
Visual disturbances, infants on extracorporeal
        membrane oxygenation and, 349
Vital signs
    maternal
        admission policies on, 171
        labor and, 172
        postpartum monitoring, 196
    neonatal, 280, 306
Vitamin A, 103t, 134t, 139–140, 351
Vitamin B$_6$, 103t, 134t
Vitamin B$_{12}$, 103t, 105, 134t, 200, 218–219
Vitamin C, 103t, 105, 133, 134t
Vitamin D
    for neonates, 294
    postpartum, 200
    preconception supplementation, 103t
    during pregnancy, 133
    for pregnant and lactating adolescents and
        women, 134t, 136
    toxicity during pregnancy, 140
Vitamin E, 103t, 134t, 140, 352, 353
Vitamin K, 103t, 134t, 140, 285
Vitamins
    neonatal supplementation, 294
    preconception supplementation, 102–103,
        103t, 105
    toxicity during pregnancy, 139–141
Voiding, neonatal
    delayed, 284b
    discharge and, 307
    parent education on, 310

Volume expanders, 268, 274
Vomiting
    neonatal illness and, 284b
    in pregnancy, 139, 219

W
Wake–sleep patterns, parent education on, 310
Wall surfaces, 56
Warfarin, 226
Warming techniques, for body temperature main-
        tenance, 270
Warning labels, on infectious materials, 527–528
Water trap cleaning, 459
Web sites
    on fetal and neonatal psychotropic drug effects,
        246
    LactMed database of drugs, 291
    on maternal retroviral therapy, 400
    for new parent education, 309–310
    as resources, 543–544
    on vaccines and immunizations, 406
Weight change
    in breastfed infants, 289–290, 289t
    greater than expected, 284b
Weight gain
    multiple gestations and, 239
    neonatal, 189b
    poor, late preterm infants and, 281
    during pregnancy, 136–137, 137t
    for preterm infants, discharge and, 374
Weight loss
    postpartum, 200
    preconception, 102
Well-being. *See* Fetal well-being
West Nile virus, 414
Whooping cough, 422–424
Windows, 56
Working
    postpartum, 208
    during pregnancy, 156–157
World Health Organization, 204, 216, 444
Wound management, 423

X
X-rays, teratogenic potential of, 142

Z
Zidovudine, 399–400, 401, 402, 403
Zinc, 104t, 135–136t
Zoonotic infections. *See* Toxoplasmosis